CARDIOVASCULAR REHABILITATION

CARDIOVASCULAR REHABILITATION
A Comprehensive Approach

EDITED BY

Lysle H. Peterson, M.D.

Director, The Houston Cardiovascular Rehabilitation Center, Houston;
Adjunct Professor of Physiology, University of Texas Health Science Center, Houston

MACMILLAN PUBLISHING COMPANY
New York

Collier Macmillan Canada, Inc.
Toronto

Collier Macmillan Publishers
London

Macmillan Publishing Company
866 Third Avenue, New York, New York 10022

Collier Macmillan Canada, Inc.

Collier Macmillan Publishers · London

Library of Congress Cataloging in Publication Data
Main entry under title:

Cardiovascular rehabilitation.

  Bibliography: p.
  Includes index
  1. Cardiacs — Rehabilitation. 2. Cardiovascular system — Diseases — Patients — Rehabilitation. I. Peterson, Lysle H. [DNLM: 1. Cardiovascular diseases — Rehabilitation. 2. Cardiovascular diseases — Therapy. WG 166 C2667]
RC682.C42 1983   616.1′206   83-22270
ISBN 0-02-394780-2

PREFACE

OBSERVANT PHYSICIANS have, for decades, espoused and practiced many of the principles utilized in cardiovascular rehabilitation. It is known widely that patients do better when encouraged to become physically active as early as medically appropriate than if permitted to remain bedridden, or sedentary. Early has become earlier and earlier, but what constitutes appropriate physical activity seems unclear to many. Should patients walk, jog, run, swim, or engage in other forms of exercise? When, how, for how long, and at what intensity should exercise be prescribed remain questionable to most physicians. Most physicians would agree that avoidance of depression, fears, anxiety, and what may be called emotional stress is good. Most busy physicians recognize, however, that it is difficult to deal effectively with the majority of these common disorders in an office practice. Few, if any, physicians would deny that a good diet, proper nutrition, and an ideal body weight are good for their patients, but how does the physician advise the patient? People do not adhere to prescribed, restrictive diets for long. If the patient is on a diet, the entire family must be on the same diet, or more than one kitchen is required. Most physicians are aware that widely publicized and promoted, or advertised, diets are faddish and temporary, soon replaced by the most recent and more highly promoted diet. Physicians are busy, and one would think that they would willingly turn their patients over to a facility that provided the right kind of exercise, took care of the psychological and nutritional problems, and did not lure patients away from them in terms of long-term care.

Extensive research on the effects of exercise has been published. Volumes have been written about the psychology of the cardiac patient, and nutrition advice abounds. Many convinced pioneers have formulated programs to provide exercise programs for patients. A lesser number have combined psychological and nutritional counseling as well. Why then, in 1983, did an editor of a recent book write, "Unfortunately, the information gathered thus far does not provide yet the desired scientific evidence that can validate the belief held by researchers in the field of the individual and social benefits they attribute to cardiovascular rehabilitation programs" (Blocker, W. P., Jr. *Rehabilitation in Ischemic Heart Disease.* S. P. Medical and Scientific Books, 1983, preface)? Why, in 1978, did Dr. Pollock say, "In his closing lecture following the 1970 Symposium on Coronary Heart Disease and Physical Fitness, Hansen concluded that large-scale application of physical conditioning in the prevention and therapy of patients with coronary heart disease could not be justified on the basis of irrefutable scientific evidence. Irrefutable evidence is still lacking and is not likely to be forthcoming in the near future" (Pollock, M. L., and Schmidt, D. H. *Heart Disease and Rehabilitation.* Houghton-Mifflin, Boston, 1979, p. 694)?

Why have so many dedicated cardiovascular rehabilitation services started and failed? Why do so relatively few physicians refer their patients to cardiovascular rehabilitation centers? Why have even some of the pioneers in the field become discouraged at the slow acceptance of dedicated cardiovascular rehabilitation? The health insurance industry has been cautious in its reimbursement practices.

There is not a simple answer to these questions. The first assumption would be that convincing, demonstrated evidence has not been sufficient to establish a widely held view that dedicated cardiovascular rehabilitation facilities provide the claimed benefits. The second assumption is that most physicians do feel that they can provide adequate rehabilitation for their patients from their offices; thus, they are not compelled to refer these patients to dedicated centers. A third assumption is that there have been few, if any, standards or guidelines for cardiovascular rehabilitation centers; hence, the field is fair game for almost anyone with the desire to conduct an array of activities of widely varying quality. Reading and listening lead me to think that those with limited or even anecdotal experience speak out, both pro and con, as often as those who work extensively in the field. It is a field where freedom of speech has certainly not been suppressed. In many cases, there has been no clear-cut differentiation made between programs for well people seeking primary prevention and body building and programs for the sick, disordered patient requiring careful medical management akin to critical care management. Programs for the healthy must be different from those for the ill, and the outcome of the same treatments will differ. The MRFIT program has created as much confusion as clarity in its concept and outcome, since the population not planned for intervention, i.e., the control group, inadvertently had much of the same intervention features as the so-called treated group. Moreover, the interventions themselves may not have been sufficient to provoke the responses that would have clarified the questions the study was designed to answer. Exercise is like treatments of most types in that too little, or the wrong kind, may be ineffective, while too much, or the wrong kind, may be dangerous.

This editor/author, then and now an enthusiast for the concept of comprehensive cardiovascular rehabilitation, made a decision six years ago to undertake the development of a dedicated, comprehensive, cardiovascular rehabilitation center. Moreover, there was awareness at that time of the fact that skepticism in the health care community as a whole exceeded enthusiasm, thus creating considerable risks for a center dependent upon adequate referrals to survive. Obviously, what was needed was an appropriate, accepted demonstration that patients with manifest cardiovascular disease, and the many coexisting disorders they suffer from, can be treated with demonstrable benefit as compared to existing modes of treatment such as the busy physician's office, or other rehabilitation centers from which such clear demonstration of benefits had been lacking.

Drawing upon both the good and bad experiences of predecessors in the field, on the often complicating and equivocal literature, and on the attitudes of the health care community, and the health insurance underwriters, a plan for a comprehensive cardiovascular rehabilitation center was drawn up and executed, resulting in the establishment of the Houston Cardiovascular Rehabilitation Center (HCRC). It was also decided that no publication of experience would be forthcoming until it appeared that an acceptable demonstration of benefits, or lack of benefits, could be achieved.

Now, almost five years later, with experience of more than 700 referred patients, 2,000 exercise stress tests, more than 30,000 hours of *one type* of exercise therapy, and with the coexisting medical, psychological, and nutritional management, it seems time to report the results. The results seem, to the authors of this book, to clearly demonstrate major benefits that most likely could not have been achieved another way.

This book, then, is written for the busy physician who would like to know how and why and indeed that a properly conducted comprehensive cardiovascular rehabilitation center can be of major benefit to his patients. This book is also written for those advising the health insurance industry that reimburses more than 80% of the cost of health care, and for the employers and public who buy the insurance and truly underwrite health care costs. This book, furthermore, is written for those who are interested in developing a cardiovascular rehabilitation center. Last, to those who are merely formulating opinions about the efficacy of diagnosis and treatment, this book is written for the students of fields of health care.

LYSLE H. PETERSON

ACKNOWLEDGMENTS

As NOTED in the Preface, the plan for the Houston Cardiovascular Rehabilitation Center (HCRC) was developed from the experience, both satisfactory and unsatisfactory, of the many pioneers in cardiovascular rehabilitation, physiology, clinical and counseling psychology, nutrition and dietetics, and clinical medicine. Some needed innovations were evident to provide and execute a plan that was comprehensive and consistent, that yielded systematic recording of data, and the analysis and collation of data.

Encouragement was needed in this expensive and risky venture. I am especially grateful to Dr. Marvin C. Schlecte, then the Medical Officer of the Texas Rehabilitation Commission, to his successor, Dr. James K. Pope, and the other leaders of that Commission. Also, I am grateful for the professional assistance given by Drs. Vincent Kitowski and William Blocker, Jr., to the residents who have rotated through the Center, and to the many physicians in the region who have shown the faith and confidence to refer their patients to the HCRC. I am grateful to Dr. E. C. Henley who formulated the initial nutrition plan and the basis for her successors; to the nurses without whom the Center could not operate, especially Cyndi Land, R.N., Liz Prather, R.N., and Mary Donadini, R.N.; to Dr. Merrill Anderson and Mary Schanler who have been responsible for the psychology and nutrition operations, and to the other HCRC staff members who make it run. Moreover, I am profoundly grateful to Mr. and Mrs. S. M. McAshan, Jr., and in addition to the Anderson Clayton Foundation, to the M. D. Anderson Foundation, to the Texas Rehabilitation Commission, the Hermann Estate Foundation, the Tenneco Corporation, and more than thirty private individuals who have contributed about one million dollars to carry out the research commitment of the Center, and to Shashi Patel, a premedical student who has devoted many hours in the computer center in the analyses of data. I am thankful to Linda Miner and Joelle Murphree for their assistance in preparing the manuscript for this book. I am certainly grateful to the other contributors to this book, and, most of all, I am grateful to my wife, Sara, who has shared the risks and work of developing the Houston Cardiovascular Rehabilitation Center and of helping report the results of its efforts.

CONTRIBUTORS

Merrill P. Anderson, Ph.D. Assistant Director, Psychological Services, Houston Cardiovascular Rehabilitation Center, Houston, Texas

Luean E. Anthony, Ph.D., R.D. Assistant Director, Dietary Department, Hermann Hospital, Houston, Texas

Donald W. Bowne, M.D., C.L.U. Vice President, Medical Services, Prudential Insurance Company, Houston, Texas

John A. Burdine, M.D. Department of Radiology, Baylor College of Medicine; Nuclear Medicine Service, St. Luke's Episcopal Hospital, Texas Children's Hospital, and Texas Heart Institute, Houston, Texas

E. Gordon DePuey, M.D. Department of Radiology, Baylor College of Medicine; Nuclear Medicine Service, St. Luke's Episcopal Hospital, Texas Children's Hospital, and Texas Heart Institute, Houston, Texas

Robert J. Hall, M.D. Director of Cardiology, St. Luke's Episcopal Hospital; Medical Director, Texas Heart Institute, Houston, Texas; Clinical Professor of Medicine, Baylor College of Medicine, and University of Texas Health Science Center, Houston, Texas

E. C. Henley, Ph.D., R.D. Director and Associate Professor, Program in Nutrition and Dietetics, School of Allied Health Sciences, University of Texas Health Science Center, Houston, Texas

Lysle H. Peterson, M.D. Director, Houston Cardiovascular Rehabilitation Center; Adjunct Professor of Physiology, University of Texas Health Science Center, Houston, Texas

Mary W. Schanler, M.S., R.D. Assistant Director, Nutritional Services, Houston Cardiovascular Rehabilitation Center, Houston, Texas

Dale W. Spence, Ed.D. Professor of Physical Education, Rice University; Visiting Professor of Physiology, Baylor College of Medicine, Houston, Texas

CONTENTS

CONTENTS

CARDIOVASCULAR
REHABILITATION

Chapter 1
INTRODUCTION, PHILOSOPHY, AND SCOPE

Lysle H. Peterson

The term "cardiovascular rehabilitation" means many things to many people. The scope, structure, and practices of cardiovascular rehabilitation centers vary widely. The pluralism of practices conducted under the designation is unusual in the field of health care. In other words, there are few types of medical service, provided to and paid for by patients and/or their insurers, that are characterized by such a variety of procedures and practices. This pluralism has caused concern and confusion among the physician community, the health insurance industry, and the general public.

Only somewhat facetiously it has been quipped that identity with cardiovascular rehabilitation is claimed from "fat farms to massage parlors." This confusion has plagued those who are concerned with providing medically sound, scientifically valid, and ethical services to an appropriate patient population largely obtained from referrals of attending physicians.

Even among physicians who have developed cardiovascular rehabilitation programs, there is pluralism in the scope of services they provide. Representatives of third-party health insurance organizations in personal discussions have stressed the need for guidelines or standards by which they might define reimbursement policies. Most practicing physicians with whom I

have spoken express the need to know the why, what, how, and when of cardiovascular rehabilitation. On the other hand, many physicians believe that they already provide cardiovascular rehabilitation from their office desks by advising their patients to exercise, lose weight, and manage emotional stress, with little or no guidance beyond the words themselves. The patient is left wondering how to exercise, how to lose weight, and how to stop worrying. The public, inundated with advertising and news media promotion of wellness, physical fitness and body building, weight and smoking control, and so forth, is confused. Should they be out in the streets jogging, adopting the latest diet fad, seeing a mental health therapist, or utilizing a commercial fitness center?

This author has visited physician-directed cardiovascular rehabilitation centers in the United States, Canada, Great Britain, Europe, Central and South America, and Asia. There is a wide variability in exercise techniques, nutritional and psychological stress-management approaches, and other aspects to be covered within this text. This variability and pluralism may be understood by considering several contributing factors.

1. Physical activity, in contrast to inactivity and bed rest, in the treatment of pathology and

illness has undergone and is still undergoing an evolution of concept and opinion. It is not that long ago that the patient with a myocardial infarction was kept at strict bed rest for a month or more. Indeed, the general concept that when a patient is ill, the place to be is in bed is deeply ingrained in the minds of most people. Early ambulation after surgery, however, has now become generally accepted. Increasingly, it is understood that sedentary living is self-generating. It is also increasingly recognized that exercise is akin to medication in that too little is ineffective and too much is harmful. Much has been learned about the effects of exercise on the patient with cardiovascular disease and on the healthy person as well, but much remains to be learned. It is clear, however, that although there is overlap, the effects of exercise on patients with cardiovascular, pulmonary, or metabolic disorders are quite different from the effects of exercise on the healthy college or professional athlete and military or NASA personnel.

2. Many rehabilitation programs feature exercise solely, neglecting the coexisting contributors to disability such as obesity and other malnutrition factors; psychological disorders such as anxiety, depression, and fears; the complexities of the many medications prescribed to cardiac patients; coexisting disorders of the neuromusculoskeletal system, which so often exist and affect ambulation; coexisting hypertension, diabetes, and so forth. In other words, the focus on exercise alone neglects the other important disorders that significantly affect disability and the outcome of exercise therapy itself.

3. Many rehabilitation programs are conducted by those who are well trained in exercise physiology but lack training in clinical medicine. At the time of writing this material, after essentially five years' experience with 710 patients with manifest cardiovascular diseases, about 25% of whom have manifestations of high-grade disease and are candidates for sudden death, this author strongly subscribes to the necessity of intensive monitoring by experienced, clinically trained personnel when patients with cardiovascular disease are being subjected to provocative exercise. To be effective, exercise must be heavy enough to provoke the so-called training effect to be discussed in this text and yet not so heavy as to be dangerous. The recent Medicare regulations governing reimbursement for cardiovascular rehabilitation stipulate that cardiovascular re-

habilitation applies to patients with diagnosed, manifest disorders and must be provided by qualified physicians in a devoted environment for defined periods of time. The American Medical Association, the American Heart Association and several of its affiliates, the American College of Cardiology, and insurance carriers have written guidelines. They all have in common a clear statement that cardiovascular rehabilitation programs caring for patients must be directed and supervised by a physician.

4. Health and wellness are "big business." As noted above, there never before has been such public interest in health as now, and such awareness that exercise, diet-nutrition, and emotional stress management play major roles in health maintenance and the prevention of disease. Commercial enterprises abound in every city, marked by an array of exercise types, generally some mix of isometric and isotonic procedures. Commercial bookstores are replete with temporarily popular and ever-changing diets, which are heavily promoted. Exercise machines and diets vary greatly, almost as fads. The streets and parks are crowded with joggers, runners, and walkers in climates ranging from hot and humid to frigid and dry, with rain and snow, hard and soft ground, and so forth. The principles of how exercise is both beneficial and harmful are not clearly understood by the public and media writers. Popular diets differ greatly in principle. Advice by psychologists, psychiatrists, and quasiprofessionals varies enormously. There are few federal, state, or local laws effectively governing these activities.

5. The literature in the field has been diverse in scope and content. The early research in exercise was conducted largely not only on a well population, but on an athletic population, or on college students, or military personnel. Many published studies of patients with cardiovascular disorders have been fragmentary and limited in scope and sample size. Much of the clinical literature on exercise is related to diagnostic exercise stress testing. Standardized exercise stress or tolerance testing began with the step test and later utilized the treadmill and bicycle ergometer. Some testing was done recumbent, some upright, and some primarily isometric, some isotonic, and some with so low a work load as to be relatively meaningless. One recent study (Sivarajan *et al.*, 1981), performed in order to ascertain the effect of early exercise on patients while still hospitalized (phase I rehabilitation), provided equivocal results because the cohort receiving exercise was

given such a low load that no effect might have been expected based upon provocative criteria. In short, the variability of published material is due in large measure to the variability of subject characteristics, procedures utilized, and population size. Indeed, the literature reflects the pluralism noted above. It is a field in which those with limited experience, but who are so inclined, feel free to express opinions.

The purpose of this text is to describe the principles of cardiovascular rehabilitation that have been shown to be appropriate for the treatment of patients with manifest, documented cardiovascular and related disorders, *from the authors' points of view and experience.* Conversely, this text does not deal primarily with so-called well-person adult fitness except as applicable to a patient population. This text, therefore, emphasizes principles and practices of medically necessary treatment as defined by the insurance industry for a certain patient population and as defined by practicing physicians for what they would, with confidence, refer their patients. In the authors' opinions, programs for ill patients requiring rehabilitation and secondary prevention differ in purpose, scope, procedures, and economics from programs for well persons desiring fitness, body building, weight loss, and primary prevention, although there is overlap in many principles. The authors have had more than casual experience with some centers that have attempted to provide their services to patients with abnormalities and at the same time to well people who desire adult fitness programs primarily for preventive and feeling-of-well-being purposes. The outcome of such dual purpose centers has not been favorable since the range of clients and the professional personnel and equipment required for each purpose is so different.

MAJOR CRITERIA FOR ESTABLISHMENT OF A CARDIOVASCULAR REHABILITATION CENTER

After careful analyses of an array of cardiovascular rehabilitation programs, after a study of the literature in the field, and after conducting a "marketing" survey among Houston area physicians and employers, as well as health insurance carriers serving the region, certain criteria, some anticipated and some not, for initiating a comprehensive cardiovascular rehabilitation center became evident. These criteria were then adopted in the creation of the Houston Cardiovascular Rehabilitation Center (HCRC) early in 1978. The major criteria are listed below, as they may help the founders of rehabilitation centers in the future.

1. A cardiovascular rehabilitation center should be *comprehensive* in the sense that the program should contain appropriate *exercise, nutrition, psychological, and medical management* involving not only the cardiovascular system but other interrelated body systems and their disorders as well, e.g., pulmonary, metabolic, neuromusculoskeletal.

2. The patients or clients in a center devoted to comprehensive cardiovascular services should be *referred* by their attending physician and/or appropriate referring agencies, such as a state rehabilitation agency, an insurance agency, or an employer, with due consideration of the attending physician. At the HCRC, the bulk of patients are referred by attending physicians, a growing number from the Texas Rehabilitation Commission (approved by a physician), by insurance (health and disability) carriers, and by employer groups. The latter two (insurance carriers and employer groups) in turn have usually worked out arrangements with attending physicians. This principle of due regard for the patient's attending physician assures a continuity of medical services for the patient and an appropriate working relationship with the attending physician that does not imperil the patient-doctor relationship.

3. The HCRC should be *free-standing* in contrast to hospital-based. There are several reasons for preferring the free-standing approach.

a. Hospital overhead was, and is, virtually always higher than free-standing overhead. Thus, the cost of services, other factors being equal, will be lower.

b. Since the patients or clients by and large will be referred, the base of referrals should be as wide as possible. In most cities with multiple hospitals, medical schools, clinical groups, and so forth, referral patterns tend to involve established constraints. For example, referrals in a hospital-based rehabilitation service will tend to be limited to the physician staff of that hospital. Cross-hospital referrals are the exception rather than the rule. A national study, based to some extent on the two American Heart Association Directories of Cardiac Rehabilitation Units (American Heart Association, 1981, 1976), conducted approximately five years apart, demonstrated a heavy casualty rate of cardiovascular rehabilitation centers primarily based in hospitals. In most cases, the referral base was not extensive enough to support the required services and associated overhead.

c. The more patients treated in a program, within certain appropriate limits, the lower the cost per patient will be, i.e., the fixed costs are divided over a larger number of patients.

d. Hospitals are a conglomerate of services, usually presided over by an executive director, to varying degrees by physician boards, and in a growing number of hospitals by remotely located proprietary corporations which own the hospitals. If any service in a hospital, such as cardiovascular rehabilitation, is not favored in comparison to other services for various reasons, then the cardiovascular rehabilitation service will be constrained and perhaps fail; i.e., it is vulnerable and often doomed before it starts. Conversely, a free-standing center can better control its own destiny. It may be noted that in earlier days, third-party insurers tended to favor in-hospital services, in part due to the often mistaken view that approval of a hospital by the Joint Commission on Hospital Accreditation guaranteed the quality of services provided by that hospital. Experience has shown that quality of service in free-standing centers may be as good as and indeed superior to in-hospital service. Many health care financial and service analysts were then and are now predicting a shift of many ancillary or ambulatory services from hospitals to free-standing units for economic reasons, without a necessary sacrifice of quality or safety. Why, it is asked, should ambulatory services be provided within facilities primarily operating in-patient services unless those services support hospital bed–related needs? Certainly, although early (phase I) rehabilitation practices may be begun while a patient is in the hospital, there is no reason that their treatment should continue in the higher cost hospital setting as the patient becomes ambulatory. The average hospital stay for myocardial infarction patients is two weeks or less with ambulatory privileges of only a few days. Most, even closed-end, ambulatory rehabilitation programs average 13 to 14 weeks. It would be economically unconscionable to extend hospital stays from 2 to 13 weeks. The free-standing center in an unusual situation may require the services of a hospital for its patients, but that is not a valid reason to locate a center within a hospital.

4. Prudent economic and management principles should be applied to the operations and pricing of the services provided.

5. To the extent possible, the HCRC was begun with the principle that, in addition to providing rehabilitation services on a fee-for-service basis, it would also serve to advance the state-of-art and science of the field through research and teaching programs. The HCRC maintains formal affiliation agreements with both The University of Texas Health Science Center at Houston and with Houston's Baylor College of Medicine. Residency programs for graduate physicians, medical, nursing, allied health, and graduate students are in effect. Research has been conducted continuously from the inception of the HCRC.

6. The HCRC is composed of two legal operating entities, formulated on sound legal, tax, and accounting advice. One is the Houston Cardiovascular Rehabilitation *Association,* which provides comprehensive cardiovascular rehabilitation on a fee-for-service basis. This is, in effect, a professional medical practice incorporated in the State of Texas. The second entity is the Houston Cardiovascular Rehabilitation *Foundation,* which is a public, nonprofit foundation for the purpose of conducting research, teaching, and eleemosynary activities under the IRS tax code 501(c)(3). The two entities operate side by side but separate economically and for accounting purposes. Both entities legally "do business as" the Houston Cardiovascular Rehabilitation *Center.* This organization is, of course, similar to that of most academic health organizations which have faculty practice plans, i.e., fee-for-service corporations or associations, and academic programs, i.e., nonprofit functions, operating side by side but separately. An important principle of this arrangement is that the costs of research or investigative work, teaching, and training are not charged to and thus borne by the patient in the fee-for-service charge.

To date, the HCRC has been in continuous operation for 53 months and has the experience of working with more than 700 patients, all with manifest cardiovascular disease and other related disorders seriously affecting their health. More than 30,000 hours of scheduled, monitored, progressive exercise sessions have been logged. More than 2,500 graded exercise tolerance (stress) tests have been performed. Fifty-three patients have been followed for more than four years; 156 patients have been followed for more than three years; 317 patients for more than two years; and 506 patients for more than one year. At present, approximately 40 patients are in the program at any given time. The mean time for patients to remain within the program has been 13.8 weeks.

Since its opening, the staff of the HCRC has consisted of a physician director, cardiovascular nurse specialists, a psychologist, nutritionists, and support office staff. During exercise sessions, described in the text, one or more cardiovascular nurse specialists and a physician are present at all times. Monitoring includes continuous electrocardiographs via telemetry, blood pressure, and continuous clinical observation. Psychological evaluation and therapy and stress management are conducted by a Ph.D. clinical/counseling, licensed psychologist. Nutritional evaluation and therapy are conducted by a Ph.D./R.D. or M.S./R.D. nutritionist. All functions are conducted under the direction and direct supervision of a qualified, licensed physician (M.D.). There is usually, in addition, a medical resident or associate physician present, and one or more exercise physiologists usually are working on research projects and interact with the staff. The medical staff (physicians and nurses) are trained and accredited in advanced life support and all staff in CPR, and a full system of advanced life support and resuscitation facilities is immediately available. Although about 25% of patients who have been treated within the program have been regarded as high risk and candidates for sudden death, as yet no resuscitation measures have been required. This safety record is regarded as a consequence of careful initial evaluation, continuous and direct monitoring of patients, and a defined methodology for prescribing and evaluating exercise protocols. The HCRC is operated in a manner similar to facilities providing critical care, e.g., the coronary care unit (CCU) and intensive care unit (ICU).

Within the past four years, about $1,000,000 has been devoted to research and development within the Houston Cardiovascular Rehabilitation Foundation. These funds have been obtained from state and federal sources, gifts from public and private foundations, and gifts of private individuals.

This textbook is intended to provide a review of the experience of the HCRC over the past 53 months along with views and information derived from the published literature. It appears evident to the authors that comprehensive cardiovascular rehabilitation provides an important, medically and scientifically sound modality for the treatment of the common and prevalent disorders of the cardiovascular system and indeed, an array of less common afflictions as well. The substantial benefits of comprehensive cardiovascular rehabilitation are documented to the extent that, when applied properly, they fulfill the criteria for any sound medical therapy as "reasonable and necessary."

There is sound evidence that most disabilities accompanying cardiovascular diseases and their associated disorders can be significantly reduced and often abolished, that the use of medications can be effectively reduced or abolished, and that morbidity in terms of subsequent visits to physicians and hospitalizations is reduced. There is growing evidence that mortality rates are favorably influenced.

The HCRC experience in Houston, known for its role in cardiovascular surgery, is that increasingly physicians are referring patients for comprehensive cardiovascular rehabilitation as step 1 in a number of circumstances in which surgery would formerly have been considered step 1.

RATIONALE FOR COMPREHENSIVE CARDIOVASCULAR REHABILITATION

One method for illustrating the overall rationale for comprehensive cardiovascular rehabilitation is provided in Figure 1-1.

This pie diagram depicts the fact that disability, to whatever degree it occurs, although arising from cardiovascular disease is usually, if not always, the result of five major factors *in addition to* the pathological damage of the disease itself. For example, the disability exhibited by a patient who has suffered a myocardial infarction, in which one or more portions of the myocardium are replaced by noncontractile scar tissue, is due not only to the fact that the patient's heart is left with less functioning myocardium, but also to other factors. Indeed, the heart is a relatively large and remarkable organ. In the majority of cases surviving infarction, enough myocardium remains to provide the patient with a heart that is capable of pumping sufficient blood to provide significant improvement in exercise tolerance and quality of life. *The cardiac's disability is usually due in large part to factors other than heart disease itself!*

In the illustrative Figure 1-1, only about 10% of the disability is due to irreversible pathology. Conversely, 90% of the disability is associated with more or less reversible disorders. The ultimate purpose of a comprehensive cardiovascular rehabilitation program is to evaluate the extent and contributions of the pieces of the pie

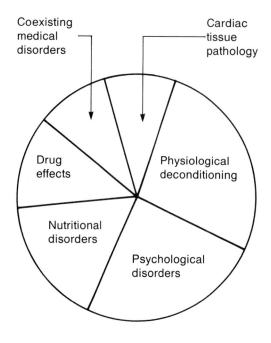

Coexisting medical disorders

Cardiac tissue pathology

Drug effects

Physiological deconditioning

Nutritional disorders

Psychological disorders

CONTRIBUTIONS TO DISABILITY

Figure 1-1. A model diagram to illustrate the major factors that disable cardiac patients. It is meant to illustrate that irreversible cardiac tissue pathology, e.g., the scarring of an infarcted area, is but one of six major factors causing disability. As noted in the text, the other five are subject to reversal or elimination with comprehensive cardiovascular rehabilitation.

illustrated in Figure 1-1 and then to reduce each slice to its minimum. In Figure 1-1, if each of the reversible components were reversed, 90% of the patient's disability would be corrected. The pieces of the disability pie are briefly discussed below and dealt with more extensively in the chapters of this text.

Physiological Deconditioning. This is present to some extent in all post–myocardial infarction and postsurgical patients after they leave the hospital. In most cases the patients were already deconditioned to some extent prior to entering the hospital, and hospitalization bed rest accelerates the rate of deconditioning. Careful medical histories reveal that many postinfarction and bypass patients have undergone increasingly easy fatigability and reduction of physical activities for months to a year or more prior to their infarction even when angina was not evident. This recallable reduction of physical activity produced a preinfarction decline in conditioning. More

generally, most patients referred to the HCRC relate a long history of sedentary life-style. Indeed, although a major interest in physical fitness has occurred in recent years, it is likely that a large majority of middle-aged and older Americans have still led relatively sedentary lives. It is well known that atherogenic vascular disease frequently begins early in life with many years of silent progression before symptoms or an acute event such as a myocardial infarction occurs.

It has been concluded that an average American up to age 50 to 55, in apparently good health but not engaged in an optimal conditioning exercise program, can achieve an average of stage VI in an exercise tolerance test using a Balke protocol, i.e., 3 miles per hour at a 12.5% grade. It will be noted in this text that the *average* male referred to the HCRC for rehabilitation achieves only stage III and is begun in exercise therapy at only 200 kpm · min^{-1} (see Chapter 6) for 30 minutes in the therapeutic exercise program. Thus, the average patient referred for rehabilitation exhibits about half of the exercise tolerance as well, but not especially conditioned, people of the same average age.

Physiological deconditioning is not regarded as a disease or pathological process. Rather, it is a normal, physiological adaptation to a sedentary life-style or, more appropriately, to reduced skeletal and cardiac muscle activity. Bed rest is often cited as an effective method of inducing physiological deconditioning in that the individual is sedentary, and the effects of gravity are largely nullified. Bed rest is the most effective method of reducing muscular activity and metabolism as a whole, except perhaps for living in a water-buoyancy state or in a weightless environment (e.g., in space). The deconditioning state begins with the initiation of bed rest and progresses with the duration of bed rest. Studies by NASA and other investigators have shown that with bed rest of the duration of most hospitalizations, i.e., 10 to 20 days, profound changes occur in the body's physiology and exercise tolerance. The maximal oxygen utilization ($\dot{V}O_2$ Max) that an individual can achieve by exercise is reduced. $\dot{V}O_2$ Max is a criterion of conditioning frequently utilized by exercise physiologists. It is directly related to exercise tolerance in that the amount of physical work achievable is proportional to and limited by the amount of oxygen that can be delivered to the metabolizing tissues, i.e., skeletal and cardiac muscle. In turn, oxygen consumption is directly and essentially linearly related to cardiac output, i.e., the delivery of oxygen to the oxygen-metabolizing muscles is via the flow of oxygen-containing blood. Cardiac output, in turn, is determined by the product of heart rate and stroke volume. When the heart has reached its limit of increasing cardiac output, oxygen supply to the tissues is limited, as is exercise level (Åstrand and Rodahl, 1977; NASA, 1980).

After 20 days of bed rest, for example, healthy young men exhibit a decline of $\dot{V}O_2$ Max of 25 to 30% together with a similar drop in maximal cardiac output. Blood volume is decreased by 10 to 20%. Reflexes, both autonomic and motor, are slowed or reduced. Studies show that a patient population of the type referred for cardiovascular rehabilitation show even greater declines in functional performance, i.e., become more severely deconditioned than healthier, younger subjects. Individuals exhibit less capacity to cope with emotional stresses, and anxiety and depression are induced more easily. Indeed, studies have shown adaptations to inactivity in most physiological and many psychological functions which amply illustrate the old saw, "If you don't use it, you lose it."

Most people, therefore, who suffer heart attacks or undergo cardiac surgery are already more or less deconditioned from years of a sedentary life-style at the time they are hospitalized. Then bed rest of about two weeks markedly accelerates the deconditioning process so that at the time the patient is considered for hospital discharge, he or she is significantly deconditioned with a low exercise tolerance, relative tachycardia, shortness of breath, easily induced sweating, and diminished temperature regulatory processes at relatively low work loads. This state is accompanied by fears, anxiety, and often depression. Since angina pectoris, arrhythmias, and ectopy are often heart-rate related, symptoms of heart disease may be more evident due to the associated tachycardia.

The symptoms and signs of physiological deconditioning both mimic and exacerbate the symptoms and signs of cardiovascular pathology. Evaluation and treatment of physiological deconditioning are essential components of comprehensive cardiovascular rehabilitation.

Psychological Disorders. It is commonly acknowledged that virtually all patients who have been faced with an event that is perceived as seriously threatening their future or life itself will suffer from psychological disorders, which further limit their functional capacity. Uncertainty, fear, anxiety, depression, denial, and loss of self-esteem are all found to be present to some degree in all cardiac patients. The extent or severity of these disorders, the effect of these disorders on functional capacity, and motivation for therapeutic compliance vary from patient to patient. These psychological disorders are usually regarded as situational rather than reflecting inherent mental illness of a pathological nature, and it is believed that unless there is significant psychopathology, they can be effectively treated by trained, experienced, clinical and counseling psychologists rather than requiring psychiatric care. In any case, psychological disorders contribute significantly to functional limitations, hence, to disability. Moreover, evaluation and reversal of these disorders should be essential components of a comprehensive rehabilitation program.

Nutrition Disorders. The average American gains 1 to 1.5 lb of body weight per year after the age of 20, due both to sedentary living and to a positive caloric balance involving a more limited caloric output and a higher caloric intake. Sixty-four per cent of HCRC-referred patients are 20% or more above their ideal body weight, which is regarded as clinically obese. Fourteen per cent have been morbidly or pathologically obese, i.e., 100 lb or 100% over their ideal weight. If fasting total cholesterol levels of 200 mg/dl, if fasting triglycerides above 100 mg/dl, and if fasting total cholesterol to HDL cholesterol ratios of <3 to 1 are regarded as ideal upper limits of cardiovascular disease risk, then 86% of the patients referred to the HCRC are above the ideal limits.

Eighteen per cent of patients referred for cardiovascular rehabilitation were insulin-dependent diabetics or exhibited sufficiently abnormal glucose tolerance tests to have been placed on oral hypoglycemic agents and/or diabetic diets.

Thirty-one per cent were moderate to severe hypertensives with at least a five-year history of hypertension prior to referral. Twenty-two per cent of these hypertensives were regarded as poorly controlled or uncontrolled with antihypertensive medications. Most of the hypertensives and 13% of the nonhypertensives were on diuretics, salt restriction, and potassium supplements. Thus, most patients referred for cardiovascular rehabilitation have some problem directly or indirectly involving nutrition and diet management. Evaluation and treatment of these problems are essential components of comprehensive cardiovascular rehabilitation.

Drug Effects. Although medications are prescribed by physicians to improve pathophysiological disorders, it must be acknowledged that most, if not all, effective medications also possess undesirable side effects. Propranolol, for example, in pharmacological, therapeutic doses frequently enhances depression, or at least a feeling described as sluggishness, diarrhea, reduced libido in both sexes, and impotence in males. It exacerbates temperature regulation, peripheral vascular, constrictive pulmonary and diabetic disorders, and congestive heart failure. As discussed in the text, the desired therapeutic effects of propranolol are a lowered heart rate and lowered blood pressure, but its effects also include reduced myocardial contractility. All of these undesirable side effects impede cardiovascular rehabilitation. It is acknowledged that antiarrhythmics are capable of producing as well as controlling arrhythmias. Antihypertensives are often accompanied by patient complaints of depressed feelings of well-being, orthostatic hypotension, and other undesirable side effects depending upon the type of antihypertensive utilized. Vasodilators are often associated with headache and gastric disturbances. One must watch for undesirable COUMADIN effects and digitalis or quinidine toxicity. Psychogenic medications possess a variety of undesirable side effects to which a rehabilitation staff must be alert. The average number of prescribed medications presumably taken by patients referred for rehabilitation is 6.4, with a range as high as 18.

Coexisting Medical Disorders. These commonly include abnormalities of the neuromusculoskeletal, metabolic, renal, pulmonary, and endocrine systems, disorders affecting the oxygen-carrying capacity of the blood, and sleep disturbances including sleep apnea. Other less common clinical problems also occur. Patients with relatively unusual problems, such as cluster headaches or myasthenia gravis, have been seen, for example, though primarily referred for cardiovascular disorders. It is unusual to see a patient referred with a primary cardiac abnormality who does not suffer from one or an array of coexisting medical problems. Reduced oxygen-carrying capacity of the

blood, chronic obstructive pulmonary disorders, disorders affecting acid-base metabolism, and ambulation efficiency problems are but a few examples of coexisting conditions that reduce functional capacities. To emphasize the effects of ambulatory efficiency, patients are told that a woman walking in high-heeled shoes may exert 20% more energy in walking at the same rate as another woman walking in low-heeled shoes which do not displace her center of gravity.

Each of these pieces of the pie illustrated in Figure 1-1, as related to the practice of comprehensive cardiovascular rehabilitation, is dealt with in this text. It is evident that each of these contributors to disability is interrelated and interacts with each other as well to further increase disability. To be effective, a cardiovascular rehabilitation center should deal with each and all of the pieces of the disability pie; hence, cardiovascular rehabilitation should be comprehensive. The staff should appreciate and be knowledgeable of the multiple factors affecting disability, their potential dangers, and their treatment. Close patient monitoring and staff interactions are essential. Expertise in clinical medicine and nursing, clinical psychology, clinical nutrition, and exercise physiology is essential. Coordination of these disciplines should be conducted by a physician with a broad understanding of this complex field.

DIFFERENCES IN PATIENT POPULATIONS

The above discussion has been intended to provide the reader with the background and philosophy which have led to experience in comprehensive cardiovascular rehabilitation as practiced by the Houston Cardiovascular Rehabilitation Center. One further comment is in order before summarizing this introductory chapter. In succeeding chapters the authors will utilize statistics derived from their own experience and that of others reported in the literature. Also, an emphasis is made on the fact that the roles of exercise, psychology, nutrition, and clinical medicine are different concerning a well, usually younger population seeking primary disease prevention, physical fitness, and body building from those for a population who are suffering from serious disease complicated by an array of coexisting conditions. Moreover, a usual experience of rehabilitation centers is that, initially at least, patients referred to them are more disabled and more ill than patients referred as the rehabilitation centers become better known. It may be said that the earlier referred patients tend to be more the therapeutic failures with referral by the physician almost as a last resort. As the rehabilitation center and the benefits it provides become better known, referrals tend to represent an earlier period in the patient's course — sooner after the myocardial infarction and surgery, sooner after symptoms are noted and workup is completed, and more often in lieu of surgery as the first consideration.

This sequence has advantages and disadvantages. The advantage is that the center's initial experience is with the difficult, complex cases, and results are often dramatic. The disadvantage is that early referral to a rehabilitation center would provide treatment at a more rational time with better patient motivation and long-term outcome. In short, a new center gains its early experience the hard way and is better prepared to deal with the array of problems that may occur at any time, but earlier referral provides earlier and larger benefits.

Another interesting aspect of the evolution of the HCRC has been the growing interest and involvement of the Texas Rehabilitation Commission, which has its counterpart in most states. Its purpose is, of course, to support rehabilitation and to some extent training for qualified individuals who are vocationally disabled. Table 1-1 lists the causes of vocational disability.

Table 1-1 THE CAUSES OF VOCATIONAL DISABILITY, AS COMPILED BY THE UNITED STATES VETERANS ADMINISTRATION, 1978*†

DISORDER	PER CENT
Cardiovascular disease	33
Rheumatic and arthritic disease	29
Orthopedic disorders	11
Nervous and mental disorders	7
Respiratory disorders	6
Visual disorders (blindness)	5
Partial or complete paralysis	4
Hearing impairment (deafness)	2
Major amputations	2

* An informal query to the Veterans Administration suggests that vocational disability due to cardiovascular disease has increased, relatively, to 36%.
† Table supplied by William P. Blocker, Jr., M.D., Chief, Rehabilitation Medicine Service, Veterans Administration Hospital, Houston, Texas.

It is evident that not only does cardiovascular disease represent the cause of more deaths than all others combined, but it is the largest cause of vocational disability as well. It has been the experience in Texas that while this is so, the case load of the Texas Rehabilitation Commission in cardiovascular rehabilitation was typically an order of magnitude lower than the probable incidence of cardiovascular-related vocational disability. This discrepancy was due largely to the rehabilitation counselors' unfamiliarity with the availability and benefits of comprehensive cardiovascular rehabilitation, and also to the lack of familiarity by referring physicians with comprehensive cardiovascular rehabilitation as well as the physicians' lack of knowledge that the Texas Rehabilitation Commission provided support for such services.

A pilot project between 1979 and 1982 supported by the Texas Rehabilitation Commission demonstrated that a high proportion (96% of compliant clients) were returned to gainful employment utilizing comprehensive cardiovascular rehabilitation. These findings, together with the cost per case, also demonstrated a high benefit/cost ratio compared to other common forms of physical and mental vocational rehabilitation. As a result, a special counselor was assigned to this task and referrals were increased.

SUMMARY

The field known as cardiovascular rehabilitation is highly varied in the manner in which it is practiced and as it is perceived by the health care and insurance communities, and by the public at large. There are many reasons for this pluralism; however, there is a certain trend underway to provide standards and guidelines of benefit to those interested in the field as providers, as physicians referring patients, as health insurers, as employers, and as the general public who, by and large, purchase health insurance. The trend includes a greater tendency for the practice of comprehensive cardiovascular rehabilitation to be conducted in devoted, free-standing centers in contrast to hospital-based centers, to identify appropriate staffing and procedural principles, and to better define appropriate candidates for comprehensive cardiovascular rehabilitation as a medically necessary practice in contrast to primary prevention, wellness, and body building programs for the well population.

The remainder of this book is structured in the following manner. *Chapter 2* (Exercise in Cardiovascular Rehabilitation: Principles) deals with the rationale for exercise tolerance testing and exercise therapy and introduces a concept found valuable in patient management and for determining when patients have achieved optimal conditioning. *Chapter 3* (Patient Responses to Exercise Tolerance Testing and Therapy) deals with representative patient experiences to which the principles defined in Chapter 2 have been applied. This chapter demonstrates benefits by case studies. *Chapter 4* deals with statistical analyses of the overall outcome of comprehensive cardiovascular rehabilitation of patients that were fully evaluated and had completed the full program and for which there is more than a six month follow-up. *Chapter 5* deals with the various types of blood pressure and heart rate responses found in exercise testing and also with the benefits of treating hypertension utilizing comprehensive cardiovascular rehabilitation. *Chapter 6* (Ergometry) deals with the principles and practice of the various ways of achieving an exercise work load and, in particular, the use of the bicycle ergometer. *Chapter 7* deals with the principles associated with the various psychological disorders usually found with patients suffering from cardiovascular disease and seen in cardiovascular rehabilitation centers. *Chapter 8* presents the experience of the HCRC, in the light of these principles, in dealing with these psychological disorders. *Chapter 9* deals with the principles of nutrition and dietetics as concerns the etiology and treatment of disorders and prevention of cardiovascular disease and its associated disorders. *Chapter 10* discusses the practices and experiences in the HCRC program relative to nutrition and dietetics.

Up to and including Chapter 10, the book has concentrated on comprehensive cardiovascular rehabilitation with emphasis on the HCRC program. It is recognized that cardiovascular rehabilitation is practiced within a much broader scope of cardiovascular disease. Thus, Dr. Robert J. Hall, an eminent and leading cardiologist, not only has an excellent overview of clinical cardiology but also, as Medical Director of the Texas Heart Institute, is at the forefront of the use of cardiovascular surgery. The manner in which patients are worked up for diagnosis, followed by the decision-making process by the cardiologist interacting with the physician referring the patient to the cardiologist, the patient himself, the surgeon, the array of others involved in diagnosis and treatment including cardiovascular rehabilitation, determines how patients are treated and what the outcome of treatment is. In other words, it is not possible to place cardiovascular rehabilitation in its perspective without an overview of the field of cardiology and the way it is practiced.

Chapters 11 and *12,* therefore, provide the broad scope not only of the diseases with which cardiovascular rehabilitation is concerned, but also of the manner in which diagnoses are made, and of the manner in which treatment decisions are made. The current status of cardiovascular surgery and its outcome regarding morbidity and mortality are reviewed. Since the use of cardiovascular nuclear medicine is rapidly becoming a major field in the diagnosis and evaluation of treatment relative to patients with cardiovascular disease, *Chapter 13* is presented.

The opinions and role of the physician within the health insurance structure are very important in the manner in which diagnosis and treatment regimens are reimbursed and thus practiced. It was evident that the opinion of a leading insurance company physician should be represented in such a book. Dr. Bowne is especially qualified, not only due to his experience as a health insurance executive and decision-maker, but also because he has led a corporate program in cardiovascular preventive medicine within his own company. *Chapters 14* and *15* represent the views of Dr. Bowne in these regards.

It is evident that the health insurance industry, commercial, nonprofit, and governmental, plays a crucial role in determining how medicine is practiced in the United States of America, now and especially in the future. The employers, as major buyers of health insurance through complex interaction with their employees and representative unions, will ultimately decide on what services they wish to pay for through their insurance carriers or through self-insurance. The taxpayers, their representatives in Congress, the Administration, and perhaps the courts will determine the role of the government and the use of tax revenues in the type of health care services that are paid for. It is gratifying that Medicare (1983) has formally recognized cardiovascular rehabilitation as a medically necessary form of treatment. It is important that patients understand the role of health insurance reimbursement for their care.

Chapter 16 summarizes and highlights the scope and principles of comprehensive cardiovascular rehabilitation and the findings during five years of its practice by the Houston Cardiovascular Rehabilitation Center.

REFERENCES

Åstrand, P.-O., and Rodahl, K. *Textbook of Work Physiology.* McGraw-Hill, New York, 1977.

Medicare Newsletter, Feb. 3, 1983.

NASA. *Proceedings of the Second Annual Meeting of the IUPS Commission on Gravitative Physiology.* Supplement to *Physiologist,* **1980,** *23,* #6.

Sivarajan, E. S.; Bruce, R. A.; Almes, M. J.; Green, B.; Laurent, B.; Lindskog, B. D.; Newton, K. M.; and Mansfield, L. W. In-hospital exercise after myocardial infarction does not improve treadmill performance. *New Engl. J. Med.,* **1981,** *305,* 357–362.

Chapter 2
EXERCISE IN CARDIOVASCULAR REHABILITATION: PRINCIPLES

Lysle H. Peterson

There are two major purposes in subjecting patients to exercise protocols. One purpose is to attempt to evaluate exercise tolerance and to reveal abnormalities of the cardiovascular system which are not evident at rest or within the patient's usual activity levels, i.e., diagnostic purpose. The other is to treat or improve abnormally limited exercise tolerance and other disorders through improvements in the underlying physiological or pathophysiological processes, i.e., treatment or therapeutic purpose.

There are many considerations, problems, and questions, some as yet unresolved, as to the type, intensity, duration, and sign or symptom markers to be utilized; as to the physiological mechanisms by which diagnostic and therapeutic achievements are obtained; and indeed, as to whether the purposes themselves are achieved. To what extent then does exercise aid diagnosis and therapy?

Studies of the sensitivity, specificity, and predictability of exercise stress testing have varied in their conclusions, but it is generally concluded that exercise stress tests are not infallible indications of the presence or absence of coronary artery disease as discussed in Chapter 11. Protocols or prescriptions for the purpose of using exercise as a therapeutic treatment vary greatly, as do the reported results. There is

controversy as to whether improvements in functional performance are primarily central (due to improvements in heart function) or peripheral (due to improved oxygen handling in the blood and/or metabolizing tissue). Some rehabilitation centers utilize multiple modes of exercise in treating each and every patient, e.g., each patient may be asked to walk, jog, or run on a track, use a bicycle ergometer and training machines, lift weights, and so on, as he moves through the rehabilitation program. Some programs leave the choice of exercise modalities to the patient. Other programs utilize primarily one repeated form of exercise, such as the stationary bicycle ergometer. Also, there are major variations from program to program in the extent of patient monitoring and the uses of physiological parameters as well as signs and symptoms to define exercise prescriptions, to judge the progress of the patient, and in the overall management of the patient during the rehabilitation program. Upper extremity versus lower extremity exercise, use of varying muscle groups, agonists and antagonists, upright or supine exercise, isotonic or isometric work—all produce different physiological responses, thus different outcomes.

Because of the extensive variability of practices of cardiovascular rehabilitation centers and the problems of interpreting and analyzing the resulting variability of results, the initial planning of the HCRC attempted to avoid variability of practices and thus achieve clearer outcomes. This decision should not be regarded so much as a criticism of other centers, many of which are pioneering efforts in the field, as it was to avoid or clarify the controversial and indistinct outcomes of variable approaches. At the time of planning the HCRC, this author would have agreed with the aforementioned statement of Dr. William P. Blocker, Jr. (1983), "Unfortunately, the information gathered thus far does not provide yet the desired scientific evidence that can validate the belief held by researchers in the field in the individual and social benefits they attribute to cardiac rehabilitation programs." Now, however, after essentially five years of experience, this author is gratified to be able to report that there is evidence to establish clearly the benefits of comprehensive cardiovascular rehabilitation. This gratification is further reinforced by continuing evidence from other centers as well.

Again, one purpose in predefining the program was to assure that consistent practices may be expected to lead to more statistically powerful results, better defined "dose-response" relationships, consistency, and replication of findings. Conversely, a program that is subject to significant variability of procedures and practices would be expected to confound analyses of experience, a problem that a number of previous rehabilitation center operators, as well as large population and multicenter trials, have reported as akin to the plague. However, attempting to establish and adhere to a predefined program increases the responsibility of making the "right" decisions in the beginning, an awesome concern.

In the introductory chapter, organizational criteria were discussed that dealt mainly with what might be called economic strategies, e.g., free-standing versus hospital-based, referral considerations, economies of scale, conducting research and teaching at no economic burden to the patients, and so on. Wrong initial decisions regarding those criteria could have resulted in economic failure of the center. The wrong initial decisions in planning and developing the diagnostic, treatment, and evaluation procedures could result in professional failure in that not only would patients be charged for inappropriate services, but also the experiences to be later analyzed in order to ascertain the effectiveness of rehabilitation could be difficult

or impossible. Poor results would further discourage the referring physicians and agencies in the emerging field of comprehensive cardiovascular rehabilitation. In this chapter the discussion will define the diagnostic and principal treatment methodologies that have been utilized.

The principal assumptions with regard to diagnostic and therapeutic purposes as related to exercise were as follows.

1. Exercise may be likened to medications or most other forms of therapy in that too little is likely to be ineffective, and too much is likely to be dangerous, and that dose-response characteristics are evident.

2. The therapeutic range between effectiveness and safety should *provoke* the intended beneficial results, and thus exercise intensity should be enough to provoke a training or conditioning effect.

3. The monitoring methods should be reliable, repeatable, and such as to permit effective and consistent handling by the staff, acceptance by the patients, and satisfactory benefit-cost relationships.

4. The measurements of exercise load and monitored parameters must be recorded accurately and consistently and utilized continuously for patient management and for evaluation of the concepts of cardiovascular rehabilitation. In other words, properly defined data should be accurately recorded and effectively utilized to manage patient therapy and provide evaluation of effectiveness.

These principles have been followed for the almost five years of the HCRC's existence, with more than 700 patients, with more than 2,500 exercise tolerance or stress tests, and with more than 30,000 hours of prescribed therapeutic exercise sessions. Some procedural variations have been introduced from time to time to improve the effectiveness of the program, but no substantial changes have been made. Thus, the methodological consistency criteria have been maintained to the degree that variability of procedures is not a significant cause of variability of results. Indeed, analyses of HCRC data and reports from the literature have been reassuring in that, were we to have the opportunity to repeat the planning and development of the HCRC rehabilitation program, no substantial or fundamental changes would be made. This belief has provided further encouragement to the authors to prepare this book.

Concerning the criteria of *effective or provocative* exercise protocols, it is concluded, and generally accepted, that to be effective, exercise therapy must be repetitive and that an optimal repetition sequence is three times per week. Although it has been shown that repetition may be reduced to two times per week with greater intensity of prescribed work load per session, this lower repetition rate applies more to younger, well individuals of athletic qualities than to patients with manifest disorders (Åstrand and Rodahl, 1977). Fatigability, convenience, compliance, and outcome itself appear to optimize for patients at three times per week.

It is also generally accepted that the training or conditioning effect is optimally achieved with a steady or constant work load sustained for 25 to 35 minutes with appropriate calisthenics and warm-up preceding the exercise and appropriate cool-down and relaxation following the exercise (Hartung, *et al.*, 1977, Pollock and Miller, 1975).

Because of the variability of response to different exercise modalities and the difficulties in monitoring patients using other exercise modalities, because the use of a bicycle ergometer is relatively independent of body weight, because the bicycle ergometer does not exert a significant, damaging mechanical stress on back and lower extremity joints relative, for example, to jogging or running, because of the advantage of repeatability and accuracy of setting exercise loads, and because long-term compliance is improved, the bicycle ergometer was chosen as the only therapeutic exercise modality to be regularly used in the HCRC program. There are exceptions for patients with exceptional problems, e.g., inability to use the lower extremities satisfactorily. Therefore, the standard exercise modality has consistently been the bicycle ergometer with a careful, periodic calibration and preventive maintenance program to assure reliability and reproducibility. The use of the bicycle ergometer as the only usual therapeutic exercise device tends to have been more the practice in European rehabilitation centers than in the United States and Canada.

PATIENTS' EXERCISE LOAD

As to the type and intensity and monitoring criteria, further discussion is warranted. The objective of therapeutic exercise is, of course, to induce the so-called training effect, i.e., to increase the physiological conditioning of the patient. To be effective, the exercise level must provoke significant cardiovascular responses. Although exercising skeletal muscle, by what-

ever means, is the *stimulus* to the conditioning process, it is the *response* of the cardiovascular system to that exercise that causes the conditioning or training effect of the cardiovascular and other systems aside from the skeletal muscle. As conditioning develops, the response of the cardiovascular system to a given skeletal muscular exercise level undergoes change, i.e., the relationship between stimulus and response changes, and these changes therefore must be monitored. Moreover, they should be monitored because they may be harmful as well as beneficial and in a given individual are not predictable. Indeed, it is the alteration of cardiovascular response to exercise intensity that indicates whether or not the conditioning effect has occurred and, as will be shown in this text, those alterations have diagnostic and therapeutic considerations beyond that of achieving the training effect itself. The argument that patients with manifest health disorders do not require monitoring in this author's experience cannot be justified.

At what level should therapeutic exercise be started? A commonly used physiological parameter to initially evaluate a patient's exercise tolerance is *heart rate*. Furthermore, a "target" heart rate frequently is utilized as a guide to home maintenance exercise level after the patient leaves the rehabilitation center program. It was initially decided that heart rate alone would not be so used in the HCRC program for evaluation or therapy.

Although the heart rate–exercise load relationship is one of the important physiological parameters of deconditioning and conditioning alike, and although it is a readily measurable entity, as a sole parameter it is not as useful as it is when combined with other observable and measurable parameters. As noted above, one of the primary purposes of exercising skeletal muscles is to provoke the training effect by increasing the work load of the heart and, in turn, cardiac oxygen demand. Although heart rate is one determinant of myocardial work and O_2 utilization, it has been shown that the *heart rate $\times$ systolic blood pressure* product correlates even better with myocardial work and oxygen consumption. Short of direct, clinically impractical measurement of myocardial oxygen consumption itself, it appears from an array of studies conducted over more than two decades that the heart rate–systolic pressure product better correlates with myocardial oxygen consumption than with heart rate or systolic blood pressure singly, or with the so-called triple product (heart rate × systolic blood pressure × systolic time interval). Moreover, the correlation holds under a variety of important clinical circumstances, e.g., whether either heart rate or systolic blood pressure is the predominant varying parameter, with isometric or isotonic work, and with patients suffering from symptomatic heart disease as well as with normal subjects, with heart pacing, and in hypertension and valve disease–produced cardiac hypertrophy. There are less reliable results and more uncertainty that the correlation holds under surgical anesthesia and with the use of certain medications, e.g., beta-blocking agents and calcium-blocking agents. Instructive references to this subject, i.e., heart rate, systolic blood pressure, and systolic time intervals, are Sarnoff et al., 1959; Lund et al., 1964; Bing, 1965; Sonnenblick et al., 1968; Jorgensen et al., 1971; Holmberg et al., 1971; Kitamura et al., 1972; Bruce et al., 1973; Goldstein and Epstein, 1973; Jorgensen et al., 1973; Braunwald, 1973; Nelson et al., 1974; Gobel et al., 1978; Kissin et al., 1980; Pickard et al., 1981; Bertrand et al., 1981. Also, the double product correlates well with the perceived effort as regards exercise work intensity (Peterson, 1983).

Double Product. Since the double product appears to be an established correlate of cardiac work and myocardial oxygen demand, and since its parameters can be measured noninvasively and with satisfactory accuracy, it was selected as the reference point regarding symptom- and/or sign-limited exercise tolerance (stress) testing and as the principal indicator for setting a provocative exercise therapy load on a day-to-day basis. It is apparent without the need for explanation that it is impractical to determine oxygen consumption, $\dot{V}O_2$, and thus maximal oxygen consumption, $\dot{V}O_2$ Max, in routine exercise tolerance testing. As discussed below, the double product also is used in the ratio of exercise work intensity to double product, which has proven to be of value and is discussed below as the Conditioning Index.

Prior to beginning exercise therapy, all patients first undergo an exercise tolerance test. The purpose is twofold: (1) to ascertain a rational initial therapeutic exercise intensity or work load, and (2) to reveal signs and/or symptoms that are likely to occur at various exercise loads, especially at maximal exercise tolerance. The Balke protocol using a treadmill is utilized as the standard procedure for several reasons. One is that the progressive stages are directly related to incremental metabolic steps. An-

other is that stages of the Balke treadmill protocol are comparable to stages of work load on a bicycle ergometer. Furthermore, the Balke protocol is easier for the patient and staff alike than other commonly used protocols (Balke and Ware, 1959; Naughton et al., 1964; Fox et al., 1971). The heart rate and systolic blood pressure normally increase directly and essentially linearly with metabolic load, hence they correspond to stages of the Balke protocol. The diastolic pressure normally does not change significantly within the range of exercise tolerance. The end-point, i.e., the stage at which the exercise tolerance test is terminated, is symptom- and/or sign-limited rather than related to a target heart rate for reasons given above. A healthy individual, who does not develop clinical signs or symptoms associated with cardiovascular or pulmonary disease, would reach an end-point at which excessive fatigue develops. This may be associated with the so-called Borg rating scale (Borg and Linderholm, 1967) as very-very hard. While Borg related the scale of perceived exertion from very-very easy to very-very hard to heart rate, this scale has been found to correlate better with the double product (Peterson and Anderson, 1983). Reaching and exceeding a double product of 300 to 350* is very-very difficult for a healthy individual.

A patient with cardiac, respiratory, or peripheral vascular disease may develop *clinically* important signs or symptoms which are interpreted by the staff monitoring the exercise tolerance test and would cause them, or indeed the patient himself, to stop the test prior to the level of perceived maximal exertion. These contraindicating signs and symptoms include those indicative of excessive myocardial ischemia (e.g., angina pectoris, arrhythmias, ST/T changes, decompensation, or failure), peripheral ischemia (e.g., claudication, dizziness), or respiratory distress (provoking increased diastolic pressure, cyanosis, dyspnea), or an excessive, dichotomous rise in systolic pressure referred to in Chapter 5 as the "hypertensive response." In effect then, the end-point of a symptom- and/or sign-limited exercise tolerance test is excessive perceived fatigue (very-very-hard) or clinical signs and/or symptoms judged to be excessive—whichever is lower.

It may be noted that, in more than 2,500 such exercise tolerance tests performed at the HCRC, no one has required resuscitation, advance life support, or hospitalization, nor have

---

* Heart rate × systolic blood pressure × 10^{-2}.

there been any sudden deaths within ten days of the test. In fact, in no patient who has been evaluated or undergone rehabilitation at the HCRC to date and died, could the death be reasonably related to the exercise tolerance test.

Relative to a practical patient concern, occasionally a patient, referred for cardiovascular rehabilitation, will note that he had received a treadmill exercise stress test from his doctor quite recently and wonders about the necessity of repeating the test. It is explained that the test is different in many respects and that the results are utilized in different ways. The HCRC staff is strongly of the opinion, after an array of exemplary experiences, that it is important to test the patients in a uniform and understood manner. Comparisons have shown that accepting the results of other tests using different protocols and end-points could have led to serious errors.

The work load associated with the highest stage reached on the initial treadmill exercise tolerance test has been used to establish the level of intensity to be used for the first exercise therapy session with a bicycle ergometer. Each stage of the treadmill exercise tolerance test lasts 3 minutes, while the bicycle ergometer therapeutic session lasts 30 minutes. Moreover, most patients find it *initially* easier to use a treadmill than a bicycle ergometer, i.e., they are more familiar with and more efficient at walking—but only for a few sessions!

The initial maximal exercise tolerance test stage, in turn, correlates with the maximal dou-ble product (see "Conditioning Index" below) and with perceived exertion. The initial therapeutic work load is arbitrarily set at 60% of the work load associated with the highest achieved exercise tolerance test utilizing the relationships described in Table 2-1.

Efficiency at performing an exercise tolerance or stress test, or in performing a therapeutic exercise activity, is important in that it affects the relationship of actual work done to the assumed work load. In other words, work loads are not usually measured with each test or therapeutic session; rather, they are assumed from preevaluations and then inferred from treadmill speed and grade or bicycle ergometer settings in everyday practice. Certainly most clinical exercise tolerance tests utilize preset protocols rather than direct measures of oxygen consumption. An example of the effect of efficiency is that an amputee may utilize 100% more oxygen in walking than a nonamputee using the same walking protocol and even with comparable conditioning. To illustrate the point to HCRC patients, it is explained, as mentioned in Chapter 1, that a woman wearing high-heeled shoes may expend as much as 20% more energy walking at three miles per hour than one wearing walking shoes which do not displace her center of gravity.

While the first day's therapeutic exercise load setting was based on 60% of the maximal load achieved on the treadmill exercise tolerance test, adjusted for any other observed condition

Table 2-1 COMPARATIVE EXERCISE VALUES

METABOLIC COST (ML O_2/KG/MIN)	METS	TREADMILL BALKE PROTOCOL % GRADE AT 3 MPH	BALKE PROTOCOL STAGE	BICYCLE ERGOMETRY (KPM · MIN^{-1}) PRE REHABILITATION	POST REHABILITATION
10.5	3	0.0	I	120	180
14.0	4	2.5	II	240	360
17.5	5	5.0	III	360	540
21.0	6	7.5	IV	480	720
24.5	7	10.0	V	600	900
28.0	8	12.5	VI	720	1080
31.5	9	15.0	VII	840	1260
35.0	10	17.5	VIII	960	1440
38.5	11	20.0	IX	1080	1620
42.0	12	22.5	X	1200	1800

Note: Table 2-1 illustrates that the Balke protocol relates metabolic cost or MET equivalents to each protocol stage. The bicycle ergometry table also illustrates the comparison of bicycle ergometer and treadmill stages for patients from HCRC findings. The difference between pre and post rehabilitation ergometry equivalents demonstrates the improvement in ergometry tolerance to a given metabolic demand. These comparative values differ somewhat from other published data (Fox, S. M.; Naughton, J. P.; and Haskell, W. L. Physical activity and the prevention of coronary heart disease. *Ann. Clin. Res.,* **1971,** *3,* 404). It must be emphasized that these values are approximations and vary with a number of factors, such as efficiency, as well as body weight. For example, a person walking inefficiently may utilize from 20 to 100% more oxygen than an efficient walker. This table represents a practical guide rather than an accurate statement under all circumstances.

that might result in risk at that level, the second or third day's settings were better correlated with a double product related to a Borg rating of hard. In other words, while the 60% of maximal work load achieved in the initial evaluation test is a reasonable starting point, it usually is adjusted upward or downward at the second or third session, depending upon the presence or absence of signs or symptoms of undue risk, perception of unnecessarily low or excessively high effort, and so forth, in order to achieve a provocative double product.

The findings of this approach again emphasize the utility of using the double product rather than heart rate as a guide to prescribing, on a day-to-day basis, a therapeutic exercise load which is effective yet safe. Moreover, as discussed earlier, double product better represents the purpose of the exercise therapy, i.e., to induce a provocative cardiac work load within the limits of safety.

An analysis of 190 male and 82 female patients who have successfully completed all phases of the rehabilitation program, and who have been followed for at least one year, documents this and other conclusions regarding comprehensive cardiovascular rehabilitation reported in this and subsequent chapters.

Drawing from these data, as they relate to the initial setting of a therapeutic exercise load, it has been found that the correlation between average maximal double product (177.8) achieved from the initial exercise tolerance test and the initial adjusted therapeutic double product adjusted for achievable but safe maximal double product was 198.8, i.e., 89%, while the average double product obtained the first day was 80% of the second or third day's adjusted load. Thus, the average patient work load was adjusted upward by 9% after the first day's experience on a bicycle ergometer which was derived from 60% of a maximal, symptom/sign-limited, treadmill exercise tolerance test. In other words, on the average, using 60% of the maximum achieved initial exercise tolerance test as a guide to setting the first therapeutic load on a bicycle ergometer, 80% of the optimal exercise therapy double product was achieved, and after adjusting for efficiency, 89% was achieved. Thus, three conclusions may be drawn. One is that using 60% of the maximal Balke exercise tolerance *test stage* achieved is a rational guide to begin a therapeutic program on a bicycle ergometer; the efficiency effect of learning to ride the bicycle ergometer is approximately 10%, achieved

usually in two to three sessions, and then an effective average training or conditioning effect can be achieved by utilizing essentially 90% of the double product occurring at the maximal exercise tolerance test stage achieved. It is also essential to recognize that there are important exceptions to these conclusions. These exceptions will be discussed in this and subsequent chapters.

As will be further emphasized, it became evident that symptoms and signs of myocardial ischemia, i.e., angina pectoris and electrocardiographic markers, do not remain constant with respect to double product. Cohort statistics and individuals used as their own controls demonstrate that the training effect or conditioning does improve the level of cardiac work and myocardial oxygen demand that can be tolerated. One of the benefits of the training or conditioning effect is that the individual is able to tolerate a higher cardiac work load and its attendant higher myocardial oxygen demand. Analyses of the HCRC experience show that the average initial exercise tolerance test maximal stage achieved using the Balke treadmill test was 3.16, while on exit it was 6.08, or virtually a doubling of treadmill-tested exercise tolerance. The related increase in double product was 21.4%, i.e., the initial average double product at the maximal stage reached was 177.8 and on exit was 226.2. Thus, a doubling of exercise tolerance was accompanied by only a 21% increase in double product, an order of magnitude difference between increase of exercise tolerance and the related cardiac work cost. The findings of the therapeutic program are even more dramatic, as will be presented in Chapters 3, 4, and 5.

Conditioning Index. Having discussed the rationale for utilizing the double product as the principal guide for day-to-day setting of the patients' exercise load on a bicycle ergometer for 30 minutes, attention is now turned to a second indicator or marker, in this case representing the manner in which the exercising patient is responding to the prescribed double product. Figure 2-1 is a *model* diagram to *illustrate* the principle of the Conditioning Index (Peterson, 1983).

Assume, for example, that a patient begins the exercise component of his cardiovascular rehabilitation program utilizing a bicycle ergometer* at a prescribed load of 150

---

* The power setting on the bicycle ergometer is represented in kpm · min⁻¹.

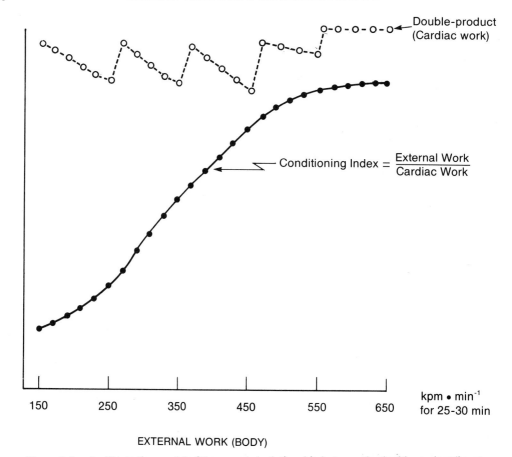

Figure 2-1. An illustrative model of the expected relationship between the double product (heart rate × systolic blood pressure at the prescribed work load) as representing cardiac work and the work load prescribed for the patient, e.g., on a bicycle ergometer. The Conditioning Index is the ratio of the prescribed exercise work load (external) to the cardiac work load as defined by the double product. See text for further discussion.

kpm · min⁻¹ for 30 minutes following a calisthenic warm-up protocol and followed by a cool-down and relaxation protocol. This exercise load will induce a double product of some value depending upon the conditioning of the patient and, as will be seen, by other important factors as well. Assuming that a training or conditioning effect occurs, the double product may then be expected to decrease with successive exercise sessions at that same prescribed bicycle ergometer (body) exercise load. At some point, in this illustrative diagram, the double product will have dropped to a level which may be regarded as too low to be optimally effective to continue to induce the conditioning effect;* again recalling that the training

*Perceived as less than hard (Borg rating) or regarding signs and/or symptoms.

or conditioning effect is related to a provocative double product rather than to the body exercise load per se. At that point, when the double product has dropped to a suboptimal level, the prescribed body work load is increased (e.g., to 250 kpm · min⁻¹) to again raise the double product to a provocative but safe level to continue the training or conditioning effect. Again, as before, the double product may be expected to progressively fall at a higher ergometer load as the training or conditioning process continues to develop.

Again, as with the previous 150 kpm · min⁻¹ work load, the new 250 kpm · min⁻¹ work load also becomes too low to induce an optimal training or conditioning effect. The prescribed body work load is then raised, in this example, to 350 kpm · min⁻¹. This same iterative, progressive process of observing the Conditioning Index and increasing the prescribed body work load to maintain the double product within a provocative but safe range is repeated *until* the body work load reaches a level at which this progressive fall in double product no longer occurs. At that point, theoretically the patient has plateaued and may not be expected to undergo significant, further progressive conditioning to the extent that it would be justifiable to further keep the patient in the structured rehabilitation program on a three-times-per-week basis. At this point the patient is exited and given a home exercise prescription based upon the plateau level achieved.

The Conditioning Index in the theoretical model illustrated in Figure 2-1 is obtained by dividing the prescribed exercise bicycle ergometer load (noted as external work) by the double product induced by that exercise load (noted as heart work). Obviously, this ratio, termed the Conditioning Index, represents the reciprocal of the heart work or myocardial oxygen demand induced by a given exercise level. The curve of the Conditioning Index illustrated in Figure 2-1 is smoothed to emphasize its S shape. The model predicts that the conditioning or training effect process will theoretically begin slowly, accelerate, level off, and plateau. It also should be noted that in this model example the tolerated exercise load is increased more than fourfold for the same average double product until a plateau is reached.

Figure 2-2 illustrates a theoretical model of the relationship of the Conditioning Index to signs and symptoms associated with myocar-

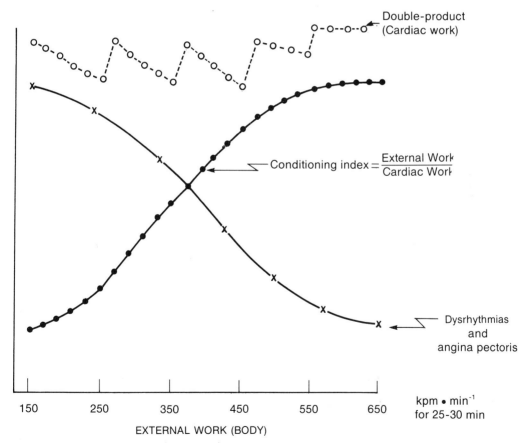

Figure 2-2. This figure is identical to that of the preceding Figure 2-1, except that a curve representing symptoms (angina pectoris) and signs (arrhythmias) of myocardial ischemia is shown to decline as the Conditioning Index rises. Studies of patients with angina pectoris and certain cardiac arrhythmias document this relationship (see text).

dial ischemia. In theory, because the Conditioning Index represents the patient's cardiac work load and myocardial oxygen demand with respect to his exercise or physical effort level, as the Conditioning Index rises, his heart will not be required to perform as much work and to utilize as much oxygen to supply the cardiac output associated with that exercise level.

At this juncture in the discussion, an important issue regarding the benefits of cardiovascular rehabilitation may be raised. The issue is whether or not the conditioning effect is accompanied by an increase in myocardial oxygen *supply* as well as by a decrease in myocardial oxygen *demand* at a given work load. It has been argued by some that a given patient exhibits the same signs and symptoms of myocardial ischemia at the same double product whether conditioned or not, i.e., when oxygen demand reaches a certain level, myocardial ischemia recurs. The HCRC experience clearly demonstrates that such is not the case.

The principle is illustrated in Figure 2-2 which diagrams a *fall* in angina and ischemia-induced arrhythmias as the Conditioning Index rises. Also, it may be noted in the model figure that the same average double product is maintained throughout the model conditioning program, but the signs and symptoms of myocardial ischemia *fall,* again, as the Conditioning Index rises. If this model is exemplified by actual patient experience, it strongly implies that myocardial oxygen supply is *increased* together with an oxygen demand decrease with respect to exercise level and its attendant cardiac output. As will be seen in Chapters 3, 4, and 5, this is amply demonstrated by an array of patient experiences.

Thus, the cardiac benefits to be expected are twofold. (1) Cardiac efficiency is increasing as the cardiac work and myocardial oxygen demand are being reduced with respect to exercise load; thus, myocardial oxygen demand is reduced. (2) Cardiac oxygen supply is increased so that at the same or greater double product, the symptoms and signs of myocardial ischemia are reduced or absent.

Because a reduction in heart rate is one component of the double product, and because beat-to-beat coronary flow is inversely related to heart rate, it may be expected that myocardial perfusion will increase as the heart rate relative to exercise load is reduced. In other words, the reduced double product implies a reduced oxygen demand, while the reduced

heart rate implies an increased supply of myocardial oxygen, apparently favoring the subendocardial portion of the heart wall.

It is generally accepted that, in the absence of occlusive coronary artery disease, coronary blood flow is adjusted to meet demand, up to physiological limits. Since the oxygen content of coronary arterial blood is discharged into the myocardium virtually to its physiological limit, an increased demand must be met by a proportional increase in flow. This, in turn, is normally achieved by a proportional decrease in coronary vascular resistance termed autoregulation. Although the stimuli to autoregulation of coronary vascular resistance are not fully understood, it is established that local metabolic factors including Po_2, Pco_2, pH, and metabolites such as adenosine and related substances, bradykinin, and so on, are involved. Moreover, innervation of the heart, especially the adrenergic beta receptors *re* norepinephrine involving stellate ganglion pathways, plays an important role and is of increasing interest with the development of beta-blocking agents. Circulating catecholamines affecting coronary artery resistance are also of importance and of interest as well in adrenergic beta-blocking agent roles. Moreover, of special interest in this discussion is the fact that coronary vascular resistance is significantly affected by the mechanical forces involved with the contractile properties of the heart wall. Thus, local metabolism related to oxygen demand, neuroendocrine influences via innervation of the heart and circulatory substances, and the mechanical properties of the heart wall within which the coronary vasculature is held, all play important, complex, and as yet not fully understood roles in control of the coronary blood flow. As noted, there is major current interest in the role of beta blockers and more recently of calcium blockers, which will be discussed at a later point in this book.

Of special interest with respect to the beneficial effects of cardiovascular conditioning is the tendency for the heart rate to slow with respect to exercise load, as the training or conditioning effect occurs. It has been shown repeatedly that the flow through the coronary vessels occurs mainly during diastole, while during systole, the vasculature is essentially choked off by the shearing and compression forces of the contracting myocardium. Indeed, retrograde coronary artery flow has been demonstrated during the isometric phase of systole. For a review of relevant literature in the field of the coronary circulation and its control, see Holmberg *et al.,* 1971; Jorgensen *et al.,* 1971; Kitamura *et al.,* 1972; Jorgensen *et al.,* 1973; Wyatt and Mitchell, 1974; Gregg, 1974; Klocke, 1976; Ball and Bache, 1976; Schaper *et al.,* 1976; Cohen *et al.,* 1977; Lambert *et al.,* 1977; Wyatt and Mitchell, 1977; Sanders *et al.,* 1978; Heaton *et al.,* 1978; Tomoike *et al.,* 1978; McElroy *et al.,* 1978; Wyatt and Mitchell, 1978; Bellamy, 1978, Jones and Roberts, 1978; St. John-Sutton *et al.,* 1978; Arnett *et al.,* 1979; Varmani and Roberts, 1979; Ellestad, 1980; Froelicher *et al.,* 1980.

From the evidence available, the working assumption of this author is that the slowing of the heart rate, in association with other events of the conditioning process, results in a beat-to-beat increase in coronary blood flow since, while systolic time remains relatively constant, there is an increased diastolic period during which most of the coronary flow during the cardiac cycle occurs. Time integration also would presumably provide a net increase in coronary flow over longer periods of time. There is evidence as well that with the slowing of the heart, there is a relatively greater increase in subendocardial flow as compared to epicardial flow.

Another related working assumption concerns the beneficial effect of propranolol which has been prescribed so widely to patients with coronary artery disease, angina, and arrhythmias. There is little or no controverting evidence that many of the beneficial actions of propranolol relate to its heart-rate-lowering effect whether through neural or circulatory catecholamine effects. It also has been shown that propranolol-induced bradycardia increases the perfusion of subendocardial areas of the heart to a greater degree than the epicardial areas (Becker, 1971). As will be discussed in more detail in Chapters 3, 4, and 16, studies of the HCRC data clearly demonstrate a view that may be summarized in the phrase, "If propranolol is good, effective exercise conditioning is better." Briefly, exercise tolerance is increased to a greater degree, and the other beneficial effects of conditioning certainly outweigh the many undesirable side effects of propranolol. Recent evidence further supports the view that improved myocardial perfusion occurs with the conditioning effect (Froelicher *et al.,* 1980).

There is much that is still unknown regarding the intricate mechanisms involving catecholamine and calcium influx effects on the heart as affected by disease, medications, and

exercise. Recently it has been shown that there is a significant increase in the density of adrenergic receptor sites in the myocytes following infarction (Mukherjee *et al.,* 1979, 1982) together with an increase in cyclic AMP catecholamines and an increase in the influx of calcium ions into the myocardial cells, with changes in Purkinje fiber activity (Corr *et al.,* 1978).

The cardiac output associated with a given total metabolic level induced by exercise does not substantially change with conditioning. Thus, as heart rate decreases, stroke volume must increase proportionately. It has been shown that this proportionate increase of stroke volume, and presumably contractility, is associated with a small increase in cardiac work and myocardial oxygen consumption compared to an increase in heart rate (Sarnoff *et al.,* 1959). Hence, it is of physiological advantage to increase the cardiac output necessary to meet exercise-metabolism demands by increasing stroke volume relative to heart rate, which is a well-demonstrated characteristic of the training or conditioning effect.

In summary, exercise tolerance is usually limited, unless by other factors such as a broken leg, by the physiological processes involved in delivering metabolic fuel and oxygen to the skeletal muscles' metabolic apparatus. This maximal oxygen consumption limit is often measured directly or assumed indirectly, and referred to as $\dot{V}O_2$ Max. The oxygen delivery system includes the respiratory system to extract oxygen from the ambient air and deliver it to the blood flowing around the alveoli. The heart's function is essentially involved in mechanically pumping the blood from the venous collecting system, through the lungs, and on to the body's metabolizing tissue. The vehicle for oxygen transport is the blood and, more specifically, the red blood cells and their contained hemoglobin. The physicochemical properties of the blood and the oxygen-utilizing tissues at the capillary level are responsible for unloading the oxygen from the blood and delivering it to the cellular metabolic processes. Moreover, there is a reordering of blood flow to other body organ systems (kidney, viscera) such that blood flow is preferentially directed to muscle, while preserving blood flow to the brain, for example.

EFFECTS OF NONCARDIAC DISORDERS

In this general, simplified sequence of exercise physiology, the reduction of exercise tolerance—symptoms of fatigue, shortness of breath, angina pectoris, and arrhythmias seen in patients with cardiovascular disease—is primarily associated with cardiac and pumping disorders rather than disorders of ventilation, oxygen-carrying capacity of the blood, or physicochemical oxygen unloading at the tissue level. However, as noted earlier, although a patient may be referred for cardiovascular rehabilitation primarily diagnosed as a cardiac disorder, he is usually also afflicted with other disorders that limit exercise tolerance and produce symptoms and signs of myocardial ischemia.

Anemia, as defined by a hemoglobin, hematocrit, or erythrocyte count > 10% lower than the laboratories' lower normal range, has been found in 9% of referred patients. Serum iron values of > 10% of the lower normal range have been found in 12% with and without accompanying changes in blood oxygen-carrying factors.

As will be discussed in Chapter 4, the mean hemoglobin, hematocrit, and serum iron values for the 272 patients referred to above were within the normal range initially and did not change significantly as a result of a virtual threefold increase in conditioning. Thus, while the patients' anemia and low serum iron levels were corrected by iron supplementation, there is no evidence from the HCRC data that there is a substantial effect of exercise conditioning on hematocrit, hemoglobin, or serum iron values. What is important, however, is that abnormalities in oxygen-carrying capacity be looked for and corrected in patients who are referred for cardiovascular rehabilitation. Indeed, several patients enjoyed resolution of angina pectoris and an improvement in exercise tolerance when their anemia was corrected.

Impaired ventilation also occurs frequently enough to warrant spirometry screening of all patients referred for cardiovascular rehabilitation. Thirteen per cent of patients referred to the HCRC exhibited significant impairment and carried diagnoses of chronic obstructive pulmonary disease associated with chronic bronchitis, asthma, and/or emphysema. These patients will be discussed further in Chapter 3.

Peripheral vascular insufficiency has been present in a few (4%) to the extent that its effects were clinically manifest. These also will be discussed in Chapter 4.

Diabetes mellitus is the most prevalent metabolic disorder seen in referred patients who might be regarded as having conditions that limit exercise tolerance through metabolic mechanisms. As has been stated, 18% of referred patients have been prescribed insulin or oral hypoglycemic agents, and 26% have had elevated fasting blood sugar levels without specific therapy except for the routine nutrition advice. It is noteworthy, as discussed in Chapter 4, that the mean fasting blood glucose levels of referred patients are normal on entering the program and do not change significantly with the threefold mean improvement in Conditioning Index.

Disorders of the bones and joints are common in the age group that has been referred for cardiovascular rehabilitation (age means for males, 52; females, 55; all, 53). Care must be taken especially with the calisthenics prior to the exercise therapy on the bicycle ergometer to adjust procedures to orthopedic problems. The bicycle ergometer exercise itself usually has not been contraindicated but indeed has proven beneficial. Care also must be exerted in using calisthenics due to the fact that some patients may undergo significant isometric stress, while others do not, while doing the same calisthenics; angina and arrhythmias may therefore occur.

Other afflictions encountered in the HCRC experience, which significantly influence the relationship of double product to prescribed exercise load, include sleep disorders, infections including influenza and even upper respiratory infections, medications, and especially emotional stress. These are conditions to which the rehabilitation staff must be alert. As will be noted in Chapter 3, the use of the Conditioning Index has proven to be of significant value in alerting the staff to such disorders while patients are in the program.

It is assumed from available data that redistribution of cardiac output and peripheral arteriovenous oxygen difference is a function of $\dot{V}O_2$ Max, i.e., essentially independent of exercise tolerance, conditioning, or disease. Apparently, these peripheral changes become even less adaptable as age increases. Certainly, they are also affected by cardiovascular medications such as adrenergic blocking, calcium-channel blocking, antianginal, and antihypertensive agents.

INITIAL EVALUATION

It is evident that the initial evaluation is a very important starting point for a comprehensive rehabilitation program. As noted above, the graded exercise tolerance test is an important component. It has been noted in the literature that the measurement of arterial blood pressure during treadmill or bicycle ergometry is difficult using the Riva-Rocci method of cuff and sphygmomanometer (Ellestad, 1980). Ellestad has stated, "The recording of blood pressure has plagued those of us doing exercise testing for a number of years, and we are still beset with problems."

We have found that the use of a relatively inexpensive Doppler flowmeter* probe increases the reliability to a satisfactory degree, and that blood pressure values are consistent among different evaluators. In addition to the exercise tolerance test as described, spirometry† is performed routinely and, when necessary, repeated following bronchodilation.

In general, the routine initial evaluation of patients referred to the HCRC includes:

1. A medical history and a physical examination with the benefit of having the background of the referring physician and hospital records whenever possible, and a nursing assessment
2. 12-lead resting and hyperventilation electrocardiograph, occasionally supplemented by a Valsalva maneuver
3. Spirometry
4. Anthropometric measurements: height, weight, and skinfold measurements
5. Fasting blood studies (SMAC 20, serum iron, and HCL cholesterol), urinalysis when necessary
6. Nutritional evaluation (see Chapter 10)
7. Psychological evaluation (see Chapter 13)

This information and related data are then compiled and made a part of the patient's permanent record, utilized as the basis of planning, executing, and evaluating the patient's program and progress through the program. The initial evaluation data are then compared with the exit and follow-up evaluation information and data.

The program itself consists of four components:

1. Exercise therapy
2. Medical therapy
3. Psychological therapy
4. Nutritional and dietary therapy

Each of these components and their outcomes are described in this and subsequent chapters.

It is important that appropriate consent

forms are provided to the patient relative to all aspects of the program, including evaluations and therapy. The patient should sign the witnessed consent forms before proceeding with any part of the program.

The following chapter provides a representative array of case studies to illustrate the principles described in this chapter.

REFERENCES

Arnett, E. N.; Isner, J. M; Redwood, D. R.; Kent, K.; Baker, W. P.; Ackerstein, H.; and Roberts, W. C. Underestimation of angiography of critical coronary arterial narrowing in life: Comparison with degree of narrowing assessed by quantitative histological examination at necropsy. *Am. J. Cardiol.,* **1979**, *43,* 343.

Åstrand, P.-O., and Rodahl, K. *Textbook of Work Physiology.* McGraw-Hill, New York, 1977.

Balke, B., and Ware, R. W. An experimental study of physical fitness of air force personnel. *U.S. Armed Forces Med. J.,* **1959**, *10,* 675.

Ball, R. M., and Bache, R. J. Distribution of myocardial blood flow in the exercising dog with restricted coronary artery flow. *Circ. Res.,* **1976**, *38,* 60–66.

Becker, L. C.; Fortwin, N. J.; and Pitt, B. Effect of ischemia and antianginal drugs on the distribution of radioactive microspheres in the canine left ventricle. *Circ. Res.,* **1971**, *28,* 263.

Bellamy, R. F. Diastolic coronary artery pressure-flow relations in the dog. *Circ. Res.,* **1978**, *43,* 92–101.

Bertrand, M. E.; LaBlanche, J. M.; Tilmat, P. Y.; Thieuleaux, F. P.; Delforge, M. R.; and Carré, A. G. Coronary sinus blood flow at rest and during isometric exercise in patients with aortic valve disease. *Am. J. Cardiol.,* **1981**, *47,* 199.

Bing, R. J. Cardiac metabolism. *Physiol. Rev.,* **1965**, *45,* 2.

Blocker, W. P., Jr. Rehabilitation in Ischemic Heart Disease. S. P. Medical and Scientific Books, New York, **1983**, preface.

Borg, G., and Linderholm, H. Perceived exertion and pulse rate during graded exercise in various age groups. *Acta Med. Scand. (Suppl.),* **1967**; *472,* 194.

Braunwald, E. Control of myocardial oxygen consumption. *Am. J. Cardiol.,* **1973**, *27,* 416.

Bruce, R. A.; Kasume, F.; and Hosner, D. Maximal oxygen intake and normographic assessment of functional aerobic impairment in cardiovascular disease. *Am. Heart J.,* **1973**, *85,* 546.

Cohen, M. V.; Yipintsoi, T.; Malhotra, A.; and Scheuer, J. Effects of exercise on coronary collateral function. *Am. J. Cardiol.,* **1977**, *39,* 262.

Corr, P. B.; Witkowski, F. X.; and Sobel, B. E. Mechanisms contributing to malignant dysrhythmias induced by ischemia in the cat. *J. Clin. Invest.,* **1978**, *61,* 9–119.

Ellestad, M. H. *Stress Testing* (Ed. 2), F. A. Davis Co., Philadelphia, 1980, pp. 20–22.

Friedman, H. S., *et al.* Acute effects of ethanol on myocardial blood flow in the nonischemia and ischemia heart. *Am. J. Cardiol.,* **1981**, *47,* 61–67.

Fox S. M.; Naughton, J. P.; and Haskell, W. L. Physical activity and the prevention of coronary heart disease. *Ann. Clin. Res.,* **1971**, *3,* 404.

---

* Vasculab, Model D-9.
† Breon, Model 2400.

Froelicher, V.; Jensen, D.; Atwood, J. E.; McKirnan, M. D.; Gerber, K.; Slutsky, R.; Battler, A.; Ashburn, W.; and Ross, J. Evidence for improvement in myocardial perfusion and function. *Arch. Phys. Med. Rehabil.,* **1980,** *61,* 517–522.

Gobel, F. L.; *et al.* The rate-pressure product as an index of myocardial oxygen consumption during exercise in patients with angina pectoris. *Circulation,* **1978,** *57,* 549.

Goldstein, R. R., and Epstein, S. E. The use of indirect indices of myocardial oxygen consumption in evaluating angina pectoris. *Chest,* **1973,** *63,* 302.

Gregg, D. E. The natural history of coronary collateral development. *Circ. Res.,* **1974,** *35,* 335–344.

Hartung, G. H.; Smolensky, M. H.; Harrist, R. B.; Rangel, R.; and Skrovan, C. Effects of varied durations of training on improvement in cardiorespiratory endurance. *J. Hum. Ergol. (Tokyo),* **1977,** *6,* 61–68.

Heaton, W. H.; Marr, K. C.; Capurro, N. L.; Goldstein, R. E.; and Epstein, S. E. Beneficial effect of physical training on blood flow to myocardium perfused by chronic collaterals in the exercising dog. *Circulation,* **1978,** *57,* 575–581.

Holmberg, S.; Serzysko, W.; and Varnauskas, E. Coronary circulation during heavy exercise in control subjects and patients with coronary heart disease. *Acta Med. Scand.,* **1971,** *190,* 465–480.

Jones, A. A., and Roberts, W. C. Quantitation of coronary artery narrowing in sudden coronary death. *Circulation,* **1978,** *58,* II133.

Jorgensen, C. R.; Kitamura, K.; Gobel, F. L.; Taylor, H. L.; and Wang, Y. Long-term precision of the N_2O method for coronary flow during heavy upright exercise. *J. Appl. Physiol.,* **1971,** *30,* 338–344.

Jorgensen, C. R.; Wang, K.; Wang, Y.; Gobel, F. L.; Nelson, R. R.; and Taylor, H. Effect of propranolol on myocardial oxygen consumption and its hemodynamic correlates during upright exercise. *Circulation,* **1973,** *48,* 1173–1182.

Kattus, A. A. Physical training and beta-adrenergic blocking drugs in modifying coronary insufficiency. In, *Coronary Circulation and Energetics in the Myocardium.* (Marchetti, G., and Toccardi, B., eds.) Karger, New York, **1967.**

Kissin, I.; Reves, J. A.; and Mardis, M. Is the rate-pressure product a misleading guide? *Anesthesiology,* **1980,** *52,* 373–374.

Kitamura, K.; Jorgensen, C. R.; Gobel, F. L.; Taylor, H. L.; and Wang, Y. Hemodynamic correlates of myocardial oxygen consumption during upright exercise. *J. Appl. Physiol.,* **1972,** *32,* 516.

Klocke, F. J. Coronary blood flow in man. *Prog. Cardiovasc. Dis.,* **1976,** *19,* 117–126.

Klocke, F. J.; Green, D. G.; Bunnell, I. L.; Roberts, D. L.; Dashkoff, N.; and Aroni, D. T. Relationship between degree of stenosis and reductoris in regional myocardial blood flow in coronary artery disease. *Clin. Res.,* **1979,** *27,* 502A.

Lambert, P. R.; Hess, D. S.; and Bache, R. J. Effect of exercise on perfusion of collateral-dependent myocardium in dogs with chronic coronary artery occlusion. *J. Clin. Invest.,* **1977,** *59,* 1–7.

Leon, A. S., and Bloor, C. M. Effects of exercise and its cessation on the heart and its blood supply. *J. Appl. Physiol.,* **1968,** *24,* 485–490.

Lund, A. S.; Taylor, S. H.; Humphreys, P. W.; Nunnelly, B. M.; and Donald, K. W. The circulatory effects of sustained voluntary muscle contraction. *Clin. Sci.,* **1964,** *27,* 229.

McElroy, C. L.; Girsen, S. A.; and Fishbein, M. C. Exercise-induced reduction in myocardial infarct size after coronary artery occlusion in the rat. *Circulation,* **1978,** *57,* 958–962.

Mosher, P.; Ross, J.; McFate, P. A.; and Shaw, R. F. Control of coronary blood flow by an autoregulatory mechanism. *Circ. Res.,* **1964,** *14,* 250–259.

Mukherjee, A.; McCoy, K. E.; Duke, R. J.; Hogan, M.; Hagler, H.; Buja, L. M.; and Willerson, J. T. Relationships between beta adrenergic receptor numbers and physiological responses during experimental canine myocardial ischemia. *Circ. Res.,* **1982,** *50,* 735.

Mukherjee, A.; Wong, T. M.; Buja, L. M.; Lefkowitz, R. T.; and Willerson, J. T. Beta adrenergic and muscarinic cholinergic receptors in canine myocardium; effects of myocardial ischemia. *J. Clin. Invest.,* **1979,** *64,* 1423.

NASA. *Proceedings of the Second Annual Meeting of the IUPS Commission on Gravitative Physiology.* Supplement to *Physiologist,* **1980,** *23,* #6.

Naughton, J.; Balke, B.; and Nagle, F. Refinements in methods of evaluation and physical conditioning before and after myocardial infarction. *Am. J. Cardiol.,* **1964,** *14,* 837.

Nelson, R. H.; Gobel, F. L.; Jorgensen, C. R.; Wang, K.; Wang, Y.; and Taylor, H. L. Hemodynamic predictors of myocardial oxygen consumption during static and dynamic exercise. *Circulation,* **1974,** *50,* 1179.

Parmley, W. W., and Tyberg, J. V. Determination of myocardial oxygen demand. In, *Progress in Cardiology.* (Yu, P. N., and Goodwin, J. F., eds.) Lea and Febiger, Philadelphia, **1976,** p. 19.

Peterson, L. H. The ratio of exercise intensity and the heart rate–systolic blood pressure product in exercise tolerance testing and physiological conditioning: The conditioning index. Submitted for publication in *J. Am. Coll. Cardiol.*

Peterson, L. H., and Anderson, M. P. Borg scale, heart rate–systolic pressure product, wellness and mood. Submitted for publication in *J. Am. Coll. Cardiol.*

Pickard, A. D.; Gordon, R.; Smith, H.; Ambrose, J.; and Meller, J. Coronary flow studies in patients with left ventricular hypertrophy of the hypertensive type. *Am. J. Cardiol.,* **1981,** *47,* 547.

Pollock, M. L., and Miller, H. S. Frequency of training as a determinant for improvement in cardiovascular function and body composition of middle-aged men. *Arch. Phys. Med. Rehabil.,* **1975,** *56,* 141–145.

Pollock, M. L., and Schmidt, D. H. Measurement of cardio-respiratory fitness and body composition in the clinical setting. *Compr. Ther.,* **1980,** 6 Suppl.

St. John-Sutton, M. G.; Frye, R. L.; Smith, H. C.; Chesbro, J. H.; and Ritman, E. L. Relation between left coronary artery stenosis and regional left ventricular function. *Circulation,* **1978,** *58,* 491–497.

Sanders, M.; White, F. C.; Peterson, T. M.; and Bloor, C. M. Effects of endurance exercise on coronary collateral flow in miniature swine. *Am. J. Physiol.,* **1978,** *234,* H614–H619.

Sarnoff, S. J.; *et al.,* Hemodynamic determinants of oxygen consumption of the heart with special reference to the tension-time index. In, *Works of the Heart* (Rosenbaum, F. F., ed.) Harper and Bros., New York, 1959.

Schaper, W.; Flameng, W.; Winkler, B.; Wristen, B.; Turschmann, W.; Neugebauer, G.; Carl, M.; and Psayk, S. Quantification of collateral resistance in acute and chronic experimental coronary occlusion in the dog. *Circ. Res.,* **1976,** *39,* 371–377.

Sonnenblick, E. H.; Ross, J.; and Braunwald, E. Oxygen consumption of the heart. Newer concepts of its multifactorial determinants. *Am. J. Cardiol.,* **1968,** *22,* 329.

Tomoike, H.; Franklin, D.; McKown, D.; Kemper, W. S.; Guberek, M.; and Ross, J., Jr. Regional myocardial dysfunction and hemodynamic abnormalities during strenuous exercise in dogs with limited coronary flow. *Circ. Res.,* **1978,** *42,* 487–496.

Varmani, R., and Roberts, W. C. Quantitation of coronary artery narrowing in clinically-isolated angina pectoris. *Am. J. Cardiol.,* **1979,** *43,* 343.

Wyatt, H. L., and Mitchell, J. H. Influences of physical training on the heart of dogs. *Circ. Res.,* **1974,** *35,* 883–889.

———. Influences of physical conditioning and deconditioning upon the coronary vasculature of dogs. *Am. J. Cardiol.,* **1977,** *39,* 262.

Chapter 3
PATIENT RESPONSES TO EXERCISE TOLERANCE TESTING AND THERAPY

*Lysle H. Peterson**

In the previous chapter, the principles and rationale for evaluating and improving the physical condition of patients referred for cardiovascular rehabilitation were discussed. Figure 2-1 (p. 18) was included to illustrate principles of certain relationships between exercise work load carried out by the patient, the response induced by the exercise work load as defined by the heart rate–systolic blood pressure product (double product), and the ratio of the exercise work load to the double product. That ratio has been named the Conditioning Index by this author.

Figure 2-2 (p. 19) was presented to illustrate the principle that, as the Conditioning Index rises, the heart is performing less work, and demanding proportionately less oxygen, in order to provide the cardiac output required by the metabolic demands of exercise. In other words, the efficiency of the heart is improved and the myocardial oxygen demand, associated with a given exercise load, is reduced as a function of the Conditioning Index. Thus, at a given exercise load, the patient's heart is less vulnerable to myocardial ischemia resulting from impaired coronary arteries.

* This chapter was written with the assistance of Cyndi M. Land, R. N., B.S.N.; Elizabeth A. Prather, R. N., B.S.N; and Mary T. Donadini, R.N.

If reduced myocardial oxygen demand were the only beneficial effect of conditioning, then it would be expected that when exercise load reached an intensity level to induce a double product that was previously associated with signs and/or symptoms of myocardial ischemia, those signs and/or symptoms would again appear. Figure 2-2, presented in the preceding chapter, illustrates the relationship that should occur if conditioning produced *both* a reduction of myocardial O_2 *demand* and an increased myocardial O_2 *supply.* With such a dual benefit, the symptoms (e.g., angina pectoris) and signs (e.g., ischemia-related arrhythmias) would decrease as the Conditioning Index increased, even though the double product were to remain the same or increase. In this chapter, the events that actually occur in patients undergoing appropriate progressive exercise are demonstrated.

It is demonstrated in this chapter that, in the actual practice of cardiovascular rehabilitation, both of these benefits do occur. Moreover, the relationships of the prescribed exercise load, the double product, and the Conditioning Index are also highly valuable in identifying factors, in addition to the training or conditioning effect, which are important in patient management in a comprehensive cardiovascular rehabilitation program. It is unusual to find, in the actual practice of cardiovascular rehabilitation, the smooth, simple, model relationships illustrated in Figures 2-1 and 2-2, although the underlying principles do apply in actual practice. In other words, the conditioning of patients involves many variables.

Everyone, including cardiac patients, has good days and bad days. It is common for people to vary, on a day-to-day basis, regarding fatigability and symptomatology, even though the reasons may not be readily evident. One of the benefits of a dedicated, structured rehabilitation program in which a patient is seen and monitored frequently and in a *consistent manner* is that much is learned that provides increased knowledge of factors that affect the patient's symptoms, signs, behavior, and performance on a day-to-day basis. In turn, these indicators can be used better to manage and provide valuable benefits to the patient in addition to the training or conditioning effect of exercise alone.

To exemplify these factors that significantly modify and modulate the day-to-day, or even week-to-week, exercise tolerance and conditioning indicators, the following case studies are presented. These case studies illustrate the variations in response to the rehabilitation process in real-life situations. Understanding this variability improves the ways in which a comprehensive rehabilitation program can manage more effectively patient problems that occur frequently, through combined psychological, medical, and nutritional therapy. Moreover, these case presentations illustrate the range of types of patients who can derive benefit from a structured, monitored, consistent, multidisciplined comprehensive rehabilitation program. The patients seen in a rehabilitation program not only vary significantly from one patient to another, but also each patient varies significantly from time to time. This fact further argues for the necessity of careful, structured, and consistent monitoring of patients on a day-to-day basis.

CASE PRESENTATIONS

Patient #314. This patient is a 49-year-old man who suffered an extensive anteroseptal infarction preceded by a sudden onset of severe substernal pain and diaphoresis. After stabilization, he underwent a cardiac catheterization and selective coronary angiography which demonstrated complete obstruction of the left anterior descending coronary artery distal to the first diagonal. An ejection fraction of 21% and marked apical dyskinesia of his left ventricle were demonstrated. He suffered complications at the catheter insertion site requiring end-to-end anastomosis of the brachial artery. He developed severe recurrent ventricular tachycardia requiring cardioversion, and his hospital course was further complicated by recurrent bouts of congestive heart failure. With medical treatment, he improved and was discharged after *one month* of hospitalization. After discharge, he did not recover satisfactory functional and systemic status and was referred for rehabilitation.

At the time of referral to the Houston Cardiovascular Rehabilitation Center (HCRC), he reported easy fatigability and shortness of breath with minimal effort. He had been instructed by the hospital staff to walk a mile per day, which he had done only intermittently because he had noted anginal symptoms and light-headedness. However, he had not taken nitroglycerin as instructed. He also had a history of long-standing hypertension treated, but only partially controlled, with diuretics. He had smoked two to three packages of cigarettes per day for more than 20 years but stopped after his infarction. He had no history of diabetes mellitus nor symptoms of peripheral vascular disease. His family history was essentially negative for cardiovascular disease except that his father was diabetic. He denied significant anxiety, depression, or sleep disturbances but did complain of financial stress and impotence. His physical examination was unremarkable except for grade II retinal changes, mild impairment of pulmonary function, a soft systolic murmur at the mitral and aortic area, and obesity. His resting blood pressure was 130/80; a resting heart rate was 72 with frequent PVCs, couplets, and occasional short bursts of ventricular tachycardia. There was ECG evidence of the previous infarction, left bundle branch block, and poor R-wave progression.

Using the Balke protocol and a treadmill exercise tolerance test, he was able to achieve stage IV (3 MPH, 7.5% grade) with marked generalized fatigue, increased unifocal PVCs and coupling, and 1 to 1.5 mm ST depression with grade II to III angina pectoris relieved by sublingual nitroglycerin.

Laboratory studies (fasting) demonstrated that the oxygen-carrying capacity of his blood was within normal limits except that his serum iron was low, i.e., 57 mEq/dl (normal range 70–105 mEq/dl). Electrolytes were normal.

Glucose, uric acid, BUN, creatinine, calcium, enzymes were normal. Total cholesterol was 196 mg/dl. HDL cholesterol was 27 mg/dl with a ratio of 7.2 to 1.

His body weight was 222½ lb relative to an estimated ideal weight of 165 ± 10%. His estimated per cent body weight as fat was 23% versus an ideal of 20%. His total daily caloric intake was 2250 with 19% as protein, 39% as carbohydrate, 42% as fat, and 0 as alcohol. His nutritional knowledge score was 60%. These nutritional factors are discussed in Chapters 4 and 5.

This patient was referred through the Texas Rehabilitation Commission and his physician in an effort to return him to gainful employment. Psychological testing predicted that he would be compliant with a comprehensive cardiovascular rehabilitation program.

His medications, on referral, were quinidine, 400 mg four times per day, isosorbide dinitrate, ˙20 mg four times per day, furosemide, 40 mg per day (which he had himself discontinued), and nitroglycerin as needed. He was not taking nitroglycerin because, he stated, it caused unpleasant headache and chest pounding.

Figure 3-1 is a computer printout of the course of prescribed exercise work load (solid line), double product (dashed line), and Conditioning Index (dotted line) over a period of 35

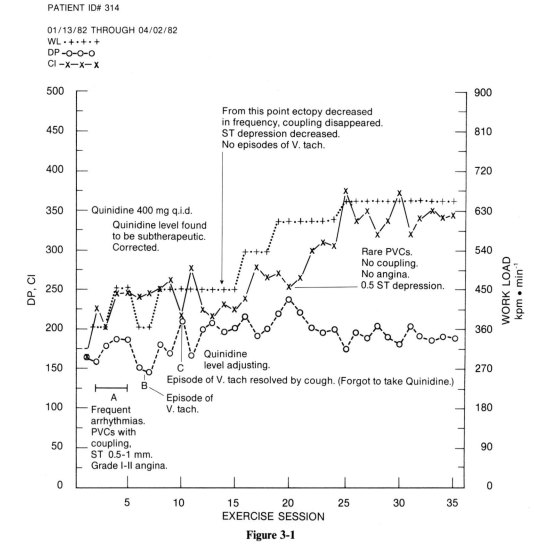

Figure 3-1

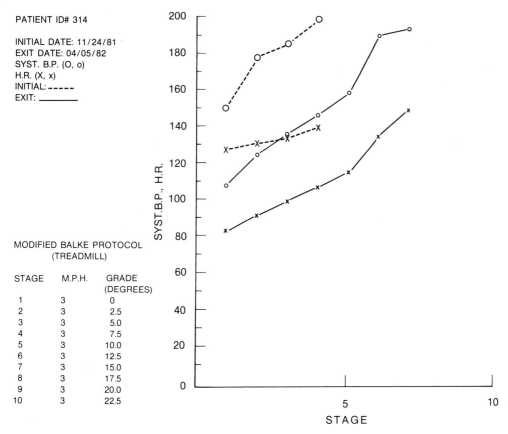

PATIENT ID# 314

INITIAL DATE: 11/24/81
EXIT DATE: 04/05/82
SYST. B.P. (O, o)
H.R. (X, x)
INITIAL: - - - - -
EXIT: _____

MODIFIED BALKE PROTOCOL
(TREADMILL)

STAGE	M.P.H.	GRADE (DEGREES)
1	3	0
2	3	2.5
3	3	5.0
4	3	7.5
5	3	10.0
6	3	12.5
7	3	15.0
8	3	17.5
9	3	20.0
10	3	22.5

Figure 3-2

scheduled exercise sessions. Several characteristics of this set of curves are noteworthy. One is that they are not smooth as in the illustrative Figure 2-1 in Chapter 2, including systematic downward progression for double product and upward progression for Conditioning Index. Nevertheless, the trends are evident. The details relating the day-to-day variability of these relations are the important aspects of practical rehabilitation.

Figure 3-2 is a computer printout of the initial dashed and exit solid exercise tolerance test of this patient. It may be noted that the upper dashed curve is the systolic blood pressure and the lower dashed curve is the heart rate obtained at each stage of the test, as noted on the abscissa.

The double product at the end-point of the initial tolerance test was 280, and, as noted above, he exhibited evident signs and symptoms of myocardial ischemia. It may be noted that, on the occasion of the exit exercise tolerance test, this patient was able to achieve stage

VII (3 MPH and 15% elevation) with a double product of 291 without arrhythmias or angina pectoris and only 0.5 mm ST depression in the electrocardiograph. The exit test was terminated due to fatigue and nonischemic leg discomfort. It is evident that the exit exercise tolerance test was extended three stages beyond the initial test and at a significantly lower systolic blood pressure and heart rate at all exercise loads during the exit test and, moreover, that the exit end-point was determined by fatigue and not by symptoms and signs of myocardial ischemia.

Returning to Figure 3-2, it may be noted that the patient was started at a therapeutic load comparable to 60% of his maximal treadmill exercise tolerance test and then moved upward to induce a resultant double product of 156 and then to 360 kpm · min^{-1} to achieve a double product of 200 with due concern for the malignant electrocardiographic history. As noted, at onset of the therapeutic program (Point *A*, Figure 3-1), this patient exhibited frequent PVCs with occasional coupling and short bursts of tachycardia, relieved by coughing, at rest and exercise, together with 0.5 to 1.0 mm ST depression and grade I to II angina relieved by nitroglycerin. At the point marked *B*, an episode of slow ventricular tachycardia occurred which was abruptly terminated by lowering the exercise load. The quinidine level was found to be below a therapeutic level and was adjusted. He had another similar episode of ventricular tachycardia at the point marked *C* which was again terminated. From that date onward, the frequency of PVCs and coupling episodes diminished, as did the angina pectoris and the ST segment depression, which had never exceeded 1 mm, but diminished to 0.5 mm. There were no further episodes of tachycardia. At the time of plateau of the Conditioning Index, this patient had increased his prescribed exercise level from the initial 260 kpm · min^{-1} to 650 kpm · min^{-1}, was asymptomatic, and exhibited little or no sign of myocardial ischemia although still maintained on a therapeutic level of quinidine. The isosorbide dinitrate was discontinued. Thus, on exit, this patient's conditioning or training effect may be summarized as shown at base of the page:

Thus, this patient leveled out at a bicycle ergometer work load level 250% higher than his initial prescribed work load. Moreover, this 2.5-fold increase in work load was accompanied by only a 6% and 5% increase in heart rate and systolic blood pressure, respectively. Hence, only a 12% increase in double product, and thus an accompanying 223% increase in Conditioning Index. It is notable that the frequent PVCs with coupling, episodes of ventricular tachycardia, 2+ mm ST depression, and angina pectoris had virtually disappeared even though the double product was higher without symptoms and signs than with the initially lower double product accompanied by signs and symptoms of myocardial ischemia. A work load of 650 kpm · min^{-1}, sustainable for 30 minutes without undue fatigue or signs or symptoms of myocardial ischemia, for someone who was hospitalized one month, discharged from the hospital three months pre-

vious to rehabilitation with an intervening total sedentary existence after a severe, complicated anteroseptal myocardial infarction and malignant arrhythmias, with significant deconditioning, must be regarded as a significant improvement. As will be noted, this is not an isolated example of dramatic benefit. Indeed, the case represents somewhat less than the average level of improvement of all patients seen at the HCRC.

On exit, this patient's only medication was a continuation of therapeutic levels of quinidine. Psychologically, while he did not represent a significantly anxious, depressed, or coronary-prone patient, his impotence had resolved, and he reported, and tests confirm, a higher coping capacity for stress. For further details, these psychological characteristics are discussed in Chapters 7 and 8.

Moreover, the patient lost 10 lb during the program and the per cent body fat dropped from 23% to 20%. He was to continue his nutrition management after exit from the program. His attendance at scheduled exercise, nutrition, psychology, and medical appointments during the program was 100%, and he has returned for all follow-up appointments. He has returned to work, and he has been diligent about maintaining his home exercise program. His latest follow-up, two years after exit from the program, demonstrated that there has been no decline in his exercise tolerance and Conditioning Index, nor has he had known recurrence of ectopy or tachycardia. An iron supplement has normalized his serum iron. Unfortunately, his home nutrition maintenance has not been as successful. His body weight has again reached 223 lb; his total cholesterol, 188; his HDL cholesterol, 31; his ratio, 6 : 1; his triglycerides, 332; and the per cent body weight as fat, 22%. The nutritionist has set a series of appointments with him, and he is currently attempting to improve his nutritional status. He is continuing steady employment without symptoms or signs of cardiac-related disorders.

Patient #427. This patient is a 49-year-old female with a long history of hypertension, who developed angina pectoris of increasing fre-

MAXIMAL EXERCISE TOLERANCE TEST STAGE	INITIAL IV	EXIT VII	CHANGE RATIO + 1.75/1
Bicycle work load (kpm · min^{-1})	260	650	+ 2.5/1
Bicycle work load, heart rate (BPM)	110	117	+ 1.06/1
Bicycle work load, systolic blood pressure	152	160	+ 1.05/1
Bicycle work load, double product	167	187	+ 1.12/1
Bicycle work load, Conditioning Index	156	348	+ 2.23/1

quency and severity with effort and emotional stress. Catheterization and selective coronary angiography demonstrated high-grade triple coronary artery disease. She underwent a quadruple aortocoronary artery bypass with temporary resolution of the angina pectoris, but with continued easy fatigability. Approximately six months postoperatively, angina pectoris with effort and stress recurred. She was again catheterized including coronary angiography, and all grafts were found to be 70 to 90% occluded, and redo-bypass was recommended. The patient's great fear of repeated surgery, and the surgeon's concern for the risk involved, led to a consensus that comprehensive cardiovascular rehabilitation should be tried as a first alternative. It may be added that this patient was under unusual emotional stress with family problems and the recent death of her husband, and she exhibited major difficulties in coping with these stresses.

On initial exercise tolerance testing she was able only to complete one out of three minutes of stage I (3 MPH, 0% grade) due as much to anxiety as to a level of exercise-provoked myocardial ischemia. She was started in therapy by simply learning to operate the bicycle ergometer. Gradually over a period of a week, she developed confidence and by the second week, she was able to sustain a work load of 180 kpm · min⁻¹ for 15 minutes, followed by increasing the time to 30 minutes. When able to sustain 30 minutes at 180 kpm · min⁻¹, her heart rate was 86; blood pressure, 142/80 mm Hg; double product, 122; and

Conditioning Index, 148. Her Conditioning Index plateaued at 227 with a work load of 320 kpm · min⁻¹, heart rate of 102, and blood pressure of 138/80 mm Hg, a double product of 141.

At 180 kpm · min⁻¹, she had exhibited an ST depression of 2 to 3 mm and grade III/V angina pectoris relieved by nitroglycerin. Prophylactic use of nitroglycerin was found to reduce and often abolish the angina pectoris but not affect the ST segment depression. As her exercise tolerance and Conditioning Index improved, the ST segment depression decreased and disappeared as did her angina pectoris.

The initial cardiac catheterization demonstrated global hypokinesis with a resting ejection fraction of 42%. No stress ejection fraction had been measured. At the time her Conditioning Index plateaued, her resting ejection fraction, determined by ventriculography, was 73% at rest and 76% with isometric stress. She has remained symptom free since her exit from the program. At the time of this writing, six months later, she is able to conduct her household and cope with the same basic stresses significantly more effectively. She is attending country-western dances at least weekly.

Figure 3-3 illustrates the electrocardiogram (lead II) at 180 kpm · min⁻¹, with a double product of 122 [427 (A)] and at 320 Kgm M/min at a double product of 141 [427 (B)].

Initially, she had been prescribed digoxin, 0.25 mg daily; nifedipine, 10 mg four times daily; propranolol, 20 mg three times daily; COUMADIN, 5 mg daily; dipyridamole, 75 mg

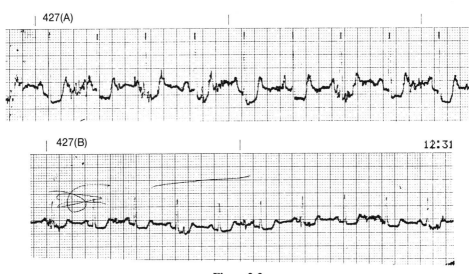

Figure 3-3

twice daily; a potassium supplement, 20 mEq daily; and an array of vitamin preparations. At the time of exit she remained on nifedipine, 10 mg daily (later discontinued), and dipyridamole, 75 mg daily. She had complained of dizziness and occasional syncope at the time of initial evaluation, which, together with many other symptoms, were regarded as of cardiac origin. After observation in the program, tests revealed the dizziness to be due to vestibular dysfunction and meclizine and isoxsuprine were prescribed with good results.

The psychologist's initial evaluation reported: "The patient is in a state of acute anxiety and depression. . . ." The exit evaluation stated: "At exit, significant reduction in anxiety and depression is apparent both clinically and psychometrically."

Patient #056. This patient was a 71-year-old male who had undergone triple coronary artery bypass surgery in 1975. Because of recurrent angina and demonstrated graft occlusion in 1976, he underwent regrafting of two of the three prior bypass grafts. His symptoms were relieved until 1979 when he again developed angina pectoris associated with emotional stress to a greater degree than with effort, though with effort as well. He also exhibited occasional episodes of bigeminy and trigeminy as well as right bundle branch block. Recatheterization revealed patent grafts, and he was referred for comprehensive cardiovascular rehabilitation. He was able to achieve stage III on the treadmill exercise tolerance test, which was terminated due to angina pectoris in the face of bundle branch block. His ejection fraction, defined by nuclear ventriculography, was 50% at rest and dropped to 38% with stress.

Figure 3-4 provides a graph of the course of this patient's rehabilitation program. He was started at 150 kpm · min^{-1}, inducing a heart rate of 68, a blood pressure of 140/86 mm Hg, a double product of 95, and a Conditioning Index of 158 (he was on propranolol, 10 mg three times daily). He complained of grade III angina, relieved by nitroglycerin, and exhibited bigeminy and trigeminy. As his Conditioning Index improved, the severity of angina decreased, as did the complex arrhythmias, first reducing to unifocal PVCs, then disappearance of the PVCs and angina pectoris. It is noteworthy that the Conditioning Index tended to vary from day to day but continued to trend upward. The declines in Conditioning Index were associated virtually always with reports from the patient of stressful family situations, confirmed by psychological interviews. It also may be noted that at the time of plateau of the Conditioning Index, the ejection fraction, determined by nuclear ventriculography, was 53% at rest and 54% with stress.

Figure 3-5 illustrates the difference between the initial and exit treadmill exercise test, i.e., from an initial end-point of stage III to an exit end-point of stage VI, discontinued due to generalized fatigue but with no complaint of angina pectoris.

This patient's therapeutic exercise level at plateau was 500 kpm · min^{-1}, at a pulse rate of 86 (propranolol had been discontinued), a blood pressure of 158/78 mm Hg, a double product of 136, and a Conditioning Index of 368. It is again noteworthy that he initially exhibited signs and symptoms at a double product of 95, while he had no such signs or symptoms at a double product of 136 at exit.

In spite of his age, this patient returned to work as a longshoreman two to three days per week and enjoyed off-shore fishing on other days. Approximately 15 months later, he returned with complaints of chest symptoms such that recurrent angina was to be ruled out. An exercise tolerance test indicated that his Conditioning Index had not declined and was virtually unchanged from the exit value. He reported that he had been diligent about continuing his maintenance exercise program at home. He did not develop chest pain at stage VI of an exercise tolerance test, at which again the end-stage was limited only by exhaustion. There was no ectopy, and recovery was uneventful. He then exercised at 500 kpm · min^{-1} on a bicycle ergometer for 30 minutes without angina or arrhythmias. However, he continued to complain of chest pain at rest and occasionally when active. His attending physician arranged for a gastrointestinal study (he had a history of peptic ulcer), which demonstrated a small hiatal hernia and cimetidine was prescribed without significant relief.

He was recatheterized, and coronary angiography demonstrated an apparent occlusion of the left anterior descending graft. It was decided to reoperate. During the surgery, it was found that the wall of the right ventricle was adhered to the retrosternal surface, and in separating the adhesive scarring, the right ventricle was irreparably ruptured and the patient died. It was revealed that the coronary grafts were patent, and that the unaffected native vessels were large and patent as well. The cause of his chest pain remains enigmatic.

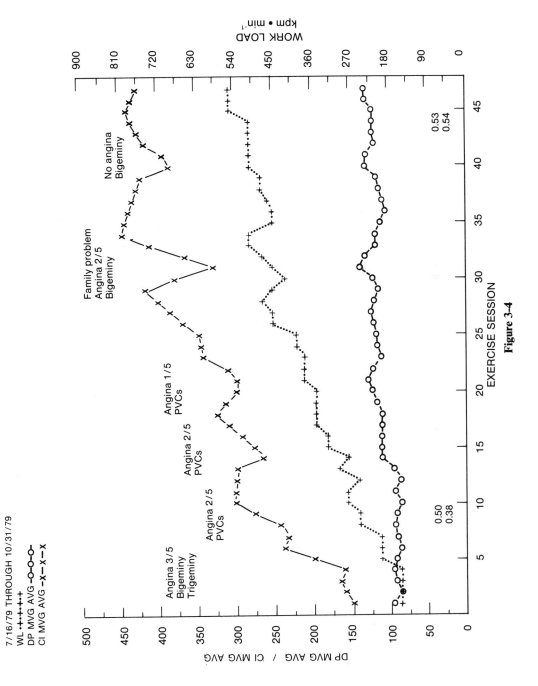

Figure 3-4

33

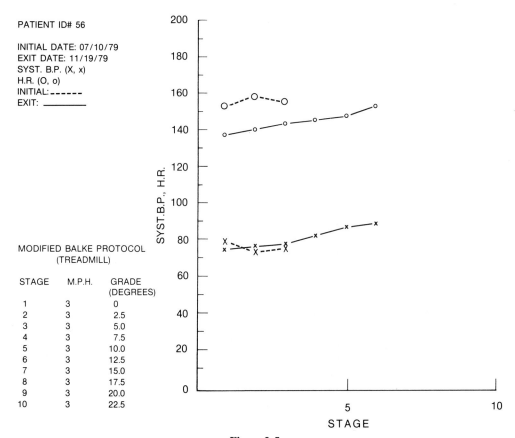

PATIENT ID# 56

INITIAL DATE: 07/10/79
EXIT DATE: 11/19/79
SYST. B.P. (X, x)
H.R. (O, o)
INITIAL: ------
EXIT: _____

MODIFIED BALKE PROTOCOL
(TREADMILL)

STAGE	M.P.H.	GRADE (DEGREES)
1	3	0
2	3	2.5
3	3	5.0
4	3	7.5
5	3	10.0
6	3	12.5
7	3	15.0
8	3	17.5
9	3	20.0
10	3	22.5

Figure 3-5

Patient #590. This patient is a 56-year-old male with a more than 10-year history of hypertension and, a rapidly resolving cerebrovascular accident followed by a left carotid endarterectomy. Subsequently, he developed bilateral, intermittent claudication followed by bilateral aortofemoral grafts. Symptoms of leg fatigue and numbness persisted. Angiographic studies revealed patent, functioning grafts with a symptom-related diagnosis of arterial spasm. During the workup, evidence via electrocardiography and nuclear ventriculography of an old apicoinferior myocardial infarction was revealed, together with hypokinesis of the apicoinferior wall but good resting global function, i.e., an ejection fraction of 53% which did not increase with stress. He was referred for cardiovascular rehabilitation relative to his medical history and due to persistent excessive fatigability with shortness of breath. He has a ++ family history of cardiovascular disease, had smoked one to two packages of cigarettes per day for 36 years and had continued to smoke. Physical examination was not remarkable. His resting blood pressure was 130/60 mm Hg bilaterally, with a resting heart rate of 86. Laboratory values (fasting) were within normal limits except for an elevated hematocrit (53.1%), hemoglobin (17.8 gm), and triglyceride level (217 mg/dl). His pulmonary function, via spirometry, revealed no significant impairment. He was only able to achieve stage II on the treadmill utilizing the Balke protocol (3 MPH, 2.5% grade) due to a rapid rise in systolic pressure to 204 mm Hg (204/76 mm Hg), with a maximum heart rate of 107, pain in both hips, and an ST depression of 2 mm but without anginal symptoms. The significance of the rapidly rising blood pressure response noted in the initial exercise tolerance test of this patient will be discussed in Chapter 5. His medications included propranolol, 10 mg twice per day, nifedipine, 10 mg four times per day, and hydroflumethiazide with reserpine, a diuretic, one tablet daily.

He was started on a bicycle ergometer work

load of 270 kpm · min⁻¹, which elicited a heart rate of 95 BMP and a blood pressure of 162/60 mm Hg, a double product of 154 with a 2-mm ST depression, and a Conditioning Index of 175. His conditioning process developed satisfactorily, and at the time he had reached a prescribed level of exercise of 600 kpm · min⁻¹, inducing a heart rate of 145 and a blood pressure of 182/60 mm Hg with little or no ST depression (<0.5 mm), he fell at home incurring a left knee injury. An arthroscopic removal of the lateral meniscus of his

left knee was performed. He was then immobilized and remained sedentary for eight and a half weeks before returning to the rehabilitation program.

On the patient's return to the program, it was necessary to reduce his prescribed work load intensity from his prior level of 600 to 360 kpm · min⁻¹, due to the deconditioning associated with the knee surgery and convalescence inactivity. At 360 kpm · min⁻¹, his heart rate was now 114, his blood pressure was 140/52, with a resulting double product of 160

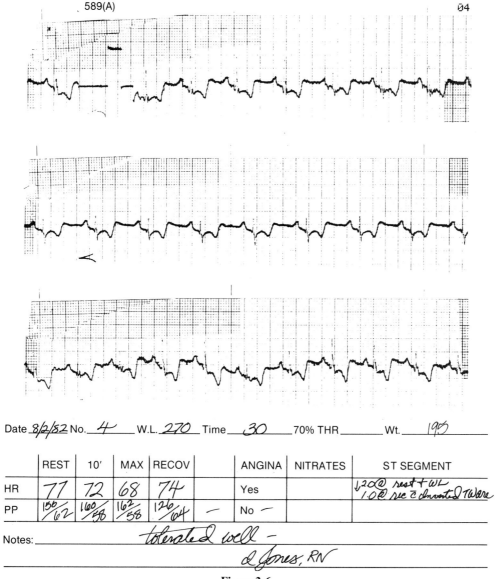

Figure 3-6

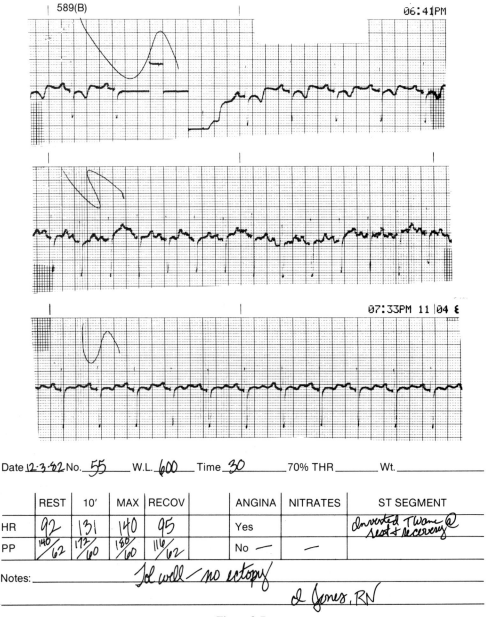

Date 12-3-82 No. 55   W.L. 600   Time 30   70% THR _____   Wt. _____

	REST	10'	MAX	RECOV		ANGINA	NITRATES	ST SEGMENT
HR	92	131	140	95		Yes		Inverted T wave @ rest + recovery
PP	140/62	172/60	180/60	116/62		No —	—	

Notes: _____ Tol well — no ectopy _____

L Jones, RN

Figure 3-7

and a Conditioning Index of 225. At this level and double product, he again exhibited 2-mm ST depression, but without anginal symptoms. His reconditioning process was then restarted and progressed well.

Figures 3-6, 3-7, and 3-8 illustrate the three conditions discussed above, i.e., the beginning of rehabilitation exercise (Fig. 3-6), the situation at the time he left the program to undergo knee surgery (Fig. 3-7), and when he returned (Fig. 3-8)]. This illustrates the fact that a patient, having achieved a high level of physiological conditioning, may regress rapidly if periodic exercise is not maintained. It should be noted that by the time this patient was forced to leave the program temporarily, he had successfully been weaned from and discontinued the use of all previously prescribed medications,

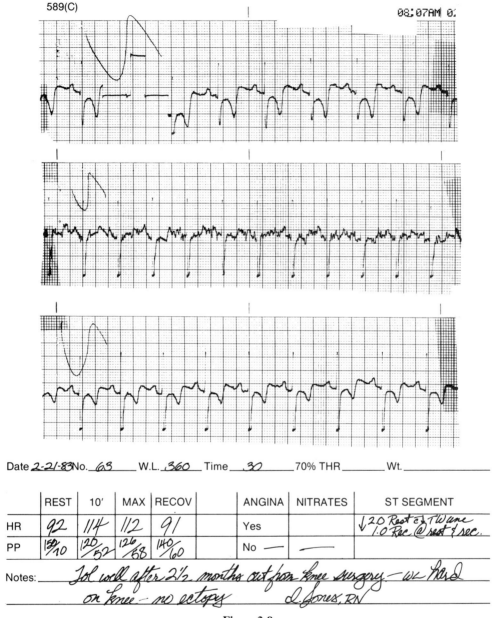

Date 2-21-83 No. 63 W.L. 360 Time 30 70% THR _____ Wt. _____

	REST	10'	MAX	RECOV		ANGINA	NITRATES	ST SEGMENT
HR	92	114	112	91		Yes		↓2.0 Rest c↓ TWave
								1.0 Rec @ rest & rec.
PP	130/10	120/52	126/68	140/60		No —	—	

Notes: _Jol well after 2½ months out from knee surgery — we hard on knee — no ectopy_   L. Jones, RN

Figure 3-8

i.e., propranolol, nifedipine, and hydroflumethiazide with reserpine. The management of medications is discussed in Chapters 4 and 16. This case again illustrates the changes in heart rate, systolic blood pressure, double product, and Conditioning Index that accompany a progressive, monitored exercise rehabilitation.

Patient #600. Case #600 is a 42-year-old fireman who had a complaint of irregular heart beat, increasing fatigability, and shortness of breath with physical effort. He reported that he was an active jogger; however, his body weight control had been unsatisfactory. The only relevant family history was that his mother suffered from hypertension. He was on no medications. He was normotensive at rest. His physical examination was unremarkable. His pulmonary function, using spirometry, exceeded applicable standards. His fasting laboratory values were well within normal and indeed within ideal limits: total cholesterol, 185 mg/dl; HDL cholesterol, 39 mg/dl, ratio 4.7 to 1; triglycerides, 98 mg/dl. His body weight was 233 lb, estimated to be 23% over his ideal body weight. His estimated per cent body fat was 27.5% versus an ideal of 20. Forty-eight per cent of his estimated caloric intake was fat. His resting and hyperventilation ECG were normal except for frequent, unifocal PVCs. He was able to achieve stage VIII (3 MPH, 17.5% elevation) on the treadmill using the Balke protocol. His maximum heart rate was 188/minute; his maximum blood pressure was 195/54 mm Hg at stage VII which fell to 174/60 in stage VIII. The test was terminated due to the fall in blood pressure, continued PVCs, and generalized fatigue. The electrocardiograph did not display ST- or T-wave changes, nor were symptoms reported. Recovery was uneventful.

A 24-hour Holter monitor* was obtained which showed 4,193 PVCs with 34 episodes of bigeminy and 268 major QRS pattern changes in QRS complexes. The variability in heart rate was from 25 to 150 beats per minute. The total 24-hour number of QRS complexes was 82,209. He was told that this degree of ectopy was associated with an increased risk, and a further evaluation with regard to coffee and alcohol use was made. He requested a repeat Holter monitoring which was not significantly different from the first.

He elected to undertake the comprehensive cardiovascular rehabilitation program. He was begun at a therapeutic exercise level of 720 kpm · min⁻¹ with an induced heart rate of 151 and a blood pressure of 180/70 mm Hg, a double product of 272, and a Conditioning Index of 298. This was accompanied by frequent, unifocal PVCs. He plateaued at a work load of 1,050 kpm · min⁻¹, at a heart rate of 156, a blood pressure of 165/78, a double product of 256, and a Conditioning Index of 410. During the progress of the program, the frequency of PVCs and coupling diminished in proportion to the rise in Conditioning Index.

On exit, a 24-hour Holter showed 73,230 total QRS complexes with 213 PVCs and one episode of bigeminy. There were 26 episodes of QRS pattern changes. At the exit exercise tolerance test, he achieved stage IX, with a maximum heart rate of 188 and a maximum blood pressure of 188/56 mm Hg with no decompen-

sation. There was a total of three PVCs during both the test and cool-down period.

His weight dropped from 233 to 188 lb; his per cent body fat, from 27.5% to 18%. The initial 47% of total calories as fat dropped to 23%. His total cholesterol dropped from 185 to 138 mg/dl; his HDL cholesterol, from 39 to 32 mg/dl. The total HDL cholesterol ratio decreased from 4.7 to 1, to 4.3 to 1. His triglycerides changed from 98 to 125 mg/dl on exit. There was no difference in hematocrit, hemoglobin or erythrocyte count.

Patient #494. This patient is a 41-year-old engineer who exhibited more frequent PVCs on Holter monitoring than that of patient #600. His case differs in other important respects as well. Without going into the details of case #494, this man also entered the program but was inconsistent in attendance, being required to be away from the city frequently for what he described as stressful business trips lasting one week or more. Moreover, this man was highly stressed in his job and at home. Initially, his exercise tolerance test was terminated at stage II due to frequent PVCs, bigeminy, and trigeminy. Nuclear ventriculography suggested early, low-grade coronary artery disease, interpreted as two-vessel equivalent. Cardiac catheterization and coronary angiography did not reveal abnormalities of the coronary arteries.

He was begun at a therapeutic exercise level of 270 kpm · min⁻¹, with persistent PVCs, bigeminy, and trigeminy. While he remained in the program, he showed signs of improvement; however, his program was interrupted so frequently for periods of one or two weeks that he would return from a stressful trip virtually back in the condition at which he started. After several such episodes, he became convinced that this intermittent approach was not of benefit and he arranged with his employer to allow him to remain in Houston until he was advised to exit the program. With compliance, he leveled off at a work load of 450 kpm · min⁻¹, and his ectopy had virtually disappeared. It should be added that he also worked consistently with the psychologist to improve his stress management capabilities.

In the case of both patients #494 and #600, nuclear ventriculography suggests the existence of low-grade, two-vessel equivalent coronary artery disease. Patient #600 did not undergo coronary angiography, however. In both cases, repeat nuclear ventriculography showed marked improvement in ventricular function

---

* Datamedix, Inc., Pecgasys Model 230.

at exit and without evidence of wall motion abnormalities as had occurred in the initial tests.

Patient #191. This case concerns an executive with a history of hypertension, diabetes mellitus, high-grade triple and left main coronary artery disease, accompanied by ischemic cardiomyopathy. The disease was so diffuse and other conditions were such that surgery was ruled out. He suffered from severe, complex arrhythmias which were difficult to control pharmacologically, and he had sustained periods of symptomatic tachycardia with rates of $200\pm$, lasting as long as two to four hours before gradually subsiding.

Initially, he was unable to complete stage I of the treadmill exercise tolerance test due to bigeminy, trigeminy, and 2.5- to 3-mm ST depression and accompanying excessive fatigue. He did not complain of angina, however. After a careful and slow beginning on an exercise

bicycle ergometer, he was able to sustain $150\ kpm\cdot min^{-1}$ for 30 minutes with an induced heart rate of 90, a blood pressure of 122/74, a double product of 110, and a Conditioning Index of 136. Figure 3-9 illustrates the accompanying ECG pattern. After a long period (36 weeks) and a careful adjustment of antiarrhythmic medications and dosages selected by trial, he was able to maintain an exercise load of $750\ kpm\cdot min^{-1}$ for 30 minutes at a pulse rate of 128, blood pressure of 158/70 mm Hg, a double product of 202, and a Conditioning Index of 356.

Although he continued to exhibit occasional to frequent PVCs with coupling, bigeminy and trigeminy and even short (three- to four-beat) bursts of ventricular tachycardia, the complexity of his arrhythmia became markedly reduced, and he has done well. He is able to maintain a full work week and enjoy weekends of golf and home gardening. On exit, he was

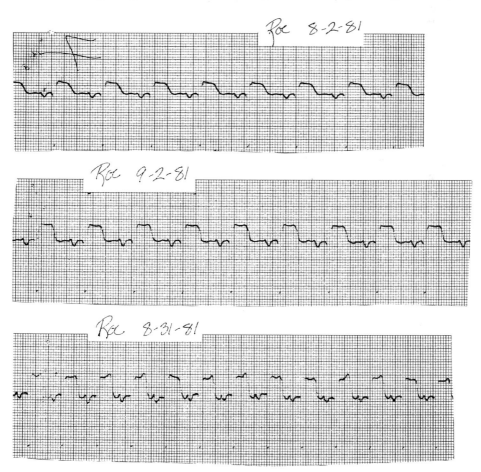

Figure 3-9

able to achieve stage IV of the exercise tolerance test at a heart rate in stage III of 136, in stage IV of 131, and a blood pressure which fell from 124/78 in stage III to 114/74 in stage IV. Nuclear ventriculography, technically difficult with a single crystal system in the presence of complex arrhythmias, was done with a multicrystal system, and the ejection fraction initially estimated at 28% had increased to 49% at rest, neither initial nor exit increasing beyond their resting levels with stress.

Patient #133. Case #133, a 54-year-old male, approximately seven years earlier had developed subacute bacterial endocarditis resulting in a tight aortic valve stenosis with regurgitation, and he underwent aortic valve replacement. The symptoms prior to surgery, including marked fatigability and shortness of breath, dyspnea, and palpitation, largely resolved following surgery until approximately six months later when he again developed general malaise, undue fatigue, and shortness of breath with low effort, e.g., one flight of steps. Palpitations at rest and with effort had recurred as well. The patient's cardiologist restudied him and found that the prosthetic valve was functioning well and his heart size was virtually normal with some left ventricular wall thickening. Nuclear ventriculography demonstrated a left ventricular ejection fraction of 82% with stress. A prior hypertension with pressures as high as 180/118 mm Hg was, at the time of restudy, averaging 160–166/90–100 mm Hg. He was referred for cardiovascular rehabilitation due to the persistent malaise, easy fatigability, palpitation, and persistent hypertension. The referring cardiologist also noted a hostility to physicians related to his expressed "bitter disappointment" over the fact that he was symptomatic following his surgery after, the patient stated, he was told that the surgery would cure his problem. The depression, anxiety, and frustration were evident! When seen, his medications included digoxin, 0.25 mg daily; crystalline warfarin sodium, 10 mg and 7.5 mg on alternate days; hydrochlorothiazide, 50 mg daily; and a potassium supplement. Propranolol, 20 mg four times per day, had been prescribed but was discontinued prior to referral.

When evaluated, he was able to achieve stage II (treadmill, Balke protocol) with a maximum heart rate of 115 and a maximum blood pressure of 180/100 mm Hg in stage I, dropping to 170/100 mm Hg in stage II.

ST depression 2 to 2.5-mm, was evident, as were frequent PVCs and generalized fatigue. He was begun on bicycle ergometer exercise therapy for 30 minutes at 150 kpm · min^{-1}, with a resulting heart rate of 93, blood pressure of 168/88, double product of 156, and a Conditioning Index of 96. His conditioning progressed to a prescribed exercise load of 525 kpm · min^{-1}, with a heart rate of 109, a blood pressure of 136/70, a double product of 156, and a Conditioning Index of 360. As the Conditioning Index rose, the ST depression, initially at 2 to 2.5 mm, but without angina, dropped to <0.5 mm, while the frequent PVCs with occasional coupling and runs of three still persisted, although having lessened. The patient exhibited manifest frustration over the persistent PVCs. Prior discussions had centered on coffee consumption which had been as much as 10 to 12 cups per day. The patient had refused to believe that coffee could be related to the occurrence of PVCs, and although he grudgingly admitted that he felt better and that his exercise tolerance had improved markedly, he remarked that doctors had repeatedly misled him. This discussion occurred on a Monday, and he demanded to know how soon the coffee-refrain effect would produce results, if indeed it did. He was told arbitrarily that by Friday of that week he should see some effect if coffee were involved. He did comply and abstained from coffee for the week; fortunately, on Friday, he exhibited only two PVCs widely dispersed in time. His initial and exit exercise tolerance tests are illustrated in Figure 3-10.

It may be noted that, at exit, in spite of a 3.5-fold increase in exercise tolerance and having become asymptomatic, his hostility toward the health profession, including the rehabilitation center, showed little sign of attenuation. He has refused follow-up and has moved out of the state. Indirect contact suggests that he is working in the mountains of a western state and has remained asymptomatic for three years.

Patient #002. Case #002 represents a 67-year-old male who had at least a 20-year history of known bradycardia (usual rate of 48 to 52 at rest) which had been diagnosed as a wandering pacemaker and as a sick sinus syndrome with at least one incident of syncope, but a pacemaker had not been prescribed. He and his referring physician thought that it would be of interest to undertake a progressive, monitored exercise therapy program prior to considering a

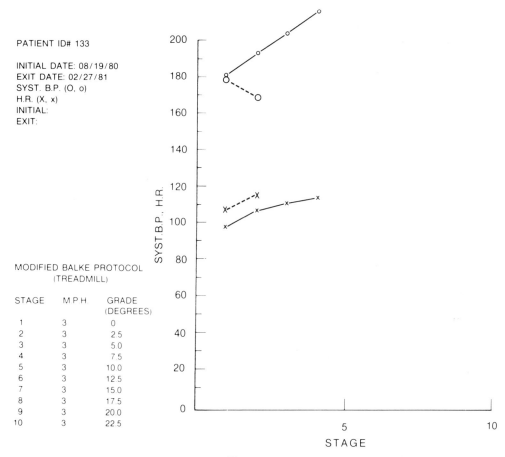

PATIENT ID# 133

INITIAL DATE: 08/19/80
EXIT DATE: 02/27/81
SYST. B.P. (O, o)
H.R. (X, x)
INITIAL:
EXIT:

MODIFIED BALKE PROTOCOL
(TREADMILL)

STAGE	M P H	GRADE (DEGREES)
1	3	0
2	3	2.5
3	3	5.0
4	3	7.5
5	3	10.0
6	3	12.5
7	3	15.0
8	3	17.5
9	3	20.0
10	3	22.5

Figure 3-10

pacemaker. At his initial exercise tolerance test, he was able to achieve stage VII with a maximal heart rate of 139 and a systolic blood pressure of 218 mm Hg at stage VII. He was begun at a therapeutic work load of 450 kpm · min^{-1}, with a heart rate of 86, a blood pressure of 180/80 mm Hg, a double product of 173, and a Conditioning Index of 260. He progressed to a work load, sustainable without undue fatigue for 30 minutes, of 900 kpm · min^{-1}, with a heart rate of 110 and a blood pressure of 156/70 mm Hg, a double product of 172, and a Conditioning Index of 523. Serial electrocardiographic studies showed a progressive improvement in his pacemaker pattern, and at Conditioning Index plateau, he did not exhibit a wandering pacemaker nor evidence of a sick sinus syndrome. He had no further symptoms of bradycardia or asystole.

Patient #302. Case #302, a 54-year-old male, was referred with a diagnosed sick sinus syndrome and a placed transvenous demand pacemaker inducing virtually all beats at a set rate of 72. At his initial exercise tolerance test, he was able to achieve stage II (3 MPH, 2.5% grade). The heart's natural pacemaker was inactive, and the paced rate remained at 72, with a systolic pressure at stage I of 180 mm Hg, which fell to 160 mm Hg at stage II. He was begun at a therapeutic work level of 270 kpm · min^{-1}, a fixed, paced heart rate of 72, a blood pressure of 156/80 mm Hg, a double product of 112, and a Conditioning Index of 241. Progressively, his work load was increased and also his native sinus pacemaker began to function after two and a half weeks still at a prescribed work load of 270 kpm · min^{-1}, but at a natural pacemaker rate of 72 to 74, a blood pressure of 148/80 mm Hg, a double product of 110, and a Conditioning Index of 245. Progressively, his therapeutic work load was increased to 650 kpm · min⁻¹ with a native pacemaker rate of 100 to 104, a blood pressure of 156–170/80 mm Hg, a double product of 156 to 170, with a Conditioning Index of 382 to 442. The initial and exit exercise tolerance tests are shown in Figure 3-11. It is evident that his demand pacemaker became unnecessary. He has completed his first year's follow-up, and with good maintenance compliance, his status has remained constant. Similar findings with primary bradyarrhythmia, wandering pacemaker, and sick sinus syndrome have been demonstrated as well in three additional cases which represent the total HCRC experience with such referrals to date.

Patient #221. This patient was, when first seen, a 50-year-old male referred for cardiovascular rehabilitation with a diagnosis of primary congestive cardiomyopathy. When first seen by the referring cardiologist, the patient was in severe congestive heart failure. He was treated as a critical patient with digitalis and zealous diuresis, to which he responded with resolution of his pulmonary edema and high-grade tachycardia. With a residual cardiomegaly, a lower grade tachycardia, poor ventricular function, an ejection fraction of 20% with global hypokinesis, and a small pericardial effusion, he was referred for comprehensive cardiovascular rehabilitation. It may be added that cardiac catheterization and selective coronary angiography revealed normal coronary arteries. The etiology of the cardiomyopathy is unknown. Alcohol intake had been reported as modest, and no severe infection had preceded the onset of the congestive failure.

At the time the patient was first seen at the HCRC, he was virtually totally disabled. He was unable to complete one minute of stage I of the treadmill exercise tolerance test. This had been his status for the prior four and a half months since his acute illness. He thus represented a stabilized full disability patient rather

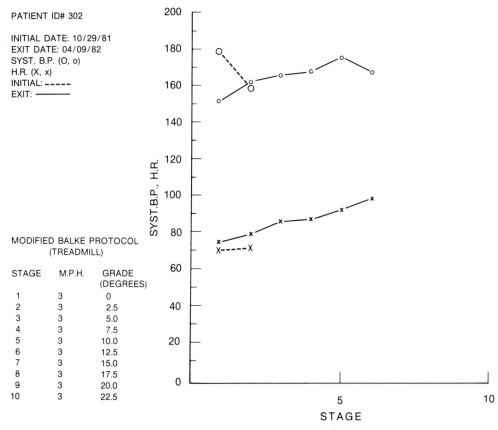

Figure 3-11

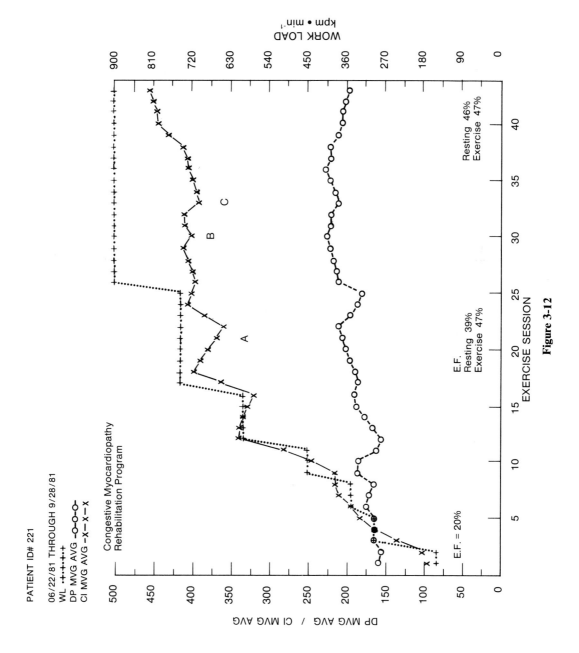

Figure 3-12

than one whose status was improving. This status also was associated with significant anxiety and depression. As an engineer-manager, he had held a high-level, responsible position. He, of course, had not worked since the onset of his acute illness and was incapable of any but a sedentary existence.

Figure 3-12 illustrates the progress achieved by this patient in the monitored, progressive cardiovascular rehabilitation program. He started the program just able to sit on the bicycle ergometer but became able to maintain a work load of 270 kpm · min^{-1} for 30 minutes with an induced heart rate of 129, a blood pressure of 129/78, a double product of 166, and a Conditioning Index of 90. As may be noted, at the end of 48 triweekly scheduled exercise sessions, of which he missed only four, he had achieved an exercise intensity level, for 30 minutes, of 900 kpm · min^{-1}, with an associated heart rate of 143, a blood pressure of 138/78 mm Hg, a double product of 197, and a Conditioning Index of 457. His heart size was normal; his ejection fraction had increased to 56% at rest and 67% with isometric stress.

A study utilizing the Beckman metabolic cart midway through the program, at the time his exercise intensity prescription had been raised from 600 to 750 kpm · min^{-1}, indicated a resting cardiac output of 4.6 liters/min; at 300 kpm · min^{-1}, 14 liters/min; and at 600 kpm · min^{-1}, 17.5 liters/min, i.e., a four-fold increase in cardiac output. These values were obtained utilizing an indirect Fick procedure. The $\dot{V}O_2$ at 300 kpm · min^{-1} was 0.971 liters/min and at 600 kpm · min^{-1} was 1.57 liters/min. It was estimated that at work loads of 300 and 600 kpm · min^{-1}, the patient was at 40% and 80%, respectively, of his aerobic capacity. The values obtained are within the ranges expected from the literature for normal, trained individuals.

The patient returned to work, first on a part-time basis after the fourteenth session with a slight decline in Conditioning Index. At the point marked *A*, an officer of his company visited his plant and gave consideration to making changes which were stressful to the patient. At points *B* and *C*, he suffered from an upper respiratory infection.

Figure 3-13 illustrates the initial and exit exercise tolerance test (Balke protocol). As noted above, initially he was unable to complete stage I; at exit he completed stage IX, i.e., 3 MPH at 20% grade. At stage IV, essentially equivalent to 1350 kpm · min^{-1}, on a bicycle ergometer, his heart rate was 167 BPM, the same as stage VIII, and his systolic blood pressure was 158 mm Hg in stage IX, having fallen from 168 at stage VIII. The test was terminated due to exhaustion. There were no ectopic nor ST changes, and recovery was uneventful. It is interesting that he achieved a level at stage VIII before sustaining a fall in systolic pressure and no increase in heart rate, which computes to virtually the same plateau Conditioning Index that he demonstrated on the bicycle ergometer for 30 minutes.

Exercise generally has been contraindicated for patients with primary congestive cardiomyopathy. The HCRC experience in prescribing exercise for such patients has been small since referrals have been few, but, as in this case, it has been demonstrated that at least in the cases referred, exercise has been shown not to be contraindicated, but indeed to be beneficial. One of the problems often encountered with such patients is psychological. Three out of six patients referred to the HCRC with congestive cardiomyopathy of unknown etiology, two with heart biopsy, dropped out of the program or were poor compliers primarily due to marked hypochondriasis and/or frank paranoid characteristics. The other three, of which this case is an example, have progressed well. Cardiomyopathy associated with coronary artery disease is more common and has responded well to exercise therapy in all cases.

Patient #623. Another apparently uncommon condition related to constrictive or obstructive left ventricle hypertrophy or cardiomyopathy is illustrated in case #623 who exhibited simultaneously significant mitral valve prolapse, high-grade triple coronary vessel disease, and status post-myocardial infarction. Studies demonstrated significant left ventricular hypertrophy and hyperkinetic wall motion with ejection of virtually all of the limited blood received during diastole. The left atrium was shown not to be unduly enlarged, but probably a mild mitral regurgitation existed. Both nuclear ventriculography and 2-D echocardiography demonstrated a 68 to 72% ejection fraction at rest with little or no increase with isometric stress. This patient achieved stage IV (3 MPH, 7.5% grade) on the initial Balke treadmill test with a maximum heart rate of 100 in stage III and stage IV and a maximal blood pressure of 180/94 mm Hg in stage IV. He was begun in therapy at a work intensity of 270 kpm · min^{-1}, inducing a heart rate of 93, a

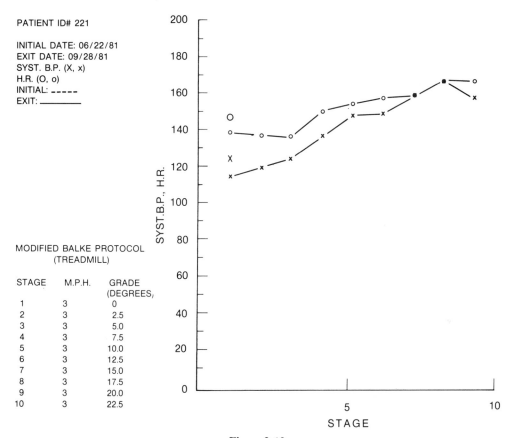

PATIENT ID# 221

INITIAL DATE: 06/22/81
EXIT DATE: 09/28/81
SYST. B.P. (X, x)
H.R. (O, o)
INITIAL: -----
EXIT: _____

MODIFIED BALKE PROTOCOL
(TREADMILL)

STAGE	M.P.H.	GRADE (DEGREES)
1	3	0
2	3	2.5
3	3	5.0
4	3	7.5
5	3	10.0
6	3	12.5
7	3	15.0
8	3	17.5
9	3	20.0
10	3	22.5

Figure 3-13

blood pressure of 154/96 mm Hg, a double product of 143, and a Conditioning Index of 189. His exercise prescription was progressively increased to 500 kpm · min^{-1} with an accompanying heart rate of 128, a blood pressure of 200/95 mm Hg, a double product of 256, and a Conditioning Index of 195. However, at a load of 500 kpm · min^{-1} and double product of 256, he developed occasional to frequent PVCs with occasional coupling which had not previously occurred below this level of work, which he perceived as highly strenuous. The work load was then reduced to 450 kpm · min^{-1}, with a heart rate of 106, a blood pressure of 180/86 mm Hg, a double product of 191, and a Conditioning Index of 236 which was accompanied by a lessening of the ectopy rate. Moreover, he exhibits occasional ectopy at rest which he had not previously shown. The pathophysiology in such a case is complex, as are the therapeutic objectives of exercise (Wyatt and Mitchell, 1974; Ballamy, 1978). The picture includes the occurrence of signs and symptoms of myocar-

dial ischemia and ventricular dysfunction when the double product reaches some, perhaps limiting, value.

Patient #502. This is a 60-year-old male who had been in relatively good health two years before referral to the HCRC when he had suffered sudden, severe chest pain with a diagnosis of acute anterior wall myocardial infarction. He was catheterized with selective coronary angiography. The right coronary artery was found to be congenitally small, with a mid-vessel 99% occlusion with filling distal collaterals. The left main vessel was calcified but without significant obstruction; the left anterior descending held 60% and 70% occlusive lesions proximal, and a distal 100% occlusion. The obtuse marginal and circumflex exhibited diffuse irregularities. The left ventricle and atrium were enlarged, and the left ventricle was hypertrophic with some pericardial effusion. There was left ventricular anterior hyperkinesis with a reported normal ejection fraction. He exhibited a first-degree AV block and exercise-related arrhythmias. He also was found to be hypertensive, hyperlipidemic, and to have gout. His medications on referral were metaprolal tartrate, 50 mg twice daily; prazosin HCL, 1 mg daily; lorazepam, 1 mg thrice daily; sulfinpyrazone HCL, 30 mg nightly; and nitroglycerin as needed. He was referred through the Texas Rehabilitation Commission because he was unemployed and fulfilled other economic and motivational criteria.

He had a positive family history of coronary heart disease. He had never smoked cigarettes and stopped smoking occasional cigars at the time of his infarction. Alcohol consumption was admitted to be mild to rare. The 25-year history of hypertension was confirmed, and clinical gout had been demonstrated eight years before. He weighed 225 lb, with an estimated ideal weight of 150 lb $\pm$ 10%; his estimated per cent body weight as fat was 28% compared to a male ideal of 20%. His fasting total cholesterol was 323; HDL cholesterol, 65, ratio 5 to 1; triglycerides, 551 mg/dl. Psychologically, he was depressed and anxious. He exhibited hostility regarding his earlier job and to the rehabilitation counselor for suggesting he return to his former job when rehabilitated.

Initially, he could only achieve stage I of the exercise tolerance test (3 MPH, 0% elevation) at a heart rate of 115 and a blood pressure of 210/120 mm Hg. The test was terminated due to the blood pressure, shortness of breath, and unsteady gait. The electrocardiograph exhibited a 1.5-mm ST depression, but he denied angina pectoris. He was begun therapeutically at 180 kpm $\cdot$ min^{-1}, inducing a heart rate of 102, a blood pressure of 190/92 mm Hg, a double product of 194, and a Conditioning Index of 93. He exhibited 1-mm ST depression, denied angina, developed occasional PVCs, and tended to decompensate toward the end of the 30-minute exercise period, i.e., his blood pressure tended to fall. His therapeutic program progressed satisfactorily. His attendance was 100%, and after 43 triweekly sessions, he plateaued at a work load of 540 kpm $\cdot$ min^{-1}, with an induced heart rate of 108, a blood pressure of 162/74 mm Hg, a double product of 175, and a Conditioning Index of 309. At this level he exhibited <0.5-mm ST depression, no evidence of a first-degree heart block, and his resting blood pressure was consistently 120–124/70–78 mm Hg without prazosin HCL and metaprolal tartrate. His weight dropped to 166 lb; his exit total cholesterol was

234 mg/dl, HDL cholesterol was 52 mg/dl, and triglycerides were 200 mg/dl. His uric acid was 3.5 mg/dl (still on sulfinpyrazone therapy).

Figure 3-14 illustrates the course of this patient's rehabilitation and Figure 3-15 compares the initial and exit exercise tolerance. One of the characteristics to be emphasized in Figure 3-14 is noted at the points marked A and B. At both of these points, a marked increase in the double product occurred at the same exercise load prior to and following the days in question. On both of the days noted as A and B, this patient had what may be characterized as a violent and threatening argument with his Texas Rehabilitation Commission counselor regarding the issue of his going back to his former employment to which he had a strong emotional aversion. This issue was resolved by interactions involving the client, the HCRC psychologist, and the TRC counselor. The man has gone back to work, the TRC case was successfully closed, and the man is satisfactorily employed. He has been diligent in maintaining his home exercise program, and follow-up evaluations have shown him to be maintaining the gains achieved during his rehabilitation program.

Patient #155. Figure 3-16 represents case #155, a 60-year-old male who had suffered an inferior myocardial infarction, followed by bilateral aortofemoral bypass due to high-grade peripheral occlusive vascular disease and claudication. This man had developed a thriving business which, when faced with his medical problems, he decided to sell. Moreover, he hoped that following his rehabilitation, he would be able to manage the company which he had developed, but then sold.

Figure 3-17 represents the initial and exit exercise tolerance test. Initially, he achieved stage IV of a treadmill test utilizing the Balke protocol at a maximal double product of 258. His initial therapeutic bicycle ergometer load was prescribed at 275 kpm $\cdot$ min^{-1}, resulting in a double product of 172 which he perceived as difficult to sustain for 30 minutes. He progressed satisfactorily, however, until the fifteenth session when, at a work load of 450 kpm $\cdot$ min^{-1}, the double product suddenly and unexpectedly rose from 192 on the fourteenth session to 263 on the fifteenth session at the same exercise load. When an unexpected rise in double product is observed, the cause is sought by a review including an interview with the patient. On the day preceding the fifteenth ses-

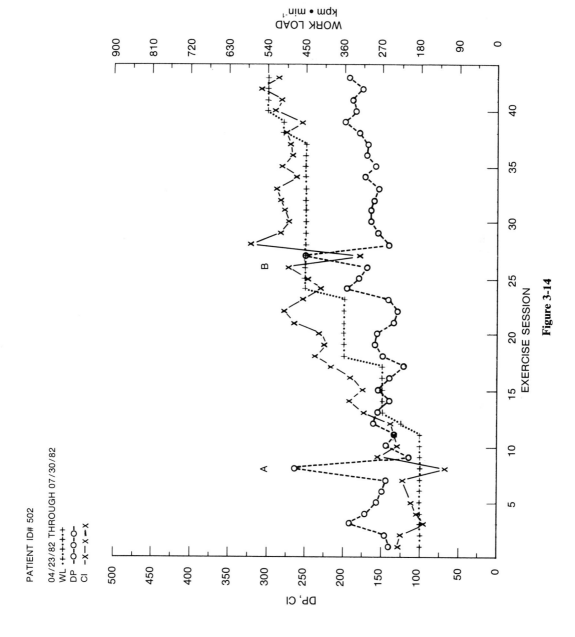

Figure 3-14

47

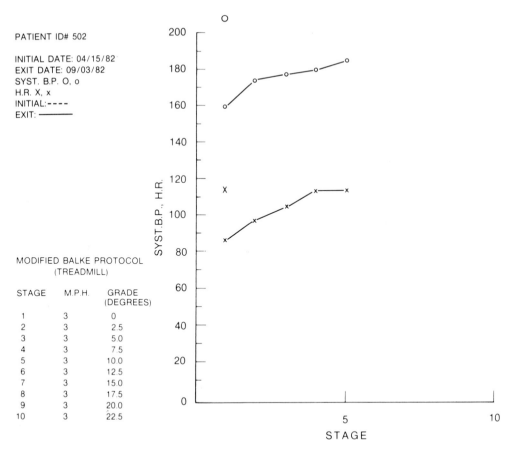

PATIENT ID# 502

INITIAL DATE: 04/15/82
EXIT DATE: 09/03/82
SYST. B.P. O, o
H.R. X, x
INITIAL:- - - -
EXIT: ————

MODIFIED BALKE PROTOCOL
(TREADMILL)

STAGE	M.P.H.	GRADE (DEGREES)
1	3	0
2	3	2.5
3	3	5.0
4	3	7.5
5	3	10.0
6	3	12.5
7	3	15.0
8	3	17.5
9	3	20.0
10	3	22.5

Figure 3-15

sion and following the fourteenth session, this patient had met with the new owner of his former company. Instead of the new owner offering the patient a contract to continue to operate the company, the new owner told the patient that he, the patient, would not be needed. This rejection was an unexpected and severe emotional shock to the patient. The results on the performance criteria are illustrated in Figure 3-16 which demonstrate that following this stressful event, his heart was working harder as judged by the rise in double product at the same exercise load, and he found the same exercise level proportionately more exhausting. This patient then underwent a series of therapeutic sessions with Dr. Merrill Anderson, the HCRC psychologist, with resolution of the acute emotional problem, and, as may be noted, the double product began to fall even as the prescribed work load was increased.

Thence, the Conditioning Index increased and proceeded upward. At session 31, the patient himself decided that he wished to drop the program due to family and business affairs. Although it was explained that his Conditioning Index had not yet plateaued, he held to his decision. He underwent an exit exercise tolerance test and the comparative results are seen in Figure 3-17, i.e., he could now achieve two additional stages to stage VI. Again, it may be noted that at each stage, except stage II, his systolic blood pressure and heart rate were substantially lower as compared to the initial test. During stage II he tripped and became anxious, but recovered. The end-point in both the initial and exit exercise tolerance tests was due to leg fatigue and cramping.

Approximately one month later, the patient called with a complaint of severe headache, and he exhibited an elevated blood pressure. He

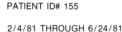

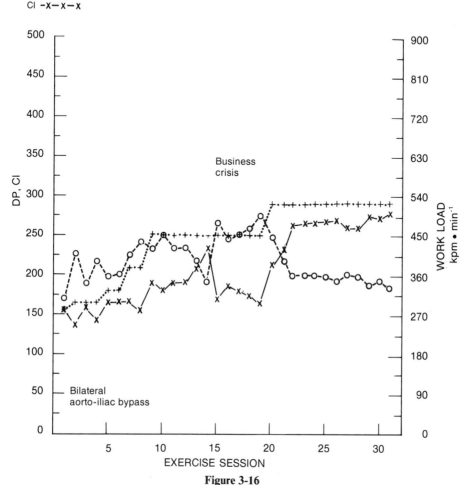

Figure 3-16

was urged to consult his attending physician, and he subsequently was seen by a neurologist with a diagnosis of cerebral aneurysm, confirmed by angiography. He was successfully treated surgically.

After recuperating from the surgery and clearance from the neurologist and attending physician, he returned to the HCRC for a modified continuation of the rehabilitation program. He already had obtained a home bicycle ergometer, and it was arranged that he would undertake a once-per-week exercise session, supervised by the HCRC, and exercise as pre-scribed the other two days per week at home.

Due to the deconditioning which had resulted from the interceding illness, hospitalization, and convalescence, he was started at 360 kpm · min^{-1}, which at this time induced a double product of 245, and Conditioning Index of 147. On this type of program, he leveled off after ten weeks at 500 kpm · min^{-1}. He has continued to retain the level of conditioning by maintaining his prescribed home exercise program.

Patient #055. Case #055 is a 58-year-old executive who had suffered an inferior wall

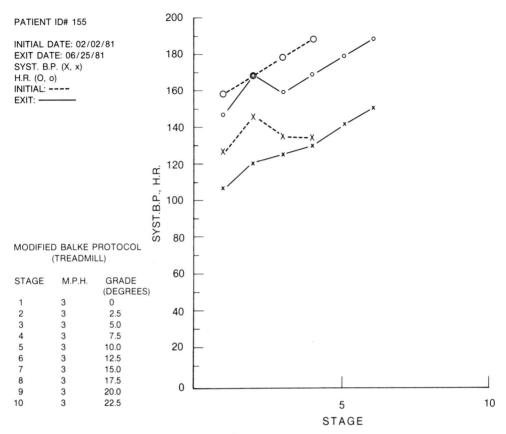

PATIENT ID# 155

INITIAL DATE: 02/02/81
EXIT DATE: 06/25/81
SYST. B.P. (X, x)
H.R. (O, o)
INITIAL: - - - -
EXIT: ———

MODIFIED BALKE PROTOCOL
(TREADMILL)

STAGE	M.P.H.	GRADE (DEGREES)
1	3	0
2	3	2.5
3	3	5.0
4	3	7.5
5	3	10.0
6	3	12.5
7	3	15.0
8	3	17.5
9	3	20.0
10	3	22.5

Figure 3-17

myocardial infarction approximately one year prior to referral for rehabilitation. He had continued to be fatigued easily and short of breath with relatively low levels of effort. He was depressed and anxious about his condition. He was overweight, 231 lb versus the recommended ideal of 185 ± 10%; the estimated per cent body weight as fat was 25% versus the recommended 20%. His total cholesterol was 395 mg/dl; HDL cholesterol, 32 mg/dl, ratio 12.3 to 1; and a triglyceride level of 356 mg/dl. His medications included propranolol, 40 mg four times daily; disopyramide phosphate, 150 mg four times daily; isorbide dinitrate, 10 mg four times daily; sulfinpyrazone and nitroglycerin as needed.

Initially, he was able to achieve stage V on the exercise tolerance test with a maximum heart rate of 114 and a maximum blood pressure of 138/64 mm Hg at stage IV, which fell to 136/66 at stage V. The test was terminated due to excessive general fatigue, progressive ST depression to 2.5 mm, and flattening T waves. He

exhibited rare PVCs and one episode of bigeminy. He complained of slight (grade I/V) tightness in his chest and chin.

He was begun at a work load of 250 kpm · min⁻¹, inducing a heart rate of 78, a blood pressure of 128/90, a double product of 100, and a Conditioning Index of 250. He was highly compliant and pressed himself and the Center staff to advance his work load, which was admittedly done more rapidly than usual, although with carefully monitored occasional nitroglycerin, and without untoward events. As indicated in Figure 3-18, he decided himself to discontinue his propranolol suddenly, in spite of warning to the contrary. The rise in double product and fall in Conditioning Index resulting from sudden discontinuation of pharmacological doses of propranolol may be noted. The marked rises in double product were accompanied by equally marked increases in perceived exertion. He was restarted on propranolol with a regaining of the sequence, then appropriately weaned from the drug. At the first point, the

PATIENT ID# 55

7/03/79 THROUGH 09/03/79
WL ·+·+·+·+
DP MVG AVG –o–o–o–
CI MVG AVG –x–x–x

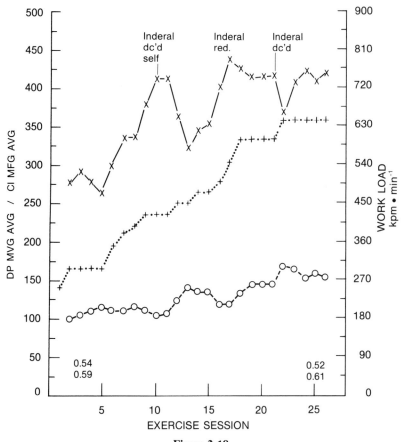

Figure 3-18

dosage was reduced by 50% and at the second point discontinued. It was decided to conduct an exercise tolerance test at the point he was established on propranolol and again when it was discontinued at essentially the same Conditioning Index. It is noteworthy from Figure 3-19 that the two courses are virtually parallel insofar as the heart rate and systolic blood pressure responses are concerned, except that he could achieve two stages more in exercise tolerance after discontinuing the propranolol.

Patient #041. Case #041, a 52-year-old male, will long be remembered at the HCRC. When referred, as one of the early referrals, this man had suffered five myocardial infarctions

and had undergone quadruple bypass surgery during the previous six years. At the time of referral, he was New York Heart Association classification IV-D. As a middle-level executive, he had lost 610 days of work prior to the year before his referral. During the prior year, he had not worked at all and was on total and permanent disability. His wife had also left her job to care for him. He had been hospitalized nine times in the previous year due to congestive heart failure. At the time of referral, his ejection fraction, obtained by nuclear ventriculography, was 18% with marked global ventricular wall hypokinesis. He exhibited a chronic sinus tachycardia of about 100 BPM. He was

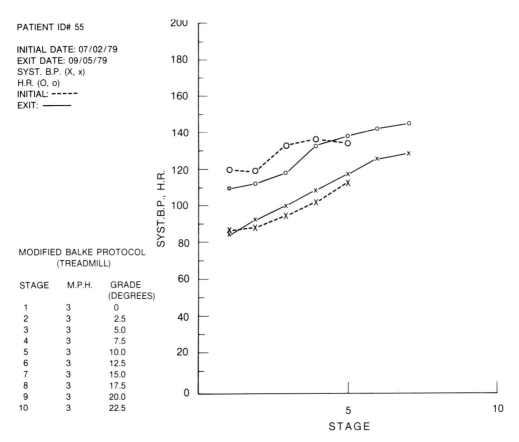

PATIENT ID# 55

INITIAL DATE: 07/02/79
EXIT DATE: 09/05/79
SYST. B.P. (X, x)
H.R. (O, o)
INITIAL: - - - - -
EXIT: ———

MODIFIED BALKE PROTOCOL
(TREADMILL)

STAGE	M.P.H.	GRADE (DEGREES)
1	3	0
2	3	2.5
3	3	5.0
4	3	7.5
5	3	10.0
6	3	12.5
7	3	15.0
8	3	17.5
9	3	20.0
10	3	22.5

Figure 3-19

hypotensive (resting blood pressure, 96–98/55–64). He was highly depressed and anxious. He could not complete stage I of the exercise tolerance test. Indeed, a 1.5 MPH brief warm-up period resulted in decompensation and a further fall in blood pressure. Recovery was uneventful, however. He suffered no angina and revealed only rare to occasional PVCs, but a 2- to 3-mm ST depression at rest. His initial total cholesterol was 310; HDL cholesterol, 15.4, ratio, 20 to 1; triglycerides, 365 mg/dl. He was approximately 20 lb over his ideal weight. The oxygen-carrying capacity of his blood was normal. His pulmonary function was significantly impaired. He had smoked two packages of cigarettes for 25 years, but had stopped two years earlier. It was estimated that this man's illness had conservatively cost $150,000 over the previous five years when hospitalization,

physician, and disability payments were considered.

After seven months and 91 scheduled exercise therapy sessions, of which he missed only 10, i.e., a 90% attendance, his exercise tolerance (30 minutes on a bicycle ergometer) had risen from effectively zero to 360 kpm · min⁻¹, with an induced heart rate of 114, a blood pressure of 122/80, a double product of 139, and a Conditioning Index of 259. His initial resting double product had been 99 with a noncalculable Conditioning Index since the 99 double product was essentially at rest. On exit, his ST segment depression was somewhat improved to 1.5 to 2 mm at work load. His resting blood pressure had normalized to 110–112/70–72 mm Hg; his resting ejection fraction became 38%, showing no change with stress. His sense of well-being had improved remarkably. He returned to work at first part time, then full time. His wife returned to work full time as well. He continued to work for 19 months when he was stricken with acute cholecystitis and cholelithiasis. He was operated upon and died one week postoperatively. The cause of death was reported as sudden death due to cardiac arrest, although his death was unattended. No post mortem was conducted.

One interesting clinical sidelight of this case is that, as noted above, he had suffered frequent episodes of congestive failure with pulmonary congestion requiring hospitalization with extensive diuresis. During the first few weeks in the program, a discussion was held with him and his wife regarding the sequence of events leading to congestive failure episodes. Briefly, on retiring and lying down, he would experience orthopnea. Both he and his wife would then become alarmed and highly anxious. This dual reaction was accompanied by increased tachycardia and a documented decline in blood pressure. It was suggested that calm relaxation, reassurance, and assuming an upright (to 70 degrees) position should be tried and frightened anxiety avoided. Apparently further episodes of congestive failure were aborted as none occurred in the next two years. Substituting calm relaxation for excitement and anxiety with the threat of a frightening episode of congestive failure appears to be rational, since stress-related tachycardia would induce increased myocardial work and oxygen demand with resulting ischemia and further ventricular failure. In addition, of course, his cardiovascular status was improving.

CONCLUSIONS

The array of case highlights presented above illustrates several important conclusions that have been drawn, to date, from the HCRC experience.

1. As a referral service, and because the referring resources of this community have been cautiously "testing" the efficiency of comprehensive cardiovascular rehabilitation, virtually the complete spectrum of cardiovascular disorders has been referred. Especially in its early years, referrals tended to reflect the relative failures or, at best, problem cases of regular office practice and treatment. Time, results, and reports from the rehabilitation center and patients alike, pointing out benefits to the referring physician, encouraged further referrals. In a sense, a cardiovascular rehabilitation center develops its own reputation since the literature has not yet apparently been widely convincing to the health profession.

Referrals to the HCRC, which have essentially doubled yearly, have been based upon case-by-case documented evidence to the referring physician and his patient of significant improvement. This has been done in an array of difficult and different types of cases, including approximately 25% who have been regarded as candidates for sudden death with high-grade coronary artery disease, severe ventricular dysfunction, and malignant arrhythmia. Over the almost five years of the HCRC experience, the case-by-case experience has collectively integrated into a sizable experience including a respectable follow-up. Again, this author feels retrospective satisfaction in having insisted on following a consistent, initially made plan for rehabilitation. Conversely, if the rationale for monitoring and documenting exercise tolerance testing and for therapeutic procedures had varied with each patient, it would have been very difficult to establish an analysis of the experiences of more than 700 patients at this time.

2. Although the cases presented above are varied, they illustrate the situations that a comprehensive cardiovascular rehabilitation center deals with in the "real" environment. These are not selected to prove benefits, but are representative examples of the overall experience of this center. In other words, 16 case studies have been presented in this chapter. An additional 16, 60, or 600 would not have altered significantly the overall conclusions which are summarized in the next chapter. The patients seen in the HCRC were not selected by the HCRC from the community; they represent what had been referred. This situation, however, has provided a splendid opportunity to apply the rationales described in this book to an array of cardiovascular disorders and to see how effective the rationales are. The patients represent an unselected sample of the problems and disorders of cardiovascular disease in a large urban community, albeit the severity of cases referred, initially at least, is skewed to the more complex medical problems. *Moreover, because most of them had been in a poor or declining status for a long time, it could not be argued that improvement was occurring in any case prior to rehabilitation.*

3. The accrued experience to date has demonstrated that all patients, without exception,

accepted for comprehensive cardiovascular rehabilitation, who complied with the program direction, improved significantly in a quantitatively documented manner. Considerable data analysis and "soul searching" preceded the writing of that seemingly audacious statement. Literally, however, the statement is true and detailed records on all patients document the conclusion. This is not to say that all referred patients benefited equally, nor were all patients referred accepted for the rehabilitation program. It may be added, however, that virtually only those who exhibited too little motivation to comply with the program or who could not exercise were not accepted. Moreover, some patients were exited even though only part of the hoped-for benefits had been achieved. The best examples of less-than-hoped-for success relate to the patients who were morbidly obese, poorly controlled, hypertensives. Although all of these patients improved their exercise tolerance and Conditioning Index by an average of 186%, and they all demonstrated some decline in resting and significant declines in exercise blood pressure, 62% left the program still significantly overweight and still hypertensive. Some referrals, after evaluation, were not accepted, some due to advanced age and organic brain syndrome, orthopedic deformities, or stroke with residual deficits such that they showed little or no promise of being able to exercise appropriately. A few were not accepted due to obvious lack of motivation. These were patients pressed by family or physician to attend the program when it was evident that the patient had little or no intention of participating effectively. Conversely, it is evident that patients with high-grade coronary artery disease, complex arrhythmias, incipient congestive heart failure, and poor myocardial function were accepted if they understood that there was a risk, that the outcome could not be guaranteed, and that after understanding these caveats, they would voluntarily and knowingly sign a consent form. The HCRC has with caution and careful monitoring, "felt its way" through a range of patients that previous published documents warned against, suggesting that exercise is contraindicated. It is agreed that certainly without close monitoring and careful patient management by a skilled staff, exercise would be contraindicated.

4. It is evident that the improvement obtained with comprehensive cardiovascular rehabilitation is not consistent with an argument that the patients were getting better anyway and would have achieved the same increases in exercise tolerance, cardiac efficiency, reduction in double product, reduced medications, optimal nutritional status, and stress management capabilities without such a program. As noted above, most of the patients seen at the HCRC had suffered their myocardial infarction or undergone their surgery, or had suffered with angina pectoris and other disorders for a year or more before being referred for cardiovascular rehabilitation. Careful history taking and review amply demonstrate that these patients had either stabilized in poor health and functional capacity or were indeed declining. As noted above, most earlier referrals had responded unsatisfactorily to office practice and often to frequent hospitalization and reworkups. It is also evident that, as the health care community has noted the performance of this center and has become better aware of a national trend as well, referrals are characterized by patients seen sooner after myocardial infarction and/or cardiovascular surgery.

5. It is evident that such an array of ill patients with such a range of disorders presents many daily management problems in addition to simply computing and executing the exercise prescription for the day. A comprehensive cardiovascular rehabilitation center should be run, as the HCRC has, as an intensive care facility. No more than eight patients are exercised simultaneously. Two nurses, each with at least five years of coronary or intensive care unit experience, before beginning work at the HCRC, are in direct control, and a trained, experienced physician is in attendance at all times. Telemetry monitoring* of the ECG is continuously maintained with appropriate alarms and automatic hard-copy recording capabilities. Blood pressures are taken and recorded before, two or more times during, and after exercise. Symptoms and other signs are monitored, evaluated, and recorded whenever they occur. All personnel are trained in advanced life support, and adequate resuscitation and life-support equipment is immediately available. Frequent and periodic staff meetings involving all staff members are held to discuss each patient in terms of his daily progress and problems as they occur.

Although it is evident that unexpected or untoward events could occur at any time, the fact that no patient has required resuscitation or immediate hospitalization within 10 days of

---

* Space Labs, 8 channel, alpha telemetry monitoring system.

attending an exercise program, with a log of more than 30,000 hours of exercise therapy and more than 2,500 symptom- and/or sign-limited exercise tolerance tests having been conducted, speaks for the policy of running the center as a critical care facility.

6. Concerning the array of disorders encountered and treated utilizing the monitoring and recording practices noted, a number of conclusions about the benefits of comprehensive cardiovascular rehabilitation can be made. These are discussed in the succeeding chapter.

It is evident by viewing the patient records from Figures 3-1 to 3-19 that the predesign of day-to-day exercise prescription is not precise. As time has gone on, however, this aspect of patient management has improved steadily. It is not possible to predict that a patient will come into the center on a given day not having slept well the previous night, having had a stressful encounter on the road between his home and the center, having experienced an unusually stressful family or job situation (the recent recession has had its impact on the center's patients with jobs threatened or lost), having forgotten to take medications, having suffered an episode of upper respiratory infection or generalized influenza, having experienced the death or serious illness of a close friend or relative, and so forth. In other words, patients come to an exercise session in many unexpected states that affect their cardiovascular status. There is an HCRC oft-repeated phrase, "If one doubts that the brain is connected to the heart, he need only work at the HCRC for one week to become convinced otherwise."

Mondays at this cardiovascular rehabilitation center reflect the weekend problems that have been noted by other observers. Instead of the weekend being a time of reduced stress, it is often one of increased stress. Underlying family frictions tend to worsen during weekends as family members are thrown more closely together for longer periods. Eating and alcoholic drinking practices tend to differ between weekdays and the weekend. Some patients abuse themselves physically in what is called avocational or recreational practices. On several occasions, patients have been given their computer printouts over several weeks and asked to identify the days in which their double products were unexpectedly high and their Conditioning Indices unexpectedly low. They are often surprised to find that these virtually all occurred on Monday. It is helpful to patients

and staff alike to understand the basis of so-called holiday depression such as is manifested more dramatically in increased suicide rates at such times as Christmas and New Year's, or when the last child leaves home.

Analyses by the HCRC staff over the years have demonstrated that certain situations account for most of the unpredicted variability in the double-product response to previously prescribed exercise work load:

1. Emotional or psychological stress, including sleep disorders
2. Forgotten medications or patient-decision medication changes (*Note:* Patients are instructed to inform the staff if the attending physician alters medications. Moreover, if the staff decides that a medication change is in order, it is done with the referring physician's concurrence)
3. Unusual physical activity conducted outside the rehabilitation center
4. Infections or other health disorders, such as diabetic complications, exacerbation of COPD such as asthma or bronchitis, influenza, URI, occult or apparent bleeding, or other causes of anemia, and so on

Conversely, it is seldom and even rare that an unexpected and otherwise undetected change is due to a worsening cardiovascular disease status.

As has been noted, there is high correlation between the individual's characteristic double product and his characteristic perception of level or intensity of effort. When the double product increases for any one of the reasons noted above, and the patient perceives a virtual equivalent increase in difficulty in maintaining the prescribed exercise work load, the staff then uses judgment as to whether or not the situation warrants maintenance or lowering of the exercise load at that time. In principle, if the increased double product is associated with contraindicating signs or symptoms, the work level is lowered.

There are few patients who are so stoic and insulated from stress or have such highly developed stress management techniques that stress-related humps and bumps in the Conditioning Index curve do not occur from time to time, and collectively, in dealing with forty patients per day, these occurrences are seen daily by the staff.

In summary: It is evident that properly prescribed and monitored exercise, together with appropriate medical, psychological, and nutritional management, provides significant benefits to a wide array of cardiovascular disease–related problems. Moreover, the methods utilized to evaluate initially the performance characteristics underlying medical disorders, medications, and psychological and nutritional disorders provide a useful and valid background for prescribing, monitoring and adjusting on a day-to-day basis a therapeutic exercise program. Experience emphasizes the conclusion that patients have good days and bad days. Thus, no rehabilitation program will experience a smooth transition from a deconditioned to an optimally conditioned state. Careful day-to-day patient management, however, modifies the patient's course in a highly beneficial manner.

REFERENCES

Ballamy, R. F. Diastolic coronary artery pressure-flow relations in the dog. *Circ. Res.,* **1978,** *43,* 92–101.

Peterson, L. H. The value of the relationships between prescribed exercise and the heart rate, systolic blood pressure product in evaluating and managing comprehensive cardiovascular rehabilitation. Submitted for publication in the *J. Am. Coll. Cardiol.*

Wyatt, H. L., and Mitchell, J. H. Influence of physical training on the heart of dogs. *Circ. Res.,* **1974,** *35,* 883–889.

Chapter 4
SUMMARIES OF DATA FROM THE
HCRC EXPERIENCE

Lysle H. Peterson

As noted previously, analysis of the responses of 274 HCRC patients to comprehensive cardiovascular rehabilitation has been completed at the time of preparing this book. These data refer to 192 males (77%) and 82 females (23%). They include all patients who were treated between 1978 and 1982, had undergone full evaluation, the full program to a Conditioning Index plateau, ten weeks of group therapy in psychology (stress management), nutrition and dietetics, and medical and physiological subjects, were exited, and have had follow-up studies. They include the entire array of types of patients seen, without selection, during the inclusive period. All have, at the time of this writing, had at least six months of follow-up. The range of conditions includes:

1. Status post – myocardial infarction
2. Status post – aortocoronary artery bypass surgery
3. Patients with documented, clinically evident coronary artery disease who had not had a documented myocardial infarction or coronary artery bypass surgery, but who were symptomatic and exhibited related disorders such as unsatisfactory exercise tolerance, angina pectoris, arrhythmias, or impaired ventricular wall function

4. Status post – aortic and/or mitral valve prosthesis, or commissurotomy surgery
5. Peripheral vascular disease, usually status post – aortic, aortofemoral, or aortoiliac grafts or bypass; and status poststroke
6. Congestive cardiomyopathy of unknown origin
7. Patients exhibiting frequent ectopy at rest and/or with exercise, usually with associated coupling, bigeminy, or trigeminy. Some had positive documentation of coronary artery disease; some had only equivocal evidence of coronary artery disease
8. Patients exhibiting primary or natural pacemaker abnormalities associated with symptomatic bradyarrhythmias

Numerically, 104 patients had undergone coronary artery bypass surgery (38%); 74 (27%) also had had one or more myocardial infarctions, and 30 (11%) had angina preceding the bypass surgery. Twelve of the 104 had also had redo – coronary artery grafting. In addition to the 104 aortocoronary artery bypass patients, two had undergone coronary artery angioplasty. Seventy-eight (28%) had suffered one or more myocardial infarctions, but had not undergone coronary artery surgery. Forty-one (15%) had angina associated with coronary artery disease, but not a documented myocardial infarction nor had undergone surgery. Fourteen (5%) exhibited high-grade ectopies, 11 (4%) status post–valve prosthesis, 6 each with cardiomyopathies and stroke, 5 with previous pacemaker bradycardias, and 2 with a diagnosis of neurocirculatory asthenia. Of this entire group, 48 (17%) had documented, clinically evident coronary artery together with coexisting clinically evident peripheral arterial disease. Moreover, 18% had diabetes or abnormal blood glucose levels, and 31% had coexisting hypertension. The average number of prescribed medications was 6.4 per patient at entry into the program. Thirteen per cent had coexisting COPD, 9% had anemias, and 12% had below normal serum iron levels.

Data analyses, to date from this number and array of patients, are given in Table 4-1

Table 4-1. DATA ANALYSES

A. AGE

	MEAN	RANGE
Males	52	(23–75)
Females	55	(32–76)
All	53	(23–76)

B. THERAPEUTIC WORK LOAD (kpm·min⁻¹)

	AT START			AT PLATEAU		
	MEAN	STD. DEV.	RANGE	MEAN	STD. DEV.	RANGE
Males	211.2	93.1	50–450	595.5	124.9	300–900
Females	154.4	61.6	50–260	379.2	120.6	150–650
All	198.8	90.1	50–450	548.4	152.6	150–900

Differences between Start and Plateau are significant at the <0.001 level.

C. HEART RATE AT WORK LOAD (Beats/min)

	AT START			AT PLATEAU		
	MEAN	STD. DEV.	RANGE	MEAN	STD. DEV.	RANGE
Males	105.4	20.9	65–180	123.7	20.4	84–190
Females	109.6	19.5	60–140	120.8	22.9	87–167
All	106.3	20.6	60–180	123.1	20.9	84–190

Differences between Start and Plateau are significant at the 0.007 level.

D. SYSTOLIC BLOOD PRESSURE AT WORK LOAD (mm Hg)

	AT START			AT PLATEAU		
	MEAN	STD. DEV.	RANGE	MEAN	STD. DEV.	RANGE
Males	140.8	27.7	90–210	152.1	19.7	108–200
Females	146.4	24.2	104–190	146.2	22.0	104–198
All	141.9	23.0	90–210	150.8	20.3	104–200

Differences between Start and Plateau significance: (Males <0.001), (Females 0.963), (All <0.001).

E. DOUBLE PRODUCT

	AT START			AT PLATEAU		
	MEAN	STD. DEV.	RANGE	MEAN	STD. DEV.	RANGE
Males	147.4	40.3	72–258	187.7	42.6	92–281
Females	159.8	42.9	62–263	178.0	48.3	106–294
All	150.1	41.0	62–263	185.6	43.8	92–294

Differences between Start and Plateau were significant at (Males <0.001), (Females 0.59), (All 0.028).

Table 4-1. (*Continued*)

F. CONDITIONING INDEX

	AT START			AT PLATEAU		
	MEAN	STD. DEV.	RANGE	MEAN	STD. DEV.	RANGE
Males	147.2	64.5	33–365	328.8	83.5	154–564
Females	98.5	39.4	31–176	220.9	75.6	104–395
All	136.6	63.1	31–365	305.3	93.0	104–564

Differences between Start and Plateau for all were <0.001.

G. DIASTOLIC PRESSURE AT LOAD

	AT START			AT PLATEAU		
	MEAN	STD. DEV.	RANGE	MEAN	STD. DEV.	RANGE
Males	80.8	14.0	58–102	79.5	10.9	66–109
Females	80.1	12.6	62– 96	76.8	9.6	64–102
All	80.1	13.1	58–102	78.9	10.2	64–109

Differences between Start and Plateau were (Males 0.390), (Females 0.141), (All 0.168).

H. RESTING SYSTOLIC BLOOD PRESSURE

(All resting values measured during postexercise recumbent relaxation period.)

	AT START			AT PLATEAU		
	MEAN	STD. DEV.	RANGE	MEAN	STD. DEV.	RANGE
Males	122.0	17.2	90–160	115.43	13.0	70–132
Females	128.0	23.6	94–150	118.87	15.5	88–138
All	123.5	18.6	90–160	116.22	13.7	70–138

Differences between Start and Plateau were significant at (Males 0.001), (Females 0.087), (All 0.001).

I. RESTING DIASTOLIC BLOOD PRESSURE

	AT START			AT PLATEAU		
	MEAN	STD. DEV.	RANGE	MEAN	STD. DEV.	RANGE
Males	80.66	11.6	54–98	75.7	8.2	58–90
Females	79.0	8.7	66–96	75.0	7.4	66–88
All	80.3	10.9	54–98	75.6	7.9	60–89.4

Differences between Start and Plateau were significant at (Males <0.001), (Females 0.013), (All 0.001).

J. RESTING HEART RATE

	AT START			AT PLATEAU		
	MEAN	STD. DEV.	RANGE	MEAN	STD. DEV.	RANGE
Males	73.0	8.5	54–92	64.5	8.0	58–86
Females	74.0	6.2	58–86	68.2	4.8	66–82
All	73.1	8.5	54–92	64.7	7.6	58–86

Differences between Start and Plateau were significant at <0.001.

Table 4-1. DATA ANALYSES (*Cont.*)

K. NUMBER OF EXERCISE SESSIONS TO PLATEAU
(three sessions per week attended.)

	MEAN DAYS	STD. DEV.	MEAN WEEKS*	RANGE (WEEKS)
Males	47.1	7.4	14.4	10.1 − 29.8
Females	38.3	8.3	11.7	10.6 − 16.4
All	45.2	7.9	13.8	10.2 − 20.6

* Average 4.33 wk/mo. Mean days/3.26 = mean weeks.

L. KILOCALORIE INTAKE

	INITIAL MEAN	STD. DEV.	EXIT MEAN	STD. DEV.
Males	1984	705	1620	602
Females	1333	374	1129	394
All	1817	699	1494	595

Differences between Initial and Exit means are significant at (Males <0.001), (Females 0.067), (All <0.001).

M. NUTRITION KNOWLEDGE

		INITIAL MEAN			EXIT MEAN	
Males	Median	60.8	$R = 85$	Median	80.83	$R = 55$
	Mode	55		Mode	80	
Females	Median	62.5	$R = 67$	Median	66.9	$R = 65$
	Mode	65		Mode	65	
All	Median	61	$R = 67-85$	Median	78.1	$R = 65-55$
	Mode	55		Mode	65	

Differences between Initial and Exit means are significant at (Males 0.123), (Females 0.655), (All 0.093).

N. WEIGHT

	INITIAL MEAN	STD. DEV.	EXIT MEAN	STD. DEV.
Males	178.9	26.8	174.6	23.6
Females	151.9	26.8	145.6	61.4
All	172.7	29.1	168.0	26.1

Differences between Initial and Exit means are significant at (Males <0.001), (Females 0.007), (All <0.001).

O. HEMOGLOBIN

	INITIAL MEAN	STD. DEV.	EXIT MEAN	STD. DEV.
Males	15.19	1.86	15.59	1.79
Females	13.93	1.42	14.09	1.29
All	14.89	1.84	15.24	1.80

Differences between Initial and Exit means are significant at (Males 0.006), (Females 0.569), (All 0.007).

Table 4-1. (*Continued*)

P. HEMATOCRIT

	INITIAL MEAN	STD. DEV.	EXIT MEAN	STD. DEV.
Males	44.96	5.23	46.1	5.5
Females	41.31	4.21	42.26	3.68
All	44.12	5.23	45.21	5.39

Differences between Initial and Exit means are significant at (Males 0.013), (Females 0.220), (All 0.005).

Q. SERUM IRON

	INITIAL MEAN	STD. DEV.	EXIT MEAN	STD. DEV.
Males	84.11	35.2	91.8	33.4
Females	57.2	23.6	70.2	28.1
All	79.14	37.36	87.86	33.33

Differences between Initial and Exit means are significant at (Males 0.128), (Females 0.191), (All 0.052).

R. CHOLESTEROL

	INITIAL MEAN	STD. DEV.	EXIT MEAN	STD. DEV.
Males	227.8	60.7	221.3	56.7
Females	253.8	65.0	234.95	75.47
All	233.6	62.36	224.32	61.19

Differences between Initial and Exit means are significant at (Males 0.186), (Females 0.107), (All 0.004).

S. TRIGLYCERIDES

	INITIAL MEAN	STD. DEV.	EXIT MEAN	STD. DEV.
Males	178.7	84.4	178.7	108.0
Females	171.8	72.8	164.2	76.4
All	177.1	84.8	175.4	101.6

Differences between Initial and Exit means are significant at (Males 0.999), (Females 0.685), (All 0.878).

T. HIGH-DENSITY LIPOPROTEIN CHOLESTEROL

	INITIAL MEAN	STD. DEV.	EXIT MEAN	STD. DEV.
Males	40.77	12.95	46.81	14.15
Females	45.65	12.84	52.57	17.83
All	42.08	12.95	48.18	15.20

Differences between Initial and Exit means are significant at (Males <0.003), (Females 0.038), (All <0.001).

U. TOTAL HIGH-DENSITY LIPOPROTEIN RATIO

	INITIAL MEAN	STD. DEV.	EXIT MEAN	STD. DEV.
Males	5.29	1.53	4.46	1.08
Females	5.31	1.51	4.27	1.29
All	5.31	1.38	4.40	1.12

Differences between Initial and Exit means are significant at (Males 0.001), (Females 0.002), (All <0.001).

Table 4-1. DATA ANALYSES (*Cont.*)

V. FASTING GLUCOSE

	INITIAL MEAN	STD. DEV.	EXIT MEAN	STD. DEV.
Males	93.91	14.58	94.30	14.61
Females	92.59	15.52	95.41	17.17
All	93.64	14.69	94.53	15.1

Differences between Initial and Exit means are significant at (Males 0.833), (Females 0.444), (All 0.590).

W. PER CENT BODY WEIGHT AS FAT

	INITIAL MEAN	STD. DEV.	RANGE	EXIT MEAN	STD. DEV.	RANGE
Males	22.6	4.6	24	21.2	3.7	20
Females	33.8	5.4	21	30.7	6.0	20
All	25.1	6.7	32	23.4	5.9	20

Differences between Initial and Exit mean values are <0.001 in all categories.

The data relative to mean therapeutic exercise load at the beginning of exercise therapy and at the time the Conditioning Index plateaued are also graphed together with the heart rates, systolic blood pressures, double products, and Conditioning Indices initially at the time of Conditioning Index plateau in the following three figures: 4-1, 4-2, and 4-3, i.e., for males, females, and the total group.

As indicated, the mean increase in bicycle ergometer exercise work load sustained without undue perceived exertion and with no dou-

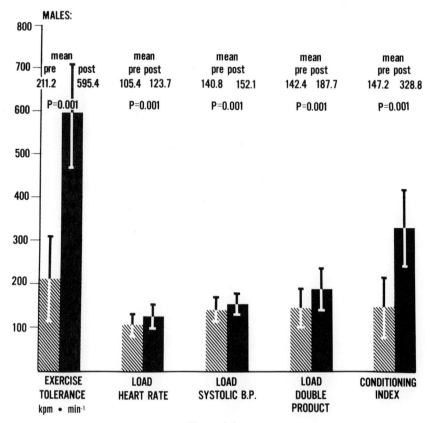

Figure 4-1

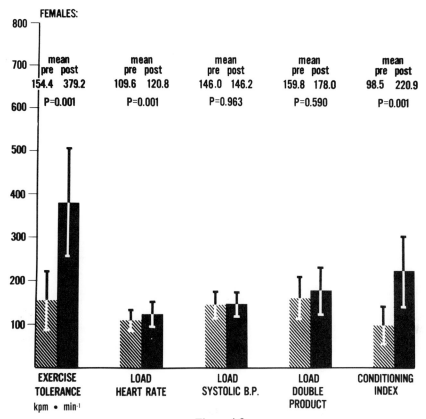

Figure 4-2

ble product exceeding 300 for 30 minutes for males was 282%, from a mean level of 211.2 initially to 595.4 kpm·min⁻¹ at Conditioning Index plateau. This increase was associated with a 14% increase in mean heart rate, a 7% increase in systolic blood pressure, thus, a 24% increase in double product. Mean exercise tolerance, therefore, increased ten times more than the double product increased, thus a mean increase of 234% in Conditioning Index. The standard deviations are shown as well on these graphs.

The females, while starting and ending at somewhat lower work levels, also showed only a slightly lower per cent improvement in exercise tolerance, i.e., a 246% increase associated with only a 10% increase in heart rate, a 0.02% (nonsignificant) increase in systolic blood pressure, a 10% (nonsignificant) increase in double product, thus a 224% increase in Conditioning Index.

The entire patient group showed an increase of 276% in therapeutic exercise tolerance with an accompanying 14% increase in heart rate, a 6% increase in systolic blood pressure, a 19%

increase in double product, and a 223% increase in Conditioning Index.

These data amply demonstrate the beneficial effects of a structured, monitored, quantitatively managed, progressive exercise therapy program. These data, illustrated by the case studies in the previous chapter, also amply demonstrate the need to combine sound medical, psychological, and nutritional management with exercise therapy. Further analyses of these data reveal certain other interesting and relevant information.

There may be a tendency to conclude that the benefits of comprehensive cardiovascular rehabilitation are age-related and that the correlation is negative, i.e., that older people do not achieve as much benefit as younger people. Analyses of the data relative to this population show that there is no significant correlation between patient age at the time of referral and the initial Conditioning Index ($P = 0.065$, i.e., nonsignificant) (correlation coefficient negative at 0.137). Moreover, at the time of Conditioning Index plateau, i.e., at exit, there was also no significant correlation of Conditioning

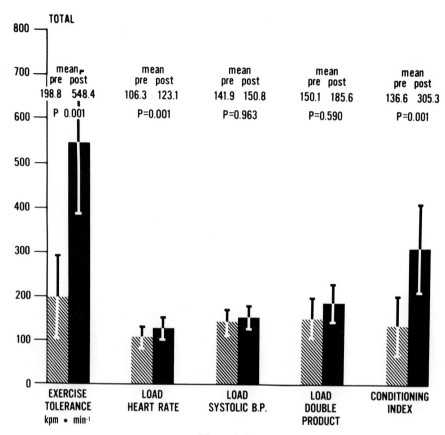

Figure 4-3

Index achieved and age ($P = 0.152$, i.e., non-significant) (correlation coefficient, 0.0934). In other words, people were ill and deconditioned at all ages and achieved similar relative benefits at all ages. The major determinants are the extent of deconditioning, the underlying pathology, coexisting disorders, and medications, rather than age.

As would be expected, the correlations of heart rate and systolic blood pressure with Conditioning Index were poor, i.e., with heart rate, the correlation coefficient was negative, 0.269, at entry, and negative, 0.330, at exit with P value $= <0.001$. With regard to systolic blood pressure and Conditioning Index, the entry correlation coefficient was negative at 0.119 ($P = 0.094$) and at exit was negative at

0.328 ($P = 0.001$). Also, as expected, the correlation of double product with Conditioning Index was low; at entry was 0.368 ($P = <0.001$), at exit was 0.314 ($P = <0.001$). Further, as expected, the correlation of Conditioning Index to work load was high; at entry, 0.796; at exit, 0.872 ($P = <0.001$).

With respect to entry and exit exercise tolerance tests, the mean initial and exit values using the conversion table from the treadmill, Balke protocol bicycle equivalent kpm · min^{-1} loads, are given in Table 4-2.

The spread in kpm · min^{-1} was:

Males <150 to 1200 kpm · min^{-1}
Females <150 to 1200 kpm · min^{-1}
All <150 to 1200 kpm · min^{-1}

Table 4-2

	ENTRY (GXT)	SD	RANGE	EXIT (GXT)	SD	RANGE
Males	603	299	1050	999	306	1650
Females	467	307	1050	810	399	1650
All	573	305	1050	957	337	1650

Table 4-3

	MALES	FEMALES	ALL
Entry	Stage IV	Stage III	Stage III+
Exit	Stages VI–VIII	Stages V to VI	Stage VI+

Table 4-3 lists the means translated back to the end stage (achieved using a treadmill and the Balke protocol). For all, an average of three stages with a range up to ten stages of improvement was accomplished.

The correlation for the entire group between the exercise tolerance work load and the therapeutic work load was found to be as follows. The correlation coefficient at entry was 0.685 ($P = <0.001$) and at exit was 0.86 ($P = <0.001$). The correlation between the exercise tolerance test results and the Conditioning Index were: the entry correlation coefficient was 0.592 ($P = 0.001$); the exit correlation coefficient was 0.667 ($P = 0.041$). Again, there were no patients who showed a decline in therapeutic or exercise tolerance levels while in the program.

Regarding correlations, it may be noted that there was also a negative correlation between the initial resting systolic and diastolic pressures and the initial Conditioning Index (negative 0.165), but a positive, although not good, correlation with the exit Conditioning Index (positive 0.227) with a $P = 0.015$. It is evident, however, that the mean resting systolic and diastolic blood pressures were significantly lower on exit than on entry (see Table 4-1). Some further correlations are also of interest.

The relationships of HDL cholesterol, exercise tolerance, and the Conditioning Index are interesting in that it has been proposed that HDL has a positive correlation with fitness. There is, however, current controversy in the literature with that view. Our findings are that there is a small, but significant increase in HDL cholesterol between entry and exit for both sexes (see Table 4-1). However, there is a poor and even negative correlation between HDL cholesterol and other measures of conditioning both at entry and exit from the program. On entry, the correlation coefficient between Conditioning Index and HDL cholesterol is *negative* 0.134, with a P value of 0.095. On exit, the correlation coefficient is also *negative* 0.1049 and the P value is 0.151.

Another parameter of current interest is the relationship between total cholesterol and HDL cholesterol. Again, there is a small, but significant difference between the entry and exit relationships of total to high-density lipo-protein ratio (see Table 4-1). On entry, the P value (0.151) between HDL cholesterol and total cholesterol is nonsignificant. Also, the correlation coefficient is poor, e.g., 0.1060. At exit, the P value is 0.031, which is of low significance, and the correlation coefficient is 0.1895, which is low.

Currently, there is also an interest in the ratio of total to HDL cholesterol as a risk factor. It has been suggested that conditioning is associated with a decline in the total-to-HDL cholesterol ratio. There is a small, but significant difference between entry and exit total:HDL cholesterol ratio, i.e., somewhat lower at exit. There is, however, a negative correlation between Conditioning Index and this ratio of 0.0311 with a P value of 0.382, i.e., nonsignificant. At exit, there is also a negative correlation coefficient of 0.0027 with a P value of 0.491, i.e., nonsignificant.

Further correlations with regard to HDL are also of interest in that the correlations with entry and exit heart rate, entry and exit systolic blood pressures, entry and exit exercise loads, and entry and exit triglyceride levels are either negative or poor, i.e., in no case was the correlation coefficient greater than 0.13.

The correlation between the exercise tolerance test (treadmill, Balke protocol) and the oxygen-carrying capacity of the blood is of some interest since Bruce et al. (1973) have suggested that a significant proportion of the benefits of exercise therapy is an improvement of this physiological parameter. It has also been noted (Goldberg, 1979), and confirmed in this center, that patients with end-stage renal disease and on dialysis, who frequently suffer from anemia, improve their anemic state with regular, structured exercise. Our data, not reported here, showed overall improvement in hemoglobin and hematocrit in this pilot subgroup study, but some patients showed little or no change.

The correlation on the entire HCRC population discussed here, i.e., 272 patients, regarding hematocrit and hemoglobin is listed in Table 4-4.

Table 4-4. BLOOD CONTENT CORRELATIONS

A. HEMOGLOBIN CORRELATED WITH CONDITIONING INDEX

	CORRELATION COEFFICIENT	P VALUE
Entry	0.256	0.005
Exit	0.185	0.033

Table 4-4. (*Continued*)

B. HEMOGLOBIN CORRELATED WITH THERAPEUTIC WORK LOAD

	CORRELATION COEFFICIENT	*P* VALUE
Entry	0.189	0.030
Exit	0.262	0.004

C. HEMATOCRIT CORRELATED WITH CONDITIONING INDEX

	CORRELATION COEFFICIENT	*P* VALUE
Entry	0.276	0.003
Exit	0.133	0.095

D. HEMATOCRIT CORRELATED WITH THERAPEUTIC WORK LOAD

	CORRELATION COEFFICIENT	*P* VALUE
Entry	0.195	0.026
Exit	0.201	0.023

Thus, although the mean hemoglobin and hematocrit values for the group are but slightly higher at exit than at entry (Table 4.1, O, P), the correlations are poor. Moreover, it has been noted that a significant number of patients who have undergone aortocoronary artery bypass surgery tend to have low hemoglobin and hematocrit. Also, a few other patients who are not postsurgical present with low hemoglobin and hematocrit. When found at initial evaluation, these patients are given iron supplements to their diets in addition to guiac testing to determine if there is a gastrointestinal bleeding source. This finding would tend to lower the initial hemoglobin and hematocrit mean values and raise the exit mean values. The exit values become normalized. When these initially anemic patients are eliminated from the data base, the change in hemoglobin and hematocrit with rehabilitation is negligible and nonsignificant.

As has been noted frequently and throughout this book, there are many factors that affect the outcome of any patient in a cardiovascular rehabilitation program. The severity of the underlying cardiovascular disease, coexisting medical disorders, the extent of initial deconditioning, psychological factors, medications, drug, alcohol, and smoking abuses, and various nutritional and diet-related problems all affect the results of the cardiovascular rehabilitation program. Thus, the data relating to such vari-

ables as oxygen-carrying capacity, plasma lipoproteins, uric acid, glucose, which show little or no consistent or mean changes, probably should not be regarded as being highly sensitive to the training or conditioning effect. Indeed, one of the study's highest HDL levels was obtained (and verified) from a patient in poor physical condition. The value was 134 mg/dl. His admitted alcohol consumption was high, 24% of his total daily caloric intake, i.e., an average of 5 to 6 oz of pure alcohol per day. As this man proceeded through the rehabilitation program, his Conditioning Index and exercise tolerance rose, while his plasma HDL level fell, associated with moderation of alcohol intake.

To prove otherwise requires tightly controlled, adequate intervention and control populations handled in a blind or double-blind fashion. Conversely, a comprehensive cardiovascular rehabilition center, whose responsibility it is to correct as many disorders and afflictions as possible, does not provide an environment for such highly controlled studies.

It is important to demonstrate what can be achieved in a comprehensive cardiovascular rehabilitation center in which as many beneficial interventions are made as can be identified and practically carried out. Moreover, in so doing, and by careful record keeping, the benefits that are achieved can be quantitatively and qualitatively identified. That is the major responsibility in demonstrating the efficacy of cardiovascular rehabilitation to the referring health care community, the third-party (insurance) reimbursement providers, and the public at large. It is evident that in spite of, or with the assistance of, many appropriate interventions, significant benefits are achieved; moreover, the causes of those major benefits are identifiable. In other words, the most significant benefits are most significant, and they can be replicated because the interventions that cause them are known.

Among the goals of comprehensive cardiovascular rehabilitation are the benefits achievable from nutritional and dietary interventions. Unfortunately, this may be one of the most difficult areas in which to achieve major benefits with regard to obesity. The group data (Table 4-1, N) show a small, but significant weight loss associated with the rehabilitation program. Overall statistics have little meaning; for example, if all patients were initially at their ideal weight and maintained their ideal weight, then the mean weight change would be effectively zero and, of course, nonsignificant. The problem is to reduce the weights of those who are overweight until, ideally, they achieve their weight goal. In the 61% who were more than 20% over their estimated ideal weight, the overall changes were found to be an initial average weight of 196 lb with a standard deviation of 30.5 lb. On exit, the average weight of these individuals was 185 lb with a standard deviation of 28.4 lb. This is an $11 \pm$ lb weight loss for this population versus a $4 \pm$ lb weight loss for the entire group. As noted before, the national experience in managing obesity is discouraging. Nevertheless, our experience is similar to other experiences (Atkinson, 1981) which can demonstrate that a comprehensive rehabilitation approach offers more hope than most types of weight-loss programs that report their data. At this center, the combined efforts of the nutritionist, psychologist, physician, and nurses seem to offer more long-term hope than other approaches so far reviewed have provided. Greater success is found in improving nutrition and diet habits in those who are not pathologically obese, although a success rate of 52% in treating obesity in general must be regarded as important.

Another important intervention is that with regard to the management of prescribed medications. It is a given fact that an important goal of cardiovascular rehabilitation is to reduce the use of prescribed medications. The major reason is that a goal of comprehensive cardiovascular rehabilitation is to provide benefits that replace the need for medications. Another goal relates to the fact that most, if not all, medications induce undesirable side effects. There are few, if any, medications that have a single-target benefit. Most produce changes throughout the body and affect most of the body's physiological and biochemical functions. Many of these effects increase the disabilities that a rehabilitation center seeks to reduce or abolish. Also, medications are expensive and add heavily to the health care costs of the nation.

On the other hand, attending physicians do attempt to balance the desirable against the undesirable effects, and the prescribing rationale should depend upon a favorable benefit balance. Thus, unless there is good reason, it would not be appropriate to change a medication. Moreover, if the patient believes that medications can indeed be substituted for comprehensive cardiovascular rehabilitation, he will often opt for the ease of taking a few pills rather than spending a few hours a week in rehabilitation and then maintaining a new lifestyle for the rest of his life.

Nevertheless, it has been the experience in this Center that most, if not all, referring physicans and their patients alike prefer to eliminate as much and as many medications as possible. The average number of prescribed medications per patient at the time of admission has been 6.4 with a range of 0–18. The bulk, i.e., those that account for more than 5% of all prescription medications surveyed, of these medications fall into 17 major categories:

1. Vasodilators, coronary (antianginal) and peripheral
2. Beta-adrenergic blocking agents
3. Digitalis preparations
4. Diuretics
5. Quinidine
6. Electrolyte (K) supplements
7. Antiarrhythmics
8. Calcium channel blockers
9. Anti-inflammatory and antiplatelet agents
10. Antidiabetic agents
11. Antihypertensive agents
12. Psychotropic agents: antidepressants, tranquilizers, sedatives, antipsychotics, psychostimulants, sleep-inducing agents
13. Antihyperuricemia agents
14. Bronchial dilators
15. Analgesics
16. Decongestants
17. Vitamins and iron supplements

These categories include 86 specific generic medications.

The average number of medications per patient was reduced 52% from 6.4 to 3.1. In 31% of the patients, all medications were eliminated. In most cases, psychotropic medications could be eliminated. Coronary vasodilators or antianginal agents were reduced or eliminated in 88% of cases; 81% of analgesics and 76% of potassium supplements were reduced or eliminated. Beta blocking agents were reduced or eliminated in 71% of cases. Sixty-four per cent of the diuretics were reduced or eliminated, as were 62% of the calcium channel blockers. Fifty-eight per cent of the antihypertensives were reduced or discontinued; 51% of antiarrhythmics were reduced or discontinued as were 34% of the antidiabetic agents. Twenty per cent of anticoagulants (COUMADIN) were reduced or discontinued. There was an increase of 18% in hyperuricemia agents prescribed.

It is evident that the staff of a comprehensive cardiovascular rehabilitation center must reasonably understand clinical pharmacology and relate it to the complexities of patient management. Chapter 16 contains a further discussion of the relationships of prescribed drugs to cardiovascular rehabilitation and provides rationale for the reductions that have been carried out.

In summary, comprehensive cardiovascular rehabilitation as exemplified by the HCRC experience can achieve a mean increase in exercise tolerance, including a wide array of patient conditions, of virtually 300%, and a comparable increase in Conditioning Index since the increases in heart rate, systolic blood pressure, and double product change proportionately less by essentially an order of magnitude, i.e., one tenth. Thus, overall, a threefold increase in exercise tolerance and the associated increase in required cardiac output is associated with but a small increase in myocardial work and oxygen consumption, and the myocardial oxygen supply is increased in proportion to the lowered heart rate at all levels of work and at rest.

Many of the other physiological and biochemical variables that have been thought to correlate significantly with physical conditioning have not been found to show high correlations; indeed, many are low or even negative. There is a poor correlation of HDL and total cholesterol/HDL ratio with physical conditioning. There is a poor correlation of changes in the oxygen-carrying capacity of the blood (hemoglobin and hematocrit) with physical conditioning. There is a small overall body weight change, but about 40% are not initially obese. There is more than twice the weight change in the obese than in the overall population. There is a significant improvement in the per cent of body weight that is fat.

An example of the problems encountered in attempting to assign significance to events is illustrated by the relationship of the % body weight estimated as fat to other variables that might affect the fat content of the body. Table 4-1.W. shows that there is a small, but statistically significant, fall in the % body weight as fat between entry and exit values for males, females, and the total population. There are very poor correlations between Conditioning Index, total plasma cholesterol, HDL plasma cholesterol, and plasma triglycerides, and the % body weight as fat. There is a *relatively* high correlation between the change in body weight for males and females (0.51 for males and 0.64 for females), but a poor correlation with the total population (0.06). Review of the scattergram for both sexes reveals that the males cluster at the high end of the relationship (high body weight and high % body weight as fat), whereas the females cluster at the low end; therefore, the total clusters toward the midrange, thus the correlation becomes poor.

The benefits of comprehensive cardiovascular rehabilitation do not correlate with age because conditions other than age play a larger role in this population in determining initial disability. The use of medications is reduced by 52%. Although there is no significant change in overall fasting blood glucose with rehabilitation, there is a significant improvement in diabetes. Again, the reason is that the number of diabetics and their fasting blood sugar do not influence the overall statistics. In Chapter 16 the summaries and conclusions are dealt with in more detail.

REFERENCES

Atkinson, R. L., and Kaiser, D. L. Nonphysician supervision of a very-low-calorie diet. Results in over 200 cases. *Int. J. Obes.,* **1981,** *5,* 237.

Bruce, R. A.; Kasume, F.; and Hosner, D. Maximal oxygen intake and normographic assessment of functional aerobic impairment in cardiovascular disease. *Am. Heart J.,* **1973,** *85,* 546.

Goldberg, A. P.; Hagberg, J. M.; Dalmez, J. A.; Haynes, M. E.; and Harter, H. R. The metabolic effects of exercise training in hemodialysis patients. *Kidney Int.,* **1980,** *18,* 754–761.

Hagberg, J. M.; Goldberg, A. P.; Ehsani, A. A.; Heath, G. W.; Dalmez, J. A.; and Harter, H. R. Exercise training improves hypertension in hemodialysis patients. *Am. J. Nephrol.,* **1983,** *3,* 209–212.

Chapter 5
VARIOUS BLOOD PRESSURE AND HEART RATE RESPONSES TO EXERCISE TESTING AND THERAPY

Lysle H. Peterson

The usual, normal response to a stepwise increase in dynamic, isotonic exercise load includes a proportional rise in heart rate and systolic blood pressure while diastolic pressure tends to remain unchanged.

The generally accepted explanation for the proportional increase in heart rate with respect to exercise load is that (1) oxygen utilization and consumption rises in proportion to the rise in aerobic metabolism of the exercising or working muscle, (2) cardiac output rises in proportion to oxygen utilization in order to supply the oxygen requirement, and (3) except for an early initial rise in stroke volume, the increased cardiac output is predominantly the resultant of a rise in pulse rate, with a stroke volume remaining relatively unchanged as exercise load increases. Thus, heart rate increase correlates well with the cardiac output which rises in proportion to the metabolic demands of increasing exercise loads.

The general explanation for the relatively direct linear relationship of systolic blood pressure to dynamic exercise load concerns the relationships between heart rate, cardiac output, and systemic peripheral resistance. The increased local metabolism of exercising muscle tends to result in locally induced peripheral vasodilation and a reduced peripheral resist-ance. Additionally, exercise is associated with reflex sympathetic vasoconstrictor inhibition and vasodilator activation of skeletal muscle that further reduces peripheral resistance. However, an important factor in limiting the net vasodilation, thus in sustaining peripheral resistance, is the mechanical compression and shearing forces of the contracting muscle. Forceful contraction of skeletal muscle (cardiac and smooth muscle as well) tends to squeeze or choke off the vasculature penetrating the muscle. Dynamic exercise, such as walking or bicycling, alternately involves agonist and antagonist muscle groups such as flexors and extensors. Hence, while one is choking off flow, in the opposite set the local and reflex vasodilation is improved and flow is enhanced. This cyclic action alternately enhances and attenuates flow to produce a net peripheral resistance.

This effect may be demonstrated easily by suddenly halting the strenuous bicycle or treadmill effort of a subject. The blood pressure, both systolic and diastolic, will suddenly drop. Indeed, this fact must be kept in mind to prevent untoward hypotensive events in patients undergoing exercise tolerance tests or therapeutic exercise sessions, and cool-down should be gradual. At the HCRC patients are reminded that race horses are never allowed to stop suddenly as they cross the finish line but are gradually slowed down.

In recalling these few general principles, many exceptions to the usual direct proportional rise of heart rate and blood pressure with exercise or metabolic load can be anticipated. One exception is, in reality, one of the normal limitations of physiological functions. No heart is capable of an unlimited increase in cardiac output. As heart rate increases beyond the range of 150 to 200 beats per minute, cardiac chamber filling time decreases at a greater rate than pumping rate increases, and cardiac output falls. Moreover, as heart rate increases, opposing relationships affecting coronary flow and myocardial perfusion come into play. Increased heart rate increases cardiac metabolism, resulting in locally induced coronary vasodilation which increases coronary blood flow. Conversely, the bulk of coronary blood flow into the myocardium occurs during diastole due, as in skeletal muscle, to the choking off of the circulation resulting from the compression and shearing forces of the contracting myocardium during systole. At some point, the coronary flow–suppressing mechanisms overtake the coronary flow–enhancing mechanisms, and myocardial perfusion declines with resulting ischemia with diminished contractility and stroke volume. The result is that a further increase of exercise level causes a fall, rather than a proportionate further increase, in arterial pressure. This is termed a decompensatory fall in systolic blood pressure as exercise tolerance testing is extended from one exercise stage to the next. This decompensation of systolic pressure may occur while the heart rate is still rising, stable, or falling. When the myocardial contractility or ionotropic property of the heart is reduced by deconditioning, disease, or medications, decompensatory systolic blood

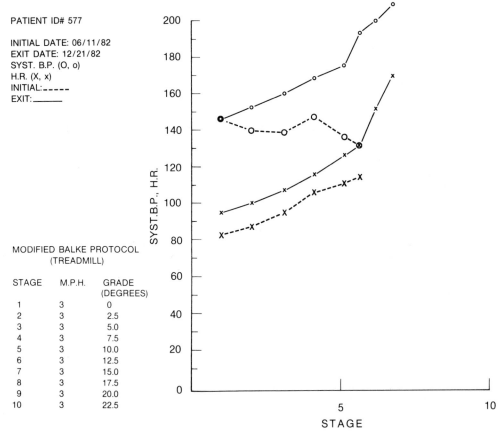

Figure 5-1

pressure response occurs at an even lower exercise intensity level. The detailed relationships between the factors enhancing and attenuating coronary blood flow as the heart rate increases are complex. There are apparently mechanical and metabolic factors that alter the distribution of the coronary circulation within areas of the heart, e.g., changes in relative distribution to subendocardial versus epicardial areas, apex, anterior, posterior, and so on. Figures 5-1 through 5-7 represent decompensatory responses seen during initial exercise tolerance testing. They also illustrate the fact that following a comprehensive cardiovascular rehabilitation program, these initial decompensatory responses are replaced by normalized blood pressure responses in which the exercise tolerance is significantly increased as well, i.e., the blood pressure range is extended.

Figure 5-1 represents a 54-year-old male, patient #577, with triple coronary artery disease, status post–myocardial infarction, sta-

tus post–triple aortocoronary artery bypass, marked hyperlipidemia, obesity, deconditioning, and psychological adjustment disorders.

Figure 5-2, a 49-year-old male, patient #290, was status post–triple coronary artery bypass, with a probable old posterior infarction, recurrent angina, chronic obstructive pulmonary disease, and deconditioning. Again, the initial decompensating response was replaced by a normal, five-stage extension of exercise tolerance with comprehensive cardiovascular rehabilitation.

Figure 5-3 represents a 49-year-old male, patient #252, also a status post–triple aortocoronary artery bypass with recurrent angina and deconditioning with chronic obstructive pulmonary disease, illustrating a decompensatory initial exercise tolerance test responding to rehabilitation in which a two-stage extension of exercise tolerance did not result in decompensation.

Figure 5-4 represents a 42-year-old female,

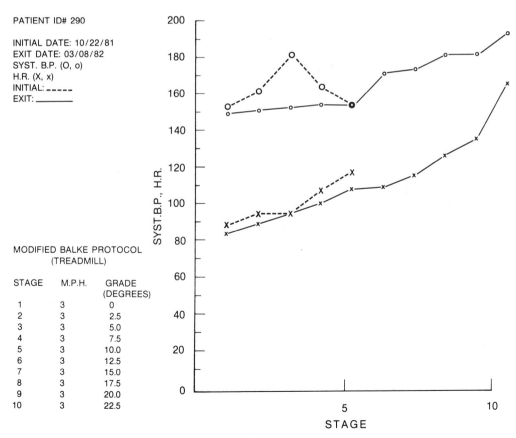

Figure 5-2

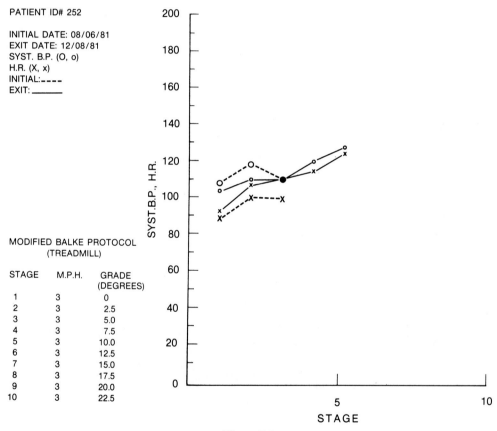

PATIENT ID# 252

INITIAL DATE: 08/06/81
EXIT DATE: 12/08/81
SYST. B.P. (O, o)
H.R. (X, x)
INITIAL: ----
EXIT: _____

MODIFIED BALKE PROTOCOL
(TREADMILL)

STAGE	M.P.H.	GRADE (DEGREES)
1	3	0
2	3	2.5
3	3	5.0
4	3	7.5
5	3	10.0
6	3	12.5
7	3	15.0
8	3	17.5
9	3	20.0
10	3	22.5

Figure 5-3

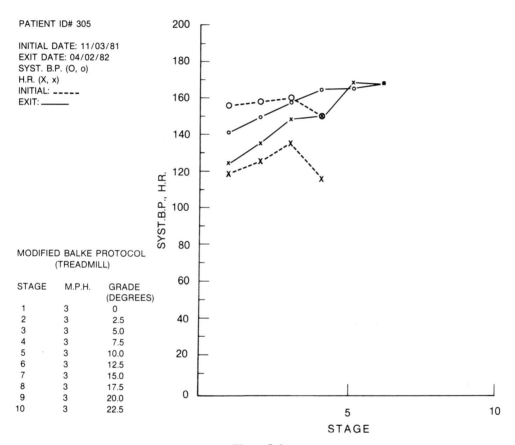

Figure 5-4

patient #305, also with high-grade triple coronary artery disease, status post–myocardial infarction, and triple aortocoronary artery bypass, recurrent angina, an insulin-dependent diabetic, hypertensive, obese, hyperlipidemic, and with emotional problems. The initial decompensation of systolic blood pressure and heart rate may be noted, whereas after rehabilitation, there was extension of exercise tolerance without a systolic blood pressure decompensation or fall in heart rate.

Figure 5-5 represents a 55-year-old male, patient #533, with a post–apicoinferior myocardial infarction, recurrent angina pectoris and arrhythmias, a quadruple aortocoronary artery bypass, again with recurrent angina and arrhythmias, severe deconditioning, hyperlipidemia, obesity, and psychological disorders. A somewhat different pre- and postrehabilitation

response of heart rate and systolic blood pressure may be observed.

Figure 5-6 is from a 36-year-old male, patient #307, who had suffered an anterior infarction, was deconditioned, hypertensive, obese, hyperlipidemic, and psychologically disordered. The initial decompensation and exit changes are noteworthy.

Figure 5-7 represents a 55-year-old male, patient #270, who suffered an inferior wall infarction, underwent a double aortocoronary artery bypass with recurrent angina pectoris followed by a single aortocoronary artery bypass repair. Again, the responses to the pre– and post–rehabilitation exercise tolerance tests are evident.

These seven examples of the so-called decompensatory systolic fall in blood pressure were apparently caused by failure of the heart to maintain an adequate stroke volume since,

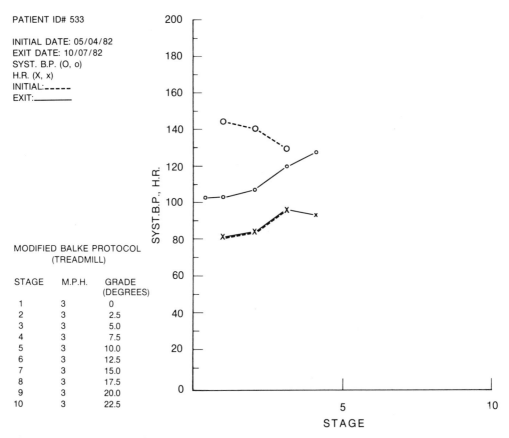

Figure 5-5

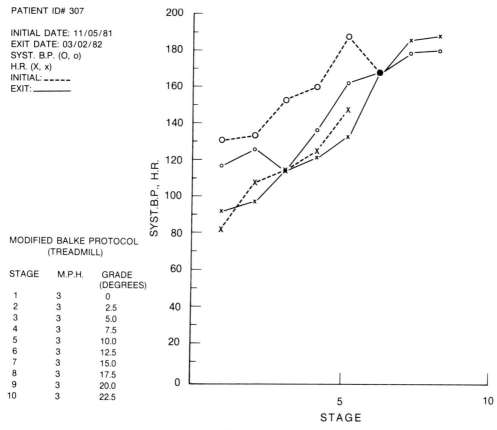

PATIENT ID# 307

INITIAL DATE: 11/05/81
EXIT DATE: 03/02/82
SYST. B.P. (O, o)
H.R. (X, x)
INITIAL: -----
EXIT: _____

MODIFIED BALKE PROTOCOL
(TREADMILL)

STAGE	M.P.H.	GRADE (DEGREES)
1	3	0
2	3	2.5
3	3	5.0
4	3	7.5
5	3	10.0
6	3	12.5
7	3	15.0
8	3	17.5
9	3	20.0
10	3	22.5

Figure 5-6

except for the patient represented in Figure 5-4, none showed a concurrent fall in heart rate or a significant fall (not shown) in diastolic pressure.

Another type of response is associated with what has been termed "the hypertensive type of response" (Peterson *et al.*, 1983). It was noted at the time exercise tolerance tests were initiated at the HCRC in 1978 that in some patients, instead of either exhibiting a relatively linear (normal) or decompensatory systolic pressure at the initial exercise tolerance test, the systolic blood pressure first rose as expected, then, with further increases in exercise load, began to rise more sharply, frequently to very high levels. Thus, there were essentially two different upward slopes of systolic blood pressure with the same stepwise increases in exercise load. Other studies relative to heart rate, blood pressure, and the aerobic threshold are

consistent with these observations (Dwyer and Bybee, 1983).

Figure 5-8 represents patient #015, who had high-grade coronary artery disease and had undergone triple aortocoronary artery bypass surgery. He had developed recurrent angina with a reoccluded graft. He was hypertensive. The dichotomous systolic blood pressure curve prior to rehabilitation may be noted. Also, it may be noted that this pattern resolved and became normal with a three-stage improvement in exercise tolerance after rehabilitation.

Figure 5-9 represents a status postinfarction in a 54-year-old hypertensive, patient #055, illustrating changes in systolic slope during the initial exercise tolerance test. Again, the curve straightened out after rehabilitation.

The responses shown in Figures 5-10, 5-11, 5-12, and 5-13, which are characterized by a marked rise in systolic blood pressure, some at

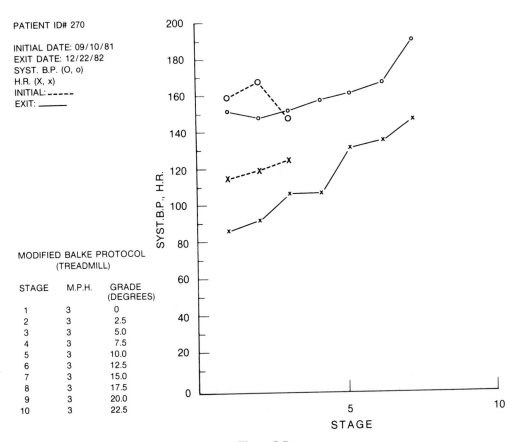

Figure 5-7

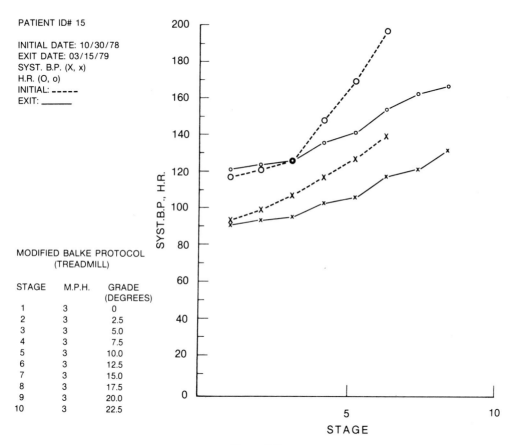

PATIENT ID# 15

INITIAL DATE: 10/30/78
EXIT DATE: 03/15/79
SYST. B.P. (X, x)
H.R. (O, o)
INITIAL: - - - - -
EXIT: _____

MODIFIED BALKE PROTOCOL
(TREADMILL)

STAGE	M.P.H.	GRADE (DEGREES)
1	3	0
2	3	2.5
3	3	5.0
4	3	7.5
5	3	10.0
6	3	12.5
7	3	15.0
8	3	17.5
9	3	20.0
10	3	22.5

Figure 5-8

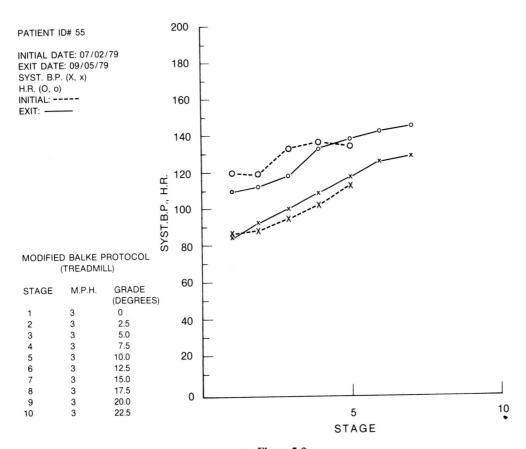

PATIENT ID# 55

INITIAL DATE: 07/02/79
EXIT DATE: 09/05/79
SYST. B.P. (X, x)
H.R. (O, o)
INITIAL: - - - - -
EXIT: ——————

MODIFIED BALKE PROTOCOL
      (TREADMILL)

STAGE	M.P.H.	GRADE (DEGREES)
1	3	0
2	3	2.5
3	3	5.0
4	3	7.5
5	3	10.0
6	3	12.5
7	3	15.0
8	3	17.5
9	3	20.0
10	3	22.5

Figure 5-9

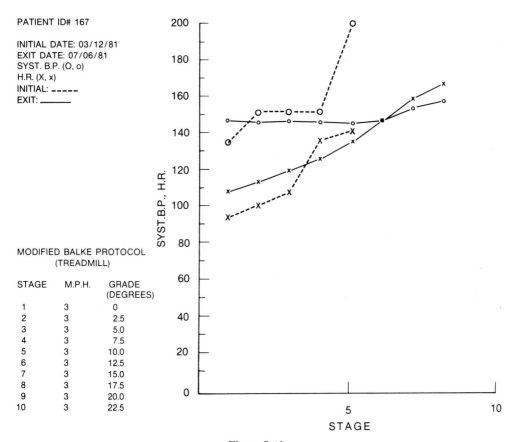

PATIENT ID# 167

INITIAL DATE: 03/12/81
EXIT DATE: 07/06/81
SYST. B.P. (O, o)
H.R. (X, x)
INITIAL: -----
EXIT: ———

MODIFIED BALKE PROTOCOL
(TREADMILL)

STAGE	M.P.H.	GRADE (DEGREES)
1	3	0
2	3	2.5
3	3	5.0
4	3	7.5
5	3	10.0
6	3	12.5
7	3	15.0
8	3	17.5
9	3	20.0
10	3	22.5

Figure 5-10

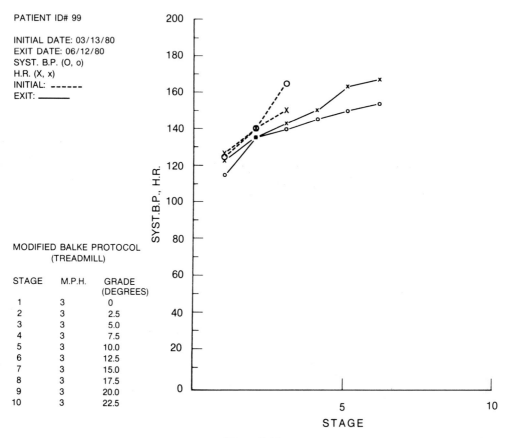

PATIENT ID# 99

INITIAL DATE: 03/13/80
EXIT DATE: 06/12/80
SYST. B.P. (O, o)
H.R. (X, x)
INITIAL: ------
EXIT: ———

MODIFIED BALKE PROTOCOL
(TREADMILL)

STAGE	M.P.H.	GRADE (DEGREES)
1	3	0
2	3	2.5
3	3	5.0
4	3	7.5
5	3	10.0
6	3	12.5
7	3	15.0
8	3	17.5
9	3	20.0
10	3	22.5

Figure 5-11

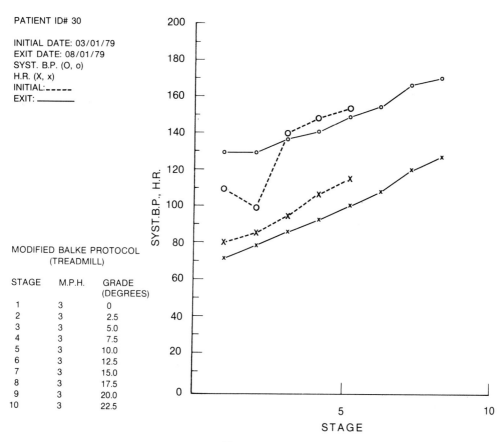

PATIENT ID# 30

INITIAL DATE: 03/01/79
EXIT DATE: 08/01/79
SYST. B.P. (O, o)
H.R. (X, x)
INITIAL:-----
EXIT: ———

MODIFIED BALKE PROTOCOL
    (TREADMILL)

STAGE	M.P.H.	GRADE (DEGREES)
1	3	0
2	3	2.5
3	3	5.0
4	3	7.5
5	3	10.0
6	3	12.5
7	3	15.0
8	3	17.5
9	3	20.0
10	3	22.5

Figure 5-12

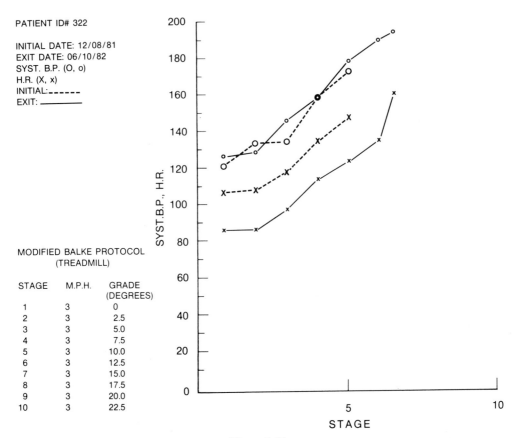

PATIENT ID# 322

INITIAL DATE: 12/08/81
EXIT DATE: 06/10/82
SYST. B.P. (O, o)
H.R. (X, x)
INITIAL: - - - - - -
EXIT: ———————

MODIFIED BALKE PROTOCOL
(TREADMILL)

STAGE	M.P.H.	GRADE (DEGREES)
1	3	0
2	3	2.5
3	3	5.0
4	3	7.5
5	3	10.0
6	3	12.5
7	3	15.0
8	3	17.5
9	3	20.0
10	3	22.5

Figure 5-13

relatively low exercise loads, if not detected may be hazardous because there is a sudden rise in double product and coronary oxygen demand and because of the vulnerability to cerebrovascular or other vascular accidents. Interestingly, the abnormal systolic pressure rise resolves with conditioning, which presumably extends the exercise load at which the anaerobic threshold occurs.

During the latter part of 1981 and into mid-1982, the HCRC had an opportunity to work with Dr. Edward Bernacki, Corporate Medical Director and Vice-President of the Tenneco Corporation in Houston, and his coworkers, on a major program the Tenneco Corporation was undertaking. Briefly, Tenneco was developing an extensive health and fitness program for its employees, numbering about 3,000 in Houston. The Tenneco plan included an employee exercise program, and employees above a certain age or who had certain medical problems were required to undergo an exercise

tolerance test. The HCRC was given the opportunity to assist in the evaluation process. A significant number who were evaluated were found to be hypertensive at rest and many, some normotensive at rest, exhibited the so-called hypertensive response to the Balke exercise tolerance test protocol.

It had been postulated that this so-called hypertensive response was associated with the shift from an aerobic to an anaerobic state and a resulting acidosis. The Tenneco Corporation then supported a study including 32 such individuals wherein the exercise tolerance test was repeated together with $\dot{V}O_2$, $\dot{V}CO_2$, and ventilation rate measurements, utilizing the Beckman metabolic cart. Briefly, in all cases, the change in slope was directly and closely correlated with the shift to the anaerobic state (Peterson et al., 1983). Additionally, six patients scheduled for comprehensive cardiovascular rehabilitation, with documented high-grade coronary artery disease of the type illustrated in

Figures 5-8 and 5-9, were similarly tested with the same result.

Figures 5-14, 5-15, and 5-16 illustrate exercise tolerance tests for three of the Tenneco group.

A third type of response may occur during both exercise tolerance tests and exercise therapy sessions, i.e., a rise in diastolic pressure. It is postulated that this variation is associated primarily with CO_2 retention such as with chronic obstructive pulmonary disease. To date, three such subjects have been studied utilizing the metabolic cart, and all have been associated with an abnormal rise in ventilating CO_2 that presumably reflects arterial P_{CO_2}. The rise in diastolic pressure is presumably associated with centrally induced peripheral vasoconstriction. It has been reported that exercise stress tests exhibiting a rise in diastolic pressure indicate a poor prognosis (Sheps *et al.*, 1977). This exercise-related rise in diastolic pressure with exercise is currently receiving further study.

Figures 5-17, 5-18, and 5-19 are composite, smoothed plots of the mean increases in systolic blood pressure, heart rate, and double product with respect to exercise work load (abscissa) prior to (hatched line) rehabilitation and following rehabilitation for the 272 HCRC patients described in Chapter 4.

Figure 5-17 demonstrates that the mean values for heart rate, pre- and postrehabilitation, for males are reduced by virtually 40% at all levels of exercise load. Moreover, the tolerated work load is extended by 282%.

Figure 5-18 demonstrates that the mean values for systolic blood pressure, pre- and postrehabilitation, for males are reduced virtually 32% over the entire range of tolerated exercise levels.

Figure 5-19 demonstrates that the double product (HR $\times$ SBP $\times 10^{-2}$) decreases virtually 34% over the entire range of exercise levels, although the nonparallel nature of the curves accentuates the product of the slighter nonpar-

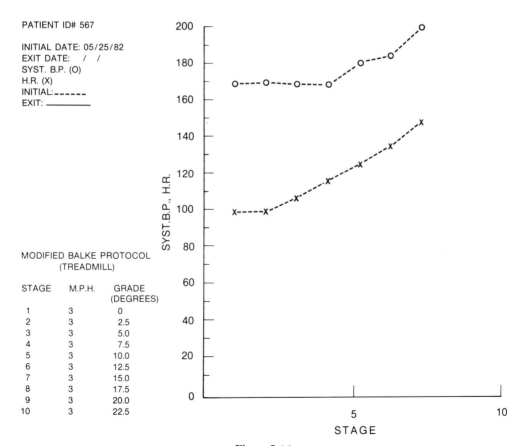

Figure 5-14

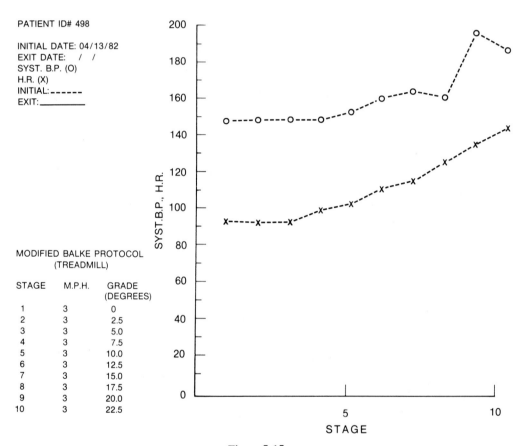

PATIENT ID# 498

INITIAL DATE: 04/13/82
EXIT DATE: /   /
SYST. B.P. (O)
H.R. (X)
INITIAL: - - - - - -
EXIT: _____

MODIFIED BALKE PROTOCOL
(TREADMILL)

STAGE	M.P.H.	GRADE (DEGREES)
1	3	0
2	3	2.5
3	3	5.0
4	3	7.5
5	3	10.0
6	3	12.5
7	3	15.0
8	3	17.5
9	3	20.0
10	3	22.5

Figure 5-15

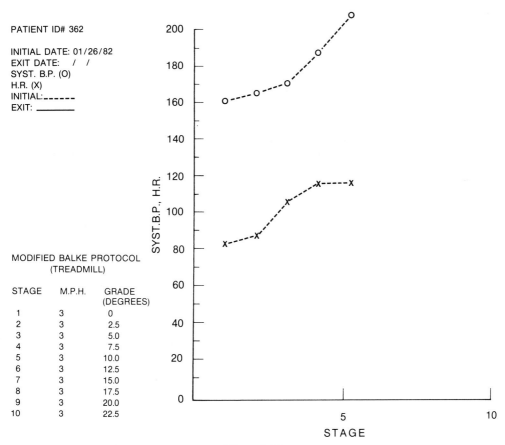

PATIENT ID# 362

INITIAL DATE: 01/26/82
EXIT DATE:　/　/
SYST. B.P. (O)
H.R. (X)
INITIAL: - - - - -
EXIT: _____

MODIFIED BALKE PROTOCOL
(TREADMILL)

STAGE	M.P.H.	GRADE (DEGREES)
1	3	0
2	3	2.5
3	3	5.0
4	3	7.5
5	3	10.0
6	3	12.5
7	3	15.0
8	3	17.5
9	3	20.0
10	3	22.5

Figure 5-16

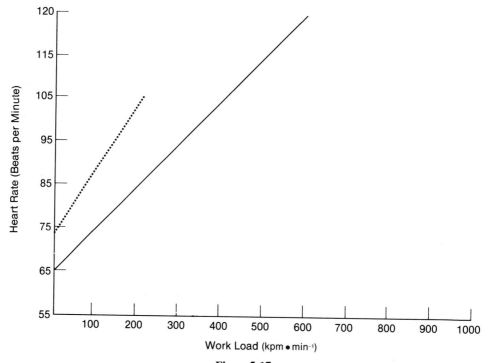

Figure 5-17

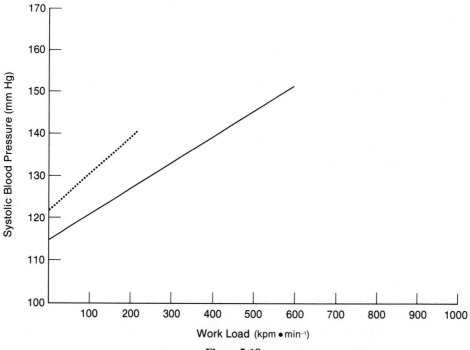

Figure 5-18

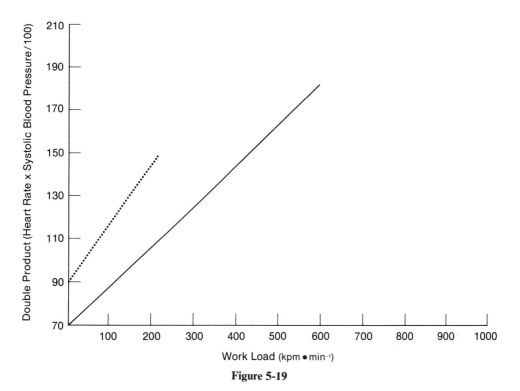

Figure 5-19

allel nature of heart rate and systolic blood pressure curves.

It is apparent from the case presentations and summary data presented within this book that blood pressure, both systolic and diastolic, declines with the conditioning process induced by structured, graded, monitored exercise. It is thus also apparent that cardiovascular rehabilitation should be an effective agent in the treatment of primary hypertension. From data obtained from the Framingham cohort (Kannel and Gordon, 1979), it was noted that for every 10% increment in relative weight, there was a 6.5-mm rise in systolic blood pressure. Declines in weight were associated with equivalent decrements. There are also studies relating emotional stress management to hypertension control. In addition, the control of sodium intake practiced in a comprehensive program of nutrition management also may involve blood pressure control.

The HCRC has now been following 87 persons with at least a five-year history of hypertension prior to referral and rehabilitation. Twenty-three have been followed for four years, 35 have been followed for three years, and 29 have been followed for two years, all of whom became normotensive (the average of

six resting blood pressures not exceeding 140/86) during this rehabilitation program or within six months of maintenance exercise after exit. Sixty-three per cent overall have remained normotensive. Of those who have remained compliant with their home exercise prescription, 71% have remained normotensive. Antihypertensive medications were discontinued with these patients. The poorest response occurred among those who were pathologically obese by definition, i.e., 100% or 100 lb over their estimated ideal body weight, although virtually all demonstrated some drop in blood pressure. Three pathologically obese patients exhibited characteristic blood pressures of 186–170/142–130 which dropped to characteristic resting levels of 158–130/112–94. These were individuals whose weight management was disappointing and who were not considered as successes in hypertension control through rehabilitation, but cardiovascular rehabilitation could be regarded as an adjunct therapy. Moreover, these three patients had been treated medically by hypertension specialists without achieving control, as may be noted from the entry pressure levels. A more detailed analysis of these patients must await a more powerful statistical analysis.

In addition to illustrating the range of types of blood pressure, heart rate, and double product responses that are induced by graded exercise, these examples, together with the standard deviations and ranges provided elsewhere, should amply demonstrate the problems in utilizing so-called predicted maximal heart rates or blood pressure as a means of evaluating exercise tolerance tests. In other words, the use of predicted maximal heart rates as guides for exercise stress testing and exercise therapy is inappropriate because of the spread or scatter. A patient may be at the predicted maximal heart rate at rest due to deconditioning, pathology, or medications, while another may never achieve the predicted maximum if under medications or under certain pathophysiological states. Moreover, the interactions of systolic and diastolic blood pressure, heart rate, and double product are highly variable. The case studies presented in this chapter further supplement those presented in Chapter 3 as demonstrated evidence of the benefits of comprehensive cardiovascular rehabilitation.

REFERENCES

Dwyer, J., and Bybee, R. Heart rate indices of the anaerobic threshold. Med. Sci. *Sports Exerc.*, **1983,** *15,* 72.

Kannel, W. B., and Gordon, T. Physiological and medical concomitants of obesity: The Framingham Study. In, *Obesity in America.* (Bray, G. A., ed.). NIH Publication, Bethesda, Md., 1979, #79,359, 125–163.

Peterson, L. H.; Spence, D. W.; and Bernacki, E. J. Hypertensive responses to exercise tolerance and their association with the anaerobic threshold. Submitted to the Journal of the American College of Cardiology, **1983.**

Sheps, D. S.; Ernst, J. C.; Franklin, W.; Briese, P. D.; and Myerberg, R. J. Diastolic blood pressure response to exercise. *Circulation,* **1977,** *55,* 153.

Chapter 6
ERGOMETRY

Dale W. Spence

There are myriad ways to exercise, and exercise machines are legion. In more sophisticated form, work machines are devices that present a means to perform regulated muscular activity, and in the process biochemical energy is converted into work and heat in different proportion depending on the efficiency of the body to perform the specific activity. In the course of chronic muscular activity of sufficient stress, physiologic adaptation will occur in the repeatedly overloaded system. It must be recognized that different forms of exercise may produce very different effects.

The work machines most commonly used in a laboratory or clinical setting include the treadmill, step, and stationary crank ergometer. Ergometers are within the family of work machines, but are of a somewhat different species from simple exercise bicycles. An ergometer is distinctive in that it is a work-measuring instrument in addition to being an exercise device; therefore, the design criteria should be stringent. The merits of different modes of exercise as used for diagnosis have been investigated and discussed extensively in the literature, but the use of various modes of exercise as used in a cardiovascular rehabilitation setting has not received the same degree of attention. There appears to be agreement that the mode

of exercise appropriate for a cardiovasuclar rehabilitation program should be dynamic, requiring minimal isometric muscular contraction. The types of dynamic exercises and devices may vary from a single type to multiple modes from program to program. On balance, the stationary crank ergometer appears to present the greatest merit for use in cardiovascular rehabilitation for a variety of reasons.

Mechanical efficiency of power produced on the ergometer is relatively independent of body weight; therefore, in longitudinal studies, which follow patient management for an extended period, fluctuations in body weight do not substantially affect the assessment of exercise tolerance. The professional worker should keep in mind that, for a given amount of ergometer work load, the metabolic demand will not vary significantly with body weight since the patient does not move his mass as in the case of treadmill walking or step exercise. The relatively immobile posture of the chest and arms during ergometric exercise is conducive to monitoring cardiovascular parameters. Accurate monitoring of the physiological response to exercise is critical in the medical management of a diseased population. The small space requirements and mobility of an ergometer permit exercise therapy to be conducted in an environmentally controlled setting, which is essential for a cardiovascular rehabilitation population. The reproducibility of load on the ergometer is highly accurate compared to nonmachine types of exercise. The exercise performed on an ergometer is expressed in standard units of power; thus, comparisons to the literature can be made. The interindividual variability of efficiency in performing ergometer exercise is relatively low (Ellestad, 1975), although not all agree on this point (Shephard, 1969). Finally, the incidence of skeletomuscular discomforts or injury is low with ergometer exercise. This is an important consideration because patient compliance to regular exercise is necessary in the cardiovascular rehabilitation process, and injuries may disallow regular exercise therapy.

TYPES OF ERGOMETERS

Ergometers may be classified according to the type of braking system integral to the device. The two general types of braking systems used on ergometers involve either mechanical or electrical loading. The mechanically loaded ergometers may be further classified according to whether they use a spring or a mass force.

Spring-loaded ergometers are usually found on the smaller, less expensive ergometers. On spring-loaded ergometers, a friction device is applied to the rotating flywheel causing a tension assembly to pivot against the resistance of a spring. The calibration tension of the spring is adjustable at the frame attachment in order to be able to vary the tension to match an external standard. The assumption with these types of devices is that the spring presents linear tension over the full range of load. Unfortunately, this assumption is not always correct with conventionally tempered springs.

The mass-loaded ergometers have a given mass securely attached to a shaft in pendulum fashion that, in turn, attaches to the tension assembly. The center of gravity of the mass is critical to the application of linear load over the complete range of load. Mass-loaded ergometers have the advantage of accuracy if properly calibrated. The principle on which this type of ergometer provides load is based on increasing tension of a friction strap applied to a rotating flywheel that creates a torsional load at the strap's attachment on an axle to which the pendulum mass is secured. With increasing tension on the strap, the axle will rotate, causing the pendulum mass to elevate equal to the torque. The index on the mass will measure the

magnitude of the load as it arcs through a scale that indicates the turning moment about the axle. The simplicity of the braking mechanism contributes to its accuracy and can be measured by the equation $N = r \times F$, where F is the applied force and r is the displacement vector from the point at which the force is applied. Appropriately, the manufacturers of ergometers have determined these variables on their particular systems.

Electrically braked ergometers are essentially dynamoelectric machines that convert mechanical energy into electrical energy by electrical induction. This type of ergometer presents a load that is independent of the rate of cranking. The calibration of the electrical ergometer is not straightforward, and there exists a possibility that the electrical components of the dynamo may be altered in the process of jarring the unit either in shipping or moving, even given that the manufacturer has correctly calculated the ergometer load data.

The advantages or, as the case may be, disadvantages of the various types of ergometers mentioned are to be considered in selecting the most suitable unit for a particular program or purpose. As has been previously addressed, the spring-loaded ergometers may present a system that does not provide linear loading in all ranges of work due to the inherent disproportionate stretch of a conventional spring mechanism. This problem can be minimized by calibrating the ergometer in the usual range that it is used. Most spring-loaded ergometers are more accurate at light work loads, the usual range of effort for a patient undergoing exercise therapy. The calibration of spring-loaded ergometers requires some careful attention and an accurate standard. The calibration procedure outlined by the manufacturer is not often practicable for most institutions nor their patients in home programs. The institution should procure a very accurate spring scale, of the small, brass, cylindrical type, such as one manufactured by Chatillon.* The calibrator should take care that the spring scale is connected at the point of attachment of the spring to the tension assembly. If the standard is attached at some other point, the calibration will be affected by a different point of leverage on the tension assembly. The smaller spring-loaded ergometers usually have limited handlebar and saddle-post adjustments. The angle of

* Model IN–15, John Chatillon & Sons, 83-30 Kew Gardens Road, Kew Gardens, NY 11415.

the saddle on the post on one type of ergometer is fixed. On another type of small ergometer, the handlebars are fixed. On both of these models, the handlebars are low and without height adjustment.

The mass-loaded mechanical ergometers present other considerations. The potential for friction fading as a braking strap absorbs heat is a probability in this type of braking system that is used by many maufacturers of ergometers. This phenomenon is lessened with larger flywheel ergometers that have more area of surface contact, thus greater heat-sinking capability of a larger metal area. The conductive properties of the flywheel metal also affect the heat-sinking capacity. Mass-loaded ergometers have the potential of becoming complex oscillators. This condition is exacerbated on small flywheel ergometers that rapidly build up microdebris of friction material and metal. In this regard, some spring-loaded ergometers oscillate extensively due to the lack of a dampening system. Some of the small-mass and/or small-flywheel ergometers lack sufficient inertial load to provide adequate momentum for the flywheel to overcome the afterload of the braking system, thus creating a progressive oscillation producing felt discomfort over time by the patient.

Electrically braked ergometers present some advantages not inherent in mechanically braked ergometers, but, on the other hand, they have some disadvantages. Electrical ergometers are not susceptible to load fade due to friction, they usually have lower noise level, the load changes are conveniently done, displays of ergometer status are clear, and the calibration has been factory determined. Conversely, they are more difficult to mount, the many controls may be confusing, they are susceptible to electrical breakdowns and power outage, they have relatively large units of incremental loading that may not be desirable in a cardiovascular population, they are difficult to calibrate without specialized equipment, and the variable load makes it difficult for deconditioned patients to maintain rotational speed when the legs tire.

CALIBRATION OF ERGOMETERS

The calibration of ergometers used in cardiovascular rehabilitation should observe the same standards as ergometers used for laboratory testing. Reproducible work load is critical with a cardiovascular rehabilitation population. The physiological response of the patient to exercise assumes a known and accurate work load for proper patient management. The day-to-day variation in the patient's exercise tolerance due to medications, moods, and a variety of unknowns presents a challenge for interpretation by the professional worker. Unreliable ergometers would seriously exacerbate the situation.

The importance of proper calibration procedures with ergometers has been addressed in an investigation that presented data on four types of ergometers (Wilmore *et al.*, 1982). The results of the study showed there was considerable calibration error with one of the mechanically braked machines, moderate error in another mechanical ergometer, moderate error but only at low-power output in an electric ergometer, and little error in an ergometer that used a mechanical system composed of hydraulics and a Prony brake to control resistance.

Calibration of mass-loaded ergometers should be performed on the load and distance the flywheel rotates per unit of time. The calibration of flywheel distance also is applicable to ergometers that use braking systems other than mass loaded. The load on mass-loaded ergometers is determined by an external weight that balances the pendulum mass of the ergometer at an even unit of measure. The calibrator should level the ergometer before conducting the calibration and should check the linearity of the range of load at which the patient will exercise. Nonlinearity of the load can be corrected by adjustment of a slug within the mass that changes the center of gravity of the weight; however, the calibrator should use this correction technique with prudence. The static calibration described above is an acceptable technique if patients are assigned specific ergometers to be used during exercise therapy, but less acceptable if they are to select ergometers randomly. A more accurate method, but requiring specialized equipment, is to calibrate the power output on the ergometer by using a dynamometer attached directly to the pedal shaft. A dynamic calibration of this sort may not be feasible for most institutions.

The calibration of distance involves measuring the flywheel rotation per unit of time, which requires that the circumference of the flywheel be determined. By measuring from the center of the flywheel axle to the center of the point of brake application, the radius can be known from which the circumference can be calculated, using the standard circumference equation. The rotational speed of the flywheel can be determined by counting the revolutions per unit of time and multipying by its circumference. A digital counter attached to the flywheel or a stroboscope greatly aids in this chore. Some ergometers have stroboscopic marks on the flywheel that allow fluorescent lights of 60-Hz frequency to calibrate time. A stopwatch and metronome are also acceptable ways of measuring time.

Upon reviewing the procedures for calibration, one may be tempted to think that it would be easier to have confidence in the manufacturer's design. In most instances this view is tenable; however, on three occasions recently, the author found considerable error in the tachometer of three ergometers from the same manufacturer. An inquiry to the company identified that the wrong ratio gear drive to the tachometer cable had been installed inadvertently. This is not to suggest that all ergometers require scrutiny. A simple comparison of the unknown calibrated ergometer with one of known calibration might be the first step. Also, calibrators by necessity will be forced to become good ergometrists. Physiological calibration by perceived exertion can be developed to a keen degree. Regarding physiological calibration, if the patient intends to obtain an ergometer for use in a structured home program, it is important that he exercise under monitored conditions on the specific machine that he will use at home. There is some probability that the patient's physiological response to a different ergometer will be somewhat unusual compared to his response to exercise on the ergometer to which he is accustomed in the clinical setting.

UNITS OF POWER USED IN ERGOMETRY

When one exercises on an ergometer, one is really doing more than work in the physics definition of the term. Since work is being done over time, the unit of measure is *power* and can be defined by $P = dW/dt$. This equation gives the instantaneous power or the rate at which work is being done at a specific moment in time. During ergometric exercise it is more meaningful to consider average power, which is the total work done per minute. Units of power that are commonly used in exercise ergometry are kilopond-meters per minute (kpm·min⁻¹) and Watts (W). A kilopond-meter is a work unit of moving one kilogram one meter, and if that work be done for one minute, then the power produced is 1 kpm·min⁻¹. Typically, power produced on an ergometer is hundreds

of times greater than this; for example, if the flywheel of the ergometer rotates 360 meters per minute, and one kilogram of load is applied to the flywheel via a friction device, then one is producing 360 kpm·min⁻¹ of power. The relationship of kpm·min⁻¹ to W is about 6 to 1 (1 W = 6.12 kpm·min⁻¹); for example, 360 kpm·min⁻¹ is approximately 60 W of power output.

Two units of measure that are designated on many ergometers are the Newton (N), a unit of load or force, and the corresponding work unit, the Newton-meter (Nm). Most ergometers designate an older unit of load or force, the kilopond (kp), which is the force acting on a 1 kilogram mass at normal acceleration of gravity (1 kp = 9.8 N or approximately 10 N). The units of N and Nm affixed on the scale of the ergometer are to be used primarily for static calibration by an external standard.

STANDARDS AND GUIDELINES FOR ERGOMETRIC EXERCISE

The following represent suggested standards and guidelines to be observed when using ergometers in cardiovascular rehabilitation programs. The first standard listed below was established by the Working Group for Ergometry of the International Council on Sports and Physical Education and approved by the IV International Seminar on Ergometry, 1981 (*Sports Med. Bull.,* Jan., 1983):

1. Standard ergometers according to the ICSPE proposals of 1965 are to be used. (Round rotating mass, 100 kg, equal diameter, with a moment of inertia of 5.55 Kgm² at equal rpm of rotating mass and crank. Different rotating mass and frequency of rotation but of the same kinetic energy may be used. Length of the crank or double-crank, 33.3 cm)
2. Flywheel of sufficient mass and diameter to achieve optimum momentum. (The weight range of flywheels of different radii is 27.5 to 41 lb on the more popular European-manufactured ergometers used in rehabilitation)
3. Ease and stability of calibration
4. Units of kpm·min⁻¹, Watts, and Newton-meters
5. Capable of 75 to 90 kpm·min⁻¹ (12 to 15 W) incremental power steps
6. Accurate tachometer
7. Crank sprocket directly connected to flywheel sprocket by single chain

8. Pedal frequency 60 rpm (±10) for cardiovascular therapy
9. Low friction load of ergometer transmission
10. Stability of load mechanism during cranking
11. Ease of maintenance and availability of parts
12. Friction device resistant to load fade
13. Durability of friction material
14. Pedal foot straps
15. Low noise level
16. Ease of mobility of unit
17. Ease of mounting
18. Lateral stability of frame and low center of gravity
19. Adjustable balance of long axis of frame
20. Accurate load scale visible and without parallax
21. Saddle positioned over crank axis
22. Adjustment of height and angle of handlebars and adjustable pitch of saddle
23. At lowest point of pedal, knee should be nearly extended when foot is horizontal
24. Anatomically correct saddle. Maximum padding and contour should consider the transverse diameter between the ischial tuberosities, and saddle horn should be sufficiently narrow
25. Durable materials and finish

REFERENCES

Åstrand, P. O., and Rodahl, K. *Textbook of Work Physiology,* 2nd ed. McGraw-Hill, New York, **1977,** pp. 335–339, 450.

deVries, Herbert A. *Physiology of Exercise for Physical Education and Athletics,* 3rd ed. Wm. C. Brown Co. Publishers, Dubuque, Iowa, **1980,** pp. 202–206.

Ellestad, M. H. *Stress Testing: Principles and Practice.* F. A. Davis, Philadelphia, **1975,** p. 55.

Exercise Testing and Training of Apparently Healthy Individuals: A Handbook for Physicians. American Heart Association, New York, **1972,** p. 17.

Fox, Edward L., and Mathews, Donald K. *The Physiological Basis of Physical Education and Athletics,* 3rd ed. Saunders College Publishing, Philadelphia, **1981,** pp. 67–69.

McKay, G. A. and Banister, E. W. A comparison of maximum oxygen uptake determination by bicycle ergometry at various pedaling frequencies and by treadmill running at various speeds. *Eur. J. Applied Physiol.,* **1976,** *35,* 191–200.

Shephard, Roy J. *Endurance Fitness.* University of Toronto Press, Toronto, **1969,** pp. 63–71.

Sports Med. Bull. American College of Sports Medicine Madison, Wis., **1983,** January, p. 11.

Wilmore, Jack H.; Constable, Stefan H.; Stanforth, Philip R.; Buono, Michael J.; Tsao, Yuan W.; Roby, Frederick B., Jr.; Lowdon, Brian J.; and Ratliff, Ronald A. Mechanical and physiological calibration of four cycle ergometers. *Med. Sci. Sports Exerc.* **1982,** *14,* 322–325.

Chapter 7

PSYCHOLOGICAL ASPECTS OF CARDIOVASCULAR DISORDERS AND REHABILITATION

Merrill P. Anderson

The large majority of patients seen at the Houston Cardiovascular Rehabilitation Center suffer some degree of disrupted psychological functioning which adversely affects their functional performance and increases the likelihood of further aggravation of the underlying disease. As is the case of other components of a comprehensive cardiovascular rehabilitation program, psychological disorders contribute both to the current disabilities and morbidity of the patients and to their long-term status as risk factors in the etiology and progress of underlying disease processes.

Psychological stress is, therefore, a central concept used in understanding the clinical status of patients entering cardiovascular rehabilitation. In a broader sense, psychological and behavioral issues are central to comprehensive cardiovascular rehabilitation as a treatment modality because the approach depends on patients' ability and willingness to initiate and maintain life-style changes in several areas, e.g., exercise, nutrition, psychological coping, and stress management. All of these changes occur in a psychosocial context that includes emotional, motivational, and social/environmental factors. Therefore, understanding, evaluation, and treatment of patients' psychological and social status are essential ingredients of a comprehensive cardiovascular rehabilitation program.

This chapter is a discussion of the Houston Cardiovascular Rehabilitation Center's experience, as well as that of others in the field as is known to this author. These experiences lead to the development of concepts and principles that improve our understanding of the psychological and behavioral aspects of cardiovascular disorders and of the rehabilitation of the victims of these disorders, and thus to the growth and progress of the field. This chapter concludes with a discussion of issues and procedures in the psychological evaluation of patients for cardiovascular rehabilitation. The following chapter discusses issues and procedures in the psychological treatment of rehabilitation patients and presents data about the effects of participation in the HCRC program on psychological functioning.

PRINCIPLES OF PSYCHOLOGICAL STRESS

Clinical Utility and the Conceptualization of Psychological Stress

Several alternative conceptualizations of the nature of psychological stress, of the mechanisms through which it affects physical health, and of the nature of adaptive and maladaptive coping are currently extant. For the practitioner, it is important to employ a criterion of clinical utility in evaluating the alternative conceptualizations of psychological stress. A conceptualization of the stress process should be useful for understanding the psychological/emotional presentation of a wide range of cases and should indicate points of intervention in these cases. Using these criteria, this writer believes that the most useful conceptualization emphasizes psychological stress as a result of the interaction between a person and the demands of his/her environment, as *perceived* by the person; i.e., similar stressors affect different individuals to varying degrees depending upon their perception of the stressor(s). Psychological stress occurs when the individual perceives that a situation involves demands or losses that he believes exceed his/her ability to satisfactorily respond. This conceptualization emphasizes the meanings that individuals assign to situations, and the ways in which they strive to achieve a balance between perceived environmental demands, perceived resources for dealing with these demands, and their own distressing emotions. This interactional approach is more clinically useful than alternative approaches because it focuses on psychological processes (e.g., thinking, emotion, and behavior) that are, in a formal sense, common to all people. Therefore, the same general concepts can be used to understand the variety of psychological/emotional responses that people have to situations.

The interactional model of psychological stress is distinguished from conceptualizations that primarily emphasize environmental factors, such as the major life-events approach (Holmes and Masuda, 1973), or from conceptualizations that primarily emphasize stable person or subject factors (e.g., trait approaches). Each of these more simplistic conceptualizations is limited in the extent to which it is clinically useful for understanding a particular patient's presentation. These conceptualizations have been drawn largely from the research literature and have been useful for characterizing large groups of people normatively, rather than for characterizing individual cases. For example, the clinical utility of the major life-events approach to psychological stress flounders on the stark fact that events do not have meanings by themselves. An event has meaning only insofar as it affects an individual with a given history in a particular circumstance, and the degree of stress experienced by an individual in response to an event is related to the meanings that he/she assigns to the event.

Clinical experience with patients at HCRC suggests that even in the potentially very stressful circumstances of myocardial infarction and heart surgery, there are wide differences among individuals in their psychological/emotional reactions. The basis of these differences is the meanings individuals assign to the events, in the context of their understanding of themselves and of their social environment. Clinically, one works with individuals. Therefore, it is important for evaluation and treatment purposes to have a perspective that recognizes the significant subjective component of psychological stress.

Trait approaches (e.g., the coronary-prone behavior pattern) are also limited in the extent to which they are clinically useful as general conceptualizations of psychological stress in cardiac patients. First, trait approaches imply a consistency of response across situations that is found by clinical experience to be the exception rather than the rule. Most individuals respond flexibly to the situations they encounter because they are continually evaluating the situation and their response to it. Therefore, any particular trait approach will be limited in the range of cases for which it is applicable. Second, stressors and thus psychological stress are common to all people and are not the sole experience of certain subgroups of individuals. For example, only about half of the patients entering the HCRC program exhibit coronary-prone tendencies (see the following chapter for data). An even smaller percentage of this group exhibits the coronary-prone pattern in full strength. Conversely, the HCRC experience is that the large majority of patients are undergoing some degree of psychological stress. Thus, the coronary-prone concept is not essentially useful in understanding the psychological stress presented by approximately half of the entering population.

In this writer's opinion, it is more clinically useful to focus on processes that are common to the range of cases one encounters. The interactional perspective of psychological stress accomplishes this goal better than its alternatives. The interactional perspective is well exemplified by the theoretical and research work of Richard Lazarus (1966, 1971), which may be summarized as follows.

The Lazarus Model of Stress and Coping

Lazarus's model of psychological stress and coping emphasizes the importance of the individual's cognitive appraisals (conscious or unconscious) of environmental demands and of resources available for dealing with demands in determining the degree of stress experienced. Initial perceptions of environmental demands are labeled as primary appraisals, and perceptions of resources as secondary appraisals. Primary appraisals can have a variety of outcomes. For example, situations can be judged as irrelevant, as benign, as favorable, or as unfavorable. Stress is the resultant of appraisals of situations as unfavorable in that they are viewed as involving threat, harm, loss, or challenge to the person. Secondary appraisals involve the individual's perception of both internal and external resources available to him/her for coping with these situations. Internal coping resources include morale, self-esteem, problem-solving skills, knowledge, and health/energy. External resources include social and material supports. Psychological stress results when the person concludes that the demands of the situation exceed available coping resources.

Appraisal processes are ongoing, and judgments change with time as the person receives new information or feedback from initial coping efforts. Thus, the cognitions related to stress are a dynamic process rather than a steady, trait condition. A situation initially appraised as threatening may be reappraised as challenging upon perceiving that initial coping efforts have been successful in moderating the potential danger. Conversely, a situation initially appraised as challenging may be appraised as threatening after realization that initial coping efforts are unsuccessful in warding off the potential danger. Changes in emotion, and in processes at the physiological and social (interpersonal) levels of analysis, may be correlated with such cognitive changes.

Coping is defined as behavioral and psychological adjustments designed to alter the subjectively perceived imbalance in the environment-person relationship (Lazarus, 1966). Coping can have two general functions, both of which lead to a realignment of the balance between perceived demands and perceived power to respond to them. *Problem-focused* coping is directed toward changing the person-environment relationship either by altering some aspect of the situation or by changing the behavioral response to it. Problem-focused coping methods tend to lead to logical and concrete steps to the resolution of the problem. *Emotion-focused* coping is directed toward keeping the experience of negative emotional states at a tolerable level. Problem-focused coping methods tend to be favored when the person believes constructive action is possible, and emotion-focused methods tend to be favored when the person believes the situation has to be accepted (Folkman and Lazarus, 1980). Most coping episodes, however, involve a mixture of both problem-focused and emotion-focused methods.

Specific coping efforts in the service of either of the two functions (goals) of coping can be classed in one of four modes: information seeking, direct action, inhibition of action, and intrapsychic processes. *Information seeking* involves searching the environment for additional knowledge on which to base appraisals of threat and coping decisions. *Direct-action* coping methods include all overt behavioral steps taken to realign the balance in a stressful transaction. The range of behaviors that could be placed in this category is broad, including, for example, such actions as expressing anger to an offending individual, taking a vacation, looking for a new job, taking medicine, exercising, and asking for help. *Inhibition of action* refers to restraint of behavior that might create or exacerbate a stressful situation. Avoidance of certain activities or situations that a person believes might involve excessive demands is a clear example of inhibition of action. Other examples include the inhibition of impulses toward angry expression, and the inhibition of potentially harmful consummatory behaviors (e.g., smoking, overeating, alcohol abuse). *Intrapsychic coping* methods refer to cognitive processes used to manage the experience of stressful emotions. The classic psychological defense mechanisms (denial, repression, projection, reaction formation, intellectualization, and so forth) fall into this category. These methods are largely emotion-focused. They involve some form and degree of self-deception that functions to reduce the level of negative emotional states.

The following points summarize Lazarus's model of stress and coping. Psychological stress is primarily related to the individual's perception of demands as exceeding available resources for coping. Coping is aimed at the adjustment of the subjectively perceived imbalance between demands and resources. Coping efforts can be problem-focused or emotion-focused and can occur in any of four modes: information seeking, direct action, inhibition of action, and intrapsychic processes.

Effectiveness of Coping

The issue of the effectiveness of coping efforts, or of the criteria against which they should be evaluated, inevitably involves value questions. Multiple criteria are available for evaluating coping effectiveness, some of which might be agreed upon by large numbers of people and others of which might be agreed upon by only a very few (e.g., a small religious sect with unusual beliefs about healing). Rather than entering into a lengthy discussion about specific criteria, this writer will suggest some general considerations relevant to the evaluation of coping effectiveness. Cost-benefit considerations and the extent of "reality" distortion are two areas of concern in evaluating coping efforts. Effective coping seems to involve balancing the need to manage negative emotional states and the need to constructively address "real" sources of threat or harm. For example, coping efforts may result in the "benefit" of manageable levels of negative emotional states. However, if this benefit is achieved through exclusive reliance on intrapsychic or self-deceptive modes (such as extreme denial), then the beneficial effects may be sadly short term, and the costs associated with the short-term relief distressingly high. For example, an individual might refuse to seek medical treatment because of anxiety-based denial of the existence or the significance of a probable medical condition. A subsequent worsening of the condition because of delays in seeking treatment would be a result of the initial coping response. Values are centrally involved in the perception of benefits and cost. If one places a high value on physical health, then coping efforts which, in the balance, lead to a maximization of health benefits will be judged effective. This is the perspective from which this chapter is written, and coping efforts will be discussed largely in terms of the cost and benefits to the individual's physical health.

IMPACT OF THE DEVELOPMENT OF CARDIOVASCULAR DISEASES ON PSYCHOLOGICAL FUNCTIONING

The major psychological reactions to serious cardiovascular disorders are states of anxiety and depression. In terms of the previously discussed model of stress and coping, these emotional states are manifestations of individuals' perceptions of threat, harm, and/or loss related to their illness and to doubts about their ability to cope satisfactorily with the situation as they perceive it. The discussion below includes the reactions of patients to such conditions as myocardial infarction (MI), heart surgery, coronary artery disease, severe hypertension, and so on. Anxiety and depression are closely intertwined in the cardiac patient, and symptoms of one rarely occur without symptoms of the other. These reactions are so predictable in some degree that their absence is of almost more diagnostic significance than their presence. A distinction is frequently made between anxiety and depression as reactions to an identifiable stressor (such as a myocardial infarction) and anxiety and depression that are more characteristic of an individual's preillness psychological functioning. The following sections discuss anxiety and depression as reactions to serious cardiovascular disorders. Factors that influence the form and severity of these reactions are discussed subsequently.

Anxiety

Anxiety is defined in the American Psychiatric Association's *Diagnostic and Statistical Manual III* (DSM III) as "a subjective state characterized by feelings of apprehension and fear related to anticipation of danger or harm from either external or internal sources" (1980). In terms of the interactional perspective of stress discussed previously, anxiety is related to perceptions of *threatening* circumstances along with doubt about ability to cope satisfactorily with them. The emotional results of this assessment of threat exceeding coping capacity are feelings of apprehension, of fear, of vulnerability, and of being overwhelmed. Experience with patients at HCRC suggests several sources from which cardiac patients typically experience threat. The most common source is the perceived heart condition itself. Patients fear further, potentially more serious, cardiac problems such as another infarction, cardiac surgery, stroke, and death. Many will deny fear of death but will focus instead on fear of pain, or on fear of invalidism. Related sources of threat are the potential disruption to the capacity for work, financial insufficiency, and uncertainty about the safe limits of physical activity. In a general sense, reactive anxiety is related to uncertainty about health status and about the future. Thus, an important aspect of the treatment of this condition in a cardiovascular rehabilitation program is appropriate education and information about health status of the patient and its implications, along with reassurance and the steady accumulation of experiences that disconfirm the patient's worst fears. Uncomplicated reactive anxiety states will generally respond well to these aspects of treatment.

Anxiety has both cognitive and somatic aspects. Cognitively, anxiety is characterized by three interrelated qualities: worry, hypervigilance, and a focus on the self. Worry can be thought of as a repetitive review or cognitive rehearsal of the sources of threat and of the imagined consequences. For example, one highly anxious post-MI patient at HCRC was obsessed with the status of his coronary arteries and studied a diagram of his coronaries, provided him by his physician following his cardiac catheterization, several times a day in order to remind himself of the location of the threatening blockages. Another patient, who was status post–coronary artery bypass surgery, had a recurring and functionally disruptive fear that his sternal sutures would pull apart. Worry typically involves an overestimate of threat and/or an underestimate of resources for coping with that threat. Overestimate of threat is apparent in the frequently encountered excessive avoidance of physical activity and in exaggerated fear reactions to physical sensations in the chest, neck, and arms. These reactions typically involve an underlying assumption that a serious cardiovascular event is only a step away. Underestimate of coping capacity is evident in expressions that the person could not handle some imagined situation. Worry is distinguished from more adaptive cognitive states such as concern and problem-oriented thinking by its repetitive, exaggerated qualities and by its failure to lead to measures that would remove the source of threat or moderate the perceived severity of it. Worry, however, can be viewed as an attempt to cope with the threat that the cardiac patient experiences. By repeatedly reviewing the sources of threat and their possible outcomes, the worrier, in a sense, is attempting to cognitively master the threat. From the patient's perspective, worrying is a way of preparing for perceived danger.

Hypervigilance is a second cognitive aspect of anxiety, and one that is closely related to worry. Most cardiac patients experience a period of heightened awareness of bodily sensations, especially in the chest, arms, neck, and abdomen. Not only are they sensitized to these sensations, but they also tend to overinterpret them as manifestations of incipient problems, which can then set up a vicious cycle of self-fulfilling expectations. The more vigilant the patient is about potential symptoms, the greater is the likelihood of discovering one, an event which then serves to reinforce the vigilance. This aspect of patients' anxiety reactions is a form of hypochondriasis in that it involves a fear of illness and an overinterpretation of or concern with bodily symptoms. However, unlike a more neurotic hypochondriasis, which is resistant to modification, this situational hypochondriasis yields relatively successfully to appropriate information and to the weight of experience and time.

A third cognitive aspect of anxiety is that attention is focused on the self, rather than on the social or material environment, to a disproportionate extent. The anxious cardiac is likely to be preoccupied with worries about health, about the future, about bodily sensations, and about physical capacities. This preoccupation is reflected in the hypochondriasis noted above and in egocentricity that may be expressed as demandingness and as apparent selfishness and insensitivity to the needs of others. As threat and uncertainty are reduced, these qualities tend to diminish in strength. Also, the experience of being with a group of people in similar circumstances tends to elicit empathy and thus to reduce egocentrism and isolation.

Anxiety also has somatic aspects. Frequent somatic symptoms associated with anxiety include increased muscular tension, insomnia, autonomic hyperactivity (increased heart rate, sweating), tics, hyperventilation, and gastrointestinal distress. Many of these symptoms can be thought of as bodily expressions of the individual's cognitive state of worry, hypervigilance, and self-preoccupation. Frequently the individual's awareness of his bodily symptoms of anxiety becomes a stimulus for further worry and hypervigilance, thus leading to a vicious cycle in which stimulus and response become indistinguishable. As symptoms become more familiar and are better understood, patients are more able to inhibit such cycles.

Sleep disturbances are especially common with patients exhibiting anxiety-based compulsive characteristics, although they are by no means restricted to this patient group. Because they are so common in the cardiovascular rehabilitation setting, they are discussed here as a related disorder. With a very few exceptions, e.g., a rare case of sleep apnea, the sleep disturbances exhibited by the cardiac rehabilitation patients seen at HCRC are understood as being related to the level of emotional distress the patient is experiencing, especially when the distress is expressed as obsessive worry. Even with patients who overtly deny emotional distress, the presence of recurrent sleep disturbance is a diagnostic sign that the patient is more distressed than he/she can, or is willing to, acknowledge. Studies of the psychological characteristics of insomniacs tend to point to relatively higher levels of anxiety, indecision, feelings of inadequacy, mild depression, and obsessive worry, compared to good sleepers (Borkovec, 1982). Interestingly, this empirically derived constellation of characteristics is a better description of the compulsive personality organization than of any other syndrome. These characteristics are hypothesized to result in greater central nervous system activation that either interferes with sleep onset or results in a subjective experience during some stages of sleep that is closer to wakefulness than to sleep (Borkovec, 1982). This hypothesis is consistent with the observation at HCRC that patients frequently attribute their sleep disturbance to intrusive cognitive activity concerning such topics as somatic sensations, the future, current concerns in other spheres of their lives, and, occasionally, specific fearful images. Fortunately, sleep disturbances tend to be reduced as the underlying situational emotional reactions are resolved. In the meantime, sleep disturbances are well controlled by appropriate medication and by psychological treatments such as progressive muscle relaxation (Borkovec, 1982).

Depression

Depression is characterized in the DSM-III (*Diagnostic and Statistical Manual-III,* 1980) as a dysphoric mood, or loss of interest or pleasure in formerly engaging activities and pastimes. The individual typically experiences feelings of sadness, discouragement, worthlessness, and/or helplessness. Depression is related to perceptions of loss of valued aspects of an individual's life, along with perceptions of diminished ability to compensate for the loss or to recover from it. Perceptions of diminished coping capacity are typically experienced as feelings of frustration, initially, and later of helplessness (Seligman, 1975). Whereas anxiety is the principal emotional issue in the acute phases of cardiac disease, depression is the primary emotional problem for the majority of patients in phase III cardiac rehabilitation. De-

pression in this circumstance can be thought of as a grief reaction with the object of the mourning being those aspects of the patient's life that he/she believes have been lost or seriously diminished.

Cardiac patients may experience a sense of loss with respect to several aspects of their lives. Commonly, they express frustration at the physical restrictions they are under or believe they will be under, and this develops into a sense of loss of valued capacity to perform, for example, physical work or sexual functioning. This may precipitate negative judgments about the self that are identical with loss of self-esteem and with feelings of worthlessness. Loss of health is another common perception among cardiacs. Before the manifestation of coronary heart disease they may have thought of themselves as being in "good health," but after the manifestation, they shift to thinking of themselves as having a condition that will be a chronic feature of their lives. Related senses of loss include a loss of autonomy, produced by the belief that they are now "patients" and must do as they are told by doctors and, to some extent, by family, and a loss of invulnerability, produced by the knowledge that they have a potentially life-threatening condition. Two additional areas in which frustration and loss are frequently experienced concern jobs and former reinforcers such as smoking and some dietary habits.

As with anxiety, depression has both cognitive and somatic aspects. Cognitively, depression involves the patient's *belief* that he/she has suffered loss and is helpless with respect to it, regardless of the factual basis of those beliefs. Patients frequently develop unrealistic and distorted beliefs about the extent of limitation they will be under, about the seriousness of their condition, about the extent to which they can help themselves, and about their self-imposed requirements for self-esteem. These distorted beliefs may be reflected in heightened self-criticism, in pessimism about the future, and in withdrawal of interest in other people and in activities. For most patients the relief of depression is identical with the modification of these distorted beliefs and with the realistic acceptance of heart disease as a feature of their lives. Common somatic aspects of depression include appetitive changes (reduced or increased), sleep disturbances (especially midnight and early morning awakening), fatigue, and loss of libido.

Resolution of reactive depression is usually

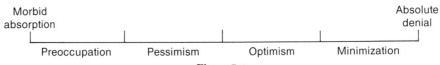

Figure 7-1

relatively rapid following involvement and progress in a comprehensive rehabilitation program, as patients' appraisals of the extent of loss become more realistic, and as the more obvious physical limitations are reduced.

Moderating Factors

This section discusses factors that influence or modulate the severity and form of the emotional reactions to cardiovascular disorders. As expected from applying the Lazarus model, individuals differ greatly in the degree to which they exhibit symptoms of anxiety and depression. Also, a given individual may vary greatly from time to time, or from situation to situation in the extent to which anxiety and depression are experienced. Two broad categories of factors that moderate the severity and form of emotional reactions are current coping efforts and the extent and quality of social resources and support.

Coping. Coping refers to the behavioral and psychological adjustments a person makes to alter the subjectively perceived imbalance between environment and person. Coping efforts can be focused on resolving a problem through instrumental action or on reducing the level of distressing emotions without changing the external situation. Coping behaviors can be categorized as occurring in one of four modes: intrapsychic, inhibition of action, information seeking, and direct action (Lazarus, 1978). Typical coping responses of cardiac patients in each mode are discussed below.

INTRAPSYCHIC COPING. The goal of intrapsychic coping efforts is the regulation of the experience of negative emotional states. This type of coping behavior is prominent in patients entering cardiac rehabilitation.

Denial is the most significant and probably the most frequently encountered example of intrapsychic coping in the cardiac rehabilitation center. Denial has been defined as "the conscious or unconscious repudiation of part or all of the total available meaning of an event to allay fear, anxiety or other unpleasant affects" (Weisman and Hackett, 1961). To understand denial (and other intrapsychic methods), it is important to reemphasize its

function. The meaning or significance of the event, in this case a manifestation of a serious cardiac condition, is altered *in order to* control the experience of stressful emotions. This writer has found it useful to conceptualize denial as one end of a continuum representing an individual's cognitive response to the significance of his cardiac condition. This continuum is depicted in Figure 7-1. The "denial" end of the continuum is represented, in the extreme, by complete rejection of the meaning of information about the cardiac status. The opposite end, termed "morbid absorption," involves excessive preoccupation with the details and significance of the cardiac status. While denial involves rejection or minimization of the fact or significance of the cardiac condition, morbid absorption involves exaggeration of the significance of the same information. Some degree of denial during the acute stages of coronary care is frequently considered an adaptive defense, as it is associated with less overt emotional distress and more rapid early recovery (Froese *et al.*, 1974).

The absolute form of denial is rarely encountered in a phase III rehabilitation program. The initial response to symptoms and even perhaps to infarction may approximate this end of the continuum, as the patient attempts to reassure himself that *nothing* is wrong. However, the power of such experiences as infarction, being in a coronary care unit, and cardiac surgery usually forces some acknowledgment of the fact of a cardiac condition. To do otherwise would require such an extreme distortion of reality as to significantly interfere with that individual's ability to function in daily living.

The form of denial more frequently encountered in a rehabilitation program involves not only minimal acknowledgment of the existence of a cardiac condition, but also substantial minimization of the significance of the condition. This degree of denial is represented on the continuum as the quadrant labeled "minimization." Because of the minimization of threat, the denier is likely to be less compliant with recommended behavioral changes for reducing risk of progression of coronary artery disease or of future infarction. Fear and a sense of threat are powerful motivators for undertaking such changes as dietary modification and weight loss, smoking cessation, regular exercise, a modified work-style, and psychological stress management. To the extent that denial is present, fear and threat are reduced, and the subjective urgency and importance of complying with recommendations in these areas is less. Conversely, the nondenying, anxious patient is likely to be highly receptive to and compliant with recommended life-style changes. The primary therapeutic task in rehabilitation with the denying patient is to obtain compliance, while with the nondenying patient, it is to reduce anxiety and depression.

Individuals whose response to their cardiac status falls into the "optimism" quadrant on Figure 7-1 typically acknowledge the fact and the significance of their health status, but do not dwell on them. They are typically hopeful, confident, and upbeat. They are unlikely to voluntarily report problems with anxiety or depression, though, if pushed, will admit to some concerns. Typically, their concerns are relatively practical and are resolved by providing appropriate information and reassurance. These patients are likely to be compliant with recommended life-style changes. Their compliance is likely to be based on a relatively pragmatic assessment of what is recommended rather than on fear and anxiety.

The "pessimism" quadrant of Figure 7-1 involves more open acknowledgment of feeling threatened, more worry about symptoms, and more doubts about recovery. These individuals are more vulnerable to periods of anxiety and of depression, but anxiety and depression are not likely to be constant features of their emotional presentation. These patients are also likely to be highly compliant with the recommendations of a cardiac rehabilitation program. Psychological interventions with this group of patients are frequently focused on managing their episodes of anxiety and depression, either through providing appropriate information to correct mistaken beliefs, or through providing emotional support and encouraging expression of feelings. In addition to specifically psychological interventions, involvement in a comprehensive rehabilitation program, per se, is a significant therapeutic agent for these patients' emotional reactions to their health status.

The region of the continuum in Figure 7-1 labeled "preoccupation" is associated with frequent and obvious symptoms of anxiety and depression. These individuals typically exaggerate the severity of their status, are hypochondriacal with respect to their somatic sensations, have sleep disturbances, and require frequent reassurance. Mistaken ideas and beliefs about their health status, about symptoms, and about prognosis are common. Typically these patients are having significant problems with depression, and the depressive issues often extend beyond coping with their health status to involve other areas of their lives and their attitudes about themselves. Potential for compliance is good with these patients, but progress in the exercise or conditioning portion of rehabilitation may be slower than with other patients because of the adverse effects of their emotional arousal on their cardiovascular functioning (see Chapter 8, pages 132–139, for a discussion of this point).

Additional intrapsychic coping methods that are frequently encountered in rehabilitation patients include the classic defense mechanisms of intellectualization, rationalization, displacement, and regression. Intellectualization refers to an absorption with the factual, technical, or conceptual aspects of an event along with a corresponding minimization of the affective meaning of the event. The intellectualizing patient typically becomes absorbed with the medical details of his/her cardiac status. He tends to analyze symptoms (angina, shortness of breath) in terms of his understanding of these details. This form of absorption differs from the absorption end of the denial continuum. With intellectualization, the absorption is with the technical aspects only, while on the denial continuum, absorption involves preoccupation with affective significance (exaggeration of the meaning). Although the intellectualizing patient believes that he/she understands his/her condition, mistaken ideas and interpretations are common because the patient actually does not have a proper context for understanding many of the details on which he/she focuses. Another reason that mistaken ideas are common is that the patient is intellectualizing for defensive purposes rather than clinical purposes. Thus, the patient's explanations are likely to be biased in favor of explanations that reduce distress. Rationalization is a similar and frequently used coping procedure involving the selection of explanations for one's behavior or symptoms that are the least likely to result in anxiety or other distressing emotions. Displacement refers to the discharging of emotions onto objects or persons other than the true source. For example, family members and physicians frequently become the objects of a patient's anger and frustration about what has happened to him. To be sure, there are circumstances in which anger and frustration with families and physicians are entirely appropriate, but often the anger is disproportionate to the actual circumstance. In these cases, the excessive aspect of the emotional expression can be considered a displacement. Regression refers to the retreat from more mature, perhaps rational, means of dealing with the world to more immature, irrational means. Common regressive behavior among cardiac patients includes excessive dependency, lowered frustration tolerance and outbursts of temper, and indulgence in a variety of consummatory behaviors such as eating, smoking, and drinking alcohol.

INHIBITION OF ACTION. Inhibition of action as a coping strategy of many cardiac patients is evident in the avoidance of physical activity and of situations that might be emotionally distressing. This avoidance is frequently designed to minimize the occurrence of symptoms such as angina pectoris or arrhythmias. Exclusive reliance on this coping mode may result in the so-called cardiac neurosis in which the individual is afraid to do much of anything for fear of exacerbating symptoms. However, continued inactivity may contribute to further physiological deconditioning, which then makes the occurrence of activity-related symptoms more likely, and a vicious cycle is created. Paradoxically, the coping strategy serves to maintain and even aggravate the very symptoms from which it was designed to protect the patient. Conversely, there are numerous instances in which choosing not to engage in certain classes of behaviors is an example of rational, problem-oriented coping. When these are informed choices based on knowledge of the relationship of activity to cardiac function, then inhibition of action can be an important component of reasonable and intelligent management of one's health. Examples of such choices include avoiding lifting or pushing heavy objects, avoiding excessive work hours, and choosing not to indulge in certain consummatory behaviors such as eating foods high in sodium or saturated fats.

INFORMATION SEEKING. Information seeking refers to the gathering of new information to answer questions about potential stressors and about ways of coping with them. Information seeking can be a highly adaptive coping strategy for cardiac patients. The kinds of information that contribute to adaptive coping include basic information about the nature and extent of their cardiac condition, explanations of their symptoms in terms of their cardiac condition, adequate rationales for recommended behavioral changes (e.g., why is smoking detrimental to your heart), explanations of the purpose of cardiac medications and of their common side effects, and explanations of expected emotional responses to their cardiac status. Judgment is always an issue in deciding how much information a particular patient requires in order to cope adaptively, but there is probably a tendency for the busy physician to err on the side of providing less rather than more information. Appropriate information and education can be powerful antidotes to anxiety and to depression, as both of these states have significant cognitive aspects that are rooted in faulty beliefs and perceptions. Although it requires more professional time and commitment, information and education are highly preferable to longer term use of tranquilizing and/or antidepressant medications. Appropriate information contributes to adaptive coping by correcting unrealistic appraisals of threat, by reducing uncertainty and thus increasing the sense of control, and by suggesting new (more appropriate) coping strategies. In terms of the Lazarus model, appropriate information serves to bring both primary and secondary appraisals into line with the objective situation.

DIRECT ACTION. Direct action refers to overt behavioral steps, such as exercising or changing dietary habits, that have coping functions with respect to subjectively perceived stressors. Direct-action coping behaviors can be highly adaptive in reducing perceived as well as actual threat and in increasing the patient's sense of competence, efficacy, or mastery with respect to illness. The patients who know what they can actively *do* about their health and emotional status are likely to experience lower levels of disruptive emotions. Positive results from direct action (e.g., progress in exercise, weight loss) are powerful inducements to a sense of personal efficacy in patients (Bandura, 1977), which is therapeutic with respect to both anxiety and depression.

Social Resources and Supports. Social resources and supports are another major category of moderators of the degree of emotional stress individuals experience following major manifestations of cardiovascular diseases. Included in this category are marital and family relations, work status, and other social contacts (acquaintances, friends). Individuals who feel secure and supported in their family relations and in their work status are likely to exhibit the least complicated situational emotional reactions. Poor social support, especially at the family level, deprives the individual of a major source of comfort, hope, and meaning and can result in more intense feelings of depression and loneliness. Good quality support has been shown to be especially helpful in buffering loss of self-esteem, which is a major aspect of depression (Billings and Moos, 1981; Pearlin *et al.,* 1981). If marital and family relations are actually conflicted, they are not only unavailable as support, but can become an additional source of stressful emotions with which the person may feel less able to cope than before the onset of the cardiac condition. Experience at HCRC is that marital and family problems have negative effects on rehabilitation progress, either through the associated elevated levels of emotional arousal that interfere with optimal cardiovascular response to exercise or through interference with compliance (e.g., irregular attendance, poor dietary habits).

Work status after a major cardiac event affects the patient's emotional state primarily through the meanings assigned to work and its alternatives. Individuals who are secure in their jobs and who feel positively about their work are generally less likely to experience severe emotional reactions. The loss of a particular job after the onset of a cardiac condition may be viewed as less threatening, and may even be welcomed, if alternative sources of esteem, satisfaction, and income are available, and if financial needs can be met. However, as with family relations, the existence of problems at work may aggravate stressful reactions in that the individual feels less able to cope with both health and work situations and begins to feel overwhelmed. If the onset of a cardiac condition threatens the individual with loss of a job which is a valued source of self-esteem, satisfaction, and/or income, then the potential for stress is much higher. For example, an individual who faces early retirement as a result of a cardiac condition has to cope not only with the uncertainties of health, but also with the frequently difficult adjustment of retirement. Such an individual may have to work hard to construct a new basis for self-esteem, identity, and meaningful involvements on a daily level. The potential for depression, especially, is very

high. The emotional stress associated with work problems can adversely affect progress in rehabilitation. Case examples of these adverse effects are presented in Chapter 8.

PSYCHOLOGICAL ASPECTS OF SECONDARY PREVENTION FOR CARDIOVASCULAR DISORDERS

Reduction of disability is the primary goal in the rehabilitation setting. Indeed, where reimbursement for therapy involves third-party insurers, reducing morbidity and disability is the only consideration. Conversely, secondary prevention is not the purpose for which insurance premiums are paid. Secondary prevention is, therefore, an important achievement, but not the one for which insurance pays. Secondary prevention is essentially risk-factor reduction, and, in practice, is an outcome of the rehabilitation goal. Intensive clinical observation at HCRC of several hundred rehabilitation patients makes it clear that psychological stress has significant effects on cardiovascular functioning, which are capable of adversely influencing progress in rehabilitation, and have the potential to contribute to progression of the underlying cardiovascular disorder. Thus, in addition to being concerned with psychological conditions that contribute to current disability, the psychologist in a cardiovascular rehabilitation setting is also concerned with psychological factors that place the person at risk for progression of disease. There has been considerable discussion in the literature about the existence of psychological risk factors for cardiovascular diseases (especially coronary artery disease), and for health and illness in general. Increasingly, there is general acceptance of the proposition that emotional stress, either chronic or acute, has significant health consequences. Evidence for psychological and emotional stress as a risk factor for cardiovascular disorders is briefly reviewed in the following sections. This begins with a discussion of the physiological mechanisms through which psychological stress is thought to confer risk, and then of the different categories of stressors that have been linked with heart disease.

Psychophysiological Mechanisms

Psychological and emotional factors affect physiological functioning in two major ways that have potential for adverse effects on cardiovascular functioning. The risk associated with emotional stress is thought to be the result of the activation of one or both of two neuroendocrine systems, the sympathetic-adrenomedullary system and the pituitary-adrenocortical system, each of which has distinct effects on the cardiovascular system (Baum *et al.,* 1982).

The sympathetic-adrenomedullary system is associated with response to acute stress, either physical or mental/emotional. The major hormonal ingredients of this reaction are the catecholamines—epinephrine and norepinephrine. These hormones potentiate several systemic changes including increased heart rate, increased blood pressure, increased circulating blood lipids, especially triglycerides, and increased platelet adhesiveness. The stress-atherosclerotic heart disease hypothesis is that chronic activation or overstimulation of this response system creates conditions favorable to the development of both hypertension and atherosclerosis. Studies have established the responsiveness of plasma levels of those hormones to emotional stress (Taggart *et al.,* 1973; Dimsdale and Moss, 1980; Frankenhauser, 1980) and the reactivity of heart rate and blood pressure to psychologically stressful situations (Light and Obrist, 1980). Triglyceride levels also have been demonstrated to be responsive to periods of intense emotional arousal (Taggart and Carruthers, 1971; Taggart *et al.,* 1973). Increased emotional stress also has been shown to be related to frequency of arrhythmias and to sudden death (Dimsdale, 1977; Rissanen *et al.,* 1978; Reich *et al.,* 1981). Finally, the sympathetic-adrenomedullary response is also stimulated by nicotine, and thus this response system is one of the mechanisms through which tobacco smoking confers cardiovascular risk (Van Lanchen, 1977).

The pituitary-adrenocortical response system is thought to be more characteristic of chronic stress conditions than of acute stress. The major hormonal products are corticosteroids which generate a wide range of defensive reactions in the body. Overactivation of this response system has been hypothesized to be related to greater susceptibility to illness in general, rather than specifically to cardiovascular conditions, through its suppressive effects on the immune response system. The major cardiovascular consequences of increased levels of corticosteroids appear to be increased sodium concentrations and thus increased fluid levels, both of which influence blood pressure.

The pituitary-adrenocortical system is the centerpiece in Selye's General Adaptation Syndrome. A brief discussion of his position and of critiques of it elucidates contemporary thinking about the elicitors of this response system.

Selye defines stress as the sum of the nonspecific physiological responses of the body to demands made on it (Selye, 1974). The primary physiological response that Selye equates with stress consists of activation of the pituitary-adrenocortical system. This response is considered nonspecific, meaning that, at this level of analysis, organisms respond in the same way to a wide variety of stimuli. Selye assumed that the common element among the eliciting stimuli is that they impose some degree of demand on the organism.

Mason (1975a, 1975b) reviewed Selye's concepts and made the following observations. In Selye's early work the classes of stressors, or evocative agents, that he studied were largely physical (cold, heat, exercise) or hormonal (adrenalin, insulin). Emotional stimuli were simply one of many classes of agents presumed capable of eliciting the stress reaction. Mason (1975b) asserts that research over the past 20 years has demonstrated "that emotional stimuli rank very high among the most potent and prevalent natural stimuli capable of increasing pituitary-adrenal cortical activity." He argues that rather than being nonspecific, Selye's stress response may be elicited largely by the single stimulus class of emotional arousal. Emotional arousal, however, can be considered a nonspecific response to a wide variety of conditions. This shifts the level in the central nervous system at which factors influencing the stress response are integrated. In other words, it implies that higher cortical processes, or psychological processes, are centrally involved in producing the hormonal response that Selye equated with stress. Mason further states that recent advances in research on the endocrine system indicate that assigning primary importance to the adrenocorticosteroids as stress hormones is probably unjustified. He suggests that the endocrine system acts in an integrated rather than a piecemeal fashion, and that the stress response is probably a complex, multihormonal affair.

While activation of the pituitary-adrenocortical system may not have as obvious and direct implications for the cardiovascular system as does the sympathetic-adrenomedullary system, the pituitary-adrenocortical activation may be important in recovery from myocardial infarction (MI). Insofar as the recovery period is stressful in a chronic way—fear, invalidism, economic uncertainty, depression, and so on —greater activation of the pituitary adrenocortical system could be hypothesized during this period. If this acts adversely on the immune response system, then one could speculate on the possible increased susceptibility to illnesses in general which could dramatically complicate recovery from a major cardiovascular event (myocardial infarction, bypass surgery). An individual easily could get into a vicious cycle of emotional stress begetting physiological changes, leading to more illness, which is more discouraging, which potentiates more emotional distress. Hence, an important variable in the rehabilitation equation may be the degree of support the person has post-MI/surgery and the quickness with which active rehabilitation efforts are undertaken, which in themselves are stress reducing.

Sources of Chronic Emotional Stress

Several categories of variables have been implicated as sources of illness-related psychological and emotional stress. This section briefly summarizes research on the relationships of cardiovascular diseases to the following categories of variables: life change, anxiety and neuroticism, coronary-prone personality, and social mobility and status incongruity.

Life Change. Historically, a major theoretical and empirical approach in the stress-illness field is the "life events" approach. The principal hypothesis is that the more major life changes a person accumulates in a given period of time, the more susceptible he/she is to health problems. "Major life changes" are defined as events that require significant changes in a person's established life pattern (Holmes and Masuda, 1973). In earlier formulations of this position, change per se was considered to be the common denominator among these events, irrespective of desirability or undesirability of the event. Thus, events involving "success" and good fortune (e.g., increased income, purchasing a new home, marriage, birth) theoretically required adjustment efforts that had relevance to health in the same way as adjustments to undesirable changes (e.g., loss of job, illness, death of loved one, legal problems). Life changes are typically assessed by having individuals indicate which events out of a list of possible events have occurred to them over a given period (usually either one or two years). The most widely used of these lists is the Social Readjustment Rating Scale (Holmes and Rahe, 1967) which consists of 43 event-items. Weights for each item were derived on the basis of ratings by a normative group of the amount of social readjustment (change) involved in the item. Mean values of these ratings were used as weights and were termed Life Change Units (LCU). Although this scale is probably the most widely used of the life-events scales, other versions are extant in the literature (Dohrenwend and Dohrenwend, 1974; Sarason et al., 1978). Beyond the published versions of these scales, individual researchers and clinicians typically modify the basic scales to fit their particular research questions or population.

At a conceptual level this approach to stress phenomena emphasizes stimulus conditions. Stress is defined by the occurrence of events of certain qualities and in sufficient quantities. The most frequently hypothesized mechanism to explain the impact of these events on health status is that significant life changes require readjustment efforts by the individual which tax him/her at a psychological and physiological level. If the readjustment period lasts long enough because of either multiplicity of changes or profundity of changes, the accumulated "wear and tear" on the individual's psychological and physiological systems is assumed to increase vulnerability to emotional problems and/or illness, presumably through the physiological mechanisms described in the previous section.

Reviews of the evidence linking life changes with manifestations of heart disease concluded that the results were provocative but unconvincing because of inconsistencies among results and methodological shortcomings, especially in the studies demonstrating positive relationships (Jenkins, 1976b). For example, Rahe and Lind (1971) found a relationship between sudden cardiac death and life change over six months preceding death compared to life changes over earlier periods. Information was obtained from the family retrospectively. However, prospective studies done by Theorell et al., (1975) found no relationship between life-change scores and incidence of myocardial infarction during the following 12 to 15 months.

Life-event studies have been criticized for their lack of comparison groups and for their frequent use of retrospective designs in which selectiveness of recall is an ever-present alternative hypothesis. Rabkin and Streuning (1976) pointed out that the positive results that have been obtained are generally weak and account for only a small proportion of the variance between change scores and illness outcomes. The Social Readjustment Rating Scale has been criticized for the assumption that desirability of events is not a relevant dimension in understanding stress-illness relationships (Mechanic, 1974). As was noted earlier in this chapter, another major criticism of research with this scale has been the failure to account for the moderating effect of individual differences in the subjective meanings people assign to the events. For example, a job promotion may be a highly valued and desired event for one individual, but for another, the new responsibilities might be seen as beyond the person's competence and as an occasion for failure and loss of esteem. Researchers in this field have introduced modifications to the basic life-event scales to accommodate these criticisms (Sarason et al., 1978; Horowitz, et al., 1979; Ross and Mirowsky, 1979).

The life-events approach recently has been criticized by Lazarus's research group, and they have developed an alternative to life-change scales. Kanner et al. (1981) argue that the life-events approach by definition focuses on the stressful nature of nonroutine, relatively infrequent events and overlooks the much more frequent and prosaic daily irritants, minor stresses, and small pleasures that characterize most people's lives. They hypothesize that the accumulation of these microstressors, or hassles, may have more significance for health and other adaptational outcomes than life events. To assess this hypothesis, they developed a 117-item list of daily irritants, the Hassles Scale, and administered it on a monthly basis for nine months to a nonclinical sample. In one study (Kanner et al., 1981), scores from the Hassles Scale were more strongly correlated with psychological symptoms than life events and remained significantly correlated after the effects of life events were partialed out. A second study (DeLongis et al., 1982) found the same pattern of results with somatic symptoms.

Kanner et al. (1981) speculate that hassles may be the mediators of the life change–health outcomes relationships reported in so many studies. In other words, major life changes may lead to a greater susceptibility to minor stressors, or to feeling hassled. This writer's experience with several hundred cardiac patients as they adjust and adapt to the "major life change" of the onset of a serious cardiovascular condition lends support to Kanner's speculation. By shifting the focus of intervention work away from major events and onto coping with the daily stresses and strains that follow from major changes, it is possible to effect greater therapeutic benefits. Daily hassles are substantially more amenable to modification through stress management or coping-oriented counseling than are life events. Major life events frequently cannot be avoided or modified.

Anxiety and Neuroticism

Many patients who present to HCRC exhibit characteristics suggesting preillness patterns of psychological adjustment that would be associated with elevated levels of anxiety and depression. These maladaptive patterns may have existed for several years prior to overt manifestation of cardiovascular disorders and may have contributed to the development of these disorders. This writer's experience with patients who already have manifest cardiovascular disorders suggests that reactive anxiety and depression are likely to be more severe and more complicated in individuals with premorbid neurotic and/or depressive adjustments. Thus, in addition to being implicated in the development of cardiovascular disorders, these characteristics may adversely affect recovery and rehabilitation.

A large number of studies link different emotional disturbances (e.g., anxiety, depression, somaticizing, nervousness, sleep disturbance, fatigue and emotional drain, alienation) to manifestations of heart disease (see Jenkins, 1976a, b for a review). Conceptually, these empirical relationships are explained relatively easily. Neuroticism (anxiety) and depression are reflections of relatively ineffective coping patterns. Applying the Lazarus model of stress and coping, they are associated with frequent primary appraisals of threat (anxiety) and of loss (depression) and secondary appraisals of insufficient resources for reducing, eliminating, or compensating for the distressing circumstances or emotions. Coping efforts among these individuals would be expected to be focused more on managing the level of distressing emotions than on solving real world problems, and more in the intrapsychic and avoidant modes than in the direct action or information-seeking modes. As a result, self-perceived problematic situations would tend to persist and new "crisis" situations would occur more frequently. The physiological response systems described in the previous section would then be activated on a more frequent and chronic basis. The stress-producing potential of major life events may be magnified with these individuals because of their propensity to infer threat and loss, to feel overwhelmed, and to use less effective coping modes.

Coronary-Prone Behavior Pattern (Type A)

The most well-established psychological and behavioral risk factor is the coronary-prone behavior pattern (CPBP) described by Friedman and Rosenman (1974). The experience at HCRC is that approximately half of the patients entering the rehabilitation program exhibit the CPBP (see Chapter 8 for data). Thus, the CPBP is an important source of chronic psychological stress affecting many rehabilitation patients. Psychological intervention in these patients should be focused on moderating these characteristics with a goal of reducing risk of progression of the underlying cardiovascular disorder, as well as of reducing a source of current disability. With respect to the latter point, coronary-prone individuals, by virtue of their propensity to stressful responses to their environments and to denial of the seriousness of their health status, frequently have their progress in rehabilitation retarded because of the adverse physiological effects of emotional arousal and because of their failure to comply with different aspects of rehabilitation (weight loss, smoking cessation). Recent major reviews of the empirical literature on the association of this pattern with cardiovascular disease all support its status as a risk factor (Jenkins, 1976a, b; Dembrowski et al., 1978; Cooper et al., 1981). The following sections briefly summarize the definition of the pattern, evidence for the link with heart disease, the proposed physiological basis of the risk, the proposed psychological basis of the pattern, and the relationship of this pattern to other categories of psychological stress.

Definition. Friedman and Rosenman (1974) define the coronary-prone pattern as "an action-emotion complex that can be observed in any person who is aggressively involved in a chronic, incessant struggle to achieve more and more in less and less time, and if required to do so, against the opposing efforts of other things or other persons." Other characteristics of the pattern include explosive, accelerated, accentuated speech patterns, self-preoccupation, a propensity to evaluate self and activities in quantitative terms, easily aroused competitiveness, divided attention (polyphasic thought), ambition, and impatience. The counterpart of the CPBP, known as type B, is less well defined. This pattern is largely defined as the absence of the coronary-prone characteristics. More positively, type B people are described as more relaxed, less competitive, less hurried, and as more appreciative of cultural, artistic, and humanistic values. Friedman and Rosenman argue that the CPBP is not a psychological *trait,* in the sense of an inferential psychological construct. Instead, it is conceived as a set of overt behaviors exhibited by some individuals in specific kinds of situations (i.e., challenging ones). Finally, the CPBP is conceptualized as a continuum of behaviors, ranging from extreme type A to extreme type B, rather than as a typology (either A or B).

Empirical Basis. The empirical basis for the CPBP as a risk factor for cardiovascular disease has been thoroughly reviewed elsewhere (Jenkins, 1976b; Dembrowski et al., 1978; Jenkins, 1978; Cooper et al., 1981). The original research establishing the association was Rosenman and Friedman's Western Collaborative Group Study (WCGS) (Rosenman et al., 1964; 1975), an eight-and-one-half-year prospective study designed to assess the risk of developing manifestations of coronary artery disease among samples of originally nonsymptomatic men who met research criteria for type A or type B. The basic result of this large-scale study was that men exhibiting the CPBP had 2.2 times the incidence of coronary artery disease symptoms than those of type B, and that this risk was independent of risk factors such as cigarette smoking and obesity. Other major studies have replicated this association at roughly the same level of risk (Quinlan et al., 1969; Shekelle et al., 1976; Kornitzer et al., 1981). Jenkins (1978) found 22 of 24 studies showed a positive association between the pattern and coronary artery disease.

Physiological Basis. The cardiovascular risk associated with CPBP is thought to be the result of excessive (more frequent and intense) arousal of the sympathetic-adrenomedullary system. Such arousal involves elevated heart rate and blood pressure, higher levels of circulation lipids (especially triglycerides), and increased platelet adhesiveness, all of which are considered contributory to atherosclerosis.

There is a body of research demonstrating higher levels of sympathetic reactivity, as indexed by these different variables in type As than in type Bs in situations hypothesized to elicit the pattern (Glass, 1977; Dembrowski *et al.*, 1979; Dembrowski *et al.*, 1981; Frankenhauser, 1980; Glass *et al.*, 1980; Gastorf, 1981). Recent research has placed more emphasis on cardiovascular and neuroendocrine reactivity as a defining aspect of the CPBP, in contrast to the more behaviorally oriented definitions used by Friedman and Rosenman. Reactivity is typically assessed by measuring physiological responsiveness (heart rate, blood pressure, catecholamines) during laboratory stress situations (e.g., video games) (Dembrowski *et al.*, 1979; Gastorf, 1981; Roskies, 1982). This strategy is based on the idea that if the risk mechanism is physiological reactivity, then focusing more explicitly on people who exhibit excess reactivity ("hot reactors") and on the environmental and psychological correlates of the reactivity may be a more precise method of approach for understanding the problem of coronary proneness. In this way, the researcher is working with a group selected more specifically for the presence of the supposed risk process, rather than with a group selected for the presence of a behavior pattern which is on average presumed to be associated with the risk process.

Psychological Basis.   This writer's experience working with patients who exhibit the CPBP is that there is probably not a unitary psychological basis for the pattern. Different psychological factors appear to underly the behavior characteristics and the reactivity in different patients. Of course, there are important commonalities among these patients, but none of them so striking as to be assumed true of all those who exhibit the pattern. A recent extensive review of the state of knowledge about the psychological basis of the CPBP concluded that the pattern essentially consists of "a collection of behaviors thought to characterize future cardiac patients" (Matthews, 1982). Clearly, a more complete understanding is needed of the psychological basis of the coronary-prone pattern, of its pathophysiological mechanisms, and of its situational correlates in order to devise meaningful, appropriate, and effective interventions.

Several conceptualizations are current in the literature about the basic psychological factors underlying coronary-prone behavior characteristics and the associated physiological reactivity. Although none of these conceptualizations has received sufficient empirical support to be generally accepted as *the* psychological basis of the pattern, they are briefly reviewed in the following paragraphs because each formulation adds something to the understanding of these patients.

Friedman *et al.* (1981) believe that the fundamental underlying psychological condition is "a basic insecurity arising from an earlier or contemporary failure to experience unconditional love and affection." The individual is thought to cope with this insecurity by exaggerated attempts to achieve and to accumulate, all in the interest of satisfying the basic insecurity. Friedman's statement is at the level of a hypothesis, however, and he does not cite empirical work in support of his belief. A significant problem with this formulation is that a basic psychological insecurity such as Friedman describes is so general a concept that it easily could be the basis for a range of patterns of psychological adjustment, rather than being unique to the coronary-prone pattern. In fact, one important psychological theorist made a similar concept (insecurity related to failure to experience unconditional love) the basic construct in his entire theory of personality (Rogers, 1951). Thus, the CPBP may be one possible outcome of this basic insecurity, but the condition is not specific to the CPBP and does not differentiate coronary-prone individuals from a wide range of other individuals.

The most extensive and systematic conceptual and empirical work on the psychological dimensions of the CPBP has been done by David Glass and his associates (Glass, 1977, 1978). Glass's primary hypothesis is that coronary-prone behaviors represent attempts to maintain control over environments that are perceived as harmful. Coronary-prone individuals' struggle for control is not only over environments but also over themselves and is reflected in characteristics such as perfectionism and suppression of negative subjective states such as fatigue. Thus, coronary-prone individuals appear externally impatient, easily frustrated and annoyed, aggressive and hard driving. Glass carries his analysis further and suggests that if the coronary-prone individual's coping efforts are not successful (i.e., control is not achieved), he/she will tend to give up and to act helpless. This writer's experience at HCRC supports Glass's emphasis on excessive needs for control over environment and over self as an important commonality among coronary-prone individuals. The transition to helplessness, however, is less evident as a common feature of the coronary-prone patients seen at HCRC. This may be related to patients' increasing sense of control over themselves as they progress through rehabilitation.

Glass (1978) speculates about the physiological aspects of this sequence of psychological coping behaviors. Sympathetic adrenomedullary arousal is hypothesized to be associated with active attempts to achieve control. However, parasympathetic dominance (especially depletion of noradrenalin) characterizes the helplessness or giving-up phase. Glass (1978) cites evidence that abrupt shifts between sympathetic and parasympathetic activity are associated with manifestations of coronary heart disease, including sudden death. Thus, coronary proneness in his conceptualization is thought to result from the effects of frequently elevated catecholamine levels and of abrupt shifts from sympathetic to parasympathetic activity.

In her review of the empirical literature relevant to Glass's conceptualizations, Matthews (1982) concluded that several studies support the basic prediction that As are more likely than Bs to respond actively to threats to their control and to succumb to helplessness when failure seems assured, although the pattern of results is not completely consistent with predictions. Less evidence is available to support the hypothesized physiological differences between As and Bs in these situations.

Another approach to conceptualizing the psychological basis of the coronary-prone pattern emphasizes the combination of a high value on productivity and ambiguous or vague standards for evaluating that productivity (Matthews, 1982), with vagueness of standards perhaps reflecting very high or perfectionistic standards. The result of these two characteristics is that As frequently find it difficult to satisfy or place limits on their need for productivity. These dynamics then may be reflected in the coronary-prone characteristics such as competitive achievement striving, impatience, and an emphasis on social comparison. Again, the HCRC experience supports this conceptualization in that difficulty with observing reasonable limits, especially on work behavior, is a common theme among many coronary-prone patients seen in rehabilitation. Evidence in support of this conceptualization, however, is limited (Matthews, 1982). It is interesting to note that Matthews has investigated developmental aspects of the coronary-prone pattern

and has found support for her conceptualization with children.

In summary, the behavioral aspects of the coronary-prone pattern and the status of the pattern as a risk factor are well established. There is relatively good agreement about the probable pathophysiological mechanisms, but important questions and inconsistencies remain to be answered. There is less agreement about underlying psychological processes, although excessive needs for control over situations and over self, and difficulty in observing reasonable limits in the context of high personal expectations for productivity appear to be important psychological commonalities among coronary-prone patients. It should be noted that the psychological basis of the CPBP has been the focus of serious research efforts for only a short period of time. After all, the CPBP has been widely accepted as a cardiovascular risk factor only within the past 10 years. A major current and future research direction emphasizes working from behaviorally induced physiological reactivity back to psychological processes. The result of this strategy may be a more precise specification of psychological processes involved in coronary risk.

Sociological Variables

Two sociological constructs that have received attention in the literature as cardiovascular risk factors are social mobility and status incongruity (Jenkins, 1976a, 1978). Social mobility refers to the number and frequency of changes in residence. Status incongruity involves exhibiting characteristics of different social classes (socioeconomic levels and subcultures in areas such as education, income, housing, and memberships). Jenkins (1976a, 1978) reviewed the empirical basis for these constructs' risk-factor status and concluded that they emerge as risk factors only under limited conditions of time, place, and other variables present and then only for certain presentations of coronary artery disease (e.g., angina pectoris). At a conceptual level, the presumed mechanism for risk with both of these constructs is increased demands on the individual for coping and adjustment, along with uncertainty and insecurity about one's psychosocial niche, both of which might contribute to more frequent and sustained experience of stressful emotional states with the associated physiological changes. The mixed empirical results suggest that the relationships involved are complex and that in moving from such distal variables as sociological constructs to patho-physiological end results, there are multiple opportunities for interaction effects to moderate or cancel the relationship. The clinical experience at HCRC is that these sociological variables are minimally useful in understanding the psychological and emotional presentation of individual patients.

Summary

The following summary statements are offered about psychosocial variables as risk factors for cardiovascular disease. The coronary-prone behavior pattern clearly emerges as the most well-established psychological risk factor. Ample amounts of research have implicated anxiety and neuroticism as correlates of some expressions of coronary artery disease, although the pattern of results is less consistent with these variables than with the CPBP. The major life-events hypothesis has received less consistent support, and the social mobility–status incongruity constructs even less.

A pattern is evident among these categories of psychological and sociological variables. The more clearly psychological variables (CPBP, anxiety, and neuroticism) are more predictive of cardiovascular status than the more sociological variables (life events, status mobility–status incongruity). A possible explanation is that the psychological variables reflect more directly the individual coping processes that would mediate the environment–health relationships posited by the sociological variables. Constructs such as anxiety and neuroticism and the CPBP may reflect specific patterns of coping with environments that place persons at risk regardless of situational conditions. The presence of certain sociological conditions (major life changes) may pose special difficulty for these individuals, but not for other individuals who exhibit alternative coping patterns that are more adaptive with respect to health outcomes.

The major final common pathway through which psychosocial variables are thought to confer risk is the neuroendocrine system. Sympathetic adrenomedullary responsiveness, especially catecholamine levels, has been correlated with psychological variables and with cardiovascular variables. A different pattern of results has been found for pituitary-adrenocortical arousal. A current research strategy in the coronary-prone area is to work from physiological responsiveness to psychological constructs, rather than the reverse, in order to identify more clearly relevant psychological processes.

Finally, an additional pathway through which psychosocial variables confer risk, but for which a more extensive review is beyond the scope of this chapter, is their influence on other health-relevant behaviors. One of the ways in which maladaptive coping influences health is through the health consequences of the coping behaviors. Insofar as behaviors such as smoking, overeating, and alcohol and other forms of substance abuse have coping functions (usually emotion-focused rather than problem-focused), they are likely to be maintained or intensified in times of emotional stress. In the neurotic or depressed individual, these behaviors can be one aspect of a total coping style that is characterized by avoidant, unproductive, short-term, and ultimately maladaptive coping. Each of these behavior patterns has specific deleterious effects on the cardiovascular system that are well recognized. Some individuals are able to gain control over these behaviors without addressing the more general style of coping, but for many others successful modification of these behaviors involves learning new, more productive coping habits. Relapse after initial gains have been achieved is a frequent problem with these behaviors. Marlatt and Gordon (1980) have studied the relapse process with smokers, alcoholics, and drug abusers and found that most relapses occur in periods of interpersonal conflict or of negative emotional states. Thus, the learning of new coping patterns appears to be an essential ingredient in both the modification and prevention of relapse of these unhealthy behavior patterns.

PSYCHOLOGICAL EVALUATION OF THE CARDIAC PATIENT

The general goal of psychological evaluation of cardiac patients entering a rehabilitation program is the identification of problems that will be targets of intervention and/or that may influence response to the rehabilitation effort. This section begins with a discussion of the major dimensions of interest in such a psychological evaluation, followed by a more specific discussion of the methods of evaluation used at HCRC.

Dimensions of Interest

The first dimension of interest is the patient's current emotional state, with particular reference to the impact of health status on current psychological functioning. A major focus in this portion of an evaluation is the presence of symptoms of anxiety and depression. Duration of symptoms and the extent to which they disrupt current functioning are important to assess. Useful information about coping styles will be gained when assessing the patient's response to the change in health status. In particular, the degree to which denial is present is a major concern. This portion of the evaluation identifies patients with immediate needs for intervention, either in the form of psychological counseling, medical counseling (i.e., providing accurate information to correct emotionally distressing misconceptions), or psychotropic medication.

The second dimension of interest is the patient's current life situation. The rehabilitation effort occurs in the context of the patient's life situation. Thus, information about home and family life and about vocational status is useful in identifying additional sources of stress, available resources, and in providing information relevant to understanding the patient's motivation for rehabilitation. Information about work and family status may be helpful in understanding the degree of situational emotional reactions to the manifestation of heart disease. In other words, the parameters of the life situation act as moderators on situational emotional reactions. In addition, information about these areas may be useful in understanding the extent of chronic emotional stress that may have preceded the manifestation of cardiovascular disorders.

A third dimension of interest is the extent to which the coronary-prone behavior pattern is present. Knowledge from such an assessment is useful in identifying severely afflicted individuals for intervention.

Personality characteristics and psychological history are a fourth dimension of interest. "Personality" refers to long-standing, general characteristics of a person such as temperament, habitual coping patterns (or defensive style), interpersonal style, and some characteristics of thought processes. Psychological history refers to key information about the person's formative years, marital history, and previous psychological problems. Information about both personality and history is helpful in understanding the psychological meaning of the patient's present circumstances, in understanding the patient's response to different aspects of the

rehabilitation program, and in designing an individual approach to treatment. A rehabilitation program is unlikely to change the basic psychological characteristics of a person with long-standing marginal or distorted functioning, but it is useful to know about such features in order to set realistic treatment goals.

A final dimension of interest is motivation. Information about factors that influence motivation is obtained when each of the preceding dimensions is assessed. Success in a cardiac rehabilitation program requires substantial motivation on the patient's part. Regular attendance at exercise and other therapy sessions clearly requires motivation, but the larger motivational question is the patient's willingness to make the effort to apply what has been learned to daily life, especially after he/she leaves the structured program. Assessment of motivation also allows the treatment team to individualize the treatment approach and to screen out the relatively few clients who are not likely to be successful candidates because of strong motivations to remain ill.

Methods of Evaluation

There are three basic approaches to psychological evaluation, two of which are traditional and one of which is more experimental. The two traditional methods are psychological tests and the clinical interview. The nontraditional method is evaluation of physiological responsiveness to psychologically challenging or stressful laboratory analogue situations.

Psychological Testing. Psychological testing has several functions in the assessment process. First, it offers a structured way to compare patients. Second, it provides quantitative data that are useful in assessing program effects. Third, test results can be used to counsel patients about their needs in the area of psychological treatment. Interpretations of psychological tests, especially standardized instruments, are dependent on an appreciation of the uses for which the test was designed and on the normative population used in the development of the test.

General considerations relevant to assembling a battery of psychological tests for use in a cardiovascular rehabilitation center are as follows. The tests should be appropriate to the population and to the kinds of treatment being considered. For example, except in special cases, projective personality testing (Rorschach, TAT) is not necessary, nor is intelligence testing. Exceptions would be when there is a question about psychopathology or when there is a question of central nervous system damage (e.g., with a stroke patient). Test selection should be guided by the dimensions of interest discussed above. The more specifically a test is aimed at a particular assessment need, the more useful it is likely to be. Tests should be selected that will be sensitive to the range of differences that will be encountered in this population. For example, a test that is designed to identify more extreme forms of psychopathology may not be sensitive to all but the most extreme differences in a population that is basically well functioning. Feedback potential to the patient is another consideration in selecting psychological tests. Tests that have face validity and that have a relatively clear focus are better than tests that appear unusual or strange, or that purport to cover a wide range of psychological characteristics. Length of time for administration is a practical consideration that should not be ignored. If testing requires over an hour for most patients, then questions about the relative benefits of information gained to costs in patients' time and effort and in staff time in scoring become relevant. Two other practical considerations are the communicability of the test results to other professionals, especially to physicians, and the individual psychologist's own clinical experience with a given instrument.

The tests used at HCRC were selected to provide information on each of the dimensions and to satisfy the general considerations discussed above. The HCRC test battery is described here as an example of how testing can be approached in the rehabilitation setting.

Two screening instruments are used at HCRC to assess anxiety and depressive symptoms. The State-Trait Anxiety Inventory (STAI) (Spielberger et al., 1970) yields a score for the presence of current anxiety symptoms (state) and for more long-standing tendencies to respond to situations with anxiety symptoms (trait). This is a widely used instrument in psychology; it has good face validity, and it is easily administered. The HCRC experience with these scales is that they yield few false positives, but many false negatives. When scores approach or exceed one standard deviation either side of the mean score of 50, the individual is very likely to be either noticeably anxious or noticeably calm and objective. However, many individuals who are experiencing current anxi-

ety symptoms will score in the midrange on these scales.

The Beck Depression Inventory (BDI) (Beck, 1967) covers 21 symptoms of depression, with each symptom represented by four or five statements describing increasingly severe manifestations of the symptom. Again, this is a widely used, easily administered, face-valid instrument. Inspection of responses allows inferences about longer standing depressive tendencies. As with the STAI, this writer's experience is that it yields few false positives, but many false negatives. The BDI has items about weight loss, fatigue, awareness of bodily symptoms, and tolerance for work. With a post–myocardial infarction or postsurgery population, these items may not reflect depression per se, but rather the individual's deliberate attempts to lose weight or the extent of deconditioning after a period of restricted activity and bed rest. If the psychologist does not inspect the responses to these items on a BDI protocol, he/she may overestimate the severity of the depressive reaction. After discounting scores in this manner, the previous statement about false positives holds. A probable explanation for the number of false negatives is the obviousness of the items. Relatively well-functioning individuals may be reluctant to endorse many of the items because of this transparency, and as a result their scores understate their reactive depression.

The Jenkins Activity Survey (JAS) (Jenkins et al., 1979) is the most widely used psychometric index of the coronary-prone behavior pattern. There are two widely accepted techniques for assessing this pattern: the JAS and the Structured Interview (SI) designed by Friedman and Rosenman. Both have proven to be valid measures of the pattern, although they tend to reflect different aspects of it. An extensive discussion of the differences between these two methods is beyond the scope of this chapter but can be found elsewhere (Dembrowski et al., 1978; Matthews, 1982). This writer selected the JAS over the SI because it yields continuous rather than categorical scores, because it more easily lends itself to pre- and post-treatment administrations, and because of its advantages as a feedback and counseling aid to clients. The JAS yields four scores, one for the overall coronary-prone pattern, and one for each of three components of the pattern: speed and impatience, job involvement, and hard driving/competitiveness.

To assess broader personality factors and to screen for psychopathology, it is useful to include in the battery a relatively standard personality measure. This author selected an abbreviated form of the Minnesota Multiphasic Personality Inventory, the MMPI-168 (Overall *et al.,* 1973) for this purpose. The MMPI-168 is comprised of the first 168 items of Form R (Overall and Gomez-Mont, 1974; Poythress, 1978) of the full-length MMPI. Considerations in selecting this were the communicability of MMPI results to a wide range of professions and the rich and deep interpretive tradition and clinical lore associated with it. Individual scale correlations with the full-length MMPI are high (in the $r = .90$s) (Overall *et al.,* 1976). However, high-point codes on the abbreviated form do not correlate as well with high-point codes on the full-length version (Hoffman and Butcher, 1975; Butcher and Tellegen, 1978), so caution must be exercised in applying "cookbook" interpretations of such pairs. Even with this caution, the MMPI-168 has proven to be a useful and sensitive measure with the cardiac population (see Chapter 8 for data). The Hypochondriasis, Depression, and to a lesser extent, Hysteria scales are responsive to the reactive emotional states typically encountered in this population. Clinically significant scores are more frequently obtained with these scales than with the STAI and BDI, and the MMPI-168 results are usually more consistent with clinical impression than results obtained with the other two instruments. Other MMPI scales, which are less frequently elevated but which do elevate with definite subgroups of this population, are those for Psychasthenia and Mania. Psychasthenia reflects anxiety, but without the somatic focus of Hypochondriasis and Hysteria. High scores imply a more compulsive, self-doubting, and guilt-ridden individual whose defenses are not successfully controlling anxiety. Psychasthenia is more of a trait anxiety than a state anxiety scale. In the cardiac population this scale is rarely elevated by itself. Elevations usually accompany higher scores on both Hypochondriasis and Depression. Individuals with this pattern are more likely to require psychotherapeutic interventions, are unlikely to exhibit denial, and in severe cases may require psychotropic medication in order to achieve satisfactory resolution of their reactive emotional states. Elevations on Mania are frequently found among individuals who are denying either the significance of their cardiac status or the extent of their concern and distress about it. Elevations on this scale are frequently accompanied by high scores on the JAS Speed/Impatience Scale. These individuals frequently have difficulty observing prudent limits in their behavior, and this typically has been characteristic of their behavior for years before their cardiac event.

The final psychometric scale used at HCRC is a version of the Holmes-Rahe Social Readjustment Scale (Holmes and Rahe, 1967). This is used to quantify the degree of stability versus instability in the individual's life situation in the spheres of health, work, home and family, personal matters, and finances. Two scores are derived. One is the Life Change Units (LCU) score which is a weighted score designed to reflect the amount of adjustment required by the major changes the person reports having experienced over the previous two years. The score makes no distinction between desirable and undesirable events and should not be thought of as reflecting emotional stress per se. Potential for stress is inferred from this score. In order to avoid this kind of inference, patients at HCRC are asked to rate the amount of emotional distress they experienced in response to the items they endorsed. This yields a self-rating score which can then be compared to the LCU score. The relationship of the LCU score to the self-rated score is clinically useful. Three general patterns occur. First, the two scores may be approximately equal, suggesting that the individual experienced emotional stress in rough proportion to the changes to which he/she had to adjust. Second, the self-rating score may be significantly lower (approaching half the LCU value). This is frequently found among individuals who are either deniers or who are exceptionally well-functioning. Typical correlates of this pattern are low scores on the STAI, BDI, and MMPI-168 anxiety and depression scales. Third, the self-rated score may be significantly higher than the LCU score (approaching double the LCU value). These individuals typically exhibit symptoms of anxiety and depression that will be clinically and psychometrically evident. Thus, by examining the relationships among the LCU and self-rating scores in the context of the other test results, the clinician can gain valuable information about the quality of coping.

Interview. Testing provides valuable information and allows standardized comparisons to be made. Testing, however, always should be considered a supplement to a thorough clinical interview. Types of information that are of interest to the psychologist in the rehabilitation setting include the following: living situation, marital and family situation, work status, financial status, emotional status, and developmental history. The kinds of information needed in each area are discussed below.

Living situation refers to the parameters of the person's home situation. How many people live at home and has this changed recently? Is this a stable or an unstable situation? Is it stressful or comfortable?

Marital and family status includes current marital situation, marital history (if changes have occurred), the ages of children, whether they live at home or independently, and the nature of the current relationship with children. Is the family a source of stability and support, or a source of concern and further stress? How has the family responded to the patient's cardiac status? Are sexual relations disrupted?

Work status includes information about the patient's current employment situation. For example, is he/she working, on medical leave of absence but returning to a known job, disabled from a former job, or unemployed? A description of the current or most recent job with a focus on duties and responsibilities, daily activities, schedule, quality of relationships with coworkers, subordinates, and superiors, and job-related stressors should be obtained. A brief vocational history is useful, especially if there have been frequent changes (if so, why), or if there has been a recent change. Future plans with respect to work are important to assess, as these may influence motivation for rehabilitation. The extent of support the individual is receiving from his employer during recuperation is relevant to understanding the stresses he/she is experiencing.

The primary issue concerning financial status is the degree of strain the patient is currently experiencing. If the person is not working, it is important to know his/her sources of income and the stability of these sources. For example, if he/she is on disability from his/her company, what per cent of full pay is he/she receiving and for how long? Have finances been a problem that preceded the change in health status?

Emotional status refers to the patient's affective reaction to his/her health status. Recency of the major cardiac event and the kind of event (e.g., MI, bypass surgery, MI and surgery,

second bypass surgery, and so on) are important facts to remember in evaluating affective state. Another relevant dimension is affective state at the time of entry to rehabilitation compared to affective state in the period shortly after the cardiac event. This dimension assumes more importance the longer the interval between the cardiac event and entry to rehabilitation. Specific areas of inquiry are symptoms of anxiety and of depression. Anxiety symptoms that are commonly encountered include hypochondriacal cardiac awareness, insomnia, activity restrictions that are fear based, thoughts of death, and nonverbal motor presentation during the interview (e.g., muscle tension, tremors, sighing, fidgeting). Frequently reported depressive symptoms include frustration, discouragement, helplessness, hopelessness, crying, sleep disturbance, loss of interest in formerly engaging activities, increased irritability, loss of self-esteem (e.g., self-critical or self-disparaging attitude), and nonverbal presentation during the interview (e.g., retarded movements and speech, crying, and so on). With both anxiety and depression, the interviewer should determine the extent to which symptoms appear related to health status per se as opposed to the effects of health on other areas (e.g., work and financial status). The extent of denial is another dimension to assess. This is especially an issue when the individual states that he/she has not had an emotional reaction to the recent change in health status. In assessing the presence of denial one must evaluate the patient's statements against the stability-instability of his/her life situation, and against such factors as previous medical history. The presence of a strong, personally meaningful religious faith affects one's evaluation of denial. And, perhaps most important, such statements should be evaluated against the individual's motivation or willingness to make changes in other risk factor areas (e.g., weight loss, smoking cessation). A final aspect of emotional reactions to assess is the kind of coping in which the patient has engaged. Has he/she coped through avoidance or inhibition of action, by gathering information (how knowledgeable is he/she?), by active problem solving, or by intrapsychic means such as intellectualization, denial, or dependency.

Developmental history refers to information about the parameters of the formative years. Examples of relevant information include birth order, siblings, parental occupation, and quality of relationship with family members. Information about the stability/instability of family life (death, divorces, marital conflict between parents) should be obtained. This kind of information is helpful in understanding patients who present with more extreme and complicated emotional symptoms. Typically, these are people who had preillness psychological adjustment problems. Knowledge about developmental background helps the psychologist in the rehabilitation setting appreciate the depth of the problem and set treatment goals accordingly.

New Directions in Psychological Evaluation

Two relatively recent developments in assessment procedures have relevance to the dimensions of interest to the psychologist working in cardiac rehabilitation and to treatment goals. The first involves a psychophysiological evaluation of cardiac patients. This is a new approach, largely restricted to research purposes, in which physiological reactivity to psychologically stressful laboratory analogue tasks is measured. The approach involves noninvasive measurement of variables such as blood pressure, heart rate, and catecholamine levels while individuals are involved in activities such as challenging video games, a difficult mental history or arithmetic quiz, the Rosenman-Friedman Structured Interview, or the cold pressor test (submerging a hand in ice water for a prescribed period). This approach to psychophysiological assessment has been used in experimental studies on the coronary-prone behavior pattern (Dembrowski et al., 1979; Dimsdale and Moss, 1980; Dembrowski et al., 1981; Gastorf, 1981; Roskies, 1982). People can be categorized as physiologically overreactive ("hot reactors") or normally reactive ("cold reactors"). This approach adds another dimension to both psychological and routine medical assessment and helps identify patients who *may* be at special risk from emotional stress. These data are not equivalent to a psychological evaluation, i.e., they do not assess current anxiety, depression, or coping capacities, and should not be considered a substitute for one. However, "hot reactors" can be targeted for exploration of psychological bases for their reactions and then for specific interventions focused on improved control and modulation of these reactions (e.g., relaxation training).

Another psychological construct that has received recent attention and is relevant to cardiovascular rehabilitation is self-motivation (Dishman et al., 1980; Dishman and Ickes, 1981). Self-motivation is defined as ". . . a behavioral tendency to persevere independent of situational reinforcements" (Dishman and Ickes, 1981). Self-motivation was designed to account for personal factors that predict adherence to programs of preventive and rehabilitation medicine, especially in the area of exercise. Dishman and Ickes (1981) reported the development and validation of a psychometric measure of the construct, the Self-Motivation Inventory (SMI). This instrument predicted adherence to exercise programs in three different settings, including a cardiac rehabilitation program. Thus, the self-motivation construct and its accompanying inventory may be clinically useful in predicting compliance with the exercise and life-style modification programs that are essential to comprehensive cardiovascular rehabilitation.

REFERENCES

Bandura, A. Self-efficacy: Toward a unifying theory of behavioral change. *Psychol. Bull.,* **1978,** *84,* 191–215.

Baum, A.; Grunberg, N.; and Singer, J. The use of psychological and neuroendocrinological measurements in the study of stress. *Health Psychol.,* **1982,** *1,* 217–237.

Beck, A. *Depression: Clinical, Experimental, and Theoretical Aspects.* Hoeber, New York, 1967.

Billings, A., and Moos, R. The role of coping responses and social resources in attenuating the stress of life events. *J. Behav. Med.,* **1981,** *4,* 139–147.

Borkovec, T. Insomnia. *J. Consult. Clin. Psychol.* **1982,** *50,* 880–896.

Butcher, J., and Tellegen, A. Common methodological problems in MMPI research, *J. Consult. Clin. Psychol.,* **1978,** *46,* 620–628.

Cooper, T.; Detre, T.; and Weiss, S. Coronary prone behavior and coronary heart disease: A critical review. *Circulation,* **1981,** *63,* 1199–1215.

DeLongis, A.; Coyne, J.; Dakof, G.; Folkman, S.; and Lazarus, R. Relationship of daily hassles, uplifts and major life events to health status. *Health Psychol.,* **1982,** *1,* 119–137.

Dembrowski, T.; MacDougall, J.; Herd, J.; and Shield, J. Effects of level of challenge on pressor and heart rate responses in Type A and B subjects. *J. Appl. Soc. Psychol.,* **1979,** *9,* 209–228.

Dembrowski, T.; MacDougall, J.; Slaats, S.; Eliot, R.; and Buell, J. Challenge induced cardiovascular response as a predictor of minor illnesses. *J. Human Stress,* **1981,** *7,* 2–5.

Dembrowski, T.; Weiss, S.; Shields, J.; Haynes, S.; and Feinleib, M. (eds.) *Coronary-Prone Behavior.* Springer Verlag, New York, **1978.**

Diagnostic and Statistical Manual III. American Psychiatric Association, Washington, D.C., **1980.**

Dimsdale, J. Emotional causes of sudden death. *Am. J. Psychiatry,* **1977,** *134,* 1361–1366.

Dimsdale, J., and Moss, J. Plasma catecholamines in stress and exercise. *JAMA,* **1980,** *243,* 340–342.

Dishman, R., and Ickes, W. Self-motivation and adherence to therapeutic exercise. *J. Behav. Med.,* **1981,** *4,* 421–438.

Dishman, R.; Ickes, W.; and Morgan, W. Self-motivation and adherence to habitual physical activity. *J. Appl. Soc. Psychol.,* **1980,** *10,* 115–131.

Dohrenwend, B., and Dohrenwend, B. *Stressful Life Events: Their Nature and Effects.* John Wiley, New York, **1974.**

Folkman, S., and Lazarus, R. An analysis of coping in a middle-aged community sample. *J. Health Soc. Behav.,* **1980,** *21,* 219–239.

Frankenhauser, M. Psychoneuroendocrine approaches to the study of stressful person-environment transactions. In, Selye, H. (ed.) *Selye's Guide to Stress Research,* Vol. 1. Van Nostrand-Reinhold, New York, **1980.**

Friedman, M., and Rosenman, R. *Type A Behavior and Your Heart.* Alfed A. Knopf, New York, **1974.**

Friedman, M.; Thoresen, C.; and Gill, J. Type A behavior: Its possible role, detection, and alteration in patients with ischemic heart disease. In, Hurst, J. (ed.), *Update V: The Heart.* McGraw-Hill, New York, **1981.**

Froese, A.; Hackett, T.; Cassem, N.; and Silverberg, E. Trajectories of anxiety and depression in denying and nondenying acute myocardial infarction patients during hospitalization. *J. Psychosom. Res.,* **1974,** *18,* 413–420.

Gastorf, J. Physiologic reaction of type A's to objective and subjective challenge. *J. Human Stress,* **1981,** *7,* 16–20.

Glass, D. *Behavior Patterns, Stress, and Coronary Disease.* Erlbaum, Hillsdale, N.J., **1977.**

———. Pattern A behavior and uncontrollable stress. In, Dembrowski, T. *et al.* (eds.) *Coronary-Prone Behavior.* Springer Verlag, New York, **1978.**

Glass, D.; Krahoff, L.; Contrada, R.; *et al.* Effect of harassment and competition upon cardiovascular and plasma catecholamine responses in Type A and Type B individuals. *Psychophysiology,* **1980,** *17,* 453–463.

Hoffman, N., and Butcher, J. Clinical limitation of three MMPI short forms. *J. Consult. Clin. Psychol.,* **1975,** *43,* 32–39.

Holmes, T., and Masuda, M. Life changes and illness susceptibility. In, Scott, J. and Senay, E. (eds.) *Separation and Depression; Clinical and Research Aspects.* American Association for the Advancement of Science, Washington, D.C., **1973.**

Holmes, T., and Rahe, R. The social readjustment rating scale. *J. Psychosom. Res.,* **1967,** *11,* 213–218.

Horowitz, M.; Wilner, N.; and Alverez, W. Impact of event scale: A measure of subjective stress. *Psychosom. Med.,* **1979,** *41,* 209–218.

Jenkins, C. Recent evidence supporting psychologic and social risk factors for coronary disease: Part 1. *N. Engl. J. Med.,* **1976a,** *294,* 987–994.

———. Recent evidence supporting psychologic and social risk factors for coronary disease: Part 2. *N. Engl. J. Med.,* **1976b,** *294,* 1033–1038.

———. Behavioral risk factors in coronary artery disease. *Annu. Rev. Med.,* **1978,** *29,* 543–562.

Jenkins, C.; Zyzanski, S.; and Rosenman, R. *Manual for the Jenkins Activity Survey.* Psychological Corp., New York, **1979.**

Kanner, A.; Coyne, J.; Schaefer, C.; and Lazarus, R. Comparison of two modes of stress measurement: Daily hassles and uplifts versus major life events. *J. Behav. Med.,* **1981,** *4,* 1–39.

Kornitzer, M.; Kittel, F.; Debacher, G.; and Dramaix, M. The Belgian Heart Disease Prevention Project: Type "A" behavior pattern and the prevalence of coronary heart disease. *Psychosom. Med.,* **1981,** *43,* 133–145.

Lazarus, R. *Psychological Stress and the Coping Process.* McGraw-Hill, New York, **1966.**

———. The concepts of stress and disease. In, Levi, L. (ed.) *Society, Stress, and Disease,* Vol. 1. Oxford University Press, London, **1971.**

———. *The Stress and Coping Paradigm.* Paper presented at the Conference on The Critical Evaluation of Behavioral Paradigms for Psychiatric Science, Bleneden Beach, Oregon, November 3–6, **1978.**

Light, K., and Obrist, P. Cardiovascular reactivity to behavioral stress in young males with and without marginally elevated casual systolic pressures: Comparison of clinic, home, and laboratory measures. *Hypertension,* **1980,** *2,* 802–808.

Marlatt, G. A., and Gordon, J. Determinants of relapse: Implications for the maintenance of behavior change. In, Davidson, P. and Davidson, S. (eds.) *Behavioral Medicine: Changing Health Lifestyles.* Brunner/Mazel, New York, **1980.**

Mason, J. A historical view of the stress field. Part 1. *J. Human Stress,* **1975a,** *1,* 6–12.

———. A historical view of the stress field. Part II. *J. Human Stress,* **1975b,** *1,* 22–35.

Matthews, K. Psychological perspectives on the Type A behavior patten. *Psychol. Bull.,* **1982,** *91,* 293–323.

Mechanic, D. Discussion of research programs on relations between stressful life events and episodes of physical illness. In, Dohrenwend, B. and Dohrenwend, B. (eds.) *Stressful Life Events: Their Nature and Effects.* John Wiley, New York, 1974.

Overall, J., and Gomez-Mont, F. The MMPI-168 for psychiatric screening. *Educ. Psychol. Meas.,* **1974,** *34,* 315–319.

Overall, J.; Higgins, W.; and Schweinitz, A. Comparison of differential diagnostic discrimination for abbreviated and standard MMPI. *J. Clin. Psychol.,* **1976,** *32,* 237–245.

Overall, J.; Hunter, S.; and Butcher, J. Factor structure of the MMPI-168 in a psychiatric population. *J. Consult. Clin. Psychol.,* **1973,** *41,* 284–286.

Pearlin, L.; Lieberman, M.; Menaghan, E.; and Mullan, J. The stress process. *J. Health Soc. Behav.,* **1981,** *22,* 337–356.

Poythress, N. Selecting a short form of the MMPI: Addendum to Faschingbauer. *J. Consult. Clin. Psychol.,* **1978,** 46, 331–334.

Quinlan, C.; Barrow, J.; and Hayes, C. *The Association of Risk Factors and Coronary Heart Disease in Trappist and Benedictine Monks.* Presented at the 42nd American Heart Association Conference on Cardiovascular Epidemiology, New Orleans, **1969.**

Rabkin, J., and Streuning, E. Life events, stress, and illness. *Science,* **1976,** *194,* 1013–1020.

Rahe, R., and Lind, E. Psychosocial factors and sudden cardiac death; A pilot study. *J. Psychosom. Res.,* **1971,** *15,* 19–24.

Reich, P.; DeSilva, R.; Lown, B.; and Murawski, B. Acute psychological disturbances preceding life-threatening ventricular arrhythmias. *JAMA,* **1981,** *246,* 233–235.

Rissanen, V.; Romo, M.; and Siltanen, P. Premonitory symptoms and stress factors preceding sudden death from ischaemic heart disease. *Acta Med. Scand.,* **1978,** *204,* 389–396.

Rogers, C. R. *Client-Centered Therapy.* Houghton Mifflin, Boston, **1951.**

Rosenman, R.; Brand, R.; Jenkins, C.; Friedman, M.; Straus, R.; and Wurm, M. Coronary heart disease in the Western Collaborative Group Study: Final follow-up experience of 8½ years. *JAMA,* **1975,** *233,* 872–877.

Rosenman, R.; Friedman, M.; Straus, R.; Wurm, M.; Kositcheck, R.; Hahn, W.; and Werthessen, N. A predictive study of coronary heart disease; the Western Collaborative Group Study. *JAMA,* **1964,** *189,* 15–22.

Roskies, E. Modifying coronary prone behavior in healthy persons. Presented at the Third Annual Meeting of the Society of Behavioral Medicine, Chicago, Ill., March, **1982.**

Ross, C., and Mirowsky, J. A comparison of life-event-weighting schemes: Change, and desirability, and effect-proportioned indices. *J. Health Soc. Behav.,* **1979,** *26,* 166–177.

Sarason, I.; Johnson, J.; and Siegel, J. Assessing the impact of life changes: Development of the life experiences survey. *J. Consult. Clin. Psychol.,* **1978,** *46,* 932–946.

Seligman, M. *Helplessness: On Depression, Development, and Death.* Freeman, San Francisco, **1975.**

Selye, H. *Stress Without Distress.* J. B. Lippincott Co., Philadelphia, **1974.**

Shekelle, R.; Schoenberger, J.; and Stamler, J. Correlates of the JAS Type A behavior pattern score. *J. Chronic Dis.,* **1976,** *29,* 381–394.

Spielberger, C.; Gorsuch, R.; and Lushene, R. *Manual for the State-Trait-Anxiety Inventory.* Consulting Psychologists Press, Palo Alto, **1970.**

Taggart, P., and Carruthers, M. Endogenous hyperlipidemia induced by emotional stress of racing driving. *Lancet,* **1971,** *1,* 303–369.

Taggart, P.; Carruthers, M.; and Someville, W. Electrocardiogram, plasma catecholamines and lipids, and their modification by axprenolol when speaking before an audience. *Lancet,* **1973,** *2,* 341–346.

Theorell, T.; Lind, E.; and Floderus, B. The relationship of disturbing life changes and emotions to the early development of myocardial infarction and other serious illnesses. *Int. J. Epidemiol.,* **1977,** *4,* 281–293.

Van Lanchen, J. Smoking and disease. In, Jowik, M.; Cullen, J.; Gutz, E.; Vogt, T.; and West, L. (eds.) *Research on Smoking Behavior.* NIDA Research Monograph 17. Rockville, Md., Dept. of Health, Education, and Welfare, **1977.**

Weisman, A., and Hackett, T. Predilection to death: Death and dying as a psychiatric problem. *Psychosom. Med.,* **1961,** *23,* 232–256.

Chapter 8
PSYCHOLOGICAL DISORDERS: GOALS, TREATMENTS, AND OUTCOMES

Merrill P. Anderson

GOALS OF PSYCHOLOGICAL INTERVENTIONS

Psychological therapy in the rehabilitation setting has four major therapeutic goals: (1) to facilitate the resolution of reactive or situational emotional states as defined in the previous chapter, (2) to encourage secondary prevention with respect to sources of chronic emotional stress, (3) to support other risk-factor reduction efforts, and (4) to enhance compliance and long-term maintenance of life-style changes in all areas of rehabilitation.

Facilitating resolution of situational emotional states refers to the reduction of disabling anxiety and/or depression and of related conditions such as denial, loss of self-esteem, and sleep disorders, which are frequently associated with cardiovascular disorders. The therapeutic task is to help people move through these common reactions as smoothly and quickly as possible. If these reactions are not resolved in a reasonable period of time, they can become chronic, more complicated, and can interfere significantly with all phases of rehabilitation. For example, fatigability and activity restrictions after myocardial infarction or bypass surgery are commonplace. Both can be frustrating and depressing. The longer they persist, the

more depressing they become, and soon depression not only contributes to but also exaggerates the fatigue. A depressive cognitive set (negative view of self, of the world, and of the future) (Beck, 1976) may develop, and there may be increased somatic complaints. Thus, a vicious cycle develops in which depression begets somatic complaints which beget more discouragement and further depression. Intervening in a chronic, complex cycle is more difficult than helping the person cope with an uncomplicated reactive emotional state. Thus, early entry into cardiovascular rehabilitation programs is highly recommended as a means of preventing the more complicated reactions from developing. In summary, a primary goal of psychological interventions during cardiovascular rehabilitation is to encourage reasonable acceptance of, or adjustment to, heart disease as a fact of life, but also to the fact that life can and does go on, and that with appropriate action, the patient may improve his/her health status and return to a more productive and higher quality of life.

The secondary prevention goal of psychological interventions involves an emphasis on what has been termed "stress management." Insofar as emotional stress is a risk factor for cardiovascular disorders, then reduction in the frequency and/or intensity of negative emotions such as anxiety, anger, and depression is one aspect of the prevention of progression of disease. Thus, psychological interventions are focused on improving the quality of coping with sources of potential emotional stress. It is important to realize that stress is not inherent either in situations or in persons. Rather, stress is a potential outcome of transactions between persons and their environments. Stress occurs when perceived environmental demands exceed perceived resources for dealing with them. So, stress-management counseling emphasizes making changes in situations, to the extent possible, but also emphasizes making changes in people's behavioral and cognitive responses to situations. For example, moderation of coronary-prone characteristics is included in stress management. Because stress-management interventions are relevant to emotional stress generally, they aid in the resolution of the situational disorders discussed in the previous paragraph, and this contributes to more rapid rehabilitation as well as to secondary prevention.

The third major goal of psychological interventions in the rehabilitation clinic is support of risk-factor modification efforts in areas such as smoking cessation and weight loss. Psychological interventions or consultations are required in these areas for two principal reasons. First, change efforts will be enriched and made more effective to the extent that they appropriately incorporate established principles of behavior modification in each area (Pechacek and Danaher, 1979; Wilson and Brownell, 1980; Lichtenstein, 1982; Brownell, 1982). Second, consummatory behaviors such as smoking, overeating, and alcohol abuse often serve coping functions. For example, overeating, drinking alcohol, and so on, may be used in the management of distressing emotions such as anxiety, anger, or depression. Successful modification of eating and smoking behavior may involve learning alternative coping behaviors (e.g., relaxation or interpersonal assertion) for use in potentially stressful situations.

The fourth major area of concern to the psychologist is compliance with therapeutic regimens and long-term maintenance of health life-style habits after departure from a structured program. This is increasingly being recognized as one of the major behavioral/psychological challenges in health care. The long-term effectiveness of a therapeutic approach such as cardiovascular rehabilitation depends on pa-

tients' ability to continue with changes made in the areas of regular exercise, weight control and dietary habits, smoking cessation, and psychological coping. Thus, the psychologist in the rehabilitation setting is concerned with enhancing compliance while the patient is in the program so that initial gains are achieved, and then with preparing the patient to cope with the problems of long-term maintenance after leaving the structured program. With respect to the latter issue, Marlatt and Gordon (1980) have developed a model of the relapse process in such habitual behaviors as smoking and alcohol abuse that has important extrapolations to cardiovascular rehabilitation. Their major points are briefly discussed in a later section of this chapter (p. 123).

TREATMENT MODALITIES

Beneficial Psychological Effects of Program Participation

There are substantial psychological therapeutic benefits that result from the fact of being involved, per se, in a comprehensive rehabilitation program. Participation in such a program is especially therapeutic with respect to emotional distress related to health status, i.e., situational anxiety and depression. The mechanisms through which these therapeutic effects occur are relatively easy to identify. The program provides patients with a structure to their efforts to improve their status. Helplessness and hopelessness are reduced as they perceive progress in an exercise program, as they meet other individuals in different stages of rehabilitation, as their understanding of what has happened to them improves, and as they become more educated about how to recognize symptoms and how to take care of themselves in the future. To a point, the more appropriate information and understanding they have about their disease and about their therapy, the less anxiety they will experience. The group cohesion and support that develop among patients in the program have powerful therapeutic potential through their effects on reducing loneliness and isolation, providing comparisons, and in maintaining motivation and effort. Perception of progress in different areas (e.g., exercise, weight loss, reduced medications) enhances the patient's hope, sense of control, and self-esteem. As functional limitations are reduced because of improved physical status, patients are able to obtain more meaningful satisfactions in daily life. In summary, if the therapeutic effects of monitored, progressive, aerobic exercise on the heart have been characterized as a "nonsurgical bypass," then the psychologically therapeutic effects of general program participation on reactive emotional states can be characterized as a nonmedicinal tranquilizer and antidepressant.

These comments are based on a significant clinical experience with patients and on the patient's own statements about therapeutic aspects of the HCRC program. Empirical data on improvements in psychological status following participation in the HCRC program are presented later in this chapter. The manner in which these data were collected, however, does not permit inferences about the contribution of the different program components (psychological, exercise, nutrition, and health education) to improvements in psychological status. Therefore, they must be considered to reflect the impact of the program as a whole on psychological functioning. They suggest that whatever therapeutic effects exercise may have are probably enhanced by the inclusion of the other program components in a comprehensive rehabilitation package that treats not just the patient's physical body, but also educates him or her about his/her care and status and treats emotional symptoms.

There is a body of research on the psychological benefits of exercise programs for post–myocardial infarction (MI) patients, with some studies showing exercise as therapeutic (Hellerstein & Horsten, 1966; Hackett and Cassem, 1973; Kavanaugh et al., 1977) and others finding no changes (Naughton et al., 1968; Plovsic et al., 1976). Stern and Cleary (1982) reported results on psychosocial outcomes from the National Exercise and Heart Disease Project (NEHDP), a large-scale study of the rehabilitative potential of exercise with myocardial infarction survivors. They found no differences between a treatment and a control group on psychological measures at intervals of six months, one year, and two years. An earlier report (Stern and Cleary, 1981), however, found beneficial psychological effects following participation in the first stage of the program protocol, a six-week, prerandomized, low-level exercise program. They speculate that this pattern of results means that exercise programs, per se, contribute to short-term reductions in anxiety and depression, but that over the longer term, they provide no additional (or measurable) psychological benefits.

Additional support for the psychological value of a combination of controlled exercise combined with medical counseling about the implications of that exercise level for daily living comes from Bandura (1982) and Ewart et al. (1980). Treadmill stress testing combined with medical counseling positively influenced post-MI patients' judgments about their ability to safely engage in physical activity. However, the protocol involved only one exercise session and only one session of medical counseling. Thus, the results can be taken only as suggestive. These effects could reasonably be expected to be magnified with patients who are involved in a more intensive exercise and counseling program, such as that provided by HCRC. Insofar as the reactive anxiety and depression following MI or heart surgery are related to uncertainty and to unrealistic assessments of post-MI or postsurgery physical limitations, then these interventions can be psychologically therapeutic.

Specifically, psychological interventions can be delivered in several modalities. Group approaches are the most frequently used, with individual counseling or psychotherapy, family and marital counseling, and psychotropic medications as additional modes. Each of these treatment modes is discussed in the following sections in the context of cardiovascular rehabilitation.

Group Approaches

Group approaches have several advantages and few limitations, which may account for their popularity in the rehabilitation of postcoronary and postbypass surgery patients. A discussion of the advantages of the group essentially involves discussing the therapeutic mechanisms of group therapy. The major therapeutic ingredient in groups for postcoronary patients is group support. This, in turn, is an umbrella term for several processes that can occur in a group but that are more difficult to specify. Examples of such processes include reduced loneliness and isolation, opportunities to care for others (as opposed to self-absorption), and increased motivation due to commitment to others. Groups offer patients a means of comparing themselves with others on any of several dimensions potentially relevant to recovery. Dimensions that are commonly mentioned by patients at HCRC include past medical history, degree of current disability or deconditioning, rate of progress in exercise, level of anxiety and/or depression, quality of coping, and degree of coronary proneness.

The comparison process is double-edged,

and patients' distress can be increased if they conclude that they compare unfavorably with others. For example, some patients become discouraged when they notice that other patients are exercising at higher work loads than they, or are advancing in their exercise work load at a faster rate. The rehabilitation staff must be alert for this kind of comparison, the potential for which is inherent in the situation, and be ready to intervene with corrective information about the uniqueness of each individual case along with support for that patient's accomplishments. In spite of the potential for unfavorable outcomes, the comparison process is therapeutic for a majority of patients.

Another advantage of the group setting is that participants have an opportunity to be helpful to others, which can serve to increase perceptions of oneself as able to contribute rather than as being a passive and receptive "patient." Patients will frequently share ideas or attitudes relevant to improved stress management, to their approach to work, to their implementation of proper dietary habits, and so on. Frequently, hearing how other patients have made changes or have implemented recommendations is more convincing and motivating than merely receiving recommendations from the professional staff. This kind of learning occurs outside formal group meetings in the interaction during exercise sessions, or before and after group meetings.

Another advantage of the group approach is the economy of effort for the professional staff. Most patient concerns are common to most patients, and the group approach allows the professional staff to take advantage of this fact. In fact, the economic consideration is one of the reasons the individual physician has difficulty doing rehabilitation in an office practice.

The major limitations of the group approach are that some individual concerns are very personal and/or embarrassing and cannot be addressed adequately in the group, and that some individuals may engage in unfavorable social comparisons. Also, occasionally a group member is disruptive because of, for example, inappropriate responses or domineering, egocentric behavior. These problems can be minimized by a skillful group leader. Individual concerns are handled easily by providing individual counseling as needed in the psychological, as well as in medical or nutritional, areas. The harmful effects of unfavorable social comparisons can be relieved by providing timely and appropriate corrective information.

The approach to psychological group therapy used at HCRC has a semistructured format in which sessions are organized topically, and the leader actively presents information and suggests exercises or structured activities pertinent to the topic of each session. The structure imposed by the leader is flexible in that discussion, self-disclosure (by patients), and group interaction are encouraged. The goal is to have an optimal mixture of structure and flexibility. Structure ensures that basic issues are covered and information is presented and provides an organizing framework from which patients can view emotional stress-management concerns. Flexibility allows the more traditional benefits of group therapy to operate. The more the group blends these two qualities of structure and flexibility, the more each quality enriches the other. The information and structured experiential activities are made more relevant and meaningful by personal discussion and self-disclosure. The structured aspect of the group helps maintain a focus and a framework within which to explore and deal with individual concerns. As should be obvious from this discussion, the clinical skill and sensitivity of the leader are critical in accomplishing the recommended blend of structure and flexibility.

There is considerable commonality among published group approaches in the topics and activities around which the sessions are organized. The topic sequence developed at HCRC is representative of other approaches, and is, therefore, presented here as an example of what is done. Unique aspects of other approaches are discussed subsequently. The HCRC stress-management group program consists of ten weekly meetings, approximately one and a half hours in length. They are led by a doctoral-level psychologist (the present writer). The topic sequence as presented below is not static and is subject to modification and evolution.

Session one introduces a framework for thinking about emotional stress and coping and explains the implications of chronic emotional arousal for physiology and health. The framework that is presented emphasizes the important role of thinking (cognitive appraisals) in the generation of emotional stress (Lazarus, 1966). The framework is presented diagramatically as a flow chart (Figure 8-1) that depicts primary and secondary appraisal processes and suggests response outcomes of different kinds of appraisals. This framework is presented in subsequent sessions to organize the discussion about weekly topics. The second

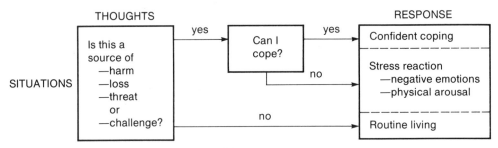

Figure 8-1

half of this first session is devoted to making a strong case for the physical health implications of chronic emotional arousal. This is the rationale for including a stress-management component in a cardiac rehabilitation program, and patients must be convinced that the quality of their coping and the degree of stress under which they operate are health issues, and that successful coping will improve their health. Accordingly, they are introduced to the basics of sympathetic-adrenomedullary arousal and its effects on cardiac work, on plasma lipid levels, and on blood platelet reactions. The implications of sustained arousal for the development of hypertension, atherosclerosis, angina, and arrhythmias are discussed.

The second session focuses on major life changes as stressors and introduces the first relaxation exercise, progressive muscle relaxation. After defining major life changes, emphasis is placed on the disruptive effects of such changes on daily habits and routines and on how such disruption contributes to potentially higher levels of frustration and stress. The discussion then turns to suggestions for improved coping during times of major life changes, with the general point being that the degree of stress actually experienced can be moderated by assuming as flexible an attitude as possible, especially in expectations for self and others. The need for more careful communication with significant others, perhaps for more anticipation and planning, and for proper sleep, exercise, and nutrition is emphasized, among other things. Progressive muscle relaxation (Jacobson, 1938; Bernstein and Borkovec, 1973) is introduced as the first of several relaxation exercises. Patients are told that it is the most fundamental and elaborate of the relaxation exercises. They are told that practicing this procedure will result in improved skill in recognizing muscle tension, which is a common accompaniment of emotional stress, in the beginnings

of the ability to deliberately release or relax such tension, and in the beginnings of their ability to use deep breathing as a relaxation skill.

Session three specifically focuses on experiences with heart disease, its disruptive effects, and on how group members have coped with them. Typically, this session involves considerable discussion and interaction among group members as they share experiences and begin to hear how others have coped. At an appropriate point in the discussion, the leader may introduce Kübler-Ross's model of the four stages of grief or mourning (Kübler-Ross, 1969), in order to emphasize to the group that their feelings can be viewed as part of a natural grief reaction to what has happened to them. This session also usually presents a good opportunity to begin introducing ideas for coping with depression. The concept of denial as a coping style also is usually introduced with appropriate warnings about the potential of denial for undermining constructive rehabilitation.

Sessions four and five in the HCRC sequence are related in that each uses the general concepts developed in session one to organize a discussion about common negative emotions: anxiety in session four and anger in session five. In each session the emotion in question is analyzed using the general framework depicted in Figure 8-1. These sessions draw heavily on cognitive-behavioral conceptualizations of anxiety (Ellis, 1962; Meichenbaum, 1977) and of anger (Novaco, 1975). These sessions are designed to increase self-awareness of the extent of either emotion, to demonstrate that one's self-appraisal processes and beliefs are involved in generating these emotions, and to introduce methods for moderating or managing them. Relaxation exercises are also practiced in each session. These are shorter than the progressive relaxation procedure introduced in session two and are based on the approach of

Arnold Lazarus (1971). These relaxation exercises emphasize suggestions of relaxation and deep breathing and involve less emphasis on muscle tension and relaxation sequences.

The coronary-prone behavior pattern is presented in session six. This session consists of a brief explanation of this behavior pattern as a risk factor, discussion of the sources of the behavior pattern, and presentation and discussion of approaches to modifying or moderating the major aspects of the pattern. Contrary to what might be expected, experience at HCRC indicates that only slightly more than half of the patients in the rehabilitation program exhibit the coronary-prone pattern, as defined by the relatively soft criterion of positive scores on the Jenkins Activity Survey Type A subscale (Jenkins *et al.,* 1979). Data bearing on this point are presented later in this chapter (p. 142). This is an important point to note because it cautions against assuming that the large majority of cardiac rehabilitation patients will fit the classic coronary-prone pattern and then designing a treatment program aimed largely at modifying these characteristics. The psychological treatment program as a whole should be aimed broadly at improved coping with emotional stress. Insofar as the program accomplishes this goal, many of the treatment modalities used by others in the field (Suinn and Bloom, 1978; Roskies, 1980; Thoresen *et al.,* 1982) to modify or moderate the major aspects of the coronary-prone pattern will be included under other topics. For example, the material presented in sessions four and five on coping with anxiety and especially with anger is highly relevant to achieving moderation of such typically coronary-prone emotions as anger, irritation, and impatience. Progressive muscle relaxation and other relaxation exercises are useful in helping coronary-prone individuals moderate their physiological reactivity when challenged. The only intervention introduced in this session that is unique to modifying coronary-prone characteristics is the idea of specific daily drills in noncoronary-prone behaviors (e.g., walking, talking, or eating slower, deliberately taking time to recall a pleasant memory, expressing affection) (Thoresen, *et al.,* 1982). Experience at HCRC suggests that the critical therapeutic event for many coronary-prone individuals is acknowledgment that these characteristics, and stress generally, constitute a risk to their health. Once they are convinced of the risk and define these characteristics as a problem, then they become more

receptive to the specific stress-management interventions. Thus, a major goal of session six is to persuade the coronary-prone members of the group that they have a problem.

Interpersonal communication and conflict-resolution skills are discussed in session seven. Emphasis is placed on the handling of interpersonal differences (e.g., preferences, moods, values, desires, tastes, priorities) through communication (assertion and listening skills), a cooperative in contrast to a competitive attitude, appropriate recognition of the underlying or central issues involved in the difference that is the current focus of disagreement, and willingness to engage in compromise. Expression of appropriate angry feelings is given special attention in the discussion of assertive communication. Role playing of assertive communications is encouraged in the session. The relaxation exercise for this session introduces mental visualization of pleasant, tranquil scenes as a means of enhancing relaxation.

Session eight presents suggestions for improving personal organization and time-management skills. The material presented is based on the system of Alan Lakein (1973) and emphasizes such activities as listing goals, setting priorities, working from daily activity lists, and breaking large projects into smaller components that can be realistically approached on a daily basis. The stress-producing qualities of being poorly organized or of being overly organized are discussed. Self-hypnosis is introduced as another type of relaxation exercise that combines the use of mental imagery and deep breathing used in previous exercises.

The ninth session focuses on psychological aspects of maintenance of the healthy life-style changes patients have been developing while in the structured rehabilitation program. The approach in this session draws on the work on relapse prevention by Marlatt and Gordon (1980). Patients are encouraged to anticipate situations that have the potential to disrupt some aspect of their new health life-style (e.g., exercise, smoking cessation, dietary habits, coping) and to develop general strategies for coping with them. They are warned of changes in motivation they may experience as they leave the structure, support, and safety of the clinic and are left to their own initiative in a different environment. With respect to exercise, they are encouraged to develop a regular schedule that becomes part of their daily or weekly routine. Goal setting and record keeping of exercise are discussed as methods of maintaining motivation. An important issue to discuss under the topic of goal setting is the difference between the process of achieving a good level of physical conditioning and the process of maintaining a good level of conditioning. The distinction to be made is that while working toward conditioning, one experiences gratification as exercise work loads are steadily increased, but that once optimal conditioning is achieved, maintenance exercise tends to remain constant and repetitive, and the sense of achievement or progress is diminished. Patients are encouraged to view the essential challenge at this point as maintaining gains already achieved rather than achieving further gains. The premium is placed on consistency of exercise. Accordingly, they are advised to set goals for themselves in terms of frequency and regularity of exercise as a part of their weekly life.

The tenth and last group session of the HCRC ten-week stress-management series is devoted to a review and summary of the major objectives of each of the sessions. Participants typically share the changes they have made over the course of the meetings, and an evaluation of the series is conducted by questionnaire.

In conducting a series of group meetings such as have just been described above, it is important to avoid the temptation to rely exclusively on didactic or lecture format. Patients should be actively involved in the discussion, either by sharing their own experiences with the topic of the day, or by reacting to the experiences of others. The leader must encourage group members to reflect on themselves with respect to each topic, to share with others, and to practice in daily life during the program suggested stress-management procedures. In short, a properly conducted stress-management group is a mix of information, activism, and assertion and is a change-oriented experience for participants.

HCRC's ten-session stress-management sequence is typical of programs described by other authors working in cardiac rehabilitation or in related fields such as modification of coronary-prone characteristics in preinfarction men. Rahe et al. (1979) used six sessions in a psychological program for postinfarction men and described the approach as largely educational and supportive. Ewart (in press) uses nine sessions in a couples counseling approach to cardiac rehabilitation. He emphasizes communication and conflict-resolution skills more than other authors, but also includes individ-ual-oriented stress-management skills such as relaxation and moderating excessively high self-standards that produce anxiety and other negative emotional states. Roskies used 14 sessions in her group treatments focused on modification of coronary-prone characteristics in preinfarction men (Roskies et al., 1978; Roskies, 1980). The major focus of their current research is reduction of physiological reactivity in type A "hot reactors." Thus, her current group treatment (Roskies, 1982) emphasizes relaxation skills and especially the application of these skills to daily life. Cognitive stress-management procedures are also included in her program of the kind recommended by Meichenbaum (1977) and Novaco (1975). The most extensive group treatment for postinfarction patients is the five-year program conducted by Friedman and his research group (Thoresen et al., 1982). As with Roskies, this program is aimed at men who exhibit the coronary-prone pattern, although men in the Friedman series have already infarcted, whereas her program was limited to those who had not. The Friedman program consists of monthly group meetings over a five-year period. The program includes every topic covered by the other group approaches and more, as well it might, given the amount of time involved. A unique aspect of the treatment program is their use of "drill books" that prescribe daily practice of specific behaviors that are incompatible with the coronary-prone pattern.

Individual Therapy

For all of the advantages and economies of group work, individual psychological counseling still has an important role in a rehabilitation program. A properly conducted group program will address and fulfill a large proportion of patient needs. However, many individuals have problems that require additional, more specifically focused, therapy. In the following sections the kinds of patients who are likely to require individual work and the level at which individual work typically occurs, i.e., whether it is counseling or psychotherapy, are discussed.

The first category of patients who require individual work are those who exhibit more severe situational reactions to their cardiac problems. Anxiety will be predominant in some, depression in others, and still others will exhibit exaggerated symptoms of each. These more severe situational reactions typically occur among certain subgroups of patients.

The first subgroup consists of individuals who are experiencing significant instability in the nonhealth spheres of their lives that is either a consequence of their health problems or that simply occurs concurrently with their health problems. Examples would be individuals whose work status is seriously jeopardized by their cardiac problems, or who were already having vocational/career problems, and for whom the onset of cardiac problems represents an additional complication. Financial strain and uncertainty frequently accompany vocational instability and can be an important source of severe situational reactions. Marital problems are frequently present with severe situational reactions. In many of these cases, the marital difficulties have preceded the cardiac problems, as opposed to patients with less severe situational reactions who may experience relatively less marital strain after major cardiac events. The reader will note that the factors discussed above are essentially the same as were discussed in the preceding chapter on psychological principles under the heading of "Moderating Factors," where they were termed "social resources and supports." The point can be summarized in the following manner. Situational emotional reactions to major cardiac events will be more severe if important sources of self-esteem, identity, and emotional security are also unstable or are in jeopardy. If such is the case, the patient is deprived of valuable sources of support and reassurance, and the relatively natural reactions to serious physical disorders interact with the reactions to the other circumstances to produce more severe disturbances.

A second category of individuals who require individual work are those characterized by psychological adjustment problems that preceded their cardiac problems. The preillness psychological adjustment problems affect the rehabilitation effort in three principal ways. First, they may contribute to more pronounced and complicated situational emotional reactions, either anxiety or depression. Second, from the secondary prevention perspective, these characteristics may contribute to future risk of cardiovascular problems because of the potential for higher levels of emotional stress associated with them. Third, they are more likely to have compliance problems with some aspect(s) of rehabilitation. Examples of the kinds of preillness adjustment problems that may require individual psychological therapy are discussed in the following paragraphs.

Long-standing depression is one of the more frequent problems encountered in the cardiac rehabilitation program. These depressed patients typically exhibit marked self-critical tendencies that are related to very high self-evaluative standards. For men, alcoholism either may be involved or may have been a factor in the past. Frequently these patients' life histories contain some significant disruptions, either during the formative years or later in life. For these people who were already depressed, the onset of cardiac problems presents an especially difficult challenge to already fragile self-esteems and to an already well-developed sense of helplessness.

Anxiety-based neurotic adjustments are another problem group. These patients typically also exhibit some depressive characteristics, but anxiety symptoms predominate. An especially common subgroup contains individuals with marked compulsive characteristics. These people typically present with obvious anxiety symptoms that are in proportion to the extent to which their excessive need for control over themselves and over their circumstances has been disrupted and frustrated by their cardiac problems. They frequently worry obsessively about small details and about events in the relatively distant future. Their worry focuses not only on their health status, but on their vocational and financial situations as well. Sleep disturbances are common, as are problems with depression. On the positive side, compulsives are generally a highly compliant group of patients. The various treatment regimens of a cardiovascular rehabilitation program seem to represent a welcome structure or framework within which they can begin to reestablish the degree of control and order with which they are comfortable. Sleep disturbances, in particular, may require medication, but also can be treated with relaxation techniques.

Hypochondriacs are a less frequent but more difficult subgroup. These individuals tend to complain of a variety of ailments, especially elaborate pain and gastrointestinal problems. Their excessive fear or preoccupation about their health usually preceded their cardiac events. Getting well for this group of patients has very different meanings than for other patients in that it involves giving up a major defense against low self-esteem and unhappiness in their lives. Thus, they tend to resist a complete recovery from all of their ailments. Characteristically, they do not have insight into the functional aspect of their somatic symptoms. Not surprisingly, they also tend to exaggerate the severity of their cardiac problems. Compliance, especially in the long term, is more difficult with these people because of the likelihood that a future somatic problem will be the occasion for cessation of exercising.

Another subgroup of patients with preillness psychological adjustment problems who may require individualized psychological interventions are those who exhibit personality disorders, as defined by the American Psychiatric Association's Diagnostic and Statistical Manual-III (1980). Personality disorders are defined as chronic characteristics of a person's behavior and functioning that cause significant subjective distress and/or impairment in some sphere of their life (e.g., interpersonal and family relationships, vocational adjustment, health). Individuals who meet the *DSM*-III diagnostic criteria for a personality disorder are relatively infrequent in the cardiac rehabilitation setting. Nonetheless, the HCRC program has had individuals who were diagnosed as exhibiting narcissistic, borderline, compulsive, and paranoid personality disorders. Most of these individuals pose problems with either compliance or in their interactions with the staff. Frequently they are demanding of special attention and consideration, and they tend to be critical of how they believe they have been treated by the staff and by other patients. One of the psychologist's major responsibilities with these patients is to help the rehabilitation team focus its efforts and not be distracted by patient behavior that is objectionable to the staff or to other patients. The psychologist must keep in mind that the major characteristics of the disordered personality are highly resistant to change. Nonetheless, some of these patients can be helped to moderate those characteristics that have deleterious effects on health. The rehabilitation team needs to be advised of management procedures that will facilitate the patient's gaining as much benefit from rehabilitation as possible. However, the psychologist must also advise the rehabilitation team of the practical limits of a patient's ability to change.

Alcoholics are another patient subcategory with longer term adjustment problems that frequently require individual interventions. Depression is a frequent concomitant to the alcohol abuse. Treatment typically involves confronting the individual about his/her alcohol use or abuse, educating him/her about the cardiovascular effects of excessive alcohol, encouraging abstinence supported by involvement in Alcoholics Anonymous, and psychological counseling focused on depression. Once the individual is abstinent, psychological counseling should continue to focus on the person's depressive tendencies as well as on relapse prevention (Marlatt and Gordon, 1980).

A final subgroup of patients with preillness adjustment problems are those whose psychological disturbance reaches psychotic proportions during their involvement in the rehabilitation program. Usually resolution of the psychotic episode has priority over other aspects of the cardiac rehabilitation program. Indeed, successful compliance with a cardiac rehabilitation program for an individual with a psychotic degree of disturbance is highly unlikely. The psychologist is involved in assessing the severity of the problem, in making recommendations for an appropriate psychiatric referral or consultation, and in providing appropriate counseling to the patient and his/her family while he is involved in the program.

A third major patient category requiring individual psychological interventions includes those who experience stressful life situations during their involvement in rehabilitation that distract them from and disrupt their rehabilitation program. Frequently these involve business or family or marital problems. The occurrence of these problems during the rehabilitation program offers the psychologist an opportunity to use the situation as an object lesson for improved coping and application of ideas from the stress-management group meetings. Counseling about these issues is frequently essential for the patient's subsequent progress in rehabilitation. Failure to resolve these kinds of problems can lead to poor compliance, and/or to an unsatisfactory response to exercise, nutritional, or medical therapy, all of which will retard the rehabilitation effort. Successful and timely resolution of these situations keeps rehabilitation progress optimally on schedule. Capitalizing on these episodes as object lessons for stress-management principles can result in convincing demonstrations to the patient (and other observing patients) of the value of attending to stress issues and of making changes in their coping style.

A fourth major patient category requiring individual attention involves individuals for whom noncompliance per se is the major initial indication of a problem. In fact, patients who are noncompliant with some aspect of the rehabilitation program (attendance at exercise, nutrition, and so on) typically exhibit one or more of the problems discussed in the preceding paragraphs. Noncompliance also can be related to logistical problems (distance to the clinic, transportation problems). Noncompliance must be confronted in a supportive manner, the reasons for it identified, and an appropriate and realistic plan for resolving the situation must be developed. Such a plan might involve specific commitments and contingencies under which continued involvement will occur; it might involve individual counseling regarding psychological/emotional issues or nutritional/weight loss issues, or it might involve adjusting the schedule of the patient's involvement at the clinic to better accommodate the demands of his/her life circumstances. Experience at HCRC suggests that noncompliance should be identified and addressed as promptly as possible in order to avoid a prolonged period of less effective treatment and to identify underlying problems and make appropriate interventions.

Counseling Versus Psychotherapy. Psychologists working in cardiac rehabilitation, like therapists in other settings, are continually faced with decisions about the proper use of their interventions. A frequent issue concerns the psychological level at which interventions are directed. This issue will be discussed by distinguishing between two different forms of individual work: counseling and psychotherapy. While there is not good agreement among psychologists about the value of such a distinction, this writer offers the distinction primarily as a means of discussing a more general point about levels of psychological intervention. Counseling focuses on current coping efforts, on behavioral change and skill development, and on education. Psychotherapy, on the other hand, focuses on emotional issues basic to personality organization such as self-acceptance and the defenses used to preserve it. Psychotherapy frequently involves exploration of the historical basis of current emotional habits, interpretation of the functional aspects of current behavior, and a more intense emotional relationship between therapist and patient.

The issue of counseling versus psychotherapy is likely to emerge with patients who exhibit preillness psychological disturbance and for whom the continuation of these psychological and emotional patterns may adversely affect their cardiovascular status. Said another way, the issue of counseling or psychotherapy tends to arise as a secondary prevention consideration. In the final analysis, the psychologist must keep the goals of the rehabilitation program clearly in mind when deciding the extent of interventions. The rehabilitation goals are the reduction of current disability and the prevention of progression of disease. Longer term psychotherapeutic involvement may be recommended for some patients in the interest of secondary prevention or if behavior problems persist that can be practically dealt with and for which there is an optimistic prognosis. The need for psychotherapy should not, however, be used as justification for keeping patients involved in a comprehensive program once they have achieved reasonable medical goals. At the same time, with all patients, counseling regarding current coping is enriched by an appreciation of the deeper emotional and cognitive bases (beliefs) of patients' overt behavioral and emotional patterns. Also, the experience of a life-threatening event such as myocardial infarction or heart surgery has the potential to confront patients with fundamental existential issues such as the reality of death and questions of meaning and values (Kübler-Ross, 1969; Becker, 1973; Yalom, 1980). Insofar as patients are grappling with these issues and the issues contribute to emotional reactions, the psychologist misses a rich opportunity for promoting personal growth by not helping patients clarify the personal meanings involved.

Psychology or Psychiatry: A Question of Emphasis. The experience at HCRC is that the psychological/emotional disorders presented by patients and the treatments required by these disorders are more consistent with a psychological than with a psychiatric professional background. There is clearly overlap between the areas of expertise claimed by the two disciplines, but important differences in emphasis exist that make psychology the more appropriate discipline for the cardiovascular rehabilitation setting. The large majority of the psychological/emotional disorders exhibited by patients are situational rather than psychogenic or psychopathological. Psychological treatment tends to be focused on emotional support, on improving current coping efforts, on adjusting to loss, on making life-style behavioral changes, and on conscious rather than unconscious factors. The primary goals of comprehensive cardiovascular rehabilitation do not include the resolution of preexisting psychopathological disorders. In fact, as has been stated earlier in this chapter, the existence of a serious (psychotic) psychological disorder frequently precludes successful involvement in a cardiovascular rehabilitation program. Insofar as psychiatry specializes in the medical treatment of more severe psychopathological disorders, there is less need for its expertise and treatment procedures. When individuals accepted into cardiovascular rehabilitation exhibit more severe disorders, a psychiatric consultation may be required, especially when there is a question of need for psychotropic medication. The experience at HCRC, however, is that such consultations are rarely needed.

WORKING WITH SPOUSES

A comprehensive approach to rehabilitation recognizes that involvement of the spouse of a cardiac patient in the therapeutic program is almost always advantageous. Reasons for their involvement include the following. First, spouses are usually a major natural source of emotional support for the cardiac patient. Frequently, spouses are unsure how to be most helpful to their stricken husband or wife. Counseling can aid them in making decisions in this area so that they can continue to provide the needed support. Second, spouses often experience situational emotional reactions similar to or related to those of their partners who have been ill. Spouses often struggle with anxiety and fears about the safety of their partner and about their proper role in his/her care. They may feel depressed about the emotional withdrawal of their husband/wife after a major cardiac event or about the ways in which the cardiac condition has affected or may affect their life-style. Adequate treatment of these conditions in spouses helps ensure that they will be able to continue providing the needed emotional support while the patient is in the program and over the long term. Third, spouses will be involved in the patient's efforts to maintain a healthier life-style; therefore, the more they understand about what is recommended and why it is recommended, the better they will be able to help the patient adhere to the program. For example, in the nutrition area, wives frequently purchase, prepare, and serve the food at home. Thus, involving them in the nutritional counseling component of cardiac rehabilitation is often critical. Also, patients are encouraged to maintain a home exercise program after they leave the structured rehabilitation program. This may involve rearrangement of family and household schedules. The more understanding and cooperation there are from the spouse, the more likely the patient is to comply. At HCRC we frequently have had wives (and husbands) join their cardiac partners in the exercise session and then continue with the joint exercising after leaving the program. In summary, spouses should be involved in a comprehensive rehabilitation program in order to facilitate their ability to provide emotional support for their partners, to give the spouses themselves needed emotional support, and to support patients' compliance with a home program of secondary prevention.

Spouses should be involved in the rehabilitation in three general ways. They can participate in group educational conferences along with their partners. At HCRC spouses are routinely encouraged to attend the series of meetings in nutrition, stress management, and medical management. This is a major means for spouses to get the information they need both to relieve their own uncertainties and to provide appropriate support to their partners. Second, counseling can be offered to spouses individually, or to the marital dyad. Typically counseling is needed when the marital relationship has been especially strained by the cardiac event and by the patient's reaction to it, or when the marital relationship was strained before the cardiac event and continues to be a source of chronic emotional stress. In the latter case, the psychologist must proceed with sensitivity to the sometimes conflicting wishes of the patient and the spouse. Issues of confidentiality may arise with respect to a spouse's inquiries about his/her partner's progress and emotional state. A third form of involvement for spouses is participation in a spouse-only support group. We have observed at HCRC that wives who accompany their husbands to the clinic tend to use the time their husbands are exercising to share with each other their respective experiences. We have noted that the wives seem to share with each other differently when they are not in their husbands' presence than when they are (for example, compared to when they are participating in educational conferences with their husbands). Thus, HCRC has begun to offer a weekly support group for spouses only. The expectation is that spouses have questions, frustrations, and emotional needs unique to their status as partners of cardiac patients to which they do not grant legitimacy because of the priority of their spouse's "patient" status. A group experience can give spouses an opportunity to hear from others in similar circumstances, can serve as a forum for learning new methods of coping and new ways of communicating, and can serve as a source of emotional support.

PSYCHOTROPIC MEDICATIONS

The experience at HCRC has been that antianxiety and antidepressant medications are rarely required to manage the emotional reactions to major cardiac events in an ambulatory, phase II and III program. Involvement in a comprehensive rehabilitation program per se (including psychological counseling) is so effective in allaying situational anxiety and depression that these medicines are not needed for the majority of patients. Many patients enter the rehabilitation program with prescriptions for antianxiety compounds (e.g., diazepam) that they may have used in the period immediately following either MI or surgery, but have discontinued by the time they enter rehabilitation. Decisions about the use of psychotropic medications always necessitate a dialogue with the program physician. At HCRC the major symptom for which antianxiety medications are prescribed is sleep disturbance, and the medicine usually prescribed is flurazepam. Typically, this is used during the initial stages of a patient's involvement in rehabilitation if sleep disturbance is present and is later discontinued. Antidepressant medications have been used at HCRC even less frequently than antianxiety agents. Tricyclic antidepressants are used only in the most severe and complicated reactions when functioning (e.g., ability to work) has been disrupted. The drug therapy should be in conjunction with psychological counseling regarding the depressive reaction. Careful consideration is advised before prescribing tricyclics to cardiac patients because of their cardiovascular effects (Jackson and Bressler, 1982). These include decreased myocardial contractility, quinidine-like effects on the cardiac conduction system, and anticholinergic effects. Thus, extreme care should be taken when prescribing tricyclics to patients already on beta-blocking drugs (e.g., propranolol) or antiarrhythmic agents (e.g., quinidine) because of the potential for adverse drug interactions.

SMOKING-CESSATION COUNSELING

Smoking cessation is a major goal of the HCRC program. Fortunately, many patients have stopped smoking by the time they enter the HCRC program. This is consistent with published results indicating that among myo-cardial infarction survivors who were smokers, 30 to 50% quit following simple medical advice to do so (Croog and Richards, 1977), and that this percentage may increase with more active counseling approaches (Burt et al., 1974). The interpretation of these comparatively high rates of cessation is relatively straightforward. People are generally more motivated to quit when they are currently experiencing, or have recently experienced, symptoms directly related to smoking. In short, fear is a powerful motivator for quitting smoking.

These observations imply that patients who have not stopped by the time they enter a cardiovascular rehabilitation program may be an especially resistant group of smokers. The HCRC experience suggests that two subgroups of patients may be involved.

"Helpless" smokers typically acknowledge the detrimental effects of smoking, but are deeply convinced that they are powerless to accomplish cessation (Pechacek and Danaher, 1979). Their lack of confidence in their personal ability to successfully stop smoking undermines motivation for initiating and especially for persisting at new efforts. Experience at HCRC suggests that individuals who fit the "helpless" smoker characterization frequently have less stable interpersonal environments (family and work) and are more likely to exhibit symptoms of impaired or less effective psychological functioning (e.g., more anxious, more depressed, less organized). The second subgroup of resistant smokers is characterized by a relative denial or minimization of the seriousness and significance of their heart disease and of the relationship of cigarette smoking to heart disease. Many patients in this group will straightforwardly assert that they simply enjoy smoking and are unwilling to stop.

The approach to smoking cessation used at HCRC is a multicomponent procedure that has much in common with many current behavioral approaches to smoking cessation (for reviews, see Pechacek and Danaher, 1979; Lichtenstein, 1982). The first step in the HCRC approach is largely educational and motivational. All entering patients are thoroughly briefed on the adverse effects of smoking on the cardiovascular system, with primary emphasis given to the stimulating effects of nicotine on the heart (e.g., increased cardiac work and oxygen demand) and to the oxygen deprivation resulting from inhalation of carbon monoxide. These presentations are factual, forceful, and unequivocal. It is useful for all patients to hear this information, as those patients who have recently quit can benefit from it as well as those who have not yet quit. The staff must remember that most recidivism in smoking occurs within one year after cessation. Thus, recent quitters are in as much need of education, motivation, and support as are current smokers. This phase of the smoking-cessation treatment is typically done in a group setting, whereas the remaining work is done on a more individualized basis.

The approach to smoking-cessation counseling that is used at HCRC is best characterized as a self-control or coping-skills approach. A variety of techniques may be used, and the patient is encouraged to take an active role in formulating his/her particular smoking-cessation strategy. Typically, the counseling begins with an analysis of the individual's smoking habit. The analysis phase should occur before the cessation attempt is begun. This phase might involve self-monitoring of cigarette consumption over a three- to five-day period, with frequency, setting, and strength of urges, all being monitored. With or without self-monitoring data, the individual is helped to identify the times of the day or situations that are especially difficult for him or her. If possible, they are encouraged to change their behavioral routine at these times (e.g., get up from the dinner table and brush teeth). They are encouraged to develop a plan for coping with urges to smoke during high-risk situations. Examples of coping skills that are frequently used include substitute oral activities (e.g., gum, toothpicks, sugarless candy, mints), deep breathing and relaxation, taking a walk, or engaging in mental imagery of the damage the cigarette is doing to the heart and lungs.

After the analysis and anticipation phases of the counseling, the individual is encouraged to develop with the psychologist a plan for actual cessation. Smokers are strongly encouraged to set a date in the near future (e.g., within a week) for quitting, and then to completely stop on that date. As a rule, abrupt cessation following the brief period of preparatory counseling described earlier is encouraged at HCRC. Some patients are unwilling, or feel unable, to follow this approach. For these individuals, alternative methods such as nicotine fading (changing to a brand with less nicotine and tar) and scheduled reduction of cigarettes may be used. If one of these methods is chosen, the period of time before abstinence is reached should be kept relatively short (e.g., two weeks maximum) in order that momentum, enthusiasm, and interest are maintained.

Once cessation has initially been achieved, the patient needs to be followed closely for several weeks in order to provide support, to help him/her develop new strategies, and especially to minimize the potential effects of any relapses. Marlatt and Gordon (1980) discuss the "abstinence violation effect" as a frequent cause of sustained relapses. They point out that abstinence is an all-or-none standard, and once it is broken, some people react as though they have failed. They become discouraged, self-critical, and lose their motivation. At HCRC individuals who have relapsed are encouraged to take a problem-solving attitude toward the incident. They are encouraged to analyze the reasons for the relapse and to develop a plan for how to cope with a similar situation in the future. Encouragement is provided, and new goals may be set.

HCRC has a unique kind of feedback available to patients who are trying to stop smoking. Because heart rate and blood pressure are monitored during every exercise session, it is frequently possible to show the newly abstinent smoker improvements in his/her exercise performance (i.e., in heart rate or blood pressure response) that correspond with the period of abstinence. Such feedback makes the beneficial effects of their effort more tangible and can be quite motivating.

HCRC does not encourage the use of aversion procedures in smoking cessation. The most widely used and researched aversion procedures are variants of the rapid smoking or satiation techniques (Lichtenstein, 1982). All of these methods involve brief periods of intense exposure to smoke and nicotine and are known to produce significant changes in heart rate, carboxyhemoglobin, blood nicotine levels, and on electrocardiograph tracings (Hall et al., 1979). There are not any reports in the literature of serious cardiovascular complications resulting from these procedures. Nonetheless, they are rarely used with cardiac patients, and HCRC does not rely on them in its smoking-cessation program.

PSYCHOLOGICAL INTERVENTIONS FOR WEIGHT LOSS: TEAMWORK WITH NUTRITION

In the HCRC program the nutritionist is the primary provider of nutritional and weight-loss counseling, but the psychologist consults with him/her on a regular basis, and the two work together with patients. This teamwork is in recognition of the significant psychological aspects of obesity and of weight-loss programming.

HCRC uses a behavior-modification approach to weight loss, along with a thorough program of nutrition education (see Chapters 9 and 10). The basic nutrition/weight-loss program is conducted in a group format, and this is supplemented by individualized counseling. The behavior-modification program for weight loss incorporates features that have been standard in behavioral weight-loss programs for over 15 years. The principal components are self-monitoring of food intake and calorie consumption, stimulus control of external cues for eating, changing the topography of eating behavior, and goal setting and reinforcement of progress. Recent reviews of the literature on the status of behavioral weight-loss programs have emphasized the importance of developing multifaceted programs for weight loss that include not only traditional behavior-modification principles and nutrition education, but also regular exercise, psychological counseling, and planning for long-term maintenance (Wilson and Brownell, 1980; Brownell, 1982).

HCRC patients already engage in regular aerobic exercise for 30 minutes, three times per week. By itself, this frequency and intensity of documented exercise distinguishes the program from many other weight-loss programs which attempt to encourage participants to exercise. Frequently, the exercises in which participants engage are of insufficient duration or intensity to achieve even mildly significant caloric expenditures, to say nothing of having appetite-suppressant effects or stimulant effects on basal metabolic rates.

The psychologist works jointly with the nutritionist in four general ways. First, the psychologist consults with the nutritionist about specific applications of behavioral principles. For example, patients who feel especially helpless about controlling their food intake may require a specially tailored behavioral program with more finely graduated steps, and with supplemental counseling focused on increasing attributions of progress to the patient's own efforts. Other patients may require more explicit behavioral contracting, perhaps to the point of a monetary deposit-refund system. Second, the psychologist can be involved when depression, anger, or frustration related to dieting threatens to undermine compliance with the weight-loss program. Depression is a well-known complication of dieting (Stunkard and Rush, 1974). It can be addressed through psychological counseling focused on cognitions and attitudes contributing to depression and through planning for alternative indulgences and satisfactions designed to offset feelings of deprivation and frustration. Third, the psychologist may work with some patients on developing ways of coping with distressing situations or with negative emotional states that are more adaptive and problem-focused than eating. For example, counseling focused on interpersonal assertiveness and communication skills can help individuals express themselves in interpersonal conflict situations in ways that may result in reduced frustration because the resolution of the situations takes their needs and preferences into consideration. Without the counseling, an individual might have felt angry about the situation, frustrated at not having his/her needs met, and depressed because of his/her passivity. Eating easily can become a safe (low anxiety), noninterpersonal mode for reducing tension associated with negative emotional states. In a similar vein, relaxation skills can be used as a means of coping with temptation situations. In short, insofar as eating may have served tension-reduction functions, then relaxation and other stress-management skills can serve as alternative, and considerably more adaptive, means of reducing emotional tension. Thus, stress-management counseling may be an important aspect of a weight-loss program, especially with patients for whom negative emotional states appear to be important cues for eating.

Finally, it is important to acknowledge that with extreme obesity the probability of a significant psychological component to the disorder increases. Eating, food, and body image have probably come to serve important dynamic roles in the individual's psychological defensive structure. The psychologist needs to work with the patient and with the nutritionist to develop a weight-loss program that takes these factors into consideration. Clearly, the research literature is not encouraging about the prospects for successful, long-term weight loss with the extremely obese. Multidimensional programs that incorporate aggressive therapies in each of the areas of dietary management, behavior modification, psychological counseling, and exercise appear to offer the best hope for whatever success can be obtained.

PHYSIOLOGIC MONITORING DURING EXERCISE AS AN INDEX OF PSYCHOLOGICAL STRESS

Peterson (1983) has developed a set of objective and quantitative measures (see Chapter 2) for managing the amount of physical work (exercise) that patients should be prescribed while they are in a rehabilitation program in order to optimize the so-called cardiovascular "training effect" and to identify an array of factors that affect cardiovascular functions. Simply stated, the method relies on the ratio of the body work (external work) performed on a bicycle ergometer or treadmill to the work performed by the heart, as assessed by the double product (heart rate × systolic blood pressure) at peak exercise load. This ratio of external work to cardiac work is called the Conditioning Index (CI). The use of this measure in exercise management is discussed in Chapter 2. Experience with this index demonstrates that it is also a sensitive method for estimating the effect of emotional stress on the cardiovascular system. Emotional stress raises cardiac work just as exercise does; either through influences on blood pressure or heart rate. Thus, day-to-day variations and longer term trends in emotional stress can reduce the CI at a given work load through the effect of the stress on heart rate, blood pressure, and arrhythmias.

The measure is helpful in management of patients' psychological status while they are in the structured rehabilitation program in the following ways. (1) Declines in the CI that are not explained by other factors such as medication changes or illness alert the staff to the possibility of ongoing emotional problems (e.g., depression, anger, sleep disturbance, family tension). By careful monitoring of the CI, the staff is frequently aware that a patient may be having a problem before the patient seeks help on his/her own initiative. Thus, the patient can be approached about the problem, and psychological counseling can be started on a timely basis. In this way, the deleterious effects of emotional stress on progress in the physical conditioning program can be minimized, and rehabilitation can proceed at an optimal rate. (2) Graphs like those in Figures 8-2 to 8-6 can be shown to patients in order to demonstrate the effects of emotional stress on their cardiovascular systems. This is a powerful form of feedback that can convince them of the importance of emotional-stress management for cardiovascular health and thereby increase their motivation for and receptiveness to psychological interventions. This form of feedback can be especially useful with patients who verbally deny the extent of emotional stress they are experiencing. (3) Resolution of specific stressful situations or improvement in general coping style (e.g., reduction in coronary-prone behaviors) are also frequently reflected by rises in the CI. This is also a powerful form of feedback about the benefits of proper stress management.

Several case examples of relationships between emotional stress and the Conditioning Index are illustrated in Figures 8-2 to 8-6. The interpretive material for each case shows how knowledge of these relationships can be used in the psychological management of patients.

Case 1: Effects of a Stressful Life Event

Figure 8-2 represents a portion of the exercise record of a man in his late 50s with a history of myocardial infarction, coronary artery bypass surgery, and hypertension. This man had not returned to work at the time of his entry to HCRC. His status vis-à-vis his employer and the circumstances under which he might return to work were emotion-laden issues for him. During the first ten weeks of his rehabilitation program, individual psychological counseling focused on consideration of his options and on ways of communicating his wishes regarding return to work to his supervisor. Point A in Figure 8-2 represents his blood pressure response when an attempt was made to increase his exercise work load, apparently prematurely. The beginnings of a positive response to the exercise is noted at B. In recognition of his progress, his exercise work load was raised at C, and for the next two sessions he began to adapt to the new work load (CI rising, cardiac work decreasing). At D the patient learned of a major reorganization within the company that would lead to the early retirement of several older employees. He was convinced that he would be one of the chosen. For the remainder of the period depicted in Figure 8-2 he did not know what the decision would be in his particular case, nor when he would hear. He expected to receive word at any time during this period and, as a result, was quite distressed and exhibited a range of symptoms of anxiety, anger, and depression. Physiologically, the predominant cause of the increased double product between sessions 32 and 45 was an average increase in systolic blood pressure of 23.2 mm Hg over the average systolic pressure for

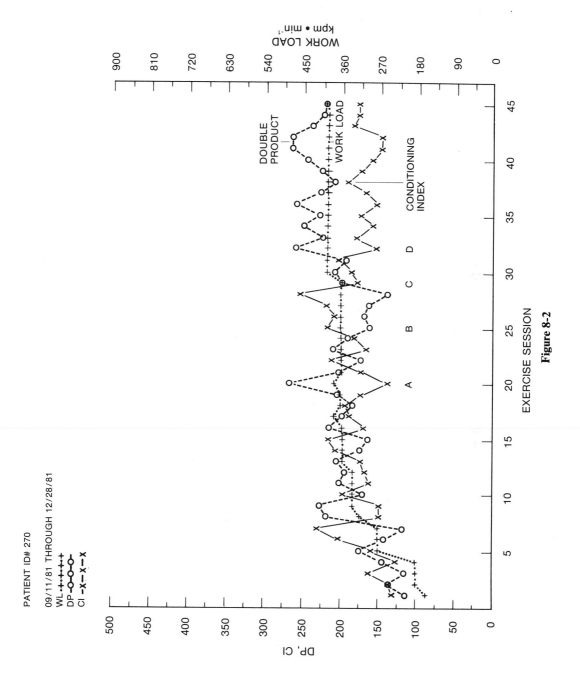

Figure 8-2

133

the previous 11 sessions (between points *A* and *D*). Heart rate also increased an average of 14 beats per minute for the same comparison periods. The gentleman learned six weeks after the last session depicted here that he would be reassigned rather than retired. He accepted the new assignment, but was not pleased with it. This case illustrates the detrimental effects of emotional stress on rehabilitation progress. Had these events not occurred, or had this individual been able to cope better (i.e., keep his emotional reactions to the events in a more moderate range), then he may have been able to sustain the progress apparent at points *B* and *C* and have achieved his exercise limit much sooner than he eventually did.

Case 2: Effects of Resolution of Stress

Figure 8-3 displays a portion of the record of a man with a history of hypertension and high-grade, three-vessel, coronary artery disease with angina. He had had a triple coronary artery bypass followed by an episode of congestive heart failure a month later. In addition, he had a history of alcohol abuse. When he entered the HCRC program the patient had not returned to work, but was eager to do so because of financial pressures. At point *A* he returned to work on a part-time basis with a reduced salary and number of sales accounts. At *B* he expressed to HCRC staff his increasing dissatisfaction with the work arrangement because of financial pressures and self-perceived loss of status. Between points *B* and *C* HCRC nurses reported alcohol on his breath during exercise. After reviewing his graph to this point, HCRC staff decided to confront the patient with the fact of his decline in progress and to explore the reasons. Point *C* represents the day of the meeting. Coincidentally, the patient's female companion called HCRC on this day to report his increasing alcohol usage over the past three weeks. The patient denied alcohol abuse, admitted to work dissatisfaction, and stated his intention to make his dissatisfaction known to his employer that day. The patient had alcohol on his breath during exercise at point *D*. He reported a stressful previous two days. He had met with his boss, but had not received an answer to his complaints. At point *E* he reported chest tightness on the previous day. This had caused anxiety about his health and sleep disturbance that night. At point *F* the patient was absent from an exercise session. Inquiry established that his request for a full reinstatement at work had been denied. His female

companion contacted HCRC to indicate that she was not going to tolerate his alcohol abuse any more. She was encouraged to come into the clinic with the patient to discuss the problem. The next scheduled exercise session the patient arrived at HCRC obviously intoxicated and accompanied by his female companion. He did not exercise due to his condition. In a private session with the HCRC psychologist he was confronted with the effects of his drinking on his relationship and on his heart. At point *G* the patient approached his employer again and was restored to his former status and responsibilities. By point *H* he reported that he had been attending Alcoholics Anonymous meetings two times per day for a week, and at point *I* he reported continued attendance at AA meetings and active participation in their program. His work situation was progressing satisfactorily. This patient was exited from the HCRC program approximately one month later at a work load of 720 kpm · min^{-1}. His job situation had improved, and he was nearing completion of AA's program. This case illustrates how these measures can indicate the presence of a stress problem, can serve as a form of feedback to the patient regarding the effects of the stress on his/her cardiovascular status, and can reflect the effects of resolution of the stress.

Case 3: Effects of Resolution of Stress

This patient (Figure 8-4) had a history of myocardial infarction, cardiac arrest and resuscitation, and triple coronary artery bypass surgery. At the time he entered the HCRC program he was dissatisfied with some aspects of his current work situation and was undecided about his future course of action. He had received offers for other positions, but was ambivalent about leaving for personal and family reasons. At point *A* this writer was briefly discussing the status of his work situation with the patient while he was exercising. A blood pressure reading taken during the conversation was unusually high, 211/120 mm Hg, so the conversation was discontinued. Another reading ten minutes later was significantly lower. Immediately after the exercise session, the reasons for the blood pressure reaction were explored in a counseling session. It developed that there had been a recent event at his place of employment that had increased his dissatisfaction and had made his ambivalence more acute. Of importance, however, the patient was very impressed by the extent of his cardiovascular response to simply talking about the situation.

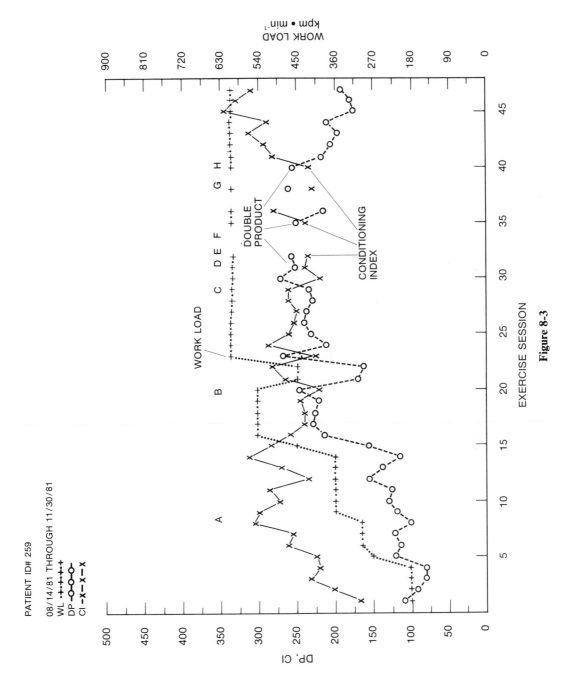

Figure 8-3

135

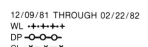

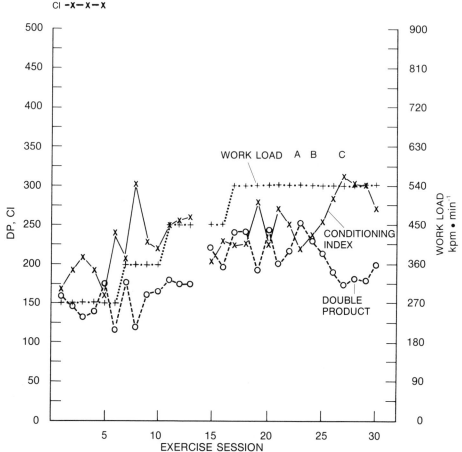

Figure 8-4

He had not realized the extent to which he was physiologically reactive and, in fact, thought of himself and appeared to others as an exceptionally relaxed, low-stress individual. He went home that night, conferred with his family, and discovered to his surprise that they were in complete support of his leaving the situation and accepting another offer. At point *B* he reported significant relief associated with his decision and described himself as beginning to let go of his emotional investment in the organization. Follow-up counseling at point *C* focused on the broader psychological issues involved in this episode in the interest of helping him learn about his own propensity to stress reactions. Subsequently, this patient was able

to apply the lesson from this episode. He realized that he was not a good judge of the degree of stress he was experiencing, so that in potentially stressful situations (e.g., overseas business trips) he insisted on a less hurried schedule and planned relaxation and recuperation periods into his schedule. This patient made the transition to another job and was exited at a work load of 720 kpm · min⁻¹.

Case 4: Extreme Physiological Reactivity

Figure 8-5 displays the record of a man with a history of myocardial infarction two years previously, hypertension, and hyperlipidemia. He had been disabled from work since his MI. His record is an example of relatively labile

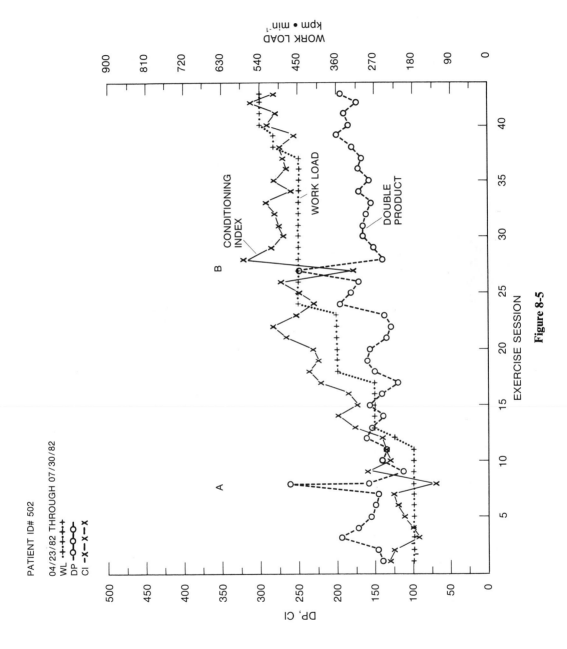

Figure 8-5

137

blood pressure in response to specific emotionally stressful episodes. Point *A* represented his heart rate and blood pressure response after a difficult time commuting to the clinic. He had missed his scheduled exercise time because of the traffic and had had to join a later exercise group. Systolic blood pressure was increased 48 mm Hg over the previous session, diastolic pressure was up 22 mm Hg, and heart rate was increased 35 beats per minute. Between points *A* and *B* the patient made exemplary progress, with his cardiac work remaining relatively constant and his CI steadily rising with increases in exercise work load. Point *B* represents a day on which he had an argument with a representative of the agency that was sponsoring his participation in the program. The argument had

occurred prior to coming into the clinic. Heart rate was elevated 43 beats per minute over the previous session, systolic pressure was up to 10 mm Hg, and diastolic pressure increased 10 mm Hg. These brief episodes did not significantly impede this man's progress through rehabilitation. Each occasion, however, was a stimulus for counseling with him about ways of coping with his reactivity (e.g., relaxation exercises) and about the emotional basis of his reaction. Following the latter incident he was counseled about his feelings toward the person with whom he had had the argument, achieved some insight into his sensitivity about receiving what he viewed as "charity," and developed alternate strategies for dealing with future interactions with the other person.

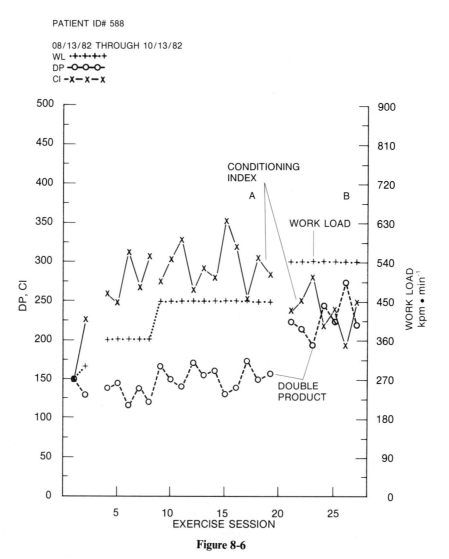

Figure 8-6

Case 5: Physiological Reactivity Mediated by Stress-Related Factors

Figure 8-6 contains the record of a man in his late 40s with a history of severe angina pectoris, hypertension, and obesity. Myocardial infarction had been ruled out. This individual's overall response to the exercise program was positive to point *A*. The drop in CI at that point was associated with three factors: a late night with out-of-town company, excessive coffee intake that morning, and a reduction in his dosage of propranolol. The next seven sessions show a pattern of rebounding from the reduced medications and adjustment to a higher exercise work load. Point *B* represents the effects of several interacting factors: Over the preceding weekend he and his teenage son had argued with the result that his son moved out the night before the exercise session, the patient had slept poorly and had drunk coffee excessively the morning of exercise, and he forgot to take his medications that morning. This last episode was the occasion for a counseling session with the nutritionist about the effects of excess caffeine and for a counseling session with the psychologist about the family situation and his response to it. Subsequent counseling focused on the need to moderate coffee and cigarette consumption, especially when he was experiencing stress from other factors.

PSYCHOLOGICAL PROFILE AND OUTCOMES: EMPIRICAL RESULTS

All patients entering the HCRC program undergo a psychological evaluation that includes a battery of psychological tests. This section reports the results of statistical analyses of the psychological test data that have been collected over a two-year period. The first set of analyses reports the psychological profile of all patients who entered the rehabilitation program over approximately a two-year period. The second set of analyses reports entry-to-exit changes on these psychological measures for patients who completed the program during that period.

The psychological tests used at HCRC are described more fully in the preceding chapter. Briefly, the test battery consists of the State and Trait Anxiety Scales (Spielberger *et al.,* 1970), the Beck Depression Inventory (Beck, 1967), the Jenkins Activity Survey (Jenkins *et al.,* 1979), the MMPI-168 (Overall *et al.,* 1973), and a version of the Holmes-Rahe Social Readjustment Rating Scale (Holmes and Rahe, 1967). MMPI-168 data are reported only for the four scales that both theory and experience indicate are most reflective of patients' psychological status during the period of involvement in rehabilitation. These scales are Hypochondriasis, Depression, Hysteria, and Psychasthenia. Hypochondriasis reflects health-related anxiety. Hysteria is an index of denial and of health-related complaints. Psychasthenia also reflects anxiety, with higher scores indicating worry, self-doubt, self-criticism, easily aroused guilt, and obsessive-compulsive characteristics. Psychasthenia is considered more of a trait anxiety than a situational anxiety scale. Results for the remaining MMPI scales are not reported here because they were generally in normal, nonclinical ranges, as would be expected with this population.

Entry Psychological Profile

The data reported in this section are based on all patients entering the HCRC program over approximately a two-year period. Thus, the population includes both successful completers and eventual dropouts. Data were analyzed in terms of a set of classification variables consisting of sex, age, medical history, and recency. Medical history refers to the primary historical reason for the referral to HCRC (e.g., MI only, bypass surgery only, both MI and bypass surgery, hypertension, angina, other cardiovascular disorders, and other medical conditions). Recency refers to the length of time from the last major medical event to entry to HCRC. Results are displayed in Table 8-1 for overall values and for the medical history and recency classifications. Sex and age yielded so few differences that they are not displayed in tabular form.

MMPI-168. Scores on the MMPI-168 are reported as standard scores with a mean of 50 and standard deviation of 10. By convention, scores of 70 and above are considered elevated and as representing increasingly severe symptoms the higher they are. For the overall intake sample, the indices of health-related anxiety (Hypochondriasis and Hysteria) and of depression were at or near 70. Thus, these scores indicate clinical levels of anxiety and depression in the entry population and can be interpreted as reflecting emotional reactions to their health status. The lower mean score on Psychasthenia is probably a function of this being more of a trait anxiety than a situational anxiety scale. The scale is probably less reflective of situational anxiety for the general sample than either Hypochondriasis or Hysteria, but is sensitive to situational anxiety in a subgroup of patients prone to anxiety from other,

Table 8-1. ENTRY PSYCHOLOGICAL PROFILE: MEAN VALUES ON PSYCHOLOGICAL TESTS

	MMPI-168				STATE ANX.	TRAIT ANX.	BDI	JAS A	JAS SI	JAS JI	JAS HD/C	RAHE LCU
	HS	D	HY	PT								
Overall sample	70.6	68.8	68.9	62.1	47.19	49.88	10.35	+2.76	+3.10	−2.24	+2.82	512
Medical history												
MI	70.7	70.4	69.7	64.4	47	50.4	8.8	2.98	1.79	−1.5	2.5	428
Surgery	74.8	72.9	71.3	65.4	51	53.5	12.5	6.50	5.9	.8	2.4	543
MI and surgery	77.6	72.5	72.4	64.7	48	49.8	12.6	1.97	4.1	−4.5	1.3	548
Major cardiac event*	73.7	71.6	70.9	64.7	48.4	51.0	10.7	3.5	3.4	−1.8	2.9	502
Others†	59.5	54.1	60.7	52.7	42.3	46.6	8.5	1.8	4.2	−4.7	−1.4	392
Recency‡												
>20 wk	69	67.9	68.8	60.7	47.2	48.8	8.1	−.45	−.38	−2.4	.62	544
21–52 wk	74.7	74.1	71.9	68.5	51.2	55.3	12.3	5.82	5.98	3.82	5.9	564
53+ wk	70.8	69.7	68.5	60.9	46.2	49.5	10.0	.62	−2.04	−5.38	7.2	479

* "Major cardiac event" includes the combined group of patients in the three categories of MI, surgery, and MI and surgery.

† "Others" include patients who had not had a major cardiac event, but who entered the program exhibiting cardiac symptoms (hypertension, angina) or risk factors (smoking, obesity).

‡ "Recency" refers to the latency from major cardiac event or onset of symptoms to entry into rehabilitation.

Table 8-2. *t*-VALUES FOR MEAN COMPARI-
SONS BETWEEN ENTERING PATIENTS
WITH MAJOR CARDIAC EVENTS (MI, CAB,
MI AND CAB) AND ENTERING PATIENTS
WITH CARDIOVASCULAR RISK FACTORS
ONLY*

	t-VALUE	α	*df*
MMPI-168			
Hypochondriasis	3.36	$p < .01$	78
Depression	4.82	$p < .01$	78
Hysteria	2.77	$p < .01$	76
Psychasthenia	2.46	$p < .05$	76
State anxiety	2.26	$p < .05$	77
Trait anxiety	1.98	$p = .05$	77
Beck Depression Inv.	1.07	N.S.	80

* Means for each test appear in Table 8-1.

more purely psychological sources (e.g., negative self-evaluations). Inspection of the scores for the different medical history categories shows that individuals with major cardiac events exhibited significantly higher scores on indices of anxiety and depression than individuals with cardiovascular risk factors only (e.g., angina, hypertension, obesity), but who had not experienced a major event. These differences were statistically significant for the four MMPI-168 scales as displayed in Table 8-2. They are consistent with expectation in that the first group has experienced a more severe trauma than the second group and should therefore exhibit higher levels of distress.

A consistent trend was observed on the recency categories for patients entering the program between 5 and 12 months after a major cardiac event to show higher levels of emotional distress than those entering either earlier or later. This trend was not statistically significant for the MMPI-168 data, although it did reach significance on other measures. The trend initially appears to be contrary to expectation, because intuition suggests that anxiety and depression would be more severe immediately following a major medical event and would then gradually diminish. This may, in fact, be the pattern for many individuals. Several interpretations of the data presented here are possible. An especially intriguing one is that the higher scores in the 5–12-month group represent anxiety and depressive reactions that have become more complicated or severe because of failure to satisfactorily recover from either MI or surgery. In other words, these people may not have been referred to rehabilitation until their recovery had already become

problematic. If this interpretation has validity, then it argues for early as opposed to later referral into rehabilitation programs as a means of encouraging prompt physical and psychological recovery and the prevention of more severe and complicated reactions.

There were not any significant differences or trends when the MMPI-168 data were analyzed by sex or by age.

Beck Depression Inventory. The guidelines suggested by Beck (1967) for interpreting scores on the BDI are as follows: 0–9, no depression; 10–15, mild depression; 16–23, moderate depression; and 24–63, severe depression. Mean BDI scores in Table 8-1 characterize the overall sample as mildly depressed, with different subgroups showing higher mean values than the overall sample, but still within the mild depression range. Patients with a history of cardiac surgery (medical history categories surgery and surgery + MI) had a significantly higher mean BDI score (12.5) than patients with a history of myocardial infarction only (8.8) ($t = 2.7$, $p < .01$, $df = 64$). Earlier entry (up to five months) into rehabilitation was associated with a significantly lower mean BDI score ($t = 2.49$, $p < .05$, $df = 32$) than later entry (5 to 12 months). The results with surgery patients and with the 5–12-month group are probably related because there is substantial overlap between the two groups of patients; i.e., surgery patients tend to be referred to rehabilitation later than myocardial infarction patients. Again, the argument can be advanced that surgery patients are not being referred for rehabilitation until their recovery has become problematic. Depression would seem especially likely in these people because their initial optimism and hope about the benefits of surgery might have been compromised by the continuation or recurrence of symptoms, with resulting discouragement, helplessness, and frustration.

State and Trait Anxiety. Scores on these scales are standard scores with a mean of 50 and standard deviation of 10. The normative population on which the standard scores are based is a population of general medical and surgical patients, as reported by Spielberger *et al.* (1970). The overall profile of incoming HCRC patients on these scales is of average levels of anxiety symptoms, compared to the norming population. Our experience with these scales over two years is that they yield few false positives, but many false negatives. In other words, they underestimate anxiety levels for many individuals. Inspection of the data from these scales for the different subgroups shows a few statistically significant differences that are consistent with patterns observed on the MMPI-168 scales and the Beck Depression Inventory. Patients with a history of major cardiac events (MI, surgery, or both) exhibited higher levels of anxiety symptoms than patients exhibiting cardiovascular risk factors only. Comparisons of means for these groups were statistically significant for State Anxiety ($t = 2.26, p < .05, df = 77$), and for Trait Anxiety ($t = 1.98, p < .05, df = 77$). Earlier entry in rehabilitation was associated with lower levels of anxiety on both scales, with the difference reaching statistical significance for Trait Anxiety ($t = 2.57, p < .01, df = 39$).

Jenkins Activity Survey. Jenkins Activity Survey (JAS) scores are reported as standard scores with a mean of 0 and a standard deviation of 10. Positive scores indicate a greater degree of coronary-prone characteristics, and negative scores a lesser degree. For the overall intake sample, mean scores on the Type A, Speed/Impatience, and Hard Driving/Competitive subscales indicate a mildly positive degree of coronary proneness. The Job Involvement subscale mean is mildly negative. Clinical experience with this subscale suggests that it has less validity than the other three scales, especially with female patients who have not been career oriented, but also with males in blue-collar and trade activities. For the entire intake sample, 60% obtained positive scores on the type A subscale, with a mean score of +8.68 for this subgroup. The mean score on this scale for the remaining 40% who obtained negative scores was −7.55. Thus, a slight majority of the intake sample exhibits the coronary-prone pattern to a moderately pronounced degree. The percentage of the sample exhibiting the coronary-prone pattern (defined somewhat arbitrarily as those with positive JAS scores) is somewhat lower than might have been expected, given that the entire sample has documented cardiac conditions. One interpretation of this is that the coronary-prone pattern is only one of several risk factors for cardiovascular disorders, and it is only one, albeit an important one, of the potential sources of emotional stress. Experience with patients at HCRC strongly indicates that high emotional stress levels occur among patients with low JAS scores as well as among those with high scores. The percentage of our sample exhibiting the coronary-prone pattern could also be an artifact of the JAS

rather than a characteristic of the population. Had we used the Rosenman-Friedman Structured Interview, a higher proportion of our sample may have been classified as coronary prone.

Reviewing the JAS data by categories in Table 8-1, there is a nonsignificant trend for the surgery-only subgroup to exhibit more pronounced coronary-prone characteristics than the other subgroups. There was also a nonsignificant trend for those entering rehabilitation between 21 and 52 weeks to exhibit a stronger coronary pattern than those entering earlier. The trend toward higher JAS scores in the 21–52-week group is not as likely to be a function of the amount of time since their major event as it is of the fact that there is substantial overlap between this group and the surgery-only subgroup, which also exhibited higher JAS scores. The only statistically significant difference on JAS scores that emerged from a series of analyses was that women had higher mean scores (7.16) than men (1.84) on the Hard Driving/Competitive subscale ($t = 2.1, p < .05$). An interpretation of this difference based on knowledge of the women included in the sample suggests that as a group they more consistently exhibited extremes of conscientiousness, perfectionism, and a high sense of personal responsibility. These qualities suggest more of the "hard driving" as opposed to the competitive element of this subscale.

Social Readjustment Rating Scale. Life Change Unit (LCU) scores for the overall sample and for the different subgroups are reported in Table 8-1. The scores reflect the sum of the LCU weights for the items endorsed as having occurred over the preceding two-year period. Note that for these patients the reporting period *includes* their major medical events so that scores reflect the impact of these events on the major spheres of their lives. Thus, these scores are not directly comparable to scores reported in other studies that reflect the period of time immediately *preceding* a major cardiac event. However, the assessment issue when the patient enters rehabilitation is the relative amount of psychosocial change he/she has experienced prior to entering rehabilitation, because these are the experiences that are most relevant to understanding the patient's emotional/psychological presentation at entry to rehabilitation. The only statistically significant difference to emerge from comparisons of LCU scores among the different subgroups was for patients 45 and under to have a higher mean score than patients 46 to 60 ($t = 2.26$, $p < .05$, $df = 77$). This difference suggests that the level of potential emotional stresses to which the younger age group was exposed was greater than the older group and perhaps contributes to an explanation for their premature problems with heart disease.

Psychological Outcomes: Entry-to-Exit Changes

When a patient leaves the HCRC program, he/she receives an exit psychological evaluation consisting of an interview and the readministration of the same psychological tests used in the initial evaluation, with the exception of the Social Readjustment Rating Scale. The latter instrument is not administered at exit because the time elapsed since the initial administration is usually too short (average of 15 weeks) for significant, meaningful changes to have occurred in scores. Thus, any changes that might be obtained would probably reflect error variance due to factors such as memory. The sample on which the analyses reported below were conducted was the subset of the intake sample who were formally exited from the program. Thus, drop-outs are not included in these analyses. All tests were t-tests for comparisons between means of correlated samples.

Table 8-3 displays the results of these analyses on the different psychological indexes for the overall sample of completers. Significant reductions occurred on every measure except the JAS-JI subscale, which has already been discussed as the least valid scale in the battery. The statistical consistency and strength of these results argue compellingly for the occurrence of clinically significant improvements in psychological functioning. To be sure, the relative

contribution of different program components to these changes cannot be determined from these data because of the lack of appropriate control conditions. Nonetheless, the results strongly indicate that involvement in a comprehensive rehabilitation program is associated with improvements in psychological status.

A frequently raised objection to conclusions based on the results of statistical analyses is that statistical significance does not equal clinical significance. The following arguments are offered in support of the clinical significance of the statistical changes displayed in Table 8-3. First, changes on MMPI-168 scales Hs, D, and Hy are all from entry scores that are at levels traditionally considered mild clinical elevations to scores that are in the nonclinical range. Less clinical significance is attached to the reductions on Psychasthenia because the mean entry score level was lower and because the magnitude of change from entry to exit was less. Second, the five remaining MMPI-168 scales (results not reported here) were all stable from entry to exit and were in a nonclinical range. Thus, the statistically significant changes that occurred on the MMPI-168 scales were specific to the scales most likely to be sensitive to the situational psychological and emotional state of rehabilitation patients. Third, Beck Depression Inventory scores went from the range associated with mild depression well into the range of no depression. The magnitude and statistical strength of this change, along with its convergence with the MMPI-168 Depression scale, point to meaningful reductions in depression. Fourth, the highly statistically significant reductions that occurred on the State and Trait Anxiety scales were somewhat unexpected because of the apparent insensitivity of

Table 8-3. ENTRY-TO-EXIT CHANGES ON PSYCHOLOGICAL MEASURES

	ENTRY	EXIT	t	α	df
MMPI-168					
HS	70.8	62.7	6.82	$p < .001$	61
D	67.4	61.5	4.13	$p < .001$	61
Hy	68.6	63.5	4.83	$p < .001$	61
Pt	61.4	57.3	2.14	$p < .036$	61
State Anxiety	46.1	42.4	3.10	$p < .003$	59
Trait Anxiety	48.9	45.0	4.16	$p < .005$	59
BDI	9.5	4.7	6.37	$p < .001$	57
JAS					
A	2.07	−1.39	2.52	$p < .001$	57
SI	2.12	−1.68	3.76	$p < .001$	57
JI	−.68	−2.99	1.06	N.S.	53
HD/C	.99	−1.94	2.49	$p < .016$	57

Table 8-4. ENTRY-TO-EXIT CHANGES ON JENKINS ACTIVITY SURVEY SUBSCALES FOR CORONARY-PRONE AND NONCORONARY-PRONE INDIVIDUALS AT ENTRY*

	POSITIVE ENTRY SCORES					NEGATIVE ENTRY SCORES				
	ENTRY	EXIT	t	α	df	ENTRY	EXIT	t	α	df
A	8.12	1.95	4.05	$p < .005$	24	−6.4	−6.5	.25	N.S.	18
SI	9.68	4.15	4.00	$p < .005$	24	−7.5	−8.4	.64	N.S.	20
HD/C	10.27	2.56	5.16	$p < .005$	27	−7.9	−7.4	.31	N.S.	18

* Coronary-proneness defined as positive JAS scores at entry.

the test to the kind of reactive anxiety symptoms presented by our patients. The fact that such highly significant changes were obtained argues for the scales' value for assessing intraindividual changes over time. If, in fact, the scale is relatively insensitive, then the changes that were observed are probably underestimates of actual reductions in anxiety symptoms.

The argument for the clinical significance of the JAS changes from entry to exit is based on the additional analyses presented in Table 8-4. For each of JAS subscales, Type A, Speed/Impatience, and Hard Driving/Competitive, two subgroups were identified: those whose entry scores were positive and those whose entry scores were negative. Means for each subgroup were computed at both entry and exit for each scale, and t-values calculated for entry-to-exit changes. As the data in Table 8-4 indicate, highly significant reductions occurred from entry to exit for the group that entered with positive scores, and no changes were observed for the group that entered with negative scores. Thus, the statistically significant results for the JAS scales reported in Table 8-3 are accounted for by the reductions that occurred among the more highly coronary-prone subgroup. The stability of the scores for the less coronary-prone group argues against a regression toward the mean interpretation of the reductions in the more coronary-prone group. The same stability of the less coronary-prone group argues against a social desirability response set (i.e., they learned what to say) as an explanation of the results.

Conclusions. The results reported above support the following conclusions. (1) Patients entering a comprehensive cardiovascular rehabilitation program exhibit, on the average, mild levels of anxiety and depression, which are largely situational. (2) The level of anxiety and/or depression is a function of medical history, with patients who have experienced major medical events (e.g., MI, surgery) exhibiting higher levels of these emotional disorders than patients who have not experienced such events, but who do have manifest cardiovascular disorders (e.g., angina, hypertension, coronary artery disease). (3) Surgery patients tend to be referred for rehabilitation later than MI-only patients, and they tend to exhibit more severe situational disorders than other patient groups. Later referrals and more serious situational disorders suggest that surgery patients are not being referred for rehabilitation until problems develop. Earlier referral to rehabilitation may be prophylactic with respect to more severe situational emotional reactions, as well as with respect to recurrent cardiovascular symptoms (e.g., angina). (4) A slight majority of entering patients exhibit the coronary-prone pattern, assessed by accepted psychometric methods. Thus, the coronary-prone behavior pattern cannot be assumed to be a pervasive characteristic of the entry population. It is important for a psychological treatment program to be oriented broadly to coping with emotional stress, whatever the source, rather than specifically to the coronary-prone pattern. (5) Situational anxiety and depression are significantly reduced during involvement in comprehensive cardiovascular rehabilitation. This conclusion is strengthened by the consistency of the results across different measures, and by patients' self-reports of improvements in each area. (6) Coronary-prone behavior characteristics were moderated to a significant degree, and these changes were specific to individuals exhibiting the coronary-prone pattern at entry. The specificity of these changes suggests that the psychological portion of the HCRC program had a causal role. Situational anxiety and depression might reasonably be expected to be affected by improvement in physical status as a result of exercise, as well as by psychological counseling. However, coronary-prone characteristics are trait variables rather than situational or reactive states, and they would not necessarily be expected to change as a result of exercise and physical improvements. Thus, the argument can be advanced that the reductions that occurred reflect the emphasis placed on psychological/emotional stress as a health concern for our patients, that this message is being heard by our patients, and that, as a result, patients' receptiveness to and motivation for psychological and life-style changes is increased. Numerous clinical examples of such life-style changes could be offered in support of these statistical results, but that would only belabor a point that has been made sufficiently well.

PSYCHOLOGIST AS MEMBER OF THE REHABILITATION TEAM

The reasons for including in the rehabilitation team a professional, skilled in dealing with psychosocial and behavioral aspects of recovery from major cardiovascular disorders, have been established in this chapter and in Chapter 7. There are several professional disciplines whose area of expertise qualifies them for working on one or another set of issues within this area. In addition to psychology, the disciplines of social work, psychiatry, rehabilitation counseling, and psychiatric nursing all have relevant training and skills. Of all of these disciplines, psychology is the most uniquely qualified to provide the range of expertise and services required. A psychologist trained in counseling or clinical psychology, and in the new specialties of health psychology and behavioral medicine, has a broader background in theories and principles of behavior and of behavior change than any other single discipline. The psychologist has training in the delivery of clinical services such as individual, marital, family, and group therapies. Only the psychologist has training in theoretical and clinical aspects of the use of psychological tests for assessment. Finally, the psychologist has better training in the principles of conducting psychological and behavioral research than the other disciplines. Thus, the psychologist has a broader general preparation for the assessment, intervention, program development, consultative, and research functions in this setting than any other single discipline.

Psychological and behavioral issues are so central to comprehensive cardiovascular rehabilitation that significant progress in the development of these as an alternative treatment for heart disease is dependent on the intimate cooperation of psychology and cardiology in the delivery of services and in research. Psychologists need not become cardiologists, and cardiologists need not become psychologists. Each discipline has knowledge and skills necessary to implement a sound, professionally responsible treatment program of this type. Matarazzo (Matarazzo *et al.,* 1982) has termed cooperation between these two disciplines *behavioral cardiology* and suggests that this be recognized as a new subspecialty under the general heading of behavioral medicine. The advantage of such recognition would be to encourage a greater degree of interdisciplinary teamwork and cross-fertilization among the different disciplines concerned with the prevention, treatment, and rehabilitation of cardiovascular illnesses. Significant progress depends on a recognition of the complex nature of these disorders, on the extent to which they are a function of behavioral factors broadly defined, and on relaxation of professional parochialism and myopia. Psychology and cardiology have much to gain from such a partnership. The population of actual and potential victims of heart disease has even more to gain.

REFERENCES

Bandura, A. Self-efficacy mechanisms in human agency. *Am. Psychol.,* **1982,** *37,* 122–148.

Beck, A. *Depression: Clinical, Experimental, and Theoretical Aspects.* Hoeber, New York, **1967.**

———. *Cognitive Therapy and the Emotional Disorders.* International Universities Press, New York, **1976.**

Becker, E. *The Denial of Death.* The Free Press, New York, **1973.**

Bernstein, D., and Borkovec, T. *Progressive Relaxation Training: A Manual for the Helping Professions.* Research Press, Champaign, Ill., **1973.**

Brownell, K. Obesity: Understanding and treating a serious prevalent, and refractory disorder. *J. Consult. Clin. Psychol.,* **1982,** *50,* 820–841.

Burt, A.; Thornley, P.; Illingworth, D.; White, P.; Shaw, T.; and Turner, R. Stopping smoking after myocardial infarction. *Lancet,* **1974,** *i,* 304–306.

Croog, S., and Richards, N. Health beliefs and smoking patterns in heart patients and their wives: A longitudinal study. *Am. J. Public Health,* **1977,** *67,* 921–929.

Diagnostic and Statistical Manual III. American Psychiatric Association, Washington, D.C., **1980.**

Ellis, A. *Reason and Emotion in Psychotherapy.* Lyle Stuart, New York, **1962.**

Ewart, C. A couples approach to stress reduction: Applications to hypertension and cardiac rehabilitation. Unpublished manuscript, Johns Hopkins University, **1981.**

Ewart, C.; Taylor, C.; and DeBusk, R. Increasing self-efficacy after heart attack: Effects of treadmill exercise.

Paper presented at the meeting of the American Psychological Association, Montreal, **1980**.

Hackett, T., and Cassem, N. Psychological adaptation to convalescence in myocardial infarction patients. In, Naughton, J. and Hellerstein, H. (eds.) *Exercise Testing and Exercise Training in Coronary Heart Disease.* Academic Press, New York, **1973**.

Hall, R.; Sachs, D.; and Hall, S. Medical risk and therapeutic effectiveness of rapid smoking. *Behav. Ther.,* **1979**, *10,* 249–259.

Hellerstein, H., and Horsten, T. Assessing and preparing the patient for return to a meaningful and productive life. *J. Rehabil.,* **1966**, *32,* 48–52.

Holmes, T., and Rahe, R. The social readjustment rating scale. *J. Psychosom. Res.,* **1967**, *11,* 213–218.

Jackson, J., and Bressler, R. Prescribing tricyclic antidepressants Part II: Cardiovascular effects. *Drug Ther.,* **1982**, *12,* 193–203.

Jacobson, E. *Progressive Relaxation.* University of Chicago Press, Chicago, **1938**.

Jenkins, C.; Zyzanski, S.; and Rosenman, R. *Manual for the Jenkins Activity Survey.* Psychological Corp., New York, **1979**.

Kavanaugh, T.; Shephard, R.; Tuck, J.; *et al.* Depression following myocardial infarction: The effects of distance running. *Ann. N.Y. Acad. Sci.,* **1977**, *301,* 1029–1037.

Kübler-Ross, E. *On Death and Dying.* Macmillan Publishing Co., Inc., New York, **1969**.

Lakein, A. *How to Get Control of Your Time and Your Life.* American Library, New York, **1973**.

Lazarus, A. *Behavior Therapy and Beyond.* New York, McGraw-Hill, **1971**.

Lazarus, R. *Psychological Stress and the Coping Process.* McGraw-Hill, New York, **1966**.

Lichtenstein, E. The smoking problem: A behavioral perspective. *J. Consult. Clin. Psychol.,* **1982**, *50,* 804–820.

Marlatt, G., and Gordon, J. Determinants of relapse: Implications for the maintenance of behavior change. In, Davidson, P. and Davidson, S. (eds.) *Behavioral Medicine: Changing Health Lifestyles.* Brunner/Mazel, New York, **1980**.

Matarazzo, J.; Connor, W.; Fey, S.; Carmody, T.; Pierce, D.; Briochetto, C.; Baker, L.; Connor, S.; and Sexton, G. Behavioral cardiology with emphasis on the family heart study: Fertile ground for psychological and biomedical research. In, Millon, T.; Green, C.; and Meagher, R. (eds.) *Handbook of Clinical Health Psychology.* Plenum Press, New York, **1982**.

Meichenbaum, D. *Cognitive-Behavior Modification: An Integrative Approach.* Plenum Press, New York, **1977**.

Naughton, J.; Bruhn, J.; and Lategola, M. Effects of physical training on physiologic and behavioral characteristics of cardiac patients. *Arch. Phys. Med. Rehabil.,* **1968**, *49,* 131–137.

Novaco, R. *Anger Control: The Development and Evaluation of an Experimental Treatment.* Lexington Books, Lexington, Mass., **1975**.

Overall, J.; Hunter, S.; and Butcher, J. Factor structure of the MMPI-168 in a psychiatric population. *J. Consult. Clin. Psychol.,* **1973**, *41,* 284–286.

Pechacek, T., and Danaher, B. How and why people quit smoking: A cognitive-behavioral analysis. In, Kendall, P. and Hollon, S. (eds.) *Cognitive-Behavioral Interventions: Theory, Research, and Procedures.* Academic Press, New York, **1979**.

Peterson, L. H. A methodological approach to provide provocative exercise intensity levels for exercise stress testing and therapy in cardiovascular rehabilitation. In preparation, **1983**.

Plovsic, C.; Turkulin, K.; Perman, Z.; *et al.* The results of exercise therapy in coronary prone individuals and coronary patients. *G. Ital. Cardiol.,* **1976**, *6,* 422–432.

Rahe, R.; Ward, H.; and Hayes, V. Brief group therapy in myocardial infarction rehabilitation: Three to four years follow-up of a controlled trial. *Psychosom. Med.,* **1979**, *41,* 229–243.

Roskies, E. Considerations in developing a treatment program for the coronary-prone (Type A) behavior pattern. In Davidson, P. and Davidson, S. (eds.) *Behavioral Medicine: Changing Health Lifestyles.* Brunner/Mazel, New York, **1980**.

———. Modifying coronary prone behavior in healthy persons. Presented at the Third Annual Meeting of the Society of Behavioral Medicine, Chicago, Ill., March, **1982**.

Roskies, E.; Spevack, M.; Surkes, A.; Cohen, C.; and Gilman, D. Changing the coronary-prone (Type A) behavioral pattern in a nonclinical population. *J. Behav. Med.,* **1978**, *1,* 210–216.

Spielberger, C.; Gorsuch, R.; and Lushene, R. *Manual for the State-Trait Anxiety Inventory.* Consulting Psychologists Press, Palo Alto, Calif., **1970**.

Stern, M., and Cleary, P. The National Exercise and Heart Disease Project: Psychosocial changes observed during a low-level exercise program. *Arch. Intern. Med.,* **1981**, *141,* 1463–1467.

———. The National Exercise and Heart Disease Project: Long-term psychosocial outcome. *Arch. Intern. Med.,* **1982**, *142,* 1093–1097.

Stunkard, A., and Rush, A. Dieting and depression reexamined: A critical review of reports of untoward responses during weight reduction for obesity. *Ann. Intern. Med.,* **1974**, *81,* 526–533.

Suinn, R., and Bloom, L. Anxiety management training for Pattern A behavior. *J. Behav. Med.,* **1978**, *1,* 25–37.

Thoresen, C.; Friedman, M.; Gill, J.; and Ulmer, D. Recurrent coronary prevention project: Some preliminary findings. *Acta Med. Scand.,* **1982**, Supplement *660,* 172–192.

Wilson, G., and Brownell, K. Behavior therapy for obesity: An evaluation of treatment outcome. *Adv. Behav. Res. Ther.,* **1980**, *3,* 49–86.

Yalom, I. *Existential Psychotherapy.* Basic Books, New York, **1980**.

Chapter 9
RATIONALE OF DIETARY MANAGEMENT IN COMPREHENSIVE CARDIOVASCULAR REHABILITATION

Luean E. Anthony, Mary W. Schanler, and E. C. Henley

Application of nutrition and dietetic principles to the field of comprehensive cardiovascular rehabilitation depends upon the extent to which this specialty can contribute to the objectives of rehabilitation. The objectives of rehabilitation that deal with people who have already developed clinically evident cardiovascular disorders are (1) to restore health and reduce disabilities to the extent possible, and (2) to provide secondary prevention in an effort to slow, or halt, the progress of an otherwise progressive pathological process. In this chapter, the role of dietary influences and nutritional disorders in the primary etiology of atherosclerotic cardiovascular disease is discussed because those principles apply and form the basis of the objectives of dietary management of the patient in a comprehensive cardiovascular rehabilitation program.

RISK FACTORS

Epidemiologic studies have formed the major approach to correlating dietary risk factors with the subsequent development of cardiovascular disease. The most studied diet-related risk factors for cardiovascular disease include hypercholesterolemia, hypertriglyceridemia, and obesity. Indirectly, diabetes mellitus and hypertension, which are affected by dietary factors, have also been implicated.

Hyperlipidemia

Hyperlipidemia is the elevation of serum cholesterol or triglycerides, or both, above an established normal range. Total serum cholesterol has long been recognized as the strongest and most consistent risk factor for atherosclerotic disease. Hyperlipidemia may occur as a secondary manifestation of another disease, e.g., diabetes mellitus or hypothyroidism, or it may result from dietary excess, a rare familial hyperlipidemia, or stress.

There is disagreement among experts as to what constitutes a normal or desirable serum cholesterol level. Hyperlipidemia is said to be present when an individual's plasma cholesterol and/or triglyceride levels exceed the 95th percentile for his or her respective age and sex distribution. Since risk of coronary heart disease is linearly related to cholesterol levels, no cutoff point separates subjects at risk from subjects free from risk. However, the use of cutoff points to classify subjects with specific types of hyperlipidemia has the advantage of focusing attention (1) on especially high-risk individuals, and (2) on certain genetically determined hyperlipidemias.

Cholesterol, triglycerides, and phospholipids are carried in the plasma bound to specific proteins. These lipoproteins, chylomicrons, low-density lipoproteins (LDL), very low-den-

147

sity lipoproteins (VLDL), and high-density lipoproteins (HDL) vary as to the amount of
proteins and fat they contain and can be identified according to their density and/or electrophoretic mobility (Figure 9-1). Intermediate
low-density lipoprotein (ILDL) is an intermediate in the conversion of VLDL to LDL and is
present in only minute amounts in the sera of
healthy persons.

The terms "hyperlipidemia," "hypercholesterolemia," and "hypertriglyceridemia" do not
indicate which lipoproteins are elevated.
Hence, it is desirable to translate hyperlipidemia into hyperlipoproteinemia. In 1967, Fredrickson, Levy, and Lees proposed a classification of hyperlipoproteinemia that was based on
the quantitative assessment of the lipoproteins.
Originally, five types were described, and, more
recently, one of these types has been subdivided
into two (Levy, *et al.*, 1974). The classification
is as follows:

Type I:	Increased chylomicrons
Type IIa:	Increased LDL
Type IIb:	Increased LDL and VLDL
Type III:	Increased ILDL
Type IV:	Increased VLDL
Type V:	Increased chylomicrons and VLDL

Each hyperlipoproteinemia may be secondary to a variety of diseases, in which case the
treatment is primarily directed to the underlying disease (LaRosa, 1977). Each may also
occur as a primary, sometimes genetically determined, abnormality. However, only a small
percentage of all patients diagnosed with coronary heart disease have a true inborn error of
lipid metabolism responsible for elevation of
lipids. In the great majority of cases of coronary heart disease, the lipid abnormality is acquired. A summary of the types of hyperlipoproteinemia is given in Table 9-1. Types I, III,

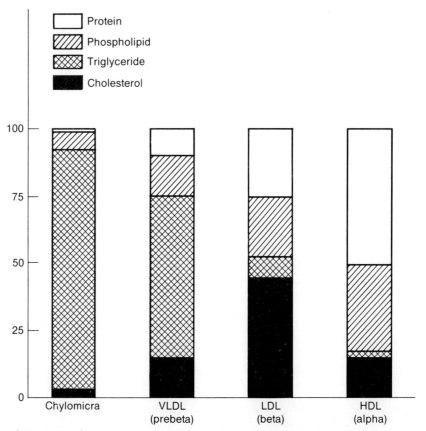

Figure 9-1.   Approximate per cent composition of lipoproteins. (Reprinted from Levy, R. I., *et al., Journal of the American Dietetic Association,* **1971,** *58,* 406.)

Table 9-1. TYPES OF HYPERLIPOPROTEINEMIA

FEATURES	TYPE I	TYPE IIa	TYPE IIb	TYPE III	TYPE IV	TYPE V
Incidence	Very rare	Common	Common	Relatively uncommon	Common	Uncommon
Lipoprotein abnormality	↑ Fasting chylomicrons	↑ LDL	↑ LDL ↑VLDI	↑ ILDL	↑ VLDL	↑ Fasting chylomicrons ↑ VLDL
Plasma cholesterol	Normal or ↑	Normal	↑	↑	Normal or ↑	Normal or ↑
Plasma triglycerides	Greatly ↑	↑	↑	↑	↑	↑ or greatly ↑
Clinical signs	Lipemia retinalis, Eruptive xanthomas, Hepatosplenomegaly, Abdominal pain, Childhood expression	Tendon and tuberous xanthomas, Xanthelasma, Juvenile corneal arcus, Accelerated coronary atherosclerosis, Severe cases detected in childhood		Palmar, tuberous, and tendon xanthomas, Accelerated atherosclerosis	Abnormal glucose tolerance, Hyperuricemia, Accelerated coronary vessel disease, Detected in adults	Lipemia retinalis, Eruptive xanthomas, Hepatosplenomegaly, Hyperglycemia, Hyperuricemia
Inheritance, if primary	Recessive	Dominant, sporadic	Dominant, sporadic	Recessive	Dominant, sporadic	Dominant, sporadic
Secondary causes	Deficiency in lipoprotein lipase, Diabetic acidosis, Hypothyroidism, Insulin-dependent diabetes, Dysgammaglobulinemia	Hypothyroidism, Nephrosis, Obstructive liver disease, Porphyria, Excess dietary cholesterol		Diabetes mellitus*, Hypothyroidism, Renal insufficiency	Diabetes mellitus, Nephrosis, Pancreatitis, Glycogen storage disease	Pancreatitis, Alcoholism, Nephrosis

* Secondary causes are rare in type III hyperlipoproteinemia.

Source: Taylor, K. B., and Anthony, L. E. *Clinical Nutrition*. McGraw-Hill, New York, 1983. Reprinted by permission of McGraw-Hill.

and V are very rare. Individuals with many of the features of type II (hypercholesterolemia) or type IV (hypertriglyceridemia) are seen more commonly.

Hypercholesterolemia

Associations between diet, serum cholesterol, and cardiovascular rates in humans were first suggested in the aftermath of World War II. The wartime food rationing in Northern Europe led to lowered total caloric intakes and a higher proportion of calories derived from carbohydrate, while diets were low in all dietary fats as well as cholesterol. Mortality from atherosclerotic disease decreased abruptly in the early years of the war and reverted to previous levels when hostilities ceased (Malmros, 1950). This provocative observation stimulated numerous studies attempting to demonstrate a causative link between dietary fat and atherosclerotic disease. To date, this goal remains elusive, and the linkage between disease causation and dietary fat intake in humans is indirect. Keys (1970) in the Seven Countries Study, based on prospective observations of 18 populations in seven countries (Finland, Greece, Italy, Japan, the Netherlands, the United States, and Yugoslavia), compared the incidence of heart disease over a ten-year period among 12,000 men who were between 40 and 59 years of age at the beginning of the study. As shown in Figure 9-2, mean rates of occurrence of heart disease varied fourfold, with the highest rates in the United States and Finland and the lowest in Japan. The rates were significantly correlated with the serum cholesterol concentration and also with the saturated fat intake of the population (Table 9-2). Other components of the diets, which included total calories, total fat, monounsaturated and polyunsaturated fats, and total protein, were not significantly correlated with the incidence of heart disease.

Epidemiological studies of migrant populations also suggest that individuals acquire the disease pattern of the host country (Keys *et al.*, 1958). A comparison of saturated fat consumption, blood lipids, and coronary-event rates in indigenous Japanese, migrant Japanese in Hawaii, and migrant Japanese in Los Angeles reveals parallel increases in all three.

In contrast to epidemiological research, studies of individuals within a single population are not as clear-cut and produce paradoxical results. Such studies have continually failed to detect a consistently significant relationship between individual intake of saturated fat, the level of plasma cholesterol, and risk of coronary heart disease. The Framingham Study reported that no statistical relationship between any of the measured dietary components (saturated fat, cholesterol, sucrose, or energy) and serum cholesterol could be shown (Kannel, 1971). The explanation for this finding may be that the dietary intake patterns are very similar in all socioeconomic groups in the United States.

Within the United States, several studies have compared various types of vegetarians with their meat-eating counterparts (Sacks *et al.*, 1975; Burslem *et al.*, 1978). Lacto-ovo-vegetarians as well as strict vegetarians whose diets are low in cholesterol and saturated fat, but relatively high in polyunsaturated fats and plant sterols, have lower plasma cholesterol levels and a lower prevalence of coronary heart disease; they also fail to show the increase in plasma cholesterol with age. This increase is regularly seen in nonvegetarians in developed societies.

Epidemiological studies have been supple-

Men 40-59, percent diet calories provided by saturated fatty acids

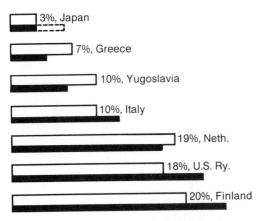

Narrow, solid bars show CHD incidence rate

Figure 9-2. Shaded bars represent the average percentage of total dietary calories provided by saturated fatty acids. Solid bars represent the 5-year incidence of coronary heart disease. White dashed bar represents emigrated Japanese. U.S. graph represents railroad workers (Ry). (Reprinted from Keys, A. [ed.]. Coronary heart disease in seven countries. *Circulation,* **1970,** *41* [Suppl. 1], 1–211, by permission of the American Heart Association.)

Table 9-2. DIETARY FAT, SERUM CHOLESTEROL, AND 10-YEAR CORONARY HEART DISEASE (CHD) MORTALITY RATE, MEN ORIGINALLY AGE 40–59, SEVEN COUNTRY STUDY*

COHORT	TOTAL FAT, % CALORIES	SATURATED FAT, % CALORIES	POLYUNSATURATED FAT, % CALORIES	SERUM CHOLESTEROL MEDIAN	SERUM CHOLESTEROL 90TH PERCENTILE	10-YEAR MORTALITY CHD	10-YEAR MORTALITY ALL
Greece	36	7	3	201	258	9	57
Yugoslavia	31	5	5	171†	219†	12†	105†
Italy	26	9	3	198	253	21	126
Rome (railroad workers)	——	——	——	207	260	22	75
United States (railroad workers)	40	18	5	236	294	57	115
Finland	37	20	3	259	323	65	167
Netherlands	40	18	5	230	291	44	125

* Keys, A. (ed.) Coronary heart disease in seven countries. *Circulation,* **1970,** *41*(Suppl.) 1–211.
† Excludes Belgrade and Slavonia.

Source: Stamler, J. In, Levy, R., *et al.* (eds.) *Nutrition, Lipids and Coronary Heart Disease.* Raven, New York, **1979.**

mented by studies in which diet has been manipulated in groups of individuals. These studies show that plasma cholesterol levels can be lowered by reducing the dietary saturated fat and cholesterol intake; this has been achieved in both institutionalized and free-living populations and in normal and hypercholesterolemic subjects (Blackburn, 1979; Diet-Heart Review Panel, 1969). Both primary prevention trials of apparently healthy men and secondary prevention trials of men who have already had a myocardial infarct or other evidence of disease, in which the amount of dietary saturated fat and cholesterol is diminished, leave no doubt that plasma cholesterol concentrations can be made to fall, but effects on coronary heart disease morbidity and mortality are equivocal. Keys *et al.* (1957) reported that gram for gram, saturated fats were twice as effective in raising the blood cholesterol as polyunsaturated fats were in lowering it, while monounsaturated fats had no effect.

Truswell (1977) has summarized what is known about the contribution of individual fatty acids in dietary triglycerides (Table 9-3). In general, saturated fatty acids have a stronger elevating effect than the cholesterol-lowering effect of linoleic acid ($C_{18:2}$), but the effect of saturated fats is due mainly to palmitic acid ($C_{16:0}$) which is more abundant in dietary fats than myristic acid ($C_{14:0}$). Fatty-acid chain length thus partly determines the activity. Saturated fatty acids containing 10 carbons or less, though saturated, do not increase plasma cholesterol. Surprisingly, stearic acid ($C_{18:0}$) has less elevating effect than palmitic acid ($C_{16:0}$).

Dietary studies of humans on the effect of dietary cholesterol or plasma lipids on plasma cholesterol levels have often produced conflicting evidence because cholesterol was not fed in a form suitable for absorption. A recent comprehensive review concluded that in healthy adults who are normolipidemic by United States standards, plasma cholesterol concentration increased as cholesterol intake increased within the range of 0 to 600 mg per day (McGill, 1979). For each additional 100 mg dietary cholesterol per 1000 Kcal, estimates of the average increase in plasma cholesterol vary from 3 to 12 mg/dl. Dietary cholesterol above about 600 mg/day produces no additional effect in most persons.

Table 9-3 EFFECTS OF DIFFERENT DIETARY FATTY ACIDS ON PLASMA CHOLESTEROL, AS DEMONSTRATED IN ACUTE EXPERIMENTS IN HUMANS

DIETARY FATTY ACID	PLASMA CHOLESTEROL
Medium-chain triglycerides, $C_{8:0}$ to $C_{10:0}$	0
Lauric, $C_{12:0}$	↑
Myristic, $C_{14:0}$	↑ ↑
Palmitic, $C_{16:0}$	↑ ↑
Stearic, $C_{18:0}$	? ↑
Oleic, $C_{18:1}$	0
Linoleic, $C_{18:2}$	↓
Other polyunsaturated	↓

Source: Adapted from Truswell, A. S. Dietary fat and cholesterol metabolism. *Bibl. Nutr. Dieta,* **1977,** *25,* 53, by permission of S. Karger AG, Basel.

Burkitt *et al.* (1974) has hypothesized that a diet deficient in fiber is one of the causes of many diseases of Western civilization, including coronary heart disease. Trowell (1972) was the first to show that rural Africans with high intake of dietary fiber have low blood cholesterol levels and a low incidence of heart disease. As the African has become semiurbanized, the incidence of coronary heart disease has increased; it is highest in the urban African (Trowell, 1972). During the African's progression through successive steps toward urbanization, the quantity of dietary fiber ingested has decreased. However, many other concomitant changes in dietary intake and life-style have occurred as well, including increased consumption of meat, saturated fat, and cholesterol. Hence, epidemiological data linking coronary heart disease (CHD) and lack of dietary fiber are circumstantial. Apart from the African, no other people have been so closely observed and no real attempt to quantify differences in fiber intake at the international level has been made. Specific studies of the effect of dietary fiber on blood cholesterol levels have neither proved nor disproved Burkitt's hypothesis. Studies have been hampered by an imprecise definition of dietary fiber (herein defined as the skeletal remains of plant cells that are resistant to hydrolysis by human digestive enzymes and includes cellulose, hemicellulose, pectin, and lignin) and the failure to distinguish between its constituents in experimental studies. However, there appears to be a pattern of results in experiments: in humans with normal blood cholesterol levels, rolled oats, Bengal gram (chickpea), and pectin are hypocholesterolemic, whereas wheat fiber, cellulose, and legumes are not (Truswell, 1977; Palumbo *et al.*, 1978). One interesting aspect of dietary fiber is its effect in diabetes mellitus. Diabetic subjects fed diets high in fiber (either as legumes, fruit, and whole grains or as guar gum or pectin) exhibit reduced blood glucose and cholesterol levels (Jenkins *et al.*, 1976). In many cases, subjects on such diets have a reduced requirement for insulin or other hypoglycemic therapy (Anderson and Ward, 1979; Simpson *et al.*, 1981).

Hypertriglyceridemia

Hypertriglyceridemia also has been associated with increased prevalence of coronary heart disease (Brown *et al.*, 1965). However, none of the evidence indicates that triglyceride levels contribute information on coronary heart disease risk independently of the other associated risk factors such as plasma cholesterol, obesity, sedentary life-style, hypertension, or impaired glucose tolerance (Rifkind *et al.*, 1979).

The influence of dietary carbohydrates on serum lipids has recently been reviewed in detail (Grande, 1974; Little *et al.*, 1979). Studies involving feeding of carbohydrates generally show that a short-term increase in the consumption of carbohydrates provokes a marked rise in plasma triglycerides (Kato *et al.*, 1973; Glueck *et al.*, 1969). Palumbo *et al.*, (1977) reported that 2 g of simple carbohydrate per kilogram of body weight had no effect on serum triglycerides, but diets containing 4 g of simple carbohydrate (predominantly sucrose) were associated with a significant rise in serum triglycerides that was greater in CHD patients than in normal controls. However, the elevation in triglycerides was short term (a few days or weeks), and the amount of sugar consumed was greater than that usually eaten by Americans.

There are divergent views regarding which type of carbohydrate is the most hypertriglyceridemic. Studies show that most population groups with a low incidence of CHD derive 65 to 85% of their total energy in the form of whole grains and potatoes which contain significant amounts of dietary fiber as well as complex carbohydrate. Current studies on the effect of fiber on the metabolism of lipids show clear indications of changes in the absorption of carbohydrate and lipid (Kritchevsky, 1977).

Alcohol also can influence plasma triglyceride levels; its effects vary with the frequency with which and the amounts in which it is consumed. Moderate social drinking can double plasma triglycerides acutely; there is a smaller effect on cholesterol (Taskinen and Nikkila, 1977). In groups of alcoholics, triglycerides are significantly elevated, but total cholesterol is not (Sirtori, *et al.*, 1972).

LDL and HDL

Generally, total cholesterol concentrations are a good reflection of LDL levels, and the high correlation between plasma cholesterol and CHD risk thus suggests that high concentrations of LDL are atherogenic. Recent epidemiological studies suggest that elevated LDL is an independent risk factor (Gordon *et al.*, 1977a; Gordon *et al.*, 1977b; Wilson *et al.*, 1980). A direct relationship between LDL concentrations and extent of coronary atherosclerosis has been shown in several angiographic studies (Naito *et al.*, 1980).

Epidemiological studies also show an inverse correlation between CHD rates and HDL levels in populations with relatively high levels of total plasma cholesterol (Rhoads *et al.*, 1976; Pooling Project Research Group, 1978). At the same time, low HDL levels may not increase risk for CHD in populations in which LDL concentrations are also low (Connor *et al.*, 1978). Thus, in the absence of relatively high LDL, mildly decreased HDL may not be particularly dangerous.

Alcoholics tend also to have high HDL levels. The association between alcohol and HDL was first recognized by Johansson and Laurell (1969). Berg and Johansson (1973), in a subsequent study, monitored the effects of beer (60 g of ethanol/day) on healthy students over a period of five weeks and noticed a slow, but significant climb in plasma HDL. They also found HDL cholesterol was increased to over 200 mg/dl in chronic alcoholics after drinking bouts (Johansson and Medhus, 1974).

Obesity

The role of obesity in atherosclerotic disease remains uncertain, despite the nearly universal recommendation that obesity should be avoided in order to reduce risk of atherosclerotic disease. Obesity appears well established as a risk factor for hypertension and diabetes, and it undoubtedly influences atherosclerosis indirectly through these mechanisms, but, in their absence, no clear association of obesity with either atherogenesis or atherosclerotic disease has been demonstrated. Keys and his associates (1972) were unable to demonstrate a significant effect of obesity on CHD when the risks attendant on elevation of blood pressure were considered. Similar findings were also reported by Massey (Chapman and Massey, 1964).

In contrast, the Framingham data demonstrated a definite and independent risk of obesity for sudden death and the development of angina pectoris in men and a smaller, more indefinite risk in women (Kannel *et al.*, 1967). In summary, although the association between obesity and the risk of CHD may operate through the effects of obesity on other risk factors, the role of obesity, per se, should not be overlooked since recent studies have found that obesity may be an independent risk factor in populations with low levels of other risk factors, e.g., Japanese men in Hawaii and in younger individuals (Kagan *et al.*, 1975; Rabkin *et al.*, 1977). Furthermore, obesity increases the work load of the heart.

Hypertension

The risk of developing CHD is strongly related to the level of blood pressure, either systolic or diastolic (Freis, 1973). As with plasma cholesterol, there is no clearly defined cutoff point below which the blood pressure can be defined as "normal." The lower the blood pressure, the lower the risk.

Of particular significance is that an elevation in mean systolic and diastolic blood pressure also correlates with relative body weight (Whyte, 1959; Kannel *et al.*, 1967). Whyte suggested that a 28-pound increase in body weight would account for an average increase in systolic pressure of 10 mm Hg and in diastolic pressure of 8 mm. Boe *et al.* (1957), who recorded the blood pressure of nearly 68,000 Norwegian men and women, found a smaller increase in blood pressure; an increase of 3 mm Hg systolic and 22 mm diastolic pressure for 10 kg of body weight. A correlation coefficient of 0.3 between systolic blood pressure and relative weight was obtained in data from the Framingham report in both sexes (Kannel *et al.*, 1967). Other data obtained on the population of Tecumseh, Michigan, produced the correlation coefficients in persons 30 to 39 years of age for both systolic (0.33) and diastolic (0.32) pressure.

Keys and his associates (1950) examined the changes in blood pressure that occur with weight loss. They found a significant decrease in blood pressure with the loss of 24 kg body weight in a group of nonobese young men undergoing semistarvation. In the Framingham Study, it was found that individuals gaining 29 or more pounds in body weight over an 11-year interval developed hypertensive levels at twice the frequency of the entire group of subjects, or four times the rate of persons whose weight was unchanged or reduced (Kannel *et al.*, 1967). This observation has been repeated in prospective studies of other populations.

When weight reduction is achieved in obese hypertensive persons, both systolic and diastolic blood pressure usually decline. Fletcher (1954) observed a group of 38 obese women whose mean blood pressure was 196/116 prior to weight reduction. With the loss of 14 or more pounds in body weight, the mean blood pressure was reduced to 163/99. Whether the reduction in blood pressure is caused by weight reduction per se, or by salt restriction resulting from caloric deprivation, is controversial. Dahl (1958) emphasized the importance of dietary sodium in a seven-month study of an obese hypertensive woman. During the first month, the patient received a daily diet containing 10 g sodium chloride (170 mEq sodium), with adequate calories to maintain her admission weight. After the first month, calories were restricted, but a daily intake of 10 g sodium chloride was continued. The patient lost 25 kg body weight over the next four and a half months, with no fall in blood pressure. After five and a half months of observation, low sodium intake (4 to 6 mg) was started and, simultaneously, her caloric intake was increased to maintain her present weight. Only after sodium chloride was restricted did her blood pressure fall ($p < 0.01$).

The blood pressure–lowering effect of weight reduction in obese hypertensives is enhanced when the diet is also sodium restricted (Dahl, 1972). Kempner, using a drastically low-sodium (10 mEq/day) rice and fruit diet, observed improvement in almost two thirds of 500 patients (Kempner, 1948). A later clinical trial by the British Medical Research Council in 1950 confirmed Kempner's studies (Medical Research Council, 1950). Grollman and his colleagues (1945) observed a marked decrease in blood pressure of six patients with essential hypertension who were treated with a more liberal diet containing 22 mEq sodium daily.

Impaired Glucose Tolerance and Diabetes Mellitus

Clinically overt diabetes mellitus is associated with a high incidence of cardiovascular disease and premature death. Prospective studies of several populations have demonstrated that hyperglycemia or impaired glucose tolerance enhances the risk of coronary disease and is independent of increases of blood pressure and serum cholesterol (Epstein, 1977; Farinaro et al., 1977). Men with glucose intolerance have almost a 50% greater chance of developing CHD than men with no evidence of glucose intolerance, whereas in women the risk is more than doubled (Shurtleff, 1974; Gordon et al., 1977c).

Early onset (type I) diabetes appears to be primarily involved in mortality from renal disease, and adult-onset (type II) is associated with death from CHD (Knowles, 1974). The Uni-

versity Group Diabetes Study was undertaken to determine if the use of hypoglycemic agents and the control of blood sugar influenced the rate of occurrence of vascular complications in patients with adult-onset diabetes (University Group Diabetes Program, 1970). A common treatment protocol was used in several centers. All patients were provided diets that were appropriate for the maintenance of body weight within 15% of desirable weight. The caloric distribution was 45% carbohydrate, 20% protein, and 35% fat. Patients were assigned to treatment groups that provided one of the following: tolbutamide, phenformin, insulin, or placebo. All efforts to control hyperglycemia as measured by fasting blood glucose levels failed to reduce mortality or morbidity from cardiovascular causes.

Adult-onset diabetes is frequently associated with obesity and hypertriglyceridemia. Weight reduction is an important part in the management of the disease and not only assists in improving diabetes control but also may be accompanied by reduction in blood pressure and/or serum lipid levels. Hence, for adult-onset diabetics, the most important aspect of treatment is calorie control and weight reduction. Until recently, most "diabetic diets" in Western industrial countries prescribed 40 to 45% of energy as carbohydrate and 40% of calories as fat. Whether the high-fat content of the diet contributed to occurrence of hyperlipidemia is conjectural. In 1979, the Committee of the American Diabetes Association on Food and Nutrition published a report which states that the dietary carbohydrate intake for insulin-dependent diabetes "should usually account for 50 to 60% of total energy intake." No comments were made concerning the amount of dietary carbohydrate to be included in the diet of insulin-independent diabetics. However, Arky, the chairman of the committee, subsequently was quoted as stating in an editorial that, "for most persons, the diet should contain 50 to 60% carbohydrate" (Nuttall, 1980).

MANAGEMENT

Since there is no single evident cause of coronary heart disease, there is no single all-encompassing treatment rationale; however, diet is the cornerstone of conventional therapy. Sometimes no other treatment is necessary. Primary efforts are aimed at (1) reducing serum lipid levels, (2) weight maintenance and/or reduction, and (3) management of other coexisting problems such as hypertension or diabetes mellitus.

A recommended individual diet varies somewhat with the particular lipoprotein that is elevated. Restricting saturated fat consumption, increasing intake of polyunsaturated fat, reducing dietary cholesterol, increasing intake of complex carbohydrate and fiber are keys to treatment of hyperlipidemia associated with elevations of cholesterol in LDL. Weight reduction, restriction of alcohol, and restriction of intake of simple sugars are the measures used for the treatment of hyperlipidemia characterized by increased concentrations of triglyceride and VLDL.

Dietary Management

A single dietary approach to all forms of hyperlipidemia, including reduced intake of energy, cholesterol, and saturated fats, is appropriate for most patients. One point cannot be overemphasized—the diet must be tailored and modified to the individual patient. It is essential to bear in mind the medical history and other factors that may require modification of the diet (e.g., presence of hypertension, patient's food preferences). The dietary prescription must be explained to a patient in terms of food products and serving sizes. Since a diet is effective only as long as the patient complies, it must not be too extreme; that is, it must be practical. A dietitian can play an important role in interpreting the prescription and adapting it to the individual and his family.

Control of personal habits, especially cigarette smoking, also should be stressed. Physical activity should be increased gradually by some form of regular exercise, such as walking, bicycling, swimming, or any other activity compatible with the patient's physical condition and personal inclinations. Research on exercise and calorie intake suggests that short-term increases in energy expenditure via moderate programmed exercise do not substantially increase or decrease overall calorie intake (Mayer, 1968). Furthermore, exercise produces energy expenditure through a direct effect on metabolic rate during the activity and by an elevation in basal metabolic rate subsequent to activity (Passmore and Johnson, 1960).

Appropriate regimens are selected from the following elements:

1. Restriction of dietary cholesterol to reduce elevated LDL levels. Dietary cholesterol is found exclusively in foods containing animal fat. Examples of foods especially rich in cholesterol are egg yolks, dairy products (cheese and whole milk), red meat, and organ meats (liver and kidney).

2. Reduction of saturated fat intake, and substitution of polyunsaturated fats. The polyunsaturated-saturated fat ratio (P:S) is raised to about 2.0. In calculating the P:S ratio, the total grams of linoleic acid in the diet are divided by the total grams of saturated fatty acids:

$$P:S = \frac{\text{Linoleic acid (g)}}{\text{Saturated fatty acid (g)}}$$

Polyunsaturated vegetable oils (corn, safflower, soybean, cottonseed) are substitued for solid shortening in cooking, and a polyunsaturated margarine is used in place of butter. Certain vegetable oils such as palm oil and coconut oil are rich in saturated fats and should be avoided.

3. Limit total fat intake to 30% total daily intake.

4. A program of weight reduction for obese patients, followed by a weight maintenance program.

5. A decrease in, or the elimination of, alcohol intake. This is an important and sometimes vital element for treatment and control of hypertriglyceridemia.

The above guidelines are consistent with the recently released dietary goals for the United States (Table 9-4) (Select Committee on Nutri-

Table 9-4. DIETARY GOALS FOR THE UNITED STATES

1. To avoid overweight, consume only as much energy (calories) as is expended; if overweight, decrease energy intake and increase energy expenditure.
2. Increase the consumption of complex carbohydrates and "naturally occurring" sugars from about 28 percent to about 48 percent of energy intake.
3. Reduce the consumption of refined and other processed sugars by about 45 percent to account for about 10 percent of total energy intake.
4. Reduce overall fat consumption from approximately 40 percent to about 30 percent of energy intake.
5. Reduce saturated-fat consumption to account for about 10 percent of total energy intake and balance that with polyunsaturated and monounsaturated fats, which should account for about 10 percent of energy intake each.
6. Reduce cholesterol consumption to about 300 mg per day.
7. Limit the intake of sodium by reducing the intake of salt (sodium chloride) to about 5 g per day (2 g sodium).

Source: Select Committee on Nutrition and Human Needs, U.S. Senate. *Dietary Goals for the United States*, 2nd ed. December **1977**.

Table 9-5. SUMMARY OF DIETS FOR HYPERLIPOPROTEINEMIAS, TYPES I TO V

	TYPE I	TYPE IIa	TYPE IIb AND TYPE III	TYPE IV	TYPE V
Diet prescription	Low fat (25–35 g)	Low cholesterol PUF increased	Low cholesterol Approximate calorie breakdown; 20% protein 40% fat 40% CHO	Controlled CHO Approximately 45% of calories Moderately restricted cholesterol	Restricted fat (30% of calories) Controlled CHO (50% of calories) Moderately restricted cholesterol
Calories	Not restricted	Not restricted	Achieve and maintain "ideal" weight, i.e., reduction diet if necessary	Achieve and maintain "ideal" weight, i.e., reduction diet if necessary	Achieve and maintain "ideal" weight, i.e., reduction diet if necessary
Protein	Total protein intake is not limited	Total protein intake is not limited	High protein	Not limited other than control of patient's weight	High protein
Fat	Restricted to 25–35 g	Saturated fat intake limited; PUF intake increased	Controlled to 40% of calories (PUF recommended in preference to saturated fats)	Not limited other than control of patient's weight (PUF recommended in preference to saturated fats)	Restricted to 30% of calories (PUF recommended in preference to saturated fats)
Cholesterol	Not restricted	As low as possible; the only source of cholesterol is the meat in the diet	Less than 300 mg (the only source of cholesterol is the meat in the diet)	Moderately restricted to 300–500 mg	Moderately restricted to 300–500 mg
Carbohydrate	Not limited	Not limited	Controlled, concentrated sweets are restricted	Controlled, concentrated sweets are restricted	Controlled, concentrated sweets are restricted
Alcohol	Not recommended	May be used with discretion	Limited to 2 servings (substituted for CHO)	Limited to 2 servings (substituted for CHO)	Not recommended

Note: PUF, polyunsaturated fat; CHO, carbohydrate.

Source: Fredrickson, D. S.; Levy, R. I.; Bonnel, M.; and Ernst, N. *Dietary Management of Hyperlipoproteinemia.* U.S. Department of Health, Education, and Welfare, National Heart and Lung Institute, Bethesda, Md., **1973.**

tion and Human Needs, 1977) and the current recommendations of the American Heart Association (Grundy *et al.*, 1982) which are based on the concept that modification of risk factors should decrease the danger of CHD.

Specific dietary guidelines for each type of primary hyperlipoproteinemia have been suggested by Fredrickson *et al.*, (1973) and are available from the National Heart and Lung Institute (Table 9-5).

The dietary goals alone cannot be used to plan diets; they must be used in conjunction with dietary guidelines, such as the Recommended Dietary Allowances (1980) in a planning scheme such as the four basic food groups or the Exchange List (American Diabetes Association and American Dietetic Association, 1976). The specifics of nutritional management as implemented at the Houston Cardiovascular Rehabilitation Center will be described in Chapter 10.

REFERENCES

American Diabetes Association and American Dietetic Association: Exchange lists for meal planning. American Diabetes Association, Chicago, **1976.**

Anderson, J. W., and Ward, K. High carbohydrate, high fiber diets for insulin-treated men with diabetes mellitus. *Am. J. Clin. Nutr.,* **1979,** *32,* 2312–2321.

Berg, B., and Johansson, B. C. Prolonged adminstration of ethanol to healthy volunteers. 3. Effects on parameters of liver function, plasma lipid concentrations and lipoprotein patterns. *Acta Med. Scand.,* **1973,** *194*(Suppl. 552), 13–20.

Blackburn, H. Diet and mass hyperlipidemia. A public health view. In, Levy, R. I., *et al.* (eds.) *Nutrition, Lipids and Coronary* Heart Disease. Raven, New York, 1979.

Boe, S.; Humberfelt, S.; and Wedervans, F. The blood pressure in a population. Blood pressure readings and height and weight determinations in the adult population of the city of Bergen. *Acta Med. Scand.,* **1957,** *321*(Suppl.), 5–336.

Brown, D. F.; Kinch, S. H.; and Doyle, J. T. Serum triglycerides in health and in ischemia heart disease. *N. Engl. J. Med.,* **1965,** *276,* 947–952.

Burkitt, D. P.; Walker, A. R. P.; and Painter, N. S. Dietary fiber and disease. *JAMA,* **1974,** *229,* 1068–1074.

Burslem, J.; Schonfeld, G.; Howard, M. A.; Weidman, S. W.; and Miller, J. P. Plasma apoprotein and lipoprotein lipid levels in vegetarians. *Metabolism,* **1978,** *27,* 711–719.

Chapman, J. M., and Massey, F. J., Jr. The interrelationship of serum cholesterol, hypertension, body weight and risk of coronary disease. *J. Chronic Dis.,* **1964,** *17,* 933–949.

Committee of the American Diabetes Association on Food and Nutrition: Special report—Principles of nutrition and dietary recommendations for individuals with diabetes mellitus. *Diabetes,* **1979,** *23,* 1027–1030.

Connor, W. E.; Cequira, M. T.; Connor, R. W.; Wallace, R. B.; Malinow, M. R.; and Casdorph, H. R. The plasma lipids, lipoproteins and the diet of the Turahumara Indians of Mexico. *Am. J. Clin. Nutr.,* **1978,** *31,* 1131–1142.

Dahl, L. K. The role of salt in the fall in blood pressure accompanying reduction in obesity. *N. Engl. J. Med.,* **1958,** *258,* 1186–1192.

——Salt and hypertension. *Am. J. Clin. Nutr.,* **1972,** *25,* 231–244.

Diet-Heart Review Panel. *Mass Field Trials of the Diet-Heart Question.* American Heart Association, New York, Monograph No. 28, **1969.**

Epstein, F. H. Hyperglycemia—A risk factor in coronary heart disease. *Circulation,* **1977,** *36,* 609–619.

Farinaro, E.; Stamler, J.; Upton, M.; Mojonnier, J.; Hall, Y.; Moss, D.; and Berkson, D. M. Plasma glucose levels: Long-term effect of diet in the Chicago coronary prevention evaluation program. *Ann. Intern. Med.,* **1977,** *86,* 147–154.

Fletcher, A. P. The effect of weight reduction upon the blood pressure of obese hypertensive women. *J. Med.,* **1954,** *91,* 331–345.

Fredrickson, D. S.; Levy, R. I.; Bonnell, M.; and Ernest, N. *Dietary Management of Hyperlipoproteinemia.* U.S. Dept. of Health, Education and Welfare, National Heart and Lung Institute, Bethesda, Md., **1973.**

Fredrickson, D. S.; Levy, R. I.; and Lees, R. S. Fat transport in lipoproteins—an integrated approach to mechanisms and disorders. *New Engl. J. Med.,* **1967,** *276,* 32–44, 94–103, 148–156, 215–224, 273–281.

Freis, E. D. Age, race, sex and other indices of risk in hypertension. *Am. J. Med.,* **1973,** *55,* 275–280.

Glueck, C. J.; Levy, M. I.; and Fredrickson, D. S. Immunoreactive insulin, glucose tolerance and carbohydrate inducibility in types II, III, IV and V hyperlipoproteinemia. *Diabetes,* **1969,** *18,* 739–747.

Gordon, T.; Castelli, W. P.; Hjortland, M. C.; Kannel, W. B.; and Dawber, T. R. High density lipoprotein as a protective factor against coronary heart disease. The Framingham Study. *Am. J. Med.,* **1977a,** *62,* 707–714.

—— Predicting coronary heart disease in middle-aged and older persons. The Framingham Study. *JAMA,* **1977b,** *238,* 497–499.

—— Diabetes, blood lipids and the role of obesity in coronary heart disease, risk for women. The Framingham Study. *Ann. Intern. Med.,* **1977c,** *87,* 393–397.

Grande, F. Sugars in cardiovascular disease. In, Sipple, H. L., and McNutt, K. W. (eds.) *Sugars in Nutrition.* Academic Press, New York, **1974,** pp. 429–440.

Grollman, A.; Harrison, T. R.; Mason, M. F.; Baxter, J.; Crampton, J.; and Reichsman, F. Sodium restriction in the diet for hypertension. *JAMA,* **1945,** *129,* 553–537.

Grundy, S. M.; Bilheimer, D.; Blackburn, H.; Brown, W. V.; Kwiterovich, P. O.; Mattson, F.; Schonfeld, G.; and Weidman, W. H.: Rationale of the diet-heart statement of the American Heart Association. *Circulation,* **1982,** *65,* 893A–854A.

Jenkins, D. J. A.; Leeds, A. R.; Wolevar, R. M. S.; Goff, D. V.; Alberti, K. G. M. M.; Gassull, M. A.; and Hockaday, T. D. R. Unabsorpable carbohydrates in diabetes: decreased post-prandial hyperglycemia. *Lancet,* **1976,** *2,* 172–174.

Johansson, B. G., and Laurell, C. B. Disorders of serum

alpha-lipoproteins after alcoholic intoxication. *Scand. J. Clin. Lab. Invest.,* **1969,** *23,* 231–233.

Johansson, B. G., and Medhus, A. Increase of plasma alpha-lipoproteins in chronic alcoholics after acute abuse. *Acta Med. Scand.,* **1974,** *195,* 273–277.

Kagan, A.; Gordon, T.; Rhoads, G. G.; and Schiffinan, J. C. Some factors related to coronary heart disease incidence in Honolulu Japanese men. The Honolulu Heart Study. *Int. J. Epidemiol.,* **1975,** *4,* 271–279.

Kannel, W. B. The disease of living. *Nutr. Today,* **1971,** *6,* 2–11.

Kannel, W. B.; Brand, N.; Skinner, J. J., Jr.; Dawber, T. R.; and McNamara, P. M. The relation of adiposity to blood pressure and development of hypertension. The Framingham Study. *Ann. Intern. Med.,* **1967,** *67,* 48–59.

Kannel, W. B.; LeBauer, E. J.; Dawber, T. R.; and McNamara, P. M. Relation of body weight to development of coronary heart disease. *Circulation,* **1967,** *35,* 734–744.

Kato, H.; Tillotson, J.; Nichaman, M.; Rhoads, G.; and Hamilton, H. Epidemiologic studies of coronary heart disease and stroke in Japanese men in Japan, Hawaii and California; Serum lipids and diet. *Am. J. Epidemiol.,* **1973,** *97,* 372–380.

Kempner, W. Treatment of hypertensive vascular disease with rice diet. *Am. J. Med.,* **1948,** *4,* 545–577.

Keys, A. (ed.): Coronary heart disease in seven countries. *Circulation,* **1970,** *41*(Suppl. 1), 1–211.

Keys, A.; Anderson, J. T.; and Grande, F. Prediction of serum cholesterol responses of man to changes of fat in the diet. *Lancet,* **1957,** *2,* 959–966.

Keys, A.; Arvanis, C.; Blackburn, H.; Van Buchem, F. S. P.; Buzina, R.; Djordevic, B. A.; Fidanza, F.; Karvonen, M. J.; Menotti, A.; Paddu, V.; and Taylor, H. L. Coronary heart disease: Overweight and obesity as risk factors. *Ann. Intern. Med.,* **1972,** *77,* 15–26.

Keys, A.; Brozek, J.; Henschel, A.; Mickelson, O.; and Taylor, H. L. *The Biology of Human Starvation.* University of Minnesota Press, Minneapolis, **1950.**

Keys, A.; Kimura, N.; Kusukawa, A.; Bronte-Steward, B.; Larsen, N.; and Keys, M. H. Lessons from serum cholesterol studies in Japan, Hawaii and Los Angeles. *Ann. Intern. Med.,* **1958,** *48,* 83–94.

Knowles, H. C., Jr. Magnitude of the renal failure problem in diabetic patients. *Kidney Int.* **1974,** *6*(Suppl. 1), 2–7.

Kritchevsky, D. Dietary fiber and other dietary factors in hypercholesterolemia. *Am. J. Clin. Nutr.,* **1977,** *30,* 979–984.

LaRosa, J. C. Secondary hyperlipoproteinemia. In, Rifkind, B. M., and Levy, R. I. (eds.) *Hyperlipidemia: Diagnosis and Therapy.* Grune & Stratton, New York, **1977.**

Levy, R. I., and Ernst, N. Diet, hyperlipidemia and atherosclerosis. In, Goodhart, R. S., and Shils, M. E. (eds.) *Modern Nutrition in Health and Disease.* Lea & Febiger, Philadelphia, **1980,** pp. 1045–1070.

Levy, R. I.; Morganroth, J.; and Rifkind, B. M. Treatment of hyperlipidemia. *N. Engl. J. Med.,* **1974,** *290,* 1295–1301.

Lipid Research Clinic Program Epidemiology Committee. Plasma lipid distribution in selected North American populations: the LRC Program Prevalence Study. *Circulation,* **1979,** *60,* 427–439.

Little, J. A.; McGuire, V.; and Derksen, A. Available carbohydrates. In, Levy, R.; Rifkind, B.; Dennis, B.; and Ernest, N. (eds.) *Nutrition, Lipids and Coronary Heart Disease.* Raven Press, New York, **1979.**

Malmros, H. The relation of nutrition to health—a statistical study of the effort of war-time on arteriosclerosis, cardiosclerosis, turberculosis and diabetes. *Acta Med. Scand.* (Suppl.), **1950,** *246,* 137–153.

Mayer, J. *Overweight: Causes, Cost and Control.* Englewood Cliffs, N.J., Prentice-Hall, **1968.**

McGill, H. C. The relationship of dietary cholesterol to serum cholesterol concentration and to atherosclerosis in man. *Am. J. Clin. Nutr.,* **1979,** *32,* 2664–2702.

Medical Research Council. The rice diet in the treatment of hypertension. *Lancet,* **1950,** *2,* 509–513.

Naito, H. K.; Greenstreet, R. L.; David, J. A.; Sheldon, W. L.; Shirey, E. K.; Lewis, R. C.; Proudfit, W. L.; and Gerrity, R. G. HDL-cholesterol concentration and severity of coronary atherosclerosis determined by cineangiography. *Artery,* **1980,** *8,* 101–112.

Nuttal, F. Q. Dietary recommendations for individuals with diabetes mellitus, 1979: summary of report from Foods and Nutrition Committee of the American Diabetes Association. *Am. J. Clin. Nutr.,* **1980,** *33,* 1311–1312.

Palumbo, P. J.; Briones, E. R.; Nelson, R. A.; and Kottke, B. A. Sucrose sensitivity of patients with coronary artery disease. *Am. J. Clin. Nutr.,* **1977,** *30,* 394–401.

Palumbo, P. J.; Briones, E. R.; and Nelson, R. A. High fiber diet in hyperlipidemia. *JAMA,* **1978,** *240,* 223–227.

Passmore, R., and Johnson, R. E. Some metabolic changes following prolonged moderate exercise. *Metabolism,* **1960,** *9,* 452–456.

Pooling Project Research Group. Relationship of blood pressure, serum cholesterol, smoking habit, relative weight and ECG abnormalities to incidence of major coronary events: final report of the pooling project. *J. Chronic Dis.* **1978,** *31,* 201–306.

Rabkin, S. W.; Mathewson, F. A.; and Hsu, P. Relation of body weight to development of ischemic heart disease in a cohort of young North American men after a 26 year observation period: The Manitoba Study. *Am. J. Cardiol.,* **1977,** *39,* 452–458.

Recommended Dietary Allowances, 9th ed. National Academy of Sciences, Food and Nutrition Board, Washington, D.C. **1980.**

Rhoads, G. G.; Gulbrandsen, C. L.; and Kagan, A. Serium lipoproteins and coronary heart disease in population study of Hawaii Japanese men. *N. Engl. J. Med.,* **1976,** *294,* 293–298.

Rifkind, B. M.; Goor, R. S.; and Levy, R. I. Current status of the role of dietary treatment in the prevention and management of coronary heart disease. *Med. Clin. North Am.,* **1979,** *63,* 911–925.

Sacks, F. W.; Castelli, W. P.; Donner, A.; and Kass, E. H. Plasma lipids and lipoproteins in vegetarians and controls. *N. Engl. J. Med.,* **1975,** *292,* 1148–1151.

Select Committee on Nutrition and Human Needs, U.S. Senate. *Dietary Goals for the United States,* 2nd ed., Washington, D. C., December, **1977.**

Shurtleff, D. Some characteristics related to the incidence of cardiovascular disease and death. The Framingham Study, 18-year follow-up. DHEW Pub. No. (NIH) 74-599, Section No. 30, Bethesda, Md. **1974.**

Simpson, H. C. R.; Lousley, S.; Geekie, M.; Simpson, R. W.; Carter, R. D.; Hockaday, T. D. R.; and Mann, J. I. A high carbohydrate leguminous fiber diet improves all aspects of diabetic control. *Lancet,* **1981,** *1,* 1–40.

Sirtori, C. R.; Agradi, E.; Mariani, C.; Canal, N.; and Frattola, L. Alcoholic hyperlipidemia. *Lancet.* **1972,** *2,* 820–821.

Taskinen, M. R., and Nikkila, E. A. Nocturnal hypertriglyceridemia and hyperinsulinemia following moderate evening intake of alcohol. *Acta Med. Scand.,* **1977,** *202,* 173–177.

Taylor, K. B., and Anthony, L. E. *Clinical Nutrition.* McGraw-Hill, New York, **1983.**

Trowell, H. Ischemic heart disease and dietary fiber. *Am. J. Clin. Nutr.,* **1972,** *25,* 926–928.

Truswell, A. S. Dietary fat and cholesterol metabolism. *Bibl. Nutr. Dieta,* **1977,** *25,* 53–63.

———— Food fiber and blood lipids. *Nutr. Rev.,* **1977,** *35,* 51–54.

University Group Diabetes Program. A study of the effects of hypoglycemic agents on the vascular complications in patients with adult onset diabetes. *J. Am. Diab. Assoc.,* **1970,** *19,* 747, 830.

Whyte, H. M. Blood pressure and obesity. *Circulation,* **1959,** *19,* 511–515.

Wilson, P. W.; Garrison, R. J.; Castelli, W. P.; Feinleib, M.; McNamara, P. M.; and Kannel, W. B. Prevalence of coronary heart disease in the Framingham Offspring Study: study of lipoprotein cholesterols. *Am. J. Cardiol.,* **1980,** 46, 649–654.

Chapter 10
THE NUTRITIONAL MANAGEMENT OF THE CARDIOVASCULAR REHABILITATION PATIENT

Mary W. Schanler, Luean E. Anthony, and E. C. Henley

A major component of comprehensive cardio-vascular rehabilitation is the provision of nutritional support services by a registered dietitian. The nutrition program includes group therapy, which is generally concerned with nutrition principles and behavior modification techniques. In addition to group therapy, individual counseling is provided in order to give specific guidelines for therapy as many patients have unique nutritional problems superimposed on the ones commonly seen in cardiovascular patients. The success of the nutrition component requires that the patient (1) gain the expertise to make appropriate eating choices which are compatible with his life-style, and (2) maintain this new regimen after exit from the program. This chapter describes the nutrition program developed at the Houston Cardiovascular Rehabilitation Center (HCRC) during the last five years.

The treatment of nutritional problems at HCRC is an ongoing counseling process focused on guiding people to make food choices that are essential for their good health. This process is integrated into the medical and psychological care of each patient. There are certain nutritional and dietary needs common to all patients, and there are needs that are specific to each individual patient. When nutritional care is integrated into a medical care program, the patient has the opportunity to learn new and more appropriate eating behaviors recommended on the basis of his medical condition. In rehabilitation, the process of evaluation is ongoing and results in a plan that is dynamic and evolving from the medical progress of the patient. The psychological support services and those of the nursing specialists add another dimension to the care process.

GOALS OF NUTRITION MANAGEMENT

The nutritional treatment of the cardiovascular patient is directed toward the primary goal of treating nutrition disorders, and secondarily of reducing identified nutritional risk factors and preventing the development of additional disabilities and risk factors. The general principles are (1) achieve and maintain ideal body weight; (2) limit fat kilocalories to 30% daily intake with 10% saturates, 10% monounsaturates, and 10% polyunsaturates; (3) limit dietary cholesterol to 300 mg/day; (4) consume 55 to 60% kilocalories as carbohydrate with emphasis on complex sources and sources containing fiber; and (5) limit sodium to 2,000 to 3,000 mg/day. The rationale for these recommendations is reviewed in Chapter

9. More specific recommendations are made in individual cases as appropriate. For example, alcohol, a source of empty calories, is discouraged in patients limiting calories for the purpose of weight loss or in patients with a history of, or currently demonstrating, hypertriglyceridemia. Patients with myocardiopathies are strongly advised to avoid alcohol completely. All of the cardiovascular patients at HCRC are encouraged to moderate the consumption of caffeine-containing beverages, and patients with cardiac arrhythmias are cautioned to avoid caffeine entirely. Included in the population at HCRC are many elderly people who have special dietary needs due to poor dentition, limited financial resources, or other chronic diseases such as diabetes. Postsurgical patients may have subclinical evidence of depleted nutritional reserves such as low ferritins or more clinically evident nutritional risk factors such as decreased subcutaneous fat stores.

INITIAL NUTRITIONAL EVALUATION

The nutritional evaluation of the patient includes nutritional assessment which is based on the physician's medical history and physical examination, the nursing assessment, the laboratory results, and the detailed diet history obtained during the dietitian's initial interview of the patient. From this assessment, recommendations and a nutritional care plan are formulated for each patient.

Nutritionally relevant information in the physician's history includes medications and present or past medical disorders that may affect the patient's nutritional status or may require nutritional therapy, such as diabetes mellitus, chronic obstructive pulmonary disease, hypertension, gastrointestinal disease, or other conditions that may alter the requirements for certain nutrients. The patient has some clinical manifestation of coronary heart disease, and most have had a myocardial infarction or coronary artery bypass surgery. The physician notes the extent of the past medical problems and course of any recent hospitalization, use of alcohol, and unusual or bizarre food habits. The physical examination reveals clinical signs of malnutrition such as obesity, hepatomegaly, decreased subcutaneous fat stores, loss of body musculature, pitting edema, or massive ascites.

The information obtained from the nursing staff's assessment of particular interest to the dietitian includes current medications, lifestyle characteristics such as smoking, activity level, and occupation. The nursing staff is re-sponsible for recording blood pressure, weight, height, and measurement of skinfold thickness using Lange skinfold calipers. The four skinfold measures (biceps, triceps, subscapular, suprailiac) are summed and used to evaluate per cent body fat (Lindner and Lindner, 1973). At the HCRC the desirable percentage body fat ranges are considered to be 16 to 20% for men and 24 to 26% for women. These appear realistic in view of the age of the population at HCRC (McArdle *et al.*, 1981).

The estimated ideal weight on individuals with a medium frame is calculated using the following formulas (Davidson, 1976):

> Men: 106 lb for the first 5 ft and 6 lb for each additional inch.
> Women: 100 lb for the first 5 ft and 5 lb for each additional inch.

The weight is adjusted for small or large frames by subtracting or adding 10%. Alternatively, the table of suggested desirable weights for heights found in the *Recommended Dietary Allowances* (The National Research Council, 1980) may be used. The per cent ideal weight is calculated by dividing the patient's actual weight by the ideal weight and multipying this number by 100.

The purpose of the dietitian's initial interview is twofold: (1) to obtain information relevant to the patient's characteristic dietary intake and the environmental factors that affect his/her dietary habits, and (2) to establish a rapport with the patient that will form a basis for future nutritional counseling. The dietitian's interview focuses on the patient's general dietary habits and on specific dietary factors that may contribute to nutritionally related risk factors (hyperlipidemia, obesity, hypertension, diabetes) or coronary artery disease. The patient is questioned about his/her present weight, the usual weight, date of maximum weight, recent changes in appetite or food intake, previous use of special diets, food aversions, intolerances and allergies, feeding problems such as use of dentures, use of nutrition supplements and vitamins, alcohol intake, and usual daily physical activity. The patient completes a food-frequency questionnaire (an example of assessment form and questions is seen in Figure 10-1). The patient's current intake is assessed by a 24-hour recall which consists of requesting him/her to remember and describe all the food and beverages consumed over the previous 24-hour period (see Figure 10-2). Lifelike food models representing specified

DIETARY ASSESSMENT FORM

Name _____   Date _____

Personal Data: Activity:
    DOB _____   Age _____   Work _____
    Ht. _____   Wt. _____   Recreation _____
    Usual wt. _____   Wt. gain or loss in past
                     month _____

    Highest Wt. _____

    Smoke _____ Packs/day _____

    Household composition _____

Food Preparation/Consumption:

    Person responsible for shopping _____

    Person responsible for menu planning _____

    Person responsible for food preparation _____

    Usual method of meat preparation _____

    No. of meals eaten away from home _____

    Carry lunch to work _____

    Times of meals each day _____

Special Diets:

    Type   Prescribed by   Duration   Results

Appetite: Hearty _____ Moderate _____ Poor _____ Anorexic _____

Cravings: _____

Influences on Diet (religion, ethnic, vegetarian):

Problem Foods and Why:

    Foods which cause . . . nausea _____ heartburn _____

    gas _____ constipation _____ diarrhea _____

Figure 10-1A

Any feeding problems (dentures, etc.) _____

Food Allergies: citrus _____ chocolate _____ grains _____ milk _____
                  seafood _____
                  other _____

Medications and Supplements: vitamins (type): _____

                               diuretics: _____

                               laxatives: _____

                               oral contraceptives: _____

                               estrogen replacement: _____

                               health foods: _____

                               other: _____

Food Frequency: How often do you consume the following foods?

Food item	No. Daily	No. Weekly	Seldom	Never	Food item	No. Daily	No. Weekly	Seldom	Never
Beef					Wh. cream				
Poultry					½ & ½				
Pork, bacon, ham					Sn. crackers chips				
Lunchmeats									
Lamb					Salad dr.				
Liver					Soft drinks				
Shellfish					Alcohol				
Fish					Coffee				
Eggs					Tea				
Cheese					Candy				
Milk					Cake				
Buttermilk					Cookies				
Yogurt					Dr.peas/beans				
Ice cream					Yellow veg.				
Bread					Gr. vegs.				
Potatoes, rice, noodles					Fruit				
					Juice				
Oleo					Bran				
Butter					Cereals				

Use of added salt: _____

Patient Nutrition Goals: _____

Comments: _____

Figure 10-1B

163

24 HOUR DIETARY RECALL:

Now, I would like for you to tell me everything you ate yesterday including coffee, tea, and sugar-free beverages:

Waking time _____   Was this usual? _____

Food & Description	Amt.	KCal	Pro Gm	Fat Gm	Carbo Gm							
_____												
_____												
_____												
_____												
_____												
_____												
_____												
_____												
_____												
_____												
_____												
_____												
_____												
_____												
_____												
_____												
_____												
_____												
_____												
_____												
_____												
_____												
_____												
_____												
Total												
% of KCal												

Was this a typical day? _____   If no, why not? _____

_____

Patient's Name: _____   Interviewer: _____

Wt. _____   Blood Pressure _____

Figure 10-2

amounts of foods help the patient describe the actual portion sizes and amounts of foods ingested. The dietitian calculates the total calories and the per cent of calories derived from protein, fat, carbohydrate, and alcohol using a combination of the following references: The Exchange system (American Diabetes Association, Inc., The American Dietetic Association, 1976), Bowes and Church's *Food Values of Portions Commonly Used* (Pennington, 1980), and *Handbook 456 — Nutritive Value of American Foods* (USDA, 1975).

In addition to obtaining precise information relevant to the patient's dietary intake, the dietitian seeks the basis of the patient's food choices. In order to facilitate modification of eating habits, the dietitian must understand the environment of the current dietary practices and the life-style of the patient, such as frequency of eating in restaurants, use of convenience foods, and involvement of the patient in menu planning and food preparation. Additionally, the reasons for these behaviors must be understood in order to plan for change. The interest and support of the family must be included in this evaluation.

Throughout the interview, the dietitian is building a relationship that will be a foundation for the future counseling process. In addition to the diet history information, the patient is encouraged to set nutritional goals during the initial dietary evaluation in order to provide some indication of the patient's perception of his nutritional problems and his priorities in terms of treatment. In some instances, the patient simply repeats his referring physician's recommendations or media information such as "avoid eggs." Often the goals are broadly stated such as "lose weight." Most people realize that their diet affects their health status but do not possess the needed specific guidelines for modification.

A written test consisting of 20 questions focusing on general nutrition principles and nutritional concepts relevant to the cardiovascular patient is completed by each patient toward the end of the dietary interview. The results are used to evaluate the patient's current knowledge of nutrition so that the dietitian has information on which to plan the counseling process. This test gives the patient an opportunity to evaluate his/her present nutritional information which may be based on popular misconceptions.

Biochemical measures of nutritional status, routinely pertinent to patients in a cardiovascular rehabilitation program, include fasting blood glucose, total serum cholesterol, HDL cholesterol, serum triglycerides, hemoglobin, hematocrit, and serum iron. Other indices such as serum potassium and albumin are routinely obtained and evaluated with respect to factors in the nursing, medical, and/or dietary histories that suggest the patient may be at increased nutrition risk.

Hypokalemia is a common side effect of chronic thiazide diuretic therapy. Serum albumin, a visceral protein, is recognized as a valuable screening indicator of nutritional status. A serum albumin of less than 3.4 g/dl in adults warrants further evaluation. Additional biochemical evaluation of anemia or other disorders may be performed if indicated by the initial report. An iron-deficiency profile (serum iron, ferritin, iron-binding capacity) is always obtained on patients with initial serum iron values below 60 mcg/dl.

Nutritional assessment is used to identify individuals at nutritional risk, provide guidelines for nutritional care, and to evaluate the patient's response to treatment. In the cardiovascular patient, the goals of nutritional assessment include the identification of the presence of nutrition-related risk factors for coronary heart disease and the evaluation of the current dietary intake. As might be expected, most of the patients seen at HCRC have at least one nutrition-related risk factor for coronary heart disease. The following risk factors are seen in at least one half of the HCRC patients: >110% ideal weight; serum cholesterol >225 mg/dl; serum triglycerides >150 mg/dl. At HCRC, the patients are given "desirable" limits of ≤200 mg/dl for serum cholesterol and ≤100 mg/dl for serum triglycerides. The desirable per cent range for body weight as fat is 16 to 20% in men and 24 to 26% in women.

Nutritional Care Plan

The results of the nutritional assessment and the nutritional recommendations for treatment (objectives) are given to each patient in an individual session with the nutritionist. The nutritionist involves the patient in setting goals with a realistic expectation of success. It is an important practical aspect that people are more motivated to attain goals they set for themselves than goals that are set without their direct involvement (Lewin, 1943). A plan to meet the patient's objectives is discussed so the patient realizes that progress (or lack of it) will be recognized. In practice, the dietitian initially may suggest limited objectives. Many principles of the dietary recommendations for patients with cardiovascular disease overlap. For example, the patient may readily agree that weight loss is indicated and agree to focus on it as an objective. Decreasing total fat intake may be another recommendation for the patient; however, the process may be incorporated into the plan for weight loss rather than emphasized as a goal in itself. The patient is encouraged to focus on short-term, achievable goals that will help to reach the long-term goal. Losing large amounts of weight often seems overwhelming. Losing one pound a week usually seems reasonable to even the most pessimistic individual. The patient is encouraged to share in the selection of strategies for achieving these goals which are based on the patient's priorities, needs, and abilities.

When the goals and objectives are formulated by patient and dietitian, the dietitian proceeds with a plan for implementing the processes needed to reach the goal. The strategies for achieving goals must be based on sound educational practices and on the patient's individual resources. Each patient at HCRC varies in terms of background, educational level, and readiness to learn. The patients represent a wide range in economic status and in previous experiences with dietary changes. As might be expected, some of the patients have been aware of their progressive cardiovascular disease and have received some nutrition counseling. Frequently, the nutrition counseling consisted of in-hospital treatment developed around acute problems and dietitian control of the diet. The concepts often need to be expanded to apply to a free-living individual who makes his/her own food choices. This is a gradual, progressive process. Some patients have previously experienced unfortunate results in attempts to lose weight by fad diets, hypnosis, gastric stapling, and other popular approaches to the problem of obesity. Others have been so distressed by their cardiac problems that they are afraid to deviate from unnecessarily rigid rules of "don'ts." Wives often seek recipes and details of implementation of prescribed diets.

TREATMENT

The methods of nutritional treatment include both group therapy and individual counseling.

Groups

Eight weekly nutrition sessions are held concurrently with weekly psychological group sessions and weekly medical group sessions. Spouses of patients are encouraged to attend the group sessions and participate in the discussions. In many families, the activities of food selection and preparation are delegated to someone other than the patient. The involvement in the program of this other person is often essential to the effective implementation of nutrition care planning. Each nutrition session has two components: (1) behavior modification therapy and (2) nutrition counseling.

The focus of the behavioral modification component is on making changes in eating habits. Behavior modification is based on the principle that behavior is controlled by stimuli in the environment. A stimulus elicits a response from an individual which is reinforced by the outcome or consequence of the response. Considerable research has been conducted over the last ten years of the effectiveness of behavior techniques in achieving weight loss (Wilson and Brownell, 1980; Foreyt et al., 1982). The program at HCRC is similar to most behavior modification programs for the treatment of obesity in that there are four main components: record keeping, restricting external cues for eating, changing the actual eating behaviors, and reinforcement of altered behavior (Wilson and Brownell, 1980). The model of behavior modification of weight control is applicable for use in producing behavioral changes in eating that bring about other desired objectives (Carmody et al., 1982). At HCRC it has been used effectively in anorexic patients to achieve weight gain. Behavior modification techniques may be used by anyone desiring to change food habits in order to select more foods appropriate for their health needs.

The nutrition counseling component of the group sessions consists of a series of topics that are based on implementation of the dietary recommendations for the cardiovascular patient. The specific content of each session is discussed below.

Group Nutrition Counseling Sequence.

Day I
- A. Nutrition for the cardiovascular patient
- B. Introduction to behavior control of weight and food habit awareness

The list of risk factors for cardiovascular disease is reviewed, and the nutrition-related ones —hyperlipidemia, obesity, hypertension, and diabetes—are discussed in the first group nutrition meeting. The general dietary principles for the management of the cardiovascular pa-

Table 10-1. GENERAL PRINCIPLES FOR THE CARDIOVASCULAR REHABILITATION PATIENT

1. Achieve and maintain ideal body weight
2. Restrict fat calories to 30% total kilocalories:
   10% saturates
   10% monounsaturates
   10% polyunsaturates
3. Limit dietary cholesterol to < 300 mg/day
4. Consume 55 to 60% kilocalories as carbohydrate with emphasis on complex carbohydrates
5. Limit sodium to 2,000 to 3,000 mg/day

tient are presented and utilized as an ongoing framework for the didactic nutritional material (Table 10-1). The patients are all given copies of *Learning to Eat* (Ferguson, 1975). The rationale and principles of behavior modification for weight control are explained. The patients are requested to keep a food diary. They are encouraged to be as specific as possible with regard to the amounts of food eaten and the methods of food preparation. Food models are used to demonstrate portion sizes so that the patient can more accurately assess quantity of food eaten. Patients with specific goals of weight loss are instructed to weigh and measure the food.

Day II
   A. Cue elimination
   B. Energy balance

Each patient's food diary is reviewed by the dietitian at the beginning of class. Any problems with instructions of the mechanics of filling it out are discussed. The importance of learning self-management techniques is emphasized. The new topic "cue elimination" is presented. The relationship of environmental cues to eating is stressed. The following suggestions for reducing the environmental cues are given:

1. Eat only in one designated place.
2. Change the habitual eating place at the table.
3. When eating, do not engage in other activities that compete with the meal (i.e., television, reading, and so forth).
4. Keep all food out of sight.
5. Keep serving dishes with additional food away from the table.

The concept of energy balance is presented. The patients calculate their estimated ideal body weight on the basis of their height. The measurement of body fat is discussed, and the patients receive the results of their skinfold measurements to determine their per cent body fat. Each patient calculates an estimate of his/her energy needs based on his/her basal metabolic rate (BMR), age, and activity using the following method:

BMR = Ideal body weight (in kg) × 24

Correction for age: Subtract 2% for every decade of age after 20

The results are increased by 30% to obtain the estimate of the total caloric requirement for these sedentary people.

The patients are usually fascinated and thus motivated by their individual calculations, and the focus turns to "What do I do to lose (or gain) weight?". The number of kilocalories needed (3,500) to gain or lose a pound is discussed.

The Exchange system (American Diabetes Association, Inc., The American Dietetic Association, 1976) is used as the basis for teaching energy composition of foods. The Exchange system provides a useful tool for the patient to use to keep variety in his or her diet and still be able to estimate the contribution of the energy nutrients. Since patients are keeping daily food diaries, the diaries provide data for patients to practice converting their food intake into the Exchange system. Patterns and menus using the Exchange system to show the ideal distribution of carbohydrate (55 to 60%), protein (10 to 15%), and fat (30%) at various calorie levels are used in class to teach patients to individualize and modify their diets. The recommended kilocalorie intake for each patient is based on the calculated energy needs adjusted for weight loss or gain. The recommended intakes for weight loss usually are approximately 1,500 kilocalories for men and 1,200 kilocalories for women.

The patients are encouraged to consider activity as a method to increase their energy expenditure and the rate of weight loss and increase their sense of well-being. The activities recommended are individualized in that they are based on each patient's exercise prescription. These patients are not able to utilize popular suggestions for increasing activity level as each individual's work load capacity varies depending on cardiac limitations. The conditioning of each patient improves over the period of monitored exercise, and each patient is advised of his/her improved capacity.

Day III
   A. Changing the act of eating
   B. Fats

The food diaries are reviewed, and the dietitian discusses the efforts of each patient to eliminate cues for eating. The next topic, "changing the act of eating," focuses on slowing the rate of eating by introducing delays such as putting the fork down after each bite.

The terms "cholesterol" and "saturated," "monounsaturated," and "polyunsaturated" fats are defined. Food sources of each type of fat are discussed, and suggestions are made to help the patients substitute polyunsaturated fats for saturated ones. The concept of a P/S ratio is discussed and food labels on food products are used to demonstrate the available information. General suggestions for low-fat cooking and recipes incorporating these principles are given. The high-fat content of fast foods is emphasized. The roles of alcohol and simple sugars in the metabolism of triglycerides are explained.

Day IV
   A. Behavior chains and alternate activities
   B. Carbohydrates

The food diaries are reviewed by the dietitian at the beginning of class. The use of exchanges is clarified. The concept that eating is a terminal response to a chain of events and that intervention early in the chain breaks the sequence of events is presented. Alternate activities may be used effectively to break the chain, and the patients are asked to identify a behavior chain in their eating patterns and plan alternate activities to substitute.

The three types of carbohydrates — simple sugars, complex carbohydrates, and fiber — are defined and grouped according to food sources. Many patients have misconceptions of the caloric content of carbohydrates. The dangers of fad diets that restrict carbohydrates are discussed. Nutritive and nonnutritive sweeteners including sugar and honey, saccharin, and aspartame are discussed. Practical suggestions for increasing fiber in the diet are given. The roles of simple sugars and alcohol in the metabolism of triglycerides are reviewed.

Day V
   A. Behavior analysis, progress
   B. Protein

The steps involved in problem solving are discussed:

   1. Observation and long-term goal definition

   2. Identification of specific small problems (short-term goal setting)
   3. Creative problem solving
   4. Decision making
   5. Feedback and evaluation

Included in this lesson are discussions of essential and nonessential amino acids, complete and incomplete proteins, animal and vegetable proteins, and the recommendations for protein in the diet. Also, in this session patients are provided with information on how to combine vegetable proteins and therefore obtain complete proteins. Practical menu suggestions for vegetarian meals are included in the class.

In order to personalize the concept of protein requirements, each patient calculates his or her own protein requirement by multiplying actual body weight in kilograms by 0.8 g. Using the Exchange system, the patients calculate the amount of protein in one day's intake listed in their food diaries and compare their actual intake with their calculated recommended requirement. Most patients are surprised to learn their intake is more than needed. Selection of low-fat, protein-rich foods is encouraged.

Throughout the five lessons thus far, patients have been reminded of the caloric content of the energy nutrients.

Day VI
   A. Preplanning
   B. Minerals

The role of planning dietary intake as a means to control food intake is discussed. The patients are directed to preplan one meal each day to focus on the planning process. Many patients find they have been planning ahead in order to keep their intake within the guidelines.

The minerals are discussed generally in terms of requirements and physiological roles. Patients are given a copy of the *Recommended Dietary Allowances* (RDA) (National Research Council, 1980), and the advised use of these recommendations is explained. The term "United States Recommended Dietary Allowance" is defined, and patients are taught to interpret food labels in terms of their own requirements. Emphasis in the class discussion is on sodium and potassium, calcium, and iron. Patients have various levels of dietary sodium restrictions, so menu patterns ranging from 2,000 mg to 3,000 mg are compared in class. Handouts with sodium and potassium content of foods are provided. Most patients are quite surprised to learn about the sodium content of fast foods and of the sodium added during processing. Samples of food labels are shown to provide examples of evaluating the sodium content of purchased foods. Many patients who are taking thiazide diuretics are delighted to know of other food sources of potassium than bananas. Patients are also encouraged to experiment with herbs and other seasonings in lieu of salt and are given a list of suggested spices and herbs to try at home. Dietary sources of iron and calcium are discussed and criteria for supplementation are given.

Day VII
    A. Energy use, Part I
    B. Vitamins

The role of activity in weight loss is one focus of this lesson. The patients are directed to record their energy expenditures as well as their intakes for one week. The concept of energy balance is reviewed and the following equation is presented:

Energy in (food) = Energy used (activity) + Storage (fat)

The patients are given suggestions for increasing their activity level as they go about their daily living.

In this class also, the patients are again referred to their copy of the RDA for a discussion of adult vitamin requirements. Many patients will ask the dietitian very early in the rehabilitation period if they need to be on a vitamin-mineral supplement. When kilocalories are restricted for weight control below 1,200 for a woman and 1,500 for a man, a vitamin-mineral supplement is advised. In addition, some patients may need specific nutrient supplements such as iron, vitamin C, or calcium. The physiological role of the vitamins, certain conditions that increase the requirement for specific vitamins, natural and synthetic vitamins, and food sources for the various vitamins are discussed.

Day VIII
    A. Energy use, Part II
    B. Problem solving: cooking, dining out, holidays

The patients' food diaries are reviewed, and their activities discussed in the final session. The energy equation is reviewed. Most of the session is focused on implementing dietary recommendations. Recipes and cooking procedures that reduce fat, sugar, and salt are given.

Suggestions for dealing with food-associated holidays are presented. Menus from various restaurants are reviewed, and patients practice selecting appropriate meals.

The patients are encouraged to maintain their new food intake when the structured group sessions end. The usual length of time spent in the monitored exercise program ranges from 12 to 15 weeks. After the group sessions are finished and while the exercise sessions continue, the dietitian and patient review the patient's progress. The patient may then request weekly individual counseling sessions, or the dietitian may suggest that the patient particiate in individual nutritional counseling. Thus, the dietitian may work with the patient during the entire rehabilitation program. Patients trying to lose weight often prefer to indefinitely continue their food diaries with the dietitian reviewing them once a week and monitoring their weight. The dietitian provides a means of support in the effort to change while the patient is gradually gaining confidence in his/her own ability to manage his/her diet. Some patients do not immediately fit into the structured program and need initial individual nutritional counseling prior to entering the series of classes. Or, more commonly, they may need intensive psychological counseling before they can focus on their diets. A few do not function in a group setting and are offered the option of individual counseling. However, these situations are quite rare; the majority of patients quickly perceive that the group environment lends emotional support for learning to change eating behaviors.

The patient's nutritional progress is monitored in various ways. The patient keeps a food diary during the eight weeks of the structured nutrition group sessions. Evaluating the patient's intake each week during the eight group counseling sessions gives prompt feedback as to the patient's progress toward desirable eating habits. Specific recommendations are given with regard to the patient's goals. The patients respond well to concrete suggestions to achieve the dietary recommendations. The weekly review encourages both the patient and the dietitian to set priorities for desired changes and allows them to incorporate them sequentially over a period of time. The opportunity to provide nutritional care during weekly reviews contrasts sharply with the experiences of many dietitians in ambulatory care settings who must assess and counsel the patient in one session and never have the opportunity for follow-up.

The patients weigh themselves prior to each exercise session and the nurse records that weight, thus revealing gain or loss of weight. In the weekly staff meeting, the nurses include weight in their progress reports. The dietitian is available for consultation with the psychologist, physician, nurse, or directly with the patient. Any patient with unexpected weight gain or specific nutritional questions is referred to the dietitian. The exercise sessions provide the opportunity for the nurses to discuss the course of treatment in detail, and often they are the first to perceive a potential problem. The psychologist, in probing for factors that are stressing the patient, may find that some of the stresses are in regard to the family interaction in dietary treatment. The dietitian can clarify the situation by offering additional information to the spouse with regard to shopping or food preparation or by suggesting alternatives to a recommendation that the patient was unable to incorporate into his environment. Most of the problems are a result of communication failure, and the effect of the input of other disciplines results in early detection and removal of obstacles in the progressive course of nutritional care. The weekly staff meeting is essential for integrating medical, psychological, and other information into the nutritional care of the patient.

The psychologist, physician, and nurse specialists all refer patients to the dietitian as nutritional problems arise. Conversely, for nonnutritional problems, the dietitian directs patients appropriately to other staff members. In some instances, the dietitian and psychologist will meet with patients jointly. This has been particularly effective for certain patients having difficulty losing weight due to family or other environmental stresses. Often the physician joins the discussions to emphasize the health problems and needs of the patient. At HCRC the patients are enrolled in a comprehensive rehabilitation program, which, in theory, may result in the patient's feeling overwhelmed at the prospect of quitting smoking, modifying his diet, and exercising in a prescribed schedule in a relatively brief time. However, in practice most, if not all, find that the basic sequential approach to dietary modification and the use of self-monitoring techniques transfer to other problem areas. Conversely, the coping mechanisms and relaxation training given by the psychologist help the patients in their efforts to change their dietary habits.

EXIT

The patient leaves the program when he/she has plateaued with regard to the conditioning process described in Chapters 2, 3, and 16 and no longer is making gains in physical conditioning. He/she then enters a home maintenance program. The exit evaluation by the dietitian provides a formal assessment of the patient's progress toward the nutritional goals and is a transition between the structured program and home maintenance. Data from a 24-hour recall are used to estimate the patient's current dietary intake. The distribution of kilocalories from each of the energy nutrients is calculated and compared to the initial calculations and the recommended distribution of protein, fat, and carbohydrate. The laboratory values obtained during the exit evaluation are compared to those obtained on initial evaluation.

A 20-question posttest similar to the initial nutrition test is completed by each patient in order to assess the patient's understanding of the nutrition principles and concepts that have been presented during the treatment program. It provides a focus for exit counseling if the patient has not understood the principles he/she needs to comply with the dietary recommendations. It also serves to evaluate the treatment program to ensure that it is focused on the desired objectives and presented with effective methods.

The patient's involvement in the dietary treatment and the progress toward defined goals is summarized and documented for the exit report by the dietitian. The patient is encouraged to maintain his/her new eating behaviors after the exit from the program.

FOLLOW-UP

The patient returns one month and three months after exit. He/she is again weighed. The patient may consult with the nutritionist, but there is usually no routine nutritional evaluation scheduled (see Chapter 16). Frequently, a member of the nursing staff will refer the patient to the nutritionist if he/she has questions, or if he/she is gaining weight. There is a formal nutritional evaluation at each successive biannual visit. In each follow-up evaluation, a 24-hour recall is taken, and an interview is structured around the patient's previous dietary problems and the progress in those areas. A problem-oriented approach is frequently helpful to patients who have deviated from the dietary modifications recommended in the program. The nutritional assessment is based on the diet therapy, the progress notes of other members of the professional staff, and the pertinent laboratory values. Any new nutritional problems warrant additional nutritional counseling for the patient.

CASE STUDY

G. S. is a 35-year-old white male who was referred for evaluation at HCRC in August for chief complaints of increasing fatigue, shortness of breath, and chest pain typical of angina. His initial evaluation revealed mild hypertension, presumptive early coronary artery disease, obesity, hyperlipidemia, grade V/VI physiological deconditioning, and moderate anxiety. He was smoking two packages of cigarettes per day.

A nutrition evaluation was conducted as part of the initial evaluation. The diet history revealed a diet with excessive calories in the form of sucrose and saturated fats. It was apparent that the patient as well as his entire family had no regular meal pattern. Most of his meals were eaten in fast-food restaurants with snacks consisting of potato chips, cookies, and other ready-to-eat items. He often omitted meals at usual times and overate at the next mealtime.

The patient stated his nutrition goal was to lose 70 lb. As this goal was desirable, the nutritional care plan contained specific approaches to weight control in addition to the usual recommendations for treatment: (1) involve his wife in nutritional counseling, (2) emphasize the behavior modification techniques to change food habits, and (3) coordinate nutrition goals with the goal for smoking cessation.

He was placed on a 1,500-calorie weight reduction diet restricting total fat, saturated fat, sugars, and alcohol. He attended all eight of the group nutrition classes and kept a food diary throughout his four-month enrollment in the monitored exercise program. His wife attended some of the classes and received nutrition counseling during the beginning phase of the patient's involvement.

The patient participated in all other components of the program. His work load was systematically increased, and he increased his exercise tolerance slightly over 200% during a five-month period. Psychological evaluation at exit revealed that he had reduced both his psychological stresses and smoking. Smoking was

reduced from two packages per day to two to no cigarettes per day.

The following is an example of those data compiled by the dietitian on each patient:

COMPARISON OF INITIAL AND EXIT DATA

	INITIAL	EXIT
Height	6′2½″	6′2½″
Weight	266 lb	219 lb
Estimated ideal weight	193 ± 10%	193 ± 10%
Per cent ideal weight	138%	113%
Per cent body weight as fat	28.5%	23.5%
Total cholesterol	240 mg/dl	204 mg/dl
Triglycerides	235 mg/dl	97 mg/dl
HDL	42 mg/dl	43 mg/dl
Estimated average daily kilocalories	3,300–3,400	1,200–1,300
Estimated % protein as kilocalorie intake	13%	22%
Estimated % carbohydrate as kilocalorie intake	27%	54%
Estimated % fat as kilocalorie intake	56%	24%
Estimated % alcohol as kilocalorie intake	4%	0%
Estimated sodium intake	7,000+ mg	2,500–3,500 mg
Estimated cholesterol intake	600 mg/day	<200 mg/day
Nutrition test score	70%	90%

REFERENCES

American Diabetes Association, Inc., The American Dietetic Association. *Exchange Lists for Meal Planning,* The American Dietetic Association, Chicago, **1976.**

Barlow, D. H., and Tillotson, J. L. Behavioral science and nutrition: A new perspective. *J. Am. Diet. Assoc.,* **1978,** *72,* 368–371.

Carmody, T. P.; Fey, S. G.; Pierce, D. K.; Connor, W. E.; and Matarazzo, J. D. Behavioral treatment of hyperlipidemia: Techniques, results and future directions. *J. Behav. Med.,* **1982,** *5,* 91–116.

Davidson, J. K. Controlling diabetes with dietary therapy. *Postgrad. Ther.,* **1976,** *59,* 114–122.

Evans, R. I., and Hall, Y. Social-psychologic perspective in motivating behavior. *J. Am. Diet. Assoc.,* **1978, 72,** 378–384.

Ferguson, J. *Learning to Eat — Behavior Modification for Weight Control.* Bull Publishing Company, Palo Alto, Ca., **1975.**

Foreyt, J. P.; Goodrick, G. K.; and Gotto, A. M. Limitations of behavioral treatment of obesity: Review and analysis. *J. Behav. Med.,* **1981,** *4,* 159–174.

Foreyt, J. P.; Mitchell, R. E.; Garner, D. T.; Gee, M.; Scott, L. W.; and Gotto, A. M. Behavioral treatment of obesity: Results and limitations. *Behav. Ther.,* **1982,** *13,* 153–161.

Gazda, G. M.; Childers, W. E.; and Walters, R. P. *Interpersonal Communication: A Handbook for Health Professions.* Aspen Systems Corp., Rockville, Md., 1982.

Glueck, C. J., and Connor, W. E. Diet-coronary heart disease relationships reconnoitered. *Am. J. Clin. Nutr.,* **1978,** *31,* 727–733.

Jones, R. J.; Turner, D.; Ginther, J.; Brandt, B.; Slowie, L.; and Lauger, G. A randomized study of instructional variations in nutrition counseling and their efficacy in the treatment of hyperlipidemia. *Am. J. Clin. Nutr.,* **1979,** *32,* 884–904.

Lewin, K. Forces behind food habits and methods of change. In, *The Problem of Changing Food Habits.* National Academy of Science, Natl. Res. Counc. Bull., Washington, D.C., **1943,** 108 (Reprinted 1964).

Lindner, P., and Lindner, D. *How to Assess Degree of Fatness.* Cambridge Scientific Industries, Cambridge, Md., **1973.**

Mahoney, M. J., and Cagguila, A. W. Applying behavioral methods to nutritional counseling. *J. Am. Diet. Assoc.,* **1978,** *72,* 372–377.

McArdle, W. D.; Katch, F. I.; and Katch, V. *Exercise Physiology: Energy, Nutrition and Human Performance.* Lea & Febiger, Philadelphia, **1981,** 368–391.

Modifications in fat content, In, *Handbook of Clinical Dietetics.* American Dietetic Association, Yale University, New Haven, **1981,** E3–E80.

Nutritive Value of American Foods in Common Units. Agriculture Handbook No. 456. Agricultural Research Service, U.S. Department of Agriculture, Washington, D.C., **1975.**

Pennington, J. A. T., and Church, H. N. *Bowes and Church's Food Values of Portions Commonly Used, 13th Edition.* J.B. Lippincott Company, Philadelphia, **1980.**

Stuart, R. B. Behavior control of overeating. *Behav. Res. Ther.,* **1967,** *5,* 357–365.

The National Research Council. *Recommended Dietary Allowances,* 9th Edition, National Academy of Sciences, Washington, D.C., **1980.**

Walker, W. J. Changing United States life-style and declining vascular mortality: Cause or coincidence? *N. Engl. J. Med.,* **1977,** *297,* 163–165.

Wilson, G. T., and Brownell, K. D. Behavior treatment for obesity: An evaluation of treatment outcome. *Adv. Behav. Res. Therap.,* **1980,** *3,* 49–86.

Chapter 11
CORONARY ARTERY DISEASE

Robert J. Hall

GENERAL

Coronary artery disease (CAD) is of epidemic proportion, responsible for over 650,000 deaths annually (Kannel, 1982). The mortality of patients with coronary heart disease increased steadily during the 1950s but reached a plateau in the 1960s. In the decade ending in 1979, CAD mortality declined more than 25% (Kannel, 1982). The occurrence of CAD increases with age, yet pathological studies from the Korean War demonstrated coronary atherosclerotic lesions in 77% of the casualties whose average age was 22 years (Enos *et al.*, 1953). Patients with CAD experience a latent period of variable duration during which there are no symptoms.

Progressive narrowing of the coronary arteries leads to impaired myocardial blood flow with resultant angina, myocardial infarction, or sudden death. Effort angina represents an imbalance between myocardial oxygen demand and coronary artery blood flow, with symptoms occurring at a level of effort expressed usually at a reproducible level of myocardial oxygen demand, as reflected by the product of heart rate and systolic blood pressure (double product). Recent data have supported the additional role of coronary vasomotor activity–spasm and platelet aggregation (Borer, 1980) in the production of rest and unstable angina, nocturnal angina, and perhaps angina occurring during the occasion of psychological or emotional stress (Maseri *et al.*, 1978; Epstein and Talbot, 1981). Short periods of myocardial ischemia occurring during attacks of angina are reversible without apparent myocardial damage, whereas prolonged myocardial ischemia results in myocardial cell death and infarction.

Current information would strongly implicate the role of superimposed thrombosis as a frequent mechanism responsible for the progression of subtotal to total atherosclerotic coronary artery occlusion (Rentrop *et al.*, 1981; Ganz *et al.*, 1981). Complete occlusion of a coronary artery usually results in varying degrees of infarction of the myocardium in the "watershed" of the occluded vessel, depending upon the presence and adequacy of preexisting collateral vessels from other nonobstructed coronary arteries. Under favorable circumstances, total coronary artery occlusion can occur without a recognizable clinical picture of infarction (Kolibash *et al.*, 1982). There may be evidence of residual myocardial damage (clinically silent infarction with electrocardiographic and wall motion abnormality), or there may be no electrocardiographic or wall motion abnormality. Coronary occlusion also can produce lesser degrees of nontransmural or subendocardial infarction or can result in an episode of prolonged coronary insufficiency producing intense myocardial ischemia but without infarction evident by ECG or enzyme elevation —the so-called "intermediate coronary syndrome." Conversely, one may observe evidence of a ventricular segmental wall motion abnormality of prior infarction at angiography, with varying degrees of subtotal occlusion of the proximal coronary artery or, at times, a normal proximal coronary artery (Kolibash et al., 1982). This would indicate that infarction may occur under certain circumstances of stress, without complete occlusion; or that transient complete occlusion, resulting from spasm and/or thrombosis precipitated the acute infarction with subsequent relaxation of spasm and spontaneous thrombolysis or recanalization of the proximally occluded coronary lumen (DeWood, et al., 1980). Our understanding of these complex interrelations of atherosclerotic coronary occlusive disease, spasm, thrombosis, and collateral supply has evolved and continues to grow since the introduction, and the widespread use, of coronary angiography.

Predictors of Survival

The determinants of long-term survival of patients with CAD has been the subject of studies for many years. Most studies, based upon coronary and ventricular angiographic staging, relate long-term survival to two factors: (1) The extent of CAD present, usually expressed as a single or multivessel involvement, and (2) the amount and severity of myocardial damage, expressed by the extent and severity of regional wall motion abnormalities, by the ejection fraction, or by the magnitude of deranged left ventricular hemodynamics (Proudfit et al., 1978; Harris et al., 1979; Mock et al., 1982; and Sanz et al., 1982). An additional determinant of long-term survival is electrical instability of the ventricular myocardium which can result in ventricular ectopy, tachycardia, and fibrillation. Although ventricular electrical instability occurs and causes death in a number of patients with an acute myocardial infarction, it is also the mechanism of sudden death in many patients with chronic CAD (Kotler et al., 1973; Kannel et al., 1975; Moss et al., 1979; Ruberman et al., 1981). Electrical instability parallels the extent of coronary disease and the magni-

tude of myocardial damage which interrelates this determinant to (1) and (2) mentioned previously (Lie and Titus, 1975; Perper et al., 1975). It is important to note that patients who experience sudden death as the first expression of CAD, or during the course of a first infarction without prior symptoms, are not considered in any of the natural history studies of symptomatic index populations staged by coronary angiography and left ventriculography.

DIAGNOSIS OF CAD

Symptoms

Coronary disease is usually diagnosed readily by the classic symptoms of angina pectoris or by recognition of the symptoms of a current or remote myocardial infarction. There is no problem in identifying angina pectoris expressed as typical retrosternal pressure pain radiating to the arm(s), recurring with a reproducible degree of exercise and relieved by rest in a 5-to-15-minute interval. Atypical isolated posterior chest, epigastric, neck, jaw, shoulder, or arm pain, or "discomfort," may be recognized less readily unless the causal and reproducible relationship to exertion, stressful events, or the postprandial state is elicited. Often the patient will deny *chest pain* only to admit a *constriction* or *tightness* in the chest, or a sense of shortness of breath with effort. At times only a vague sense of profound weakness, and perhaps some dyspnea, is the only expression of effort-induced coronary insufficiency. Inordinate fatigue, albeit mostly nonspecific, is a common expression of severe CAD; and I have seen fatigue, irritability, and personality aberrancies on occasion precede a first infarction as the only symptoms.

Angina is considered unstable when symptoms occur with increasing frequency and with little provocation, at rest, or awaken the patient from sleep. Although one half of the patients who present with an acute infarction report no history of prior angina, the others will have had chronic stable angina, chronic angina with recent increase and an unstable pattern, or recent new onset angina (Harper et al., 1979).

Physical Examination

The examination usually reveals few or no abnormalities. Presence of a corneal arcus, especially in a younger patient, is suggestive of atherosclerotic disease (Rosenman et al., 1974), as is a horizontal skin crease on the ear pinna (Frank, 1973; Haft et al., 1979). Similarly, there may be pulse discrepancies or arterial bruits associated with concomitant peripheral arterial atherosclerosis. Varying degrees of obesity and systemic hypertension are common. The heart is usually normal in size, and the point of maximal intensity is normal in position. A presystolic atrial sound (S_4) is nearly always present and is commonly palpable. The patient's anxiety concerning the physical examination occasionally may provoke rest angina during which time the clinician may appreciate augmentation of the fourth sound, new appearance of an early diastolic filling sound (S_3), and, occasionally, a blowing apical holosystolic or late systolic murmur of mitral regurgitation—all of which disappear promptly after administration of a sublingual nitroglycerin tablet. Visible and palpable evidence of dyskinesia of the ventricle also may be observed transiently in the area of the chest at, above, or medial to the apex during spontaneous angina, especially if the patient is positioned in a semi–left lateral position. Facial anxiety, pallor, and diaphoresis may be additional clues to spontaneous angina during the examination. In the presence of a current or remote myocardial infarction, ventricular enlargement, visible and/or palpable dyskinesia, and/or dyssynergia, a third heart sound and mitral regurgitation are not uncommon; and in the presence of advanced myocardial dysfunction, features of left or biventricular failure may be prominent.

Electrocardiogram

In patients with angina without infarction, results of the resting electrocardiogram (ECG) are usually normal, although atrial abnormalities (P-wave notching or definite evidence of left atrial enlargement) may be present; and, if hypertension coexists, ECG evidence of left ventricular hypertrophy is likely to be present. The transient ECG pattern of "subendocardial injury" (diffuse horizontal ST-segment depression) accompanies spontaneous anginal attacks or induced ischemia during diagnostic exercise testing; and variable degrees of ST depression may be present at rest, in the absence of digitalis or left ventricular hypertrophy in some patients, especially in those with more advanced CAD. Episodes of rest angina may be accompanied by either ST-segment depression or elevation (Maseri et al., 1978), and transient recurrent episodes of ST elevation may accompany both symptomatic and asymptomatic periods of myocardial ischemia due to vasospastic

angina (Prinzmetal or variant angina) (Prinzmetal et al., 1959; Braunwald, 1981; Brown, 1981; Kirshenbaum et al., 1981). Such episodes may occur secondary to coronary vasospasm without coronary occlusive disease or in association with varying degrees of atherosclerotic coronary occlusive disease (Brown, 1981) and are commonly accompanied by ventricular ectopy, ventricular tachycardia, sinus bradycardia, and varying degrees of atrioventricular block. Ventricular fibrillation and sudden death may occur (Brown, 1981). These disturbances are recognized most often by means of continuous hospital electrocardiographic monitoring or dynamic ambulatory ECG (Holter) monitoring records. At present, there is ample evidence suggestive that recurrent rest angina in patients with CAD is often, if not always, due to vasospastic changes superimposed upon fixed atherosclerotic coronary artery lesions (Kirshenbaum et al., 1981).

In the presence of a remote, or current, acute myocardial infarction, classic ECG changes are evident (Savage et al., 1977). Nontransmural or subendocardial infarction may be accompanied by only ST- and T-wave changes with elevated cardiac enzyme levels, usually to a level less than that of a classic transmural infarction. An episode of prolonged coronary insufficiency without infarction may be manifested by localized T-wave inversion (ischemic T changes) of hours' or several days' duration with minimal or, more commonly, without laboratory evidence of elevated serum myocardial enzyme levels. Right bundle branch block will not obscure the recognition of an acute or an old myocardial infarction. Recognition of an infarction, however, in the presence of a left bundle branch block is difficult, and the presence of a Q deformity usually is not diagnostic.

Chest Roentgenogram

Most patients with CAD have a normal chest roentgenogram. The cardiac size and silhouette may be altered by preexisting left ventricular hypertrophy, usually due to coexisting hypertension or valvular heart disease or by current or remote myocardial infarction. One or even several remote infarctions may not appreciably alter the size of the cardiac silhouette, unless there is sufficient myocardial damage to cause formation of a left ventricular aneurysm or dilatation of the left ventricular chamber which ultimately would produce not only cardiac enlargement but the additional features of congestive failure. These include an increase in pulmonary venous markings and, at times, pulmonary edema. When left ventricular failure is long standing and severe, pulmonary hypertension results with secondary right heart enlargement and failure.

Noninvasive Diagnostic Testing: Exercise Stress Testing

In most instances, the diagnosis of CAD is readily made by the recognition of classic angina or by clinical and electrocardiographic confirmation of current or prior myocardial infarction. Various methods of exercise testing have been developed to elicit the presence of occult coronary disease in asymptomatic populations and to clarify the etiology of atypical chest pain syndromes. Progressive accumulation of knowledge about exercise test results in patients with CAD makes it clear that the character of the response to exercise may be predictive of the extent of CAD and, to certain degrees, the prognosis (Ellestad and Wan, 1975; Goldschlager *et al.*, 1976; McNeer *et al.*, 1978).

The efficacy of any test in identifying the presence of a disease state in a test population is expressed as *sensitivity* (the percentage of times the test result is positive when the disease state is present), *specificity* (the percentage of individuals with an abnormal test who have the disease state), and *relative risk* of an abnormal test (the risk of having the disease state if the test result is abnormal as compared to having the disease state if the test response is normal) (Table 11-1). As with all forms of testing, it has long been appreciated that both false-positive as well as false-negative tests may result when exercise testing is used in the detection of CAD. Recently, the application of Bayes' theorem to exercise test results has been appreciated (Ep-

stein, 1980). Simply stated, exercise testing, with a known frequency of false-positive responses, yields widely disparate predictive accuracy when applied to younger populations in which the prevalence of CAD is low, in contrast to older populations in which the prevalence of CAD is progressively higher. Although application of Bayes' theorem (Kannel, 1982) to exercise testing for CAD is relatively recent, its principles have long been understood in the clinical interpretation of the symptom of chest pain. In a relatively young population in which CAD is infrequent, chest pain is usually suggestive of diverse etiologies other than CAD. The converse is true in an older population, perhaps in part explaining the relative high specificity attributable to the history alone in the diagnosis of CAD. This, nonetheless, is not meant to detract from the value of a careful history, especially as it establishes a distinctive pattern and the reproducibility of a pain syndrome to some specific provocation, usually a certain magnitude of physical effort.

Exercise testing was first used to measure the overall condition of the circulatory system, with observation made of the pulse rate and blood pressure response to a calibrated amount of effort (Master, 1935). The amount of effort was standardized to the number of ascents and descents over steps of a standard height at a prescribed rate of speed. Provocation of classic angina during the test and recognition of electrocardiographic ST-segment depression during the period immediately following exercise led to popularization of the Master two-step exercise test for identifying CAD in an asymptomatic population or confirming the diagnosis in the presence of atypical or confusing symptoms (Mattingly, 1962; Robb and Marks, 1967). Prognostication of life survival or coronary events was derived from such testing of asymptomatic groups (Arnow and Cassidy, 1975). At the same time the diagnostic importance of *linear ST depression* was recognized, in contrast to *junctional depression* with an up-sloping ST segment, which bore little predictive value to the existence of CAD (Mattingly, 1962). A shortcoming of the Master two-step exercise test, as it was originally employed, consisted of electrocardiographic recording before and after, but not during, the exercise period.

Further simplification and standardization of exercise testing ensued with the use of the motorized treadmill or a stationary bicycle to graduate and calibrate the exercise load deliv-

---

Table 11-1. EFFICACY OF DIAGNOSTIC TESTING

$$\text{Sensitivity} = \frac{\text{TP}}{\text{TP} + \text{FN}} \times 100$$

$$\text{Specificity} = \frac{\text{TN}}{\text{FP} + \text{TN}} \times 100$$

$$\text{Predictive value} = \frac{\text{TP}}{\text{TP} + \text{FP}} \times 100$$

$$\text{Relative risk} = \frac{\text{TP}}{\text{TP} + \text{FP}} \bigg/ \frac{\text{FN}}{\text{TN} + \text{FN}}$$

TP = True positive (abnormal test result with disease state).
FN = False negative (normal test result with disease state).
TN = True negative (normal test result without disease state).
FP = False positive (abnormal test result without disease state).

ered. Simultaneous development of improved ECG lead and recording systems has facilitated ECG monitoring during the period of exercise as well as during the recovery period. Current electrocardiographic exercise-testing techniques, with either a treadmill or upright bicycle ergometry, usually include a 12-lead ECG (placement of the limb lead electrodes is modified to positions on the trunk to circumvent limb motion artifact), multichannel ECG recording, and cathode-ray oscilloscopic ECG monitoring, as well as indirect cuff sphygmomanometry for periodic recording of blood pressure. Although the risk of exercise testing in an asymptomatic population is low, the risk increases slightly as more patients with known CAD are tested. A review of 170,000 tests from 73 centers disclosed 16 fatal and 40 nonfatal complications associated with exercise testing, a mortality of 10 deaths per 100,000 tests and a morbidity rate of 24 instances per 100,000 tests (Rochmis and Blackburn, 1971). Other large series, totaling more than 41,000 patients, disclosed a combined mortality of 2.4 per 100,000 patients and a morbidity rate of 17 per 100,000 patients (Sheffield and Reeves, 1965; Bruce *et al.*, 1968; Kattus *et al.*, 1968; Ellestad *et al.*, 1969; Doyle and Kinch, 1970; Jelinek and Lown, 1974; McHenry *et al.*, 1974). Among 35,300 patients who underwent exercise stress testing during a period of 10 years in our laboratory, three patients sustained a myocardial infarction, and one patient died after the test.

Test safety is enhanced by careful evaluation of the patient before, and close monitoring of the patient and physiological variables during, the test procedure. Most exercise-testing facilities, including ours, require a signed, informed consent from the patient before the test. A brief history is obtained and pertinent examination is performed before the test, with particular attention paid to any change in symptoms tht may have occurred since the prior assessment. A baseline 12-lead ECG is recorded before the test, and the results are *compared* with previously recorded ECGs to ascertain whether any change has occurred. The ECG is then recorded with the patient in the standing position and again after 30 seconds of hyperventilation. Both maneuvers, especially the latter, may produce a nonspecific ST-segment shift unrelated to exercise stress which serves as the baseline with which stress-induced changes are compared. Various graded exercise test protocols are followed (Table 11-2), which vary mainly in the length of time at each level and

the rapidity with which the patient is advanced to higher levels.

We employ the Bruce protocol in which the grade and walking speed are advanced in three-minute stages. The ECG, displayed oscilloscopically, is monitored continuously during the rest, and an ECG record is made each minute during exercise and recovery. The blood pressure is also recorded each minute. A symptom-limited maximal exercise test has been used in healthy men (Bruce *et al.*, 1980); or the test may be terminated after achieving either 85 to 90% (submaximal test) or 100% of the maximum predicted heart rate for the individual (Table 11-3). The test is terminated earlier if the patient develops generalized physical or leg exhaustion, unusual dyspnea, progressive angina (usually 2+ severity on a scale of 1+ to 3+), an inappropriate rise or a fall of systolic blood pressure with progressive exercise, significant arrhythmia (frequent ventricular ectopy, especially if of multiform morphology or in volleys of three or more beats, or rapid supraventricular tachycardia), or linear ST-segment depression 2 mm below that recorded in the control tracings. The test should also be terminated if the patient shows signs of circulatory insufficiency, i.e., pallor or clammy perspiration. Exercise-induced ST-segment elevation may occur in leads reflecting Q waves of a prior infarction and is of no particular diagnostic significance. ST-segment elevation during exercise in a patient with a normal resting ECG signifies serious transmural ischemia and should prompt immediate termination of the test. Such ST-segment elevation has been associated with either exercise-induced coronary vasospasm (Specchia *et al.*, 1981; de Servi *et al.*, 1981; Waters *et al.*, 1982) or high-grade proximal fixed coronary occlusive disease (Longhurst and Kraus, 1979; Dunn *et al.*, 1981).

Exercise ECG tests are considered positive for CAD if exercise results in horizontal or down-sloping ST-segment depression 1 mm or more below the baseline during exercise or in the postexercise ECG recordings. When the control ECG demonstrates abnormal ST depression, additional exercise-induced depression of 1.5 to 2 mm is required for a positive test. False-positive ST-segment depression occurs in the presence of left ventricular hypertrophy, digitalis ingestion, or hypokalemia — conditions known to alter the ST segment. Less readily understood are false-positive tests in some individuals with the mitral valve prolapse

Table 11-2. OXYGEN REQUIREMENTS FOR STEP, TREADMILL, AND BICYCLE ERGOMETER*

FUNCTIONAL CLASS	METS	O₂ REQUIREMENTS ML O₂/KG/MIN	STEP TEST — NAGLE-BALKE-NAUGHTON† (2-min stages, 30 steps/min; step height increased 4 cm q 2 min) Height (cm)	TREADMILL — BRUCE‡ (3-min stages) mph / % gr	TREADMILL — KATTUS** (3-min stages) mph / % gr	TREADMILL — BALKE†† % grade at 3.4 mph	TREADMILL — BALKE†† % grade at 3 mph	BICYCLE ERGOMETER†† For 70-kg body weight kgm/min
Normal and I	16	56.0				26		
	15	52.5				24		
	14	49.0			4 / 22	22		
	13	45.5		4.2 / 16		20		1500
	12	42.0	40		4 / 18	18	22.5	1350
	11	38.5	36			16	20.0	1200
	10	35.0	32	3.4 / 14	4 / 14	14	17.5	1050
	9	31.5	28			12	15.0	900
	8	28.0	24		4 / 10	10	12.5	750
	7	24.5	20	2.5 / 12	3 / 10	8	10.0	600
II	6	21.0	16			6	7.5	450
	5	17.5	12	1.7 / 10	2 / 10	4	5.0	300
III	4	14.0	8			2	2.5	150
	3	10.5	4				0.0	
	2	7.0						
IV	1	3.5						

Note: Oxygen requirements increase with work loads from bottom of chart to top in various exercise tests of the step, treadmill, and bicycle ergometer types.

* From *Exercise Standards Book,* © American Heart Association, 1979. Reproduced with permission.

† Nagle, F. S.; Balke, B.; and Naughton, J. P. Gradational step tests for assessing work capacity. *J. Appl. Physiol.,* **1965,** *20,* 745–748.

‡ Bruce, R. A.; Kusmi, F.; and Hosmer, D. Maximal oxygen intake and nomographic assessment of functional aerobic impairment in cardiovascular disease. *Am. Heart J.,* **1973,** *85,* 546.

** Kattus, A. A.; Jorgensen, C. R.; Worden, R. E.; Alvaro, A. B. S-T segment depression with near-maximal exercise in detection of preclinical coronary heart disease. *Circulation,* **1971,** *41,* 585–595.

†† Fox, S. M.; Naughton, J. P.; Haskell, W. L. Physical activity and the prevention of coronary heart disease. *Ann. Clin. Res.,* **1971,** *3,* 404.

Table 11-3. AGES AND MAXIMAL HEART RATE (MHR)*†

AGE	MHR	AGE	MHR	AGE	MHR
20	200	37	185	54	171
21	199	38	184	55	171
22	198	39	183	56	170
23	197	40	182	57	170
24	196	41	181	58	169
25	195	42	180	59	168
26	194	43	180	60	168
27	193	44	180	61	167
28	192	45	179	62	167
29	191	46	177	63	166
30	190	47	177	64	165
31	190	48	177	65	164
32	189	49	176	66	163
33	188	50	175	67	162
34	187	51	174	68	161
35	186	52	173	69	161
36	186	53	172	70	160

* Mean maximum heart rates used as a guide for determining approximate end-point of stress.

† From Ellestad, M. H. *Stress Testing: Principles and Practice,* 2nd ed. F. A. Davis Co., Philadelphia, **1980**, p. 160.

syndrome (Gardin *et al.*, 1980) and in some apparently otherwise normal individuals. Although exercise-induced ST-segment depression has diagnostic significance in the presence of a right bundle branch block, the presence of a left bundle branch block invalidates interpretation of ST-segment shift secondary to exercise (Orzan *et al.*, 1978). If the exclusions cited previously are observed, especially if the resting ECG is normal, specificity of abnormal ST depression exceeds 90%. Sensitivity, however, is as low as 50% in patients with single-vessel disease, 70% in patients with double-vessel disease, and 90% in patients with triple-vessel CAD (Garcia *et al.*, 1975).

The predictive value of the ECG-exercise test for CAD, or any noninvasive and hence less-than-perfect diagnostic test, is dependent upon the present likelihood of the presence of the disease (Bayes' theorem) (Epstein and Talbot, 1981). In young asymptomatic individuals with low pretest likelihood of CAD, the predictive value of the test is low, and the false-positive ratio is high. Hence, the test has limited value in such groups of individuals. Nevertheless, even in asymptomatic individuals, the predictive value of exercise testing increases when the pretest likelihood of CAD is increased by the concomitant existence of other risk factors (Bruce *et al.*, 1980). In general, for predictive purposes, exercise testing is not indicated in asymptomatic men without other risk factors.

However, such testing may serve to establish a baseline of functional performance and limitations for comparisons with subsequent testing.

If the exercise ECG test is viewed solely as an epidemiological tool, the shortcomings in sensitivity are bothersome. If, however, the test is used as a functional measure of the residual perfusion abnormality to the viable myocardium in a patient known to have CAD, the test has considerable clinical value. Various investigators (Ellestad and Wan, 1975; McNeer *et al.*, 1978) have related positivity of the test at progressively lower exercise levels to a proportionately less favorable outcome, based upon the occurrence of subsequent coronary events or death (Figure 11-1). In the latter study (McNeer *et al.*, 1978), individuals with CAD could be subdivided into low- and high-risk subsets based upon certain exercise test endpoints. Most patients with a positive test in stage I or II of the Bruce protocol had significant CAD, with the majority demonstrating three-vessel or left main CAD. A low-risk subset of patients was identified who were able to exercise to stage IV or were able to achieve a maximum heart rate of 160 beats per minute or more, and/or had a negative exercise test. This subset had such a favorable actuarial survival that aggressive therapy to enhance survival did not appear justified. Patients with exercise limitations in stage I or II, or who had low heart rates below 120 beats per minute had a poor prognosis and were candidates for more aggressive therapy (Figure 11-2). ST-segment depression persisting past eight minutes into the recovery period, as well as onset of ST depression in the first three minutes of the test, has also been correlated with a high frequency of multivessel or left main CAD (Goldschlager *et al.*, 1976). Failure to achieve an appropriate increase in heart rate with exercise (chronotropic incompetence) (Ellestad and Wan, 1975) or, more important, a decrease of blood pressure with continuing exercise is indicative of the existence of CAD and, in the latter circumstance, usually severe CAD (Bruce *et al.*, 1959; Thompson and Kelemen, 1975; Morris *et al.*, 1978). It is apparent that it is no longer appropriate to designate an ECG exercise test as only positive or negative. The test must be characterized by the duration and stage of the testing achieved, the peak heart rate and blood pressure reached, the percentage of predicted maximum heart rate achieved, the development of angina and ST-segment changes reached and their time of occurrence, and the duration of

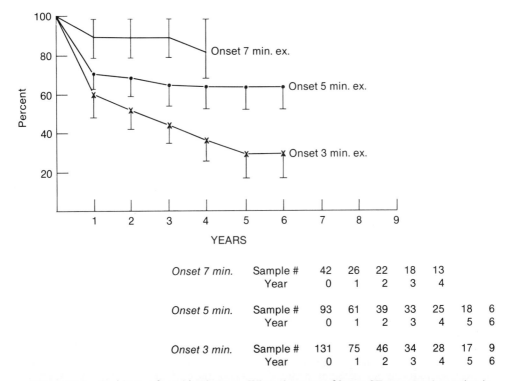

Onset 7 min.	Sample #	42	26	22	18	13		
	Year	0	1	2	3	4		
Onset 5 min.	Sample #	93	61	39	33	25	18	6
	Year	0	1	2	3	4	5	6
Onset 3 min.	Sample #	131	75	46	34	28	17	9
	Year	0	1	2	3	4	5	6

Figure 11-1. Incidence of combined events. When the onset of 2-mm ST-segment depression is at 3 min or before, the prognosis is significantly worse than when it is manifested first at 5 mins. When ST depression is first manifested at 7 mins, which is near peak capacity, the incidence of coronary events is only slightly greater than those with a negative test. (From Ellestad, M. H., and Wan, M. K. C. Predictive implication of stress testing: Follow-up of 2700 subjects after maximum treadmill stress testing. *Circulation,* **1975,** *51,* 363–369. By permission of the American Heart Association, Inc.)

ST changes into the recovery period (Dagenais *et al.,* 1981). Production of ventricular ectopy during exercise also denotes significant exercise-induced myocardial ischemia (Goldschlager *et al.,* 1973). Used in a knowledgeable fashion, the exercise ECG test can provide a great deal of functional and prognostic information for evaluating patients with CAD.

Exercise Testing Soon After Myocardial Infarction. Exercise testing recently has been employed in the predischarged phase of patients with *uncomplicated* myocardial infarctions (Epstein *et al.,* 1982). With a protocol modified both in duration and total work load, the patients' response can be tested to levels of exercise which they have either already achieved in the hospital or can be expected to progressively achieve upon discharge from the hospital. Such objective testing has considerable value, reassuring to both the patient and the physician. Provocation of arrhythmias or

angina enables the physician to better prescribe antiarrhythmic and antianginal therapy upon discharge of the patient. Additionally, it has been demonstrated that production of an ischemic ST-segment abnormality by this modified exercise challenge early in the postinfarction period distinguishes a high- from a low-risk subset with nearly a tenfold difference of mortality in the first year after infarction. This high-risk subset of patients should undergo further invasive testing to determine the best methods of subsequent management.

Nuclear Cardiology (see Chapter 13)

Exercise tests employing radionuclide isotopes are also used extensively in the evaluation of patients with CAD. Myocardial perfusion imaging utilizes the intravenous injection of thallium-201 at peak levels of exercise to demonstrate stress-induced myocardial perfusion defects (Ritchie, 1982). Radionuclide an-

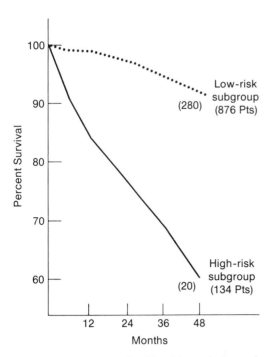

100

90

Percent Survival

80

70

60

Low-risk
subgroup
(280) (876 Pts)

High-risk
subgroup
(20) (134 Pts)

12   24   36   48

Months

Figure 11-2. Cumulative life-table survival rates in low- and high-risk subgroups. Numbers in parentheses represent the number of patients followed for 48 months. Numbers in brackets represent the number of patients in each subgroup. Low-risk subgroup includes patients with a negative test or exercise duration $\geq$ stage IV and/or a maximum heart rate $\geq$ 160. High-risk subgroup includes patients with a positive test and exercise duration $<$ stage III. (From McNeer, J. C.; Margolis, J. R.; Lee, K. L.; *et al.* The role of the exercise test in the evaluation of patients for ischemic heart disease. *Circulation,* **1978,** *57,* 64–70. By permission of the American Heart Association, Inc.)

giograms, using ^{99m}technetium pertechnetate-labeled red blood cells, can be generated by the first transit method or by the equilibrium gated blood pool technique (Asinger *et al.,* 1981). These techniques permit evaluation of ventricular function characterized by global function (ejection fraction and volumes) and by segmental wall motion. Stress-induced abnormalities are indicative of reversible myocardial ischemia. Both myocardial perfusion imaging and radionuclide angiographic exercise stress testing have higher sensitivity and specificity in diagnosing the presence of CAD than exercise electrocardiographic testing alone (Ritchie, 1982; Strauss and Boucher, 1982). Although the concept of pretest probability of CAD is also applicable to radionuclide exercise testing,

it is suggested that the sensitivity and specificity of thallium perfusion imaging are preserved even when the pretest likelihood of CAD is low (Ritchie, 1982). Although more expensive than conventional ECG exercise testing, radionuclide exercise testing provides a considerable contribution when the standard ECG stress test is indeterminate and when there are major abnormalities in the resting ECG that make interpretation of changes due to exercise difficult. Both methods of radionuclide exercise testing, but especially gated blood pool ventriculography, also have definite limitations in patients with left bundle branch block (Rowe *et al.,* 1982). Radionuclide exercise testing can be useful in characterizing functional significance of coronary artery stenosis, the severity of which is indeterminate by coronary angiography.

Echocardiography

M-mode echocardiographic imaging of the heart has distinct limitations in patients with CAD, a disease characterized by segmental wall motion abnormalities. Global abnormalities, as well as those of the interventricular septum and the posterior wall, may be identified (Popp, 1982). Two-dimensional (2-D) echocardiography imaging, however, yields considerable information about the segmental wall motion in patients with CAD (Henry, 1982). Hypokinetic, akinetic, and dyskinetic areas can be identified with reasonable ease in the 75% of the patients who have a satisfactory echo window. Intracavitary thrombi can be identified with considerable confidence (Asinger *et al.,* 1981; Stratton *et al.,* 1982; Visser *et al.,* 1983). Recognition of changes in wall motion after an intervention such as coronary artery bypass is also possible (Rubenson *et al.,* 1982). Recently 2-D echo imaging has been used successfully to identify segmental wall deterioration with exercise in patients with CAD. Although this form of exercise testing has not undergone the extensive evaluation that has been applied to the standard ECG-treadmill test and exercise-radionuclide tests, it holds promise for the future.

INVASIVE DIAGNOSTIC TESTING

The technique of selective coronary angiography, which permits direct visualization of the lumen of the coronary arteries (Sones and Shirey, 1962), opened a new era in the understanding and treatment of patients with CAD. Coronary angiography, coupled with left ventriculography for assessing left ventricular function, provides strong information of prognostic importance and the standards by which noninvasive testing techniques are compared.

Cardiac Catheterization and Coronary Angiography

Although many laboratories confine studies to retrograde arterial catheterization of the left ventricle and selective coronary angiography, simultaneous venous catheterization can provide considerable additional information concerning right heart, pulmonary artery, and pulmonary wedge pressures. Continuous monitoring of left ventricular filling pressure, as reflected by the pulmonary pressure, also adds to the safety of coronary angiography, especially in patients with unstable angina (Salem et al., 1979). Arterial catheterization is accomplished by brachial artery cut-down (Sones, 1959) or by percutaneous needle and guide-wire entry into the femoral artery (Seldinger, 1953; Judkins, 1967). Retrograde catheter passage through the aortic valve allows measurement of left ventricular pressure and the cine recording of the left ventricular angiogram by opacification of the chamber with a contrast medium containing iodine. The roentgenographic images most commonly are recorded on 35-mm cine film at 30 to 60 frames per second, using a high-gain image intensifier x-ray tube. Biplane ventriculographic imaging in the right anterior and left anterior oblique projections provides the most information about global and regional left ventricular wall motion and permits each left ventricular segment to be characterized as normal, hypokinetic, akinetic, or dyskinetic. The systolic and diastolic volumes of the ventricle can be measured (Dodge et al., 1960) and the overall ejection fraction of the left ventricle calculated (Dodge, 1974). Left ventriculography also provides information about the presence and the degree of mitral regurgitation, which may coexist with CAD as a consequence of dysfunction or infarction of a papillary muscle or of the ventricular myocardium at its base. The left and right coronary arteries are then selectively catheterized and opacified by hand injections of small amounts of contrast medium and cine filmed in multiple views. The coronary angiogram essentially is a lumenogram and demonstrates the distribution, extent, and severity of narrowing and/or occlusion of the coronary artery and provides information about coronary collateral flow. X-ray tube configurations permitting cranial-caudal angulation significantly improve visualization of the left main

and proximal left anterior descending coronary arteries, as well as the branches of the right coronary artery at the crux, by eliminating overlap of vessels created by conventional frontal and oblique views which cause difficulty in interpretation (Bunnell et al., 1973; Lesperance et al., 1974; Sos et al., 1974; Gomes et al., 1982). The importance of quality television video monitoring of every injection and the facilities for instant video playback cannot be emphasized strongly enough. These factors are paramount in achieving superior diagnostic studies.

Occlusion of the coronary arteries is characterized by location, extent, and degree of diameter narrowing, usually expressed as a percentage of reduction of lumen diameter compared to an uninvolved adjacent segment of the vessel (AHA Committee Report, 1975). (Note that a 50% diameter narrowing is equivalent to a 75% cross-sectional reduction of lumen area.) The eccentric character of many atherosclerotic lesions requires that diseased segments be evaluated in several views since oval or slitlike lesions may appear different when viewed in two projections perpendicular to each other. It is also important for the angle of the x-ray beam to be as near perpendicular to the coronary vessel as possible; otherwise, a short segmental narrowing can be obscured by overlap of the adjacent normal vessel. Cranial-caudal angulation facilitates obtaining perpendicular views of the proximal left coronary system. Although coronary atherosclerosis has a major segmental distribution, with a propensity for lesions to occur in the proximal portions of the coronary arteries, the process is frequently diffuse, and the ratio of narrowed segment to an "apparent" normal segment may underestimate the extent and degree of luminal obstruction (Zir et al., 1976; Arnett et al., 1979). Conversely, in a small percentage of coronary angiograms studied, varying degrees of ectasia and aneurysmal dilation of the major proximal coronary vessels are noted (Markis et al., 1976), usually with areas of interspersed narrowing, often creating a "sausage-link" pattern. In these circumstances, quantitating the severity and functional significance of individual points of narrowing can be difficult, and the tendency for overlap of the tortuous ectatic segment can interfere with the proper identification of short segmental occlusive lesions.

The coronary anatomy is subject to a considerable variation in vascular distribution. The right coronary artery (RCA), as it courses around the right atrioventricular groove, usually gives off a vessel to the sinoatrial node and several other vessels which supply the free wall of the right ventricle. The RCA is considered "dominant" if it gives origin to the posterior descending coronary artery at the inferior atrioventricular crux, a condition that prevails in approximately 90% of patients studied. Additionally, there is usually a moderate-size posterior left ventricular branch of the RCA serving a portion of the inferior wall of the left ventricle beyond the crux. At times, the RCA is "superdominant" and gives origin to a cascade of three or four branches supplying a considerable portion of the inferolateral portion of the left ventricle.

The left main coronary artery is short and divides quickly into the left anterior descending and circumflex coronary arteries. The former gives off prominent septal perforator branches and, usually, several diagonal branches. The circumflex coronary artery usually gives off several arcuate marginal branches supplying the lateral and posterior wall of the left ventricle. In 10% of individuals, the left coronary system is "dominant," and a large circumflex coronary artery continues in the left atrioventricular groove to the crux and gives origin to the posterior descending coronary artery. The RCA under these circumstances is a small vessel with only right ventricular branches and does not contribute to the supply of blood to the left ventricular myocardium. A codominant system is present when both the right and the circumflex coronary arteries supply a vessel along the posterior interventricular groove.

Atherosclerotic narrowing can vary from minor luminal irregularities, through all degrees of vessel narrowing, to total occlusion of a vessel. When a coronary artery is completely occluded, the vessel distal to the occlusion is almost invariably opacified by one of several collateral routes—albeit at a slower rate, and usually with less density, than normal. Collateral vessels may bridge around an obstruction, filling the distal vessel in a prograde manner, or more commonly, the obstructed vessel is filled retrogradely during opacification of the remaining intact ipsilateral vessels or upon injection of contrast medium into the contralateral coronary artery. Although most of the collateral connections are too small for imaging, there are frequent examples in which large tortuous collateral vessels are visualized over the atria, around the atrioventricular groove, through the atrial or ventricular septum, or

anteriorly across the right ventricular outflow tract. In our experience collateral filling of a vessel, distal to a narrowed segment, is *never observed angiographically* unless the proximal obstruction is total or subtotal (95% or greater narrowing).

Although total obstruction of a coronary artery is usually accompanied by a major left ventricular wall motion abnormality distal to the obstruction, on many occasions the regional wall motion may be normal or the abnormality is minimal. In these latter instances, narrowing and ultimate total occlusion of the coronary artery apparently progressed gradually, permitting collateral flow to develop and maintain normal or near-normal viability of the distal recipient myocardial bed. In other patients, a single proximal occlusion is accompanied by a large area of akinesia with serious left ventricular thinning or actual dyskinesia (aneurysm). In these latter circumstances, progression to total occlusion must have occurred during a short period, providing little time for collateral circulation to develop and preserve myocardial viability beyond the point of obstruction. Even in these patients, subsequent angiography demonstrates that the occluded vessel beyond the point of obstruction is almost invariably opacified by collateral flow, albeit such collateral flow developed too slowly to protect the viability of the myocardium. In other patients, a major wall motion abnormality of prior infarction may exist in the distribution of a narrowed, yet still patent, coronary artery. Infarction and consequent production of regional wall motion abnormality in these circumstances occurred either as the result of high metabolic demand beyond a relatively severe atherosclerotic restriction, or as the consequence of transient total obstruction due to thrombosis or spasm with return of prograde flow after spontaneous thrombolysis, recanalization, or relaxation of spasm. Recent knowledge gained from angiography performed soon after the onset of myocardial infarction (De Wood *et al.*, 1980), and from the acute intracoronary thrombolysis studies, lends support to the suggestion that total coronary artery occlusion in the early hours of an evolving myocardial infarction is the most frequent finding (Ganz *et al.*, 1981; Mathey *et al.*, 1981; Merx *et al.*, 1981; Rentrop *et al.*, 1981).

Dissolution of the occluding thrombus by early postinfarction intracoronary adminstration of a thrombolytic agent frequently reestablishes prograde flow past a residual, usual high-grade, atherosclerotic lesion. These interventional procedures designed to preserve ischemic myocardium are currently under research, and further experience is required to establish their ultimate role in the management of patients within the early hours of an acute myocardial infarction (Swan, 1982). Intracoronary administration of nitroglycerin before the infusion of a thrombolytic agent has proven that coronary spasm is not the cause of total coronary occlusion in most patients studied in the early hours after the onset of an infarction.

The possible etiologic role of spasm prior to the onset of thrombotic occlusion presently is unknown. Patients with the syndrome of Prinzmetal's vasospastic angina with normal arteries may experience a subsequent myocardial infarction (Braunwald, 1981). Similarly, there are patients with evidence of infarction, both by clinical and angiographic studies, who are found to have normal or near-normal coronary arteries by means of coronary arteriography (Ciraulo et al., 1983). Both of these circumstances are suggestive that vasospasm alone, in certain patients, can be the mechanism of total coronary occlusion of sufficient duration to produce myocardial infarction.

Progressive coronary atherosclerotic narrowing with intermittent and variable rates of progress, superimposed spasm, and acute thrombosis of the residual lumina all play an interrelated (although incompletely understood) role in infarction of the myocardium (Borer, 1980; Olvia, 1981). These processes, coupled with collateral development which can provide myocardial protection, determine the extent of resultant myocardial damage that follows complete occlusion of a coronary vessel. The important and preeminent role of coronary angiography during the last two decades in our progressive understanding of these mechanisms cannot be overemphasized.

MANAGEMENT OF PATIENTS WITH CORONARY ARTERY DISEASE

General

The treatment of patients with CAD has undergone major changes in the past three decades. The goals of treatment include (1) relief of symptoms, (2) prevention, insofar as possible, of the first or subsequent myocardial infarctions that result in a progressive decrease of the myocardial contractile reserve, (3) rehabilitation of the patient to as full and productive a life-style as possible, and (4) prolongation of life. The mechanisms available to achieve these goals include (1) identification and elimination of risk factors known to play a role in the development of coronary atherosclerosis and probably in the rate of progression, (2) treatment directed at optimizing the myocardial oxygen demand/coronary blood flow ratio, (3) treatment directed, when indicated, at improving myocardial function, and (4) recognition and management of serious ventricular arrhythmias which may lead to sudden death.

Risk Factors

The male sex, systemic hypertension, a family history of CAD, diabetes mellitus, hyperlipidemia, and cigarette smoking have been demonstrated to be risk factors in the development of CAD (Brand et al., 1976), with an increasing frequency of CAD in population subsets having proportionately more risk factors. Although it is suggested that recognition of the role of these risk factors and a widespread professional and community effort to modify them have resulted in the recorded decline in CAD mortality in the United States in the last 15 years (Kannel and Thom, 1979), a cause-and-effect role remains unsubstantiated. The genetic risk factor, among the strongest, is presently beyond modification; although its recognition should serve as a strong incentive to the progeny to practice vigorous risk-factor detection and modification.

Cessation of cigarette smoking has been shown to reduce risk of subsequent events (Doyle et al., 1964; Gordon et al., 1974; Borhani, 1977). Control of hypertension has reduced the risk of death, predominantly from stroke, but clear evidence of its efficacy in the secondary prevention of subsequent myocardial infarction is not available presently (Multiple Risk Factor Intervention Trial, 1982). Control of patients with diabetes mellitus, with either insulin or the oral hypoglycemic agents, has not appeared to lessen the occurrence or complications of atherosclerosis (University Group Diabetes Program, 1979). Hyperlipidemia, especially hypercholesterolemia, has been incriminated in atherogenesis and CAD for a number of years (Shekelle et al., 1981). Although dietary modification is relatively effective at reducing serum cholesterol levels in many patients (Frederickson et al., 1974), a number of pharmacological agents also have been developed, the prime action of which has been to lower serum lipids, cholesterol, or triglyceride levels (Gotto, 1978). Although achieving reduced levels of blood lipids, many of these agents have produced undesirable side effects when used during a longer period of time (Levy and Rifkind, 1977); and in the secondary prevention trials, clear-cut evidence of reduced CAD mortality and morbidity has not been established (Oliver, 1978; Profstfield and Gotto, 1982). Regression of atherosclerotic arterial lesions has been demonstrated in animal models, but angiographically documented regression of human atherosclerosis is limited (Malinow, 1981).

Modification of the level of physical activity has become popular in the treatment of patients with CAD during the last decade. There is no question that achieving an enhanced level of physical fitness results in many favorable alterations in both cardiovascular and total body function. These include, among others, reduced body weight, heart rate, blood pressure, and lipid levels, and improved overall circulatory efficiency such that equivalent exercise levels can be achieved at the lower heart rate. These effects reduce myocardial oxygen demand and modify symptoms, permitting greater work levels with decreased or even complete elimination of angina and/or symptoms of myocardial insufficiency. Nonetheless, there are no secondary prevention or angiographic studies that demonstrate either reduction of morbidity or mortality, or regression of coronary arteriographic lesions in patients who follow an exercise program (Fischell, 1981; Milvy and Siegel, 1981; Pickering, 1981).

The role of stress, long touted as a contributing factor to the etiology, progression, morbidity, and mortality of CAD, is equally elusive (Frank *et al.*, 1978). The influence of stress in altering lipid levels and coagulability has been demonstrated in a number of studies, and behavior modification directed at reducing stress has been used to treat patients with CAD (Friedman and Rosenman, 1974; Ornish *et al.*, 1983). Proof that such modification of behavior influences the risk of CAD, however, is not available.

The relationship between the use of oral contraceptives and cardiovascular disease in women also has been explored. The use of oral contraceptive agents by some women, especially those over 35 years of age who also smoke cigarettes, results in considerable increase in the risk of cardiovascular disease (Stadel, 1981).

Clinical studies are still lacking that confirm the efficacy of attempts to control most of the risk factors in the secondary prevention of CAD. The convincing evidence of the role of these factors in the cause of atherogenesis, however, has provided strong impetus for aggressive risk-factor modification, not only as a mechanism for primary prevention but also in the secondary management of patients with CAD. Considering the many years involved in the development of atherosclerosis during which the risk factors are active, it is not surprising that it has been difficult to demonstrate the efficacy of secondary prevention following short periods of risk modification. The present inability to document results should not discourage aggressive pursuit of risk-factor management in the treatment of these patients. Most risk-factor modification can be performed at no physical hazard and little expense to the patient, provides clear-cut and measurable salutary effects, and usually requires only persistently firm physician direction and patient compliance to be effective. Failure of these latter two components is the major difficulty with this form of treatment. This is especially true in the current era when ingestion of a pill to produce some particular beneficial effect is easier and less demanding of personal sacrifice on the part of the patient.

Optimizing Myocardial Oxygen Demand/ Coronary Blood Flow Ratio

The time-honored method of decreasing myocardial oxygen demand, invariably discovered by most patients with chronic angina, is self-imposed limiting of physical activity. Until other methods of therapy became available, reducing the level of physical activity constituted the only treatment available for angina pectoris. Similarly, from a purely mechanical standpoint, the most effective method of increasing coronary blood flow is by aortocoronary bypass surgery, transluminal balloon coronary angioplasty, or intracoronary thrombolysis (Swan, 1982). These procedures provide immediate restoration of coronary arterial flow to the myocardium by means of bypassing or reducing a high-grade or total coronary occlusive lesion. The efficacy of aortocoronary bypass in reestablishing flow is beyond dispute, and its role in the treatment of patients with CAD will be considered subsequently.

DRUG THERAPY
Nitroglycerin

Nitroglycerin has been used in the treatment of patients with angina for more than a century, but its mechanism of action has been the subject of controversy. For years, the prevailing role of nitroglycerin was believed to be that of a coronary vasodilator. Subsequently the beneficial effects resulting from peripheral venous and arteriolar dilatation, predominantly the former, were recognized (Mason and Braunwald, 1965; DeMaria et al., 1974). Reducing preload and, to a lesser degree, afterload effectively decreases ventricular volume, wall tension, and consequently the work of the myocardium (Lee et al., 1970). After nitroglycerin is given to patients with CAD, exercise is accomplished at a lower rate-pressure product and can be continued to a higher level before the onset of angina. The rate-pressure product at the onset of angina, however, is similar to that of the untreated state (Robinson, 1968; Lee et al., 1970; Goldstein et al., 1971). These observations are consistent with the beneficial effects of nitroglycerin (and nitrates in general) being dependent upon favorable alteration of the hemodynamic determinants of myocardial oxygen demand, rather than upon improved myocardial perfusion per se. It has been demonstrated, however, that nitroglycerin does dilate coronary collateral vessels, especially in patients with angina. Results of experimental studies indicate intracoronary nitroglycerin may protect ischemic myocardium in border zones of an acute infarction, thereby reducing infarct size (Goldstein et al., 1974; Hirshfeld et al., 1974). Direct coronary vasodilatation by nitroglycerin of vessels that were seriously occluded with atherosclerotic lesions has been considered unlikely. Current appreciation of the role of spasm in normal epicardial coronary vessels, as well as in those with varying degrees of atherosclerotic occlusive lesions, has widened our understanding of the total efficacy of the vasodilator agents (Epstein and Talbot, 1981; Olvia, 1981). It is likely that the beneficial results of nitroglycerin are due to a combination of effects upon both the peripheral vascular bed and direct coronary vasodilatation.

The buccal mucosal membrane has been the route used most widely for the administration of nitroglycerin. A longer effect, 8 to 12 hours, has been achieved with orally ingested sustained-release capsules of nitroglycerin. Based upon reported transcutaneous absorption of nitroglycerin by workers in munitions factories, administration of nitroglycerin in ointment form (Taylor et al., 1976; Mikolich et al., 1980), and recently in sustained-release adhesive bandages, allows 6 to 24 hours of sustained vasodilator drug effectiveness via the percutaneous route. The sustained reduction of pre-load and afterload by nitroglycerin makes this a useful agent for treatment of patients with myocardial insufficiency as well as angina pectoris. Continuous intravenous infusion of nitroglycerin in buffered solution has been effective in controlling refractory angina (Buxton et al., 1980; Mikolich et al., 1980), and selective intracoronary injection during coronary angiography, balloon angioplasty, and ergonovine provocative testing for Prinzmetal's angina has relieved coronary spasm promptly in patients with both diseased and normal vessels (Buxton et al., 1980).

Long-Acting Nitrates

These agents have been used in the treatment of patients with angina for many years, even though their efficacy following oral ingestion has been questioned intermittently. Some of the early reports substantiating the efficacy of these agents were based upon improved performance during exercise testing, as determined by symptoms and ST-segment changes. Subsequent experience (Franciosa et al., 1974; Williams et al., 1977) with a balloon tip flotation catheter, used to record pulmonary capillary pressures and cardiac output, demonstrated the hemodynamic efficacy of larger oral doses of isosorbide dinitrate (similar to those of sublingual nitroglycerin and intravenous nitroprusside) in reducing both preload and afterload. The efficacy of larger doses of oral isosorbide dinitrate in postponing the time of onset and decreasing the severity of angina has been documented in carefully conducted treadmill exercise testing (Thadani et al., 1980).

Calcium-Channel Blocking Agents (Calcium-Entry Blocking Agents)

A chemically heterogenous group of pharmaceuticals, including verapamil, nifedipine and diltiazem (in use outside the United States for more than a decade), have the unique property of blocking the slow transmembrane calcium-transport channels (Ellrodt et al., 1980; Calcium-Entry Blockers in Coronary Artery Disease, 1982). Blockade of the slow calcium channel has interesting pharmacological effects upon the atrioventricular node, arteriolar smooth muscle cells, and myocardial cells (Table 11-4). The action on the atrioventricular node, slowing conduction time, a property displayed particularly by verapamil, has beneficial effects in terminating paroxysmal supraventricular tachycardia and slowing the ventricular rate in patients with atrial flutter or fibrillation.

Table 11-4. CARDIOVASCULAR EFFECTS OF CALCIUM-CHANNEL-ENTRY BLOCKERS

	VERAPAMIL	DILTIAZEM	NIFEDIPINE
Heart rate	↑ ↓	↓	↑ ↑
AV conduction	↓ ↓	↓	↑
Coronary dilatation	↑ ↑	↑ ↑ ↑	↑ ↑ ↑
Myocardial contractility	↓	○	↑
Peripheral arterial dilatation	↑ ↑	↑	↑ ↑ ↑

All of these agents block calcium entry into arteriolar smooth muscle cells which produces a vasodilatory, or antivasoconstrictor, effect. Because of individual pharmacological variability, nifedipine has little or no slowing effect upon atrioventricular node conduction and, consequently, appears to have relatively pure coronary and peripheral vasodilator properties. These agents were first used successfully in the treatment of patients with Prinzmetal's vasospastic angina (Curry *et al.*, 1978; Solberg *et al.*, 1978; Goldberg *et al.*, 1979; Heupler and Proudfit, 1979; Antman *et al.*, 1980). Their efficacy in reducing symptoms in patients with atherosclerotic coronary artery occlusive disease with both unstable and stable angina pectoris has subsequently become established (Cardens, 1975; Moskowitz *et al.*, 1979; Hecht *et al.*, 1981; Mueller and Chahine, 1981; Frishman and Somberg, 1982). Whether the antianginal effect in this setting is due to a coronary and/or peripheral vascular effect, or negative inotropic action, is not clarified (Frishman and Somberg, 1982).

Nifedipine also reduces systemic blood pressure and may have a role as an antihypertensive agent (Beer *et al.*, 1981). Verapamil (ISOPTIN, CALAN), available in both parenteral and oral forms), nifedipine (PROCARDIA in the United States and ADALAT in other areas of the world), and diltiazem (CARDIZEM) are approved for use. All of these compounds share, to a varying degree, the property of decreasing left ventricular contractility (Antman *et al.*, 1980), although effects on cardiac output and ejection fraction are variable, presumably the result of interplay between direct and reflex phenomena (Singh *et al.*, 1980). This property is most notable with verapamil and is the basis for its use in patients with hypertropic cardiomyopathy (Rosing *et al.*, 1979). The role of decreased left ventricular contractility in the relief of angina

as well as in the production of adverse sequelae in some patients remains to be clarified. The calcium-entry blockers also may serve a role in the preservation of ischemic myocardium after coronary occlusion (Ellrodt *et al.*, 1980).

Beta-Adrenergic Blocking Drugs

The widespread use and favorable influence of the beta-adrenergic blocking agents (betablockers) upon hypertension, angina, and longterm survival in patients with CAD, as well as upon those with a number of noncardiac conditions, highlight one of the major therapeutic advances of this century. In the short time since 1948, when the original pioneering work on adrenergic neurotransmitters began (Ahlquist, 1948), a large number of beta-adrenergic blocking drugs have evolved. These agents differ chemically, have varying beta-blocking potency, vary in cardioselectivity, demonstrate differing partial agonist activity (intrinsic sympathomimetic effect), demonstrate variable membrane-stabilizing activity (quinidine-like effect, although this effect is probably not operative at therapeutic doses, and the antiarrhythmic property of these agents is more likely related to beta-blockade per se), and display variable pharmacokinetic properties (Frishman, 1979; Thadani *et al.*, 1979) (Table 11-5). Propranolol (*Inderal*), until recently the only beta-blocker approved for use in the United States, has been used widely in the management of patients with hypertension, angina, and arrhythmias. Propranolol does not have cardioselective properties and is contraindicated when bronchospastic problems coexist. Metoprolol (*Lopressor*) and atenolol (*Tenormin*) are relatively cardioselective. Low lipid solubility, with perhaps lower resultant concentration in brain tissue, is a property of atenolol, nadolol, and timolol. Timolol (*Blocadren*) and pindolol (*Visken*), the beta-blockers most

Table 11-5. PHARMACOKINETIC PROPERTIES OF BETA-ADRENORECEPTOR BLOCKING DRUGS

DRUG	SYNONYMS	RELATIVE PATENCY	RELATIVE CARDIOSELECTIVITY	PARTIAL AGONIST ACTIVITY
Atenolol	*Tenormin*	1	+	0
Metoprolol	*Lopressor, Betaloc*	1	+	0
Nadolol	*Corgard*	1	0	0
Pindolol	*Visken*	6	0	+++
Propranolol	*Inderal*	1	0	0
Timolol	*Blocadren*	6	0	±

recently released for use in the United States, have considerably higher potency per milligram than propranolol, and pindolol possesses sympathomimetic activity. This property allows less risk of provoking excessive bradycardia and may provide some degree of protection from bronchospasm in patients intolerant of propranolol (Frishman, 1979). Propranolol and metoprolol are subject to extensive obligatory presystemic, hepatic "first-pass" elimination. This first-pass elimination decreases as higher doses are employed, suggesting saturation of the hepatic elimination process. As a consequence, wide variability of plasma concentrations is seen in patients who received similar doses. Likewise, there is a major difference between the oral and intravenous dosage of these agents (Frishman, 1979). Atenolol, nadolol (*Corgard*), timolol, and pindolol are excreted by the kidneys. Atenolol and nadolol have a long plasma half-life and may be effective in single daily dosages (Frishman, 1980) (Table 11-6).

The beta-blockers slow the pulse rate, lower blood pressure, and decrease myocardial contractility, thereby reducing myocardial oxygen requirements both at rest and during exercise. The antianginal properties of the beta-blockers appear to result from the blunting of the catecholamine-induced increase in heart rate, blood pressure, and myocardial contractility in response to exercise, thus permitting greater effort tolerance with a lower myocardial oxygen requirement (Jorgenson *et al.*, 1973). Patients with CAD treated with beta-blockers demonstrate improved treadmill performance, and they can achieve a higher total body work load before the onset of angina. The rate-pressure product at the onset of angina, however, is usually somewhat lower than in the untreated state (Robin *et al.*, 1967; Amsterdam *et al.*, 1971; Jorgenson *et al.*, 1973), suggesting in-

Table 11-6. PHARMACOKINETICS OF ORAL β-ADRENERGIC-BLOCKING AGENTS*

PHARMACOKINETIC EFFECT	DRUG					
	ATENOLOL	METOPROLOL	NADOLOL	PINDOLOL	PROPRANOLOL	TIMOLOL
Extent of absorption (%)	~50	>95	~30	>90	>90	>90
Extent of bioavailability (% of dose)	~40	~50	~30	~90	~30	75
Interpatient variations in plasma levels	Fourfold	Tenfold	Sevenfold	Fourfold	Twentyfold	Sevenfold
β-blocking plasma concentration	0.2–0.5 µg/ml	50–100 ng/ml	50–100 ng/ml	50–100 ng/ml	50–100 ng/ml	5–10 ng/ml
Protein binding (%)	<5	12	~30	57	93	~10
Lipophilicity†	Low	Moderate	Low	Moderate	High	Low
Elimination half-life (hours)	6–9	3–4	14–24	3–4	3.5–6	3–4
Predominant route of elimination	RE‡ (mostly unchanged)	HM**	RE	RE (~40% unchanged)	HM	RE (~20% unchanged) and HM
Active metabolites	No	No	No	No	Yes	No

* From Frishman, W. H. Beta-adrenergic blockade in clinical practice. *Hosp. Pract.*, **1980,** September, 57–68.
† Determined by the distribution ratio between octanol and water.
‡ RE denotes renal excretion.
** HM denotes hepatic metabolism.

creased myocardial oxygen supply is not a major factor in the beneficial effect of these agents. Beta-blockers and the nitrates are additive in their effect on stable angina pectoris — beta-blockers, by limiting the increase in myocardial oxygen requirement associated with exercise and emotion, and nitrates, predominantly by venodilatation and reduction of heart size and wall tension.

The precise mechanism of the antihypertensive effect of the beta-blockers is unclear but in large part appears to result from reduced cardiac output and systemic flow. Other postulated mechanisms involved in lowering blood pressure include a central nervous system effect, reduced renin production by the kidney, decreased plasma volume and reduced peripheral arterial resistance, a mechanism shared to some degree by the cardioselective beta-blockers, but, more important, by those with partial agonist activity such as pindolol (Frishman and Silverman, 1979). The magnitude of any of these effects varies from one beta-blocking agent to another.

The beta-blockers also decrease platelet adhesion and aggregation, probably mediated by their direct effect upon membranes. This action suggests another potentially beneficial role of the beta-blockers in the treatment of patients with CAD (Frishman and Silverman, 1979).

The beta-blockers together with nitrates and, more recently, the calcium-channel-blocking agents, have become the foundation for the medical management of patients with CAD. These agents control the symptoms of CAD, increase work capacity, and in many patients permit a satisfactory quality of life, exercise capacity, and ability to continue gainful employment.

Although beta-blockers are known to be compatible with the nitrates, experience combining beta-blocking drugs with the calcium-channel-blockers is limited (*FDA Drug Bull.,* 1982; Gerstenblith et al., 1982); and there is risk of myocardial depression and congestive failure especially with, but not limited to, the combination with verapamil (Gillmer and Kark, 1980; Chew *et al.,* 1981; Robson and Vishwanath, 1981; Subramanian *et al.,* 1982).

Randomized studies have demonstrated decreased mortality in patients with acute myocardial infarction who are treated with beta-blockers (Hjalmarson *et al.,* 1981). Initiation of the drugs after myocardial infarction has resulted in a decreased mortality during a period of several years (Norwegian Multicenter Study Group, 1981; Beta Blocker Heart Attack Trial Research Group, 1982; Hampton, 1982).

Adverse Effects of the Beta-Blockers

The pharmacological effects of the beta-blockers, generally advantageous to patients with CAD, may also have undesirable consequences (Frishman *et al.,* 1979). Depression of myocardial contractility may result in cardiac enlargement and myocardial failure, especially when a considerable degree of myocardial dysfunction preexists. Increased peripheral vascular resistance may be a component of heart failure induced by a beta-blocker and may be less prominent with cardioselective agents (Vaughan-Williams *et al.,* 1973). Beta-blockers with intrinsic sympathomimetic activity may also circumvent this problem. All beta-blockers slow atrioventricular conduction, and this effect is advantageous in patients with arrhythmias of supraventricular origin. Beta-blockade can cause excessive atrioventricular slowing in patients with intrinsic AV node pathology, resulting in high degrees of AV block (Conolly *et al.,* 1976). Drugs with intrinsic sympathomimetic effect do not depress atrioventricular conduction.

In any patient with asthma or bronchospasm, propranolol is contraindicated; and the beta-blockers must be used with caution in any patient with chronic obstructive lung disease. Agents with greater cardioselectivity such as metoprolol or atenolol may be tolerated better (Skinner *et al.,* 1976). Cardioselectivity is dose related and not absolute; consequently, larger doses of cardioselective agents may also produce undesirable bronchospasm.

Patients with peripheral vascular disease depend to some degree upon beta-adrenergic stimulation, and beta-blocking agents may lead to worsening of Raynaud's phenomena, increased claudication, and even progression to gangrene (Rodger *et al.,* 1976).

Beta-blockers may cause hypoglycemic episodes, and patients with diabetes dependent upon insulin should receive beta-blockers with caution since the manifestations of, and responses to, hypoglycemia are beta-adrenergic-mediated (Lloyd-Mostyn and Oram, 1975). Recognition of the early manifestations of hypoglycemia may consequently be blunted severely.

Beta-blockers, especially those that are highly soluble in lipids, such as propranolol, can cause nightmares, vivid dreams, and depression (Waal, 1967) (at times so severe the drug must be discontinued), as well as lesser degrees of mental lethargy and fatigue. These latter symptoms are sufficiently nonspecific that differentiating the effects of the drug from those of the underlying disease process or situational depression is difficult. It is likely that all factors are operative to varying degrees in different patients and may prompt a change to an agent with partial agonist effect or to one which does not cross the blood-brain barrier. Impotence is also a frequent complaint of male patients taking beta-blocking agents.

If renal insufficiency coexists or develops, the dosage of those agents excreted by the kidney (atenolol, nadolol, pindolol, timolol) must be reduced. An unusual oculomucocutaneous syndrome (Wright, 1975), an immunological syndrome involving the skin, eyes, ears, and peritoneum has been reported with the administration of practolol (Waal-Manning, 1975), resulting in curtailment of its use.

So universal with the administration of beta-blockers, sinus bradycardia hardly warrants inclusion with observed side effects. Heart rates as low as 48 to 50 per minute at rest and inability to exceed rates of 90 to 100 per minute with graded exercise is the mark of effective beta-blockade. Patients with sinus bradycardia of this degree are almost always asymptomatic, as are those with occasional resting heart rates as low as 40 per minute, and do not require cessation of therapy. An occasional patient will be intolerant to even low dosages of propranolol, experiencing inordinate symptomatic bradycardia and orthostatic hypotension. Drugs with intrinsic sympathomimetic activity do not lower the resting rate to the same degree as does propranolol.

Beta-Blockade Withdrawal

Following abrupt cessation of beta-blocker therapy, reduced exercise tolerance has been noted in patients with angina. Platelet hyperaggregability has been demonstrated, angina may become unstable, and an increased incidence of coronary events has been reported (Frishman et al., 1978; Nattel et al., 1979). An enhanced sensitivity develops to beta-adrenergic stimuli, with onset in 2 to 6 days (average of 4) after beta-blocker withdrawal, persisting from 3 to 13 days (average of 6). Beta-blocker therapy should be discontinued gradually and cautiously in patients with CAD. Discontinuation of beta-blockers before cardiac or noncardiac surgery, a practice that was common in the early days of aortocoronary bypass, is no longer

advocated (Slogoff et al., 1978). Continuation to the time of cardiac, or noncardiac, surgery has resulted in smoother endotracheal intubation and anesthetic induction; less reactive hypertension, tachycardia, and arrhythmias; and decreased risk of complications such as increased angina, infarction and even death. To prevent the withdrawal syndrome, we reinstitute beta-blockers orally on the first day after aortocoronary bypass and generally continue use for four to six weeks. Since institution of this practice, the incidence of arrhythmias, particularly atrial flutter or fibrillation, has been reduced by 50% in the postoperative period following aortocoronary bypass.

Treatment of Patients with Myocardial Failure

The consequence of prior myocardial infarction, especially multiple infarctions, is myocardial insufficiency and congestive heart failure. Treatment consists of sodium restriction and diuretic and digitalis administration. Vasodilator therapy, to lower preload and afterload, decreases symptoms and increases the patient's tolerance for activity, although the long-term efficacy of vasodilator therapy is not established (Franciosa et al., 1974). The angiotensin-converting enzyme inhibitor, captopril (which reduces peripheral vascular resistance that is directly related to the control of plasma renin activity) (Cohn and Levine, 1982), has been found to exert a prolonged and favorable effect in patients with normotensive, resistant congestive heart failure (Fouad et al., 1982; LeJemtal et al., 1982).

NATURAL HISTORY OF CORONARY ARTERY DISEASE

Early clinical studies characterized the natural history of CAD from the time angina was identified. In the early twentieth century, the recorded survival from the onset of angina until death ranged from 3 to 10 years (Reeves et al., 1974). Subsequent clinical series, however, revealed an annual mortality of approximately 4 to 7% per year, although one series of young soldiers experienced only a 2.5% annual mortality (Reeves et al., 1974). These observers noted a wide range of annual mortality (5 to 16% per year) dependent upon the presence or absence of electrocardiographic abnormalities, cardiac enlargement, or congestive failure (Reeves et al., 1974). One of the first studies relating survival to coronary angiographic findings identified the important relationships of survival to the extent, and the number, of coronary arteries obstructed (Friesinger *et al.*, 1970).

Several studies conducted before 1974, relating angiographic staging to survival, revealed an average annual mortality of 2.2, 6.8 and 11.4% for patients with one-, two-, and three-vessel disease, respectively (Reeves *et al.*, 1974). These studies also corroborated the increased mortality with cardiac enlargement or congestive failure. A single large series of patients who underwent coronary angiography between 1963 and 1965 were followed for more than 10 years (Proudfit *et al.*, 1978). Receiving medical therapy only, patients with one-, two-, three-vessel, and left main coronary artery disease had an average annual mortality of 4.1, 7, 12.5, and 12.6%, respectively (Figure 11-3). Patients with single-vessel disease involving the left anterior descending coronary artery experienced a higher mortality than those with either circumflex or right coronary disease, with the

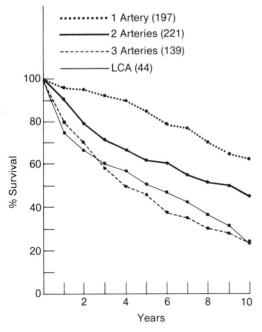

Figure 11-3. Survival curves for arteries obstructed. Mortality for single artery, 4.1%/yr; two arteries, 7%/yr; three arteries, 12.5%/yr; left main artery, 12.6%/yr. Survival at 10 years: single artery, 62.9%; two, 45.4%; three, 23.4%; left main artery, 22.5%. (From Proudfit, W. L.; Bruschke, A. V. T.; and Sones, F. M., Jr. Natural history of obstructive coronary artery disease: Ten year study of 601 nonsurgical cases. *Prog. Cardiovasc. Dis.,* **1978,** *21,* 53. By permission)

latter patients at lowest risk. Patients with a normal left ventriculogram experienced an annual mortality of only 4.6%, while those with severe left ventricular dysfunction experienced a 15% average annual mortality during the first three years, with only 11% surviving at 10 years. The unfavorable influence of progressive degrees of left ventricular impairment was evident in each patient subset, based upon the number of diseased coronary arteries. These data contain some patients who may not have been satisfactory for surgical bypass, and medical therapy with beta-blocking drugs was not available during the period studied.

A more recent report has detailed the follow-up of 1,214 patients managed medically during the beta-blocker era (Harris *et al.*, 1979). Although the assignment to medical or surgical management was not random, it was based upon the decision of the attending physician and the patient. The seven-year survival of patients managed medically was 65%, an average annual attrition of 5% per year; attrition was 1.6, 3, 7.2, and 12.6% per year for patients with one-, two-, three-vessel and left main coronary artery disease (Figure 11-4). It was important that 504 of the total 1,214 patients who had normal left ventricular contraction experienced only a 2.2% annual attrition; for those with one-, two-, three-vessel, and left main disease, attrition was 0.6, 1.6, 3.6, and 10%. Those with moderate left ventricular dysfunction experienced a 6% annual attrition. These data stress the important role of abnormal left ventricular function on survival (Figure 11-5). In each subset the presence of progressive angina, or abnormal ventricular hemodynamics, decreased late survival significantly (Harris *et al.*, 1979).

Survival of over 20,000 patients managed medically has been reported from the coronary artery surgery study (CASS) conducted by the National Heart, Lung and Blood Institute (Mock *et al.*, 1982). The findings are comparable to the previous cited study with survival related to the number of diseased vessels, involvement of the left main coronary artery, and the degree of impairment of the left ventricular function. In both of these studies, left ventricular function was a more important predictor of survival than the number of diseased vessels.

Assignments of patients into low- and high-risk categories also has been based upon noninvasive characteristics. Several investigators (Bruce *et al.*, 1959; Thompson and Kelemen, 1975; Morris *et al.*, 1978) have noted the fre-

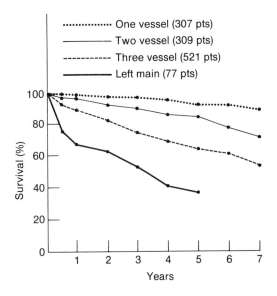

Figure 11-4. Cumulative survival rates in patients with one-, two-, three-vessel, and left-main coronary disease. (From Harris, M. B.; Phil, D.; Harrell, F. E.; *et al.* Survival in medically treated coronary artery disease. *Circulation,* **1979,** *60,* 1259–1269. By permission of the American Heart Association, Inc.)

quent finding of severe CAD, often left main coronary artery disease, when exertional hypotension is induced during stress testing. The frequency of subsequent coronary events (Ellestad and Wan, 1975) and late survival (McNeer *et al.,* 1978) also has been correlated with the response to electrocardiographic exercise stress testing. A positive ST-segment ischemic response was predictive of subsequent coronary events, progression of angina, myocardial infarction, or death (Ellestad and Wan, 1975). The time of onset of ischemic ST-segment depression was a particularly potent predictor of subsequent coronary events, with a significantly worse prognosis when

2-mm ST-segment depression was manifest within the first five minutes of exercise testing (Ellestad and Wan, 1975). In another study of patients with known CAD, those whose treadmill test was negative or who achieved a maximum heart rate of 160 per minute and/or stage IV of the Bruce protocol had a one-year survival of 98% and a four-year survival of 93% and were characterized as low risk. A high-risk cohort had a positive test and exercise duration of only stage I or II of the Bruce protocol. These individuals had less than 60% survival at four years (McNeer *et al.,* 1978). Similarly, the results of submaximal electrocardiographic exercise testing performed prior to the discharge of

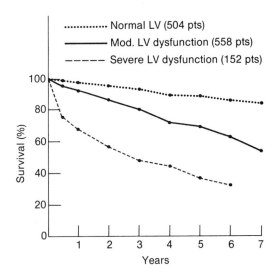

Figure 11-5. Cumulative survival rates related to the overall left ventricular (LV) contraction pattern. Moderate LV dysfunction is an abnormal but not diffusely abnormal contraction pattern. Severe LV dysfunction is a diffusely abnormal LV contraction pattern. (From Harris, M. G.; Phil, D.; Harrell, F. E.; *et al.* Survival in medically treated coronary artery disease. *Circulation,* **1979,** *60,* 1259–1269. By permission of the American Heart Association, Inc.)

patients with an uncomplicated myocardial infarction have been correlated with late survival. Patients with an ischemic ST-segment response experienced an annual mortality of 19%, while those with a negative response had a one-year mortality of only 2.6% (Epstein *et al.*, 1982).

There are additional clinical presentations that give clues to the probable natural history. Patients requiring hospitalization with unstable angina but without infarction were followed prospectively after discharge (Gazes *et al.*, 1973). At three months, the incidence of infarction was 21% with a resulting mortality of 10%. The mortality at one year was 18% and at two years, 25%. The subset of patients who had recurrent ischemic episodes with accompanying ST-segment changes during hospitalization experienced a 43 and 53% one- and two-year mortality (Gazes *et al.*, 1973).

The most devastating event in the course of ischemic heart disease is acute myocardial infarction, not only from the standpoint of the high mortality associated with this event but also due to the consequences, in the survivors, of injury and destruction of a variable amount of left ventricular myocardium. The degree of myocardial injury is, as already indicated, a strong predictor of postinfarction survival. A reasonable estimate of the mortality of patients who have acute myocardial infarction is 40% during the first 30 days. Fifty per cent of the deaths occur within the first several hours and approximately 70 to 80% within the first 24 hours of the onset of the infarction (Fulton *et al.*, 1969; Armstrong *et al.*, 1972). Survivors of an acute myocardial infarction experience a first-year mortality of 10%, with most of the deaths occurring in the first six months. There is an annual mortality of 3 to 5% after the first year (Humphries *et al.*, 1979). Other characteristics of the postinfarction survivor can be identified that have strong influence on subsequent mortality. Adverse predictors of late survival include an ejection fraction below 30%, triple-vessel disease (27% mortality at 30 months), and a prior myocardial infarction. Patients with and without serious ventricular arrhythmias, on 24-hour electrocardiographic monitoring, experienced, respectively, a 29 and 11% mortality at 30 months (Humphries *et al.*, 1979). The value of assessing the postinfarction patient by means of radionuclide ventriculography, 24-hour ambulatory electrocardiographic monitoring, and submaximal treadmill exercise testing to predict subsequent risk is evident. Further invasive evaluation by coronary angiography is indicated in the high-risk subsets.

Patients summarized from nine reports who had sustained a subendocardial or nontransmural infarction experienced an in-hospital mortality of 11% which was equal to or slightly less than the mortality of patients with transmural infarction in the same institutions (Levy *et al.*, 1981). The mortality after discharge, however, was similar to and, in some reports, worse than that of patients who had had a transmural infarction (Levy *et al.*, 1981). Clearly, nontransmural infarction is not a benign entity and usually indicates extensive underlying CAD (Aintablian *et al.*, 1978; Schulze *et al.*, 1978). Patients who have sustained a nontransmural infarction frequently have persistent in-hospital angina or even proceed to experience a complete transmural infarction. The annual mortality after discharge in the cumulated report (Levy *et al.*, 1981) ranged from 10 to 16%, and sudden death was frequent. Persistent angina and recurrent infarction were frequent in the survivors (Cannon *et al.*, 1976; Fabricius-Bjerre *et al.*, 1979). Patients who have sustained a nontransmural infarction frequently have only limited myocardial damage, yet often have extensive coronary artery disease, and are at continued risk for a subsequent catastrophe.

Another subset of patients deserves attention. This group is composed of individuals who are hospitalized with symptoms suggesting acute infarction, but who do not develop serial enzyme or electrocardiographic changes suggestive of myocardial necrosis, i.e., patients in whom myocardial infarction has been ruled out. This subset of patients, many of whom have suffered an episode of prolonged coronary insufficiency without discernible infarction, includes a number of individuals at high risk. A two-year follow-up study of patients in whom myocardial infarction was ruled out revealed the same incidence of total events (22%), death, and subsequent infarction, as in a comparable group of patients followed after infarction. The incidence of sudden death in a two-year period was 9% compared to 7% in the postinfarction patients (Schroeder *et al.*, 1980). Similar to patients with nontransmural infarction, patients who have had an acute ischemic event without infarction include many who have extensive CAD and are at high risk of a subsequent event.

Survivors of out-of-hospital sudden death syndrome represent a subgroup who are also at high risk. When documented by electrocardiographic data soon after the patient's collapse, this event is usually found to be due to ventricular fibrillation (Cobb *et al.*, 1975). Although coronary disease is the most common underlying pathology, ventricular fibrillation is the consequence of a new acute transmural myocardial infarction in the minority (19%) of patients (Cobb *et al.*, 1980). Mortality at 24 months was 40% for those who did not, compared to 20% for those who did, sustain a new transmural infarction (Cobb *et al.*, 1980). Recurrence of the sudden cardiac death syndrome was eleven times as frequent in the former group, and even higher if there was a history of a prior infarction or congestive heart failure (Cobb *et al.*, 1980). Angiographic study of survivors of out-of-hospital sudden death revealed severe CAD in 94% of the patients studied, multivessel disease in 61%, and ventricular contraction abnormalities in 70%. Among the patients studied, anatomy with potential for complete revascularization was present in 54% and for incomplete revascularization in 39% (Weaver *et al.*, 1976).

It is evident that the natural history of CAD is determined strongly by the extent of the vessels affected by coronary disease, the amount of myocardium damaged, and the occurrence of serious ventricular arrhythmias. Medical therapy with the beta-blocking drugs appears to be altering the natural history of stable angina (Multicenter International Study, 1975; Norwegian Multicenter Study Group, 1981; Beta Blocker Heart Attack Trial Research Group, 1982; Hampton, 1982). Whether the calcium-channel blockers will also favorably influence long-term survival is unknown at this time. The decision process used in evaluating patients with CAD, and in planning short- and long-term therapy, must take these factors into consideration; and since coronary disease is progressive, these decisions must be periodically reassessed.

Coronary Bypass Surgery

Surgical bypass of proximal high-grade coronary artery occlusive lesions has the immediate benefit of restoring direct aortocoronary blood flow to underperfused areas of the myocardium. The techniques, results, and indications will be considered in the following chapter.

REFERENCES

Ahlquist, R. P. A study of the adrenotropic receptors. *Am. J. Physiol,* **1948,** *153,* 586–600.

Aintablian, A.; Hamby, R. I.; Weisz, D.; *et al.* Results of aortocoronary bypass grafting in patients with subendocardial infarction: Late follow-up. *Am. J. Cardiol.,* **1978,** *42,* 183–186.

American Heart Association Committee Report. A reporting system on patients evaluated for coronary artery disease. *Circulation,* **1975,** *51,* 7.

Amsterdam, E. A.; Hughes, J. L.; Mansour, E.; *et al.* Circulatory effects of practolol: Selective cardiac beta adrenergic blockade in arrhythmias and angina pectoris (abstr.). *Clin. Res.,* **1971,** *19,* 109.

Antman, E.; Muller, J.; Goldberg, S.; MacAlpin, R.; *et al.* Nifedipine therapy for coronary artery spasm: Experience in 127 patients. *N. Engl. J. Med.,* **1980,** *302,* 1269–1273.

Armstrong, A.; Duncan, B.; Oliver, M. T.; *et al.* Natural history of acute coronary heart attacks: A community study. *Br. Heart J.,* **1972,** *34,* 67.

Arnett, E. N.; Isner, H. M.; Redwood, D. R.; *et al.* Coronary artery narrowing in coronary heart disease: Comparison of cineangiographic and necropsy findings. *Ann. Intern. Med.,* **1979,** *91,* 350–356.

Arnow, W. W., and Cassidy, J. Five-year follow-up of double Master's test, maximal treadmill stress test, and resting and post-exercise apexcardiogram in asymptomatic persons. *Circulation,* **1975,** *52,* 616–618.

Asinger, R. W.; Mikell, F. L.; Elsperger, J.; *et al.* Incidence of left ventricular thrombosis after acute transmural myocardial infarction. *N. Engl. J. Med.,* **1981,** *305,* 297–302.

Beer, N.; Gallegos, I.; Cohen, A.; *et al.* Efficacy of sublingual nifedipine in the acute treatment of systemic hypertension. *Chest,* **1981,** *79,* 571–574.

Beta Blocker Heart Attack Trial Research Group. A randomized trial of propranolol in patients with acute myocardial infarction. I. Mortality results. *JAMA,* **1982,** *247,* 1707–1714.

Borer, J. S. Unstable angina: A lethal gun with an invisible trigger. *N. Engl. J. Med.,* **1980,** *302,* 1200–1202.

Borhani, N. O. Primary prevention of coronary heart disease: A critique. *Am. J. Cardiol.,* **1977,** *40,* 251.

Brand, J. R.; Rosenman, R. H.; Sholtz, R. I.; and Friedman, M. Multivariate prediction of coronary heart disease in the Western Collaborative Group Study compared to the findings of the Framingham Study. *Circulation,* **1976,** *53,* 348.

Braunwald, E. Coronary artery spasm: Mechanisms and clinical relevance. *JAMA,* **1981,** *246,* 1957–1960.

Brown, G. G. Observations linking the clinical spectrum of ischemic heart disease to the dynamic pathology of coronary atherosclerosis. *Arch. Intern. Med.,* **1981,** *141,* 716–722.

Bruce, R. A.; Cobb, L. A.; Katsura, S.; *et al.* Exertional hypotension in cardiac patients. *Circulation,* **1959,** *19,* 543.

Bruce, R. A.; Hornsten, T. R.; and Blackmon, J. R. Myocardial infarction after normal responses to maximal exercise. *Circulation,* **1968,** *38,* 552.

Bruce, R. A.; DeRouen, T. A.; Hossack, K. F.; *et al.* Value of maximal exercise tests in risk assessment of primary coronary heart disease events in healthy men: Five years' experience of the Seattle Heart Watch Study. *Am. J. Cardiol.,* **1980,** *46,* 371–378.

Bunnell, I. L.; Greene, D. G.; Tandon, R. N.; and Arani,

D. T. The half-axial projection. A new look at the proximal left coronary artery. *Circulation,* **1973,** *48,* 1151.

Buxton, A.; Goldberg, S.; Hirshfeld, J. W.; Wilson, J.; et al. Refractory ergonovine-induced coronary vasospasm: Importance of intracoronary nitroglycerin. *Am. J. Cardiol.,* **1980,** *46,* 329–334.

Calcium-entry blockers in coronary artery disease. Proceedings of a symposium held in San Francisco, California, March 19, 1981. *Circulation,* **1982,** *65* (Suppl. I), 59. (Introduction by Jay N. Cohn, M.D.)

Cannon, D. S.; Levy, W.; and Cohen, L. S. The short and long term prognosis of patients with transmural and non-transmural myocardial infarction. *Am. J. Med.,* **1976,** *61,* 452–458.

Cardens, P. Effect of intravenous verapamil on exercise tolerance and left ventricular function in patients with severe exertional angina pectoris. *Eur. J. Cardiol.,* **1975,** *2,* 443.

Chew, C. Y. C.; Hecht, H. S.; Collett, J. T.; et al. Influence of severity of ventricular dysfunction on hemodynamic responses to intravenously administered verapamil in ischemic heart disease. *Am. J. Cardiol.,* **1981,** *47,* 917–922.

Ciraulo, D. A.; Bresnahan, G. E.; Frankel, P. S.; et al. Transmural myocardial infarction with normal coronary angiogram and with single vessel obstruction: Clinical-angiographic features and five-year follow-up. *Chest,* **1983,** *83,* 196.

Cobb, L. A.; Baum, R. S.; Alvarez, H.; and Schaffer, W. A. Resuscitation from out-of-hospital ventricular fibrillation: 4 year follow-up. *Circulation,* **1975,** *51, 52* (Suppl. III), 223.

Cobb, L. A.; Werner, J. A.; and Trobaugh, G. B. Sudden cardiac death. I. A decade's experience with out-of-hospital resuscitation. *Mod. Concepts Cardiovasc. Dis.,* **1980,** *19,* 31.

Cohen, M. V.; Sonnenblick, E. H.; and Kirk, E. S. Comparative effects of nitroglycerin and isosorbide dinitrate on coronary collateral vessels and ischemic myocardium in dogs. *Am. J. Cardiol.,* **1976,** *37,* 244–249.

Cohn, J. N., and Levine, T. B. Angiotensin-converting enzyme inhibition in congestive heart failure: The concept. *Am. J. Cardiol.,* **1982,** *48,* 1480–1483.

Conolly, M. E.; Kersting, F.; and Dollery, C. T. The clinical pharmacology of beta-adrenoceptor-blocking drugs. *Prog. Cardiovasc. Dis.,* **1976,** *19,* 203.

Curry, R. C.; Pepine, C. J.; and Conti, R. Refractory variant angina treated with perhexilene maleate: Results in 14 patients (abstr). *Circulation,* **1978,** *58,* (Suppl. II), 693.

Dagenais, G. R.; Rouleau, J. R.; Christen, A.; et al. Survival of patients with strongly positive exercise electrocardiogram. *Circulation,* **1981,** *65,* 452–456.

DeMaria, A. N.; Vismara, L. A.; Auditore, K.; et al. Effects of nitroglycerin on left ventricular cavity size and cardiac performance determined by ultrasound in man. *Am. J. Med.,* **1974,** *57,* 754.

de Servi, S.; Falcone, C.; Gavazzi, A.; et al. The exercise test in variant angina: Results in 114 patients. *Circulation,* **1981,** *64,* 684–688.

DeWood, M.; Spores, J.; Notske, R.; et al. Prevalence of total coronary occlusion during the early hours of transmural myocardial infarction. *N. Engl. J. Med.,* **1980,** *303,* 897–902.

Dodge, H. T. *Hemodynamic Aspects of Cardiac Failure. The Myocardium: Failure and Infarction.* H. P. Publishing Co., New York, **1974,** pp. 70–79.

Dodge, H. T.; Sandler, H.; Ballew, D. W.; and Lord, J. D., Jr. The use of biplane angiocardiography for the measurement of left ventricular volume in man. *Am. Heart J.,* **1960,** *60,* 762.

Doyle, J. T.; Dawber, T. R.; Kannel, W. B.; et al. The relationship of cigarette smoking in coronary heart disease. The second report of the combined experience of the Albany, N. Y. and Framingham, Mass. studies. *JAMA,* **1964,** *190,* 886.

Doyle, J. T., and Kinch, S. H. The prognosis of an abnormal electrocardiographic stress test. *Circulation,* **1970,** *41,* 545.

Dunn, R. F.; Freedman, B.; Kelly, D. T.; et al. Exercise-induced ST segment elevation in leads V_1 or aV_L. *Circulation,* **1981,** *63,* 1357–1363.

Ellestad, M. H.; Allen, W.; Wan, M. C. K.; and Kemp, G. L. Maximal treadmill stress testing for cardiovascular evaluation. *Circulation,* **1969,** *39,* 517.

Ellestad, M. H., and Wan, M. K. C. Predictive implication of stress testing: Follow-up of 2700 subjects after maximum treadmill stress testing. *Circulation,* **1975,** *51,* 363–369.

Ellrodt, G.; Chew, C. Y. C.; and Singh, B. N. Therapeutic implications of slow-channel blockade in cardiocirculatory disorders. *Circulation,* **1980,** *62,* 669–679.

Enos, W. F.; Holmes, R. H.; and Beger, J. Coronary disease among United States soldiers killed in action in Korea. *JAMA,* **1953,** *152,* 1090.

Epstein, S. E. Implications of probability analysis on the strategy used for noninvasive detection of coronary artery disease. *Am. J. Cardiol.,* **1980,** *46,* 491–499.

Epstein, S. E.; Palmeri, S. T.; and Patterson, R. E. Evaluation of patients after acute myocardial infarction. *N. Engl. J. Med.,* **1982,** *307,* 1487–1492.

Epstein, S. E., and Talbot, T. L. Dynamic coronary tone in precipitation, exacerbation and relief of angina pectoris. *Am. J. Cardiol.,* **1981,** *48,* 797–803.

Fabricius-Bjerre, N.; Munkvad, M.; and Knudsen, J. B. Subendocardial and transmural myocardial infarction: A five year survival study. *Am. J. Med.,* **1979,** *98,* 176–184.

FDA Drug Bull., April, **1982,** *12* (1), 1–3. New angina drugs.

Fischell, T. Running and the primary prevention of coronary heart disease. *Cardiovasc. Rev. Rep.,* **1981,** *2,* 238–244.

Fouad, F. M.; Terazi, R. C.; Bravo, E. L.; et al. Long-term control of congestive heart failure with captopril. *Am. J. Cardiol.,* **1982,** *49,* 1489–1496.

Franciosa, J. A.; Mikulek, E.; Cohn, J. N.; et al. Hemodynamic effects of orally administered isosorbide dinitrate in patients with congestive heart failure. *Circulation,* **1974,** *50,* 1020.

Frank, K. A.; Heller, S. S.; Kornfeld, D. S.; et al. Type A behavior pattern and coronary angiographic findings. *JAMA,* **1978,** *240,* 761.

Frank, S. T. Aural sign of coronary artery disease. *N. Engl. J. Med.,* **1973,** *289,* 327–328.

Frederickson, D. S.; Levy, R. I.; Bonnell, M.; and Ernst,

N. Dietary management of hyperlipoproteinemia. DHEW Publ. No. (NIH), Washington, D.C., **1974**, pp. 75–110.

Friedman, H., and Rosenman, R. H. *Type A Behavior and Your Heart.* Alfred A. Knopf, New York, **1974.**

Friesinger, G. C.; Page, E. E.; and Ross, R. S. Prognostic significance of coronary arteriography. *Trans. Assoc. Am. Physicians,* **1970,** *83,* 75.

Frishman, W. H. Clinical pharmacology of the new beta-adrenergic blocking drugs. Part I. Pharmacodynamic and pharmacokinetic properties. *Am. Heart J.,* **1979,** *97,* 663–670.

———Beta-adrenergic blockade in clinical practice. *Hosp. Prac.* **1982,** September, *17,* 58–67.

Frishman, W. H.; Christodoulou, J.; Weksler, B.; et al. Abrupt propranolol withdrawal in angina pectoris: Effects on platelet aggregation and exercise tolerance. *Am. Heart J.,* **1978,** *95,* 169.

Frishman, W., and Silverman, R. Clinical pharmacology of the new beta-adrenergic blocking drugs. Part 2. Physiologic and metabolic effects. *Am. Heart J.,* **1979,** *97,* 797–807.

Frishman, W.; Silverman, R.; Strom, J.; et al. Appraisal and reappraisal of cardiac therapy: Clinical pharmacology of the new beta-adrenergic blocking drugs. Part 4. Adverse effects. Choosing a β-adrenoreceptor blocker. *Am. Heart J.,* **1979,** *98,* 156–262.

Frishman, W. H., and Somberg, J. Comparative effects of calcium-entry blockers and long-acting nitrates in the therapy for angina pectoris. *Cardiovasc. Rev. Rep.* **1982,** *10,* 1435–1443.

Fulton, M; Julian, D. C.; and Oliver, M. F. Sudden death and myocardial infarction, American Heart Association Monograph No. 27, Research in acute myocardial infarction. *Circulation,* **1969,** *40* (Suppl. IV), 182.

Ganz, W.; Buchbinder, N.; Marcus, H.; et al. Intracoronary thrombolysis in evolving myocardial infarction. *Am. Heart J.,* **1981,** *101,* 4–13.

Garcia, E.; Nasrallah, A.; Goussous, Y.; and Hall, R. J. The treadmill exercise test: Diagnostic accuracy in coronary artery disease. In Norman, J. C. (ed.) *Coronary Artery Medicine and Surgery: Concepts and Controversies.* Appleton-Century-Crofts, New York, **1975,** pp. 216–220.

Gardin, J. M.; Isner, J. M.; Ronan, J. A.; et al. Pseudoischemic "false positive" ST segment changes induced by hyperventilation in patients with mitral valve prolapse. *Am. J. Cardiol.,* **1980,** *45,* 952–958.

Gazes, P. C.; Mobley, E. M., Jr.; Faris, H. M., Jr.; et al. Preinfarctional (stable) angina—a prospective study: Ten year follow-up. Prognostic significance of electrocardiographic changes. *Circulation,* **1973,** *48,* 331.

Gerstenblith, G.; Auyang, P.; Achuff, S. C.; et al. Nifedipine in unstable angina: A double blind randomized trial. *N. Engl. J. Med.,* **1982,** *306,* 885–889.

Gillmer, D. J., and Kark, P. Pulmonary edema precipitated by nifedipine. *Br. Med. J.,* **1980,** *284,* 1420–1421.

Goldberg, S.; Reichek, N.; Wilson, J.; et al., Nifedipine in the treatment of Prinzmetal's (variant) angina. *Am. J. Cardiol.,* **1979,** *44,* 804–810.

Goldschlager, N.; Cake, D.; and Cohn, K. Exercise-induced ventricular arrhythmias in patients with coronary artery disease. Their relation to angiographic findings. *Am. J. Cardiol.,* **1973,** *31,* 434–440.

Goldschlager, N.; Seizer, A.; and Cohn, K. Treadmill stress tests as indicators of presence and severity of coronary artery disease. *Ann. Intern. Med.,* **1976,** *85,* 277–286.

Goldstein, R. E.; Rosing, D. R.; Redwood, D. R.; et al. Clinical and circulatory effects of isosorbide dinitrate. *Circulation,* **1971,** *43,* 629–640.

Goldstein, R. E.; Stinson, E. B.; Scherer, J. L.; et al. Intraoperative coronary collateral function in patients with coronary occlusive disease. *Circulation,* **1974,** *49,* 298–308.

Gomes, A. S.; Esposito, V. A.; Grollman, J. H., Jr.; and O'Reilly, R. J. Angled views in the evaluation of the right coronary artery. *Cathet. Cardiovasc. Diagn.* **1982,** *8,* 71.

Gordon, T.; Kannel, W. B.; McGee, D.; and Dawber, T. R. Death and coronary attacks in men after giving up cigarette smoking. A report from the Framingham study. *Lancet,* **1974,** *2,* 1345.

Gotto, A. M., Jr. Drug treatment of hyperlipidemia. *Mod. Med.,* February 15, **1978,** *15,* 92.

Haft, J. I.; Gonnella, G. R.; Kirtane, J. S.; and Anastasiades, A. Correlation of ear crease sign with coronary arteriographic findings. *Cardiovasc. Med.,* August, **1979,** *4,* 861–867.

Hampton, J. R. Should every survivor of a heart attack be given a β-blocker? *Br. Med., J.,* **1982,** *285,* 33–36.

Harper, R. W.; Kennedy, G.; DeSanctis, R. W.; et al. The incidence and pattern of angina prior to acute myocardial infarction: A study of 577 cases. *Am. Heart J.,* **1979,** *97,* 178–183.

Harris, M. B.; Phil, D.; Harrell, F. E.; et al. Survival in medically treated coronary artery disease. *Circulation,* **1979,** *60,* 1259–1269.

Hecht, H. S.; Chew, C. Y. C.; Burnam, M. H.; et al. Verapamil in chronic stable angina: Amelioration of pacing-induced abnormalities of left ventricular ejection fraction, regional wall motion, lactate metabolism and hemodynamics. *Am. J. Cardiol.,* **1981,** *48,* 536.

Henry, W. L. Evaluation of ventricular function using two-dimensional echocardiography. *Am. J. Cardiol.,* **1982,** *49,* 1319–1323.

Heupler, F. A., and Proudfit, W. L. Nifedipine therapy for refractory coronary arterial spasm. *Am. J. Cardiol.,* **1979,** *44,* 798–803.

Hirshfeld, J. W., Jr.; Borer, J. S.; Goldstein, E. E.; et al. Reduction in severity and extent of myocardial infarction when nitroglycerin and methoxamine are administered during coronary occlusion. *Circulation,* **1974,** *49,* 291–299.

Hjalmarson, A.; Herlitz, J.; Malek, I.; et al. Effect on mortality of metoprolol in acute myocardial infarction: A double-blind randomized trial. *Lancet* **1981,** *2,* 823–826.

Humphries, J. O.; Taylor, G.; Mellits, E. D.; et al. Predictions of clinical course after survival of myocardial infarction. *Trans. Am. Clin. Climatol. Assoc.,* **1979,** *91,* 128.

Jelinek, M. V., and Lown, B. Exercise stress testing for exposure of cardiac arrhythmia. *Prog. Cardiovasc. Dis.,* **1974,** *16,* 497.

Jorgenson, C. R.; Wang, K.; Gobel, F. L.; et al. Effect of

propranolol on myocardial oxygen consumption and its hemodynamic correlates during upright exercise. *Circulation*, **1973**, *48*, 1173–1182.

Judkins, M. P. Selective coronary arteriography. I. A percutaneous transfemoral technic. *Radiology*, **1967**, *89*, 815.

Kannel, W. B. Meaning of the downward trend in cardiovascular mortality. *JAMA* **1982**, *247*, 877–880.

Kannel, W. B.; Boyle, J. T.; McNamara, P.; Quickenton, P.; and Gordon, T. Precursors of sudden coronary death: Factors related to the incidence of sudden death. *Circulation*, **1975**, *51*, 606.

Kannel, W. B., and Thom, T. J. Implications of the recent decline in cardiovascular mortality. *Cardiovasc. Med.*, **1979**, *4*, 983–997.

Kattus, A. S.; Hanafee, W. N.; Lingmise, W. P.; *et al.* Diagnosis, medical and surgical management of coronary insufficiency. *Ann. Intern. Med.*, **1968**, *69*, 115.

Kirshenbaum, H. D.; Ockene, I. S.; and Alpert, J. S. The spectrum of coronary artery spasm. *JAMA*, **1981**, *246*, 354–359.

Kolibash, A. J.; Bush, C. A.; Wepsic, R. A.; *et al.* Coronary collateral vessels: Spectrum of physiologic capabilities with respect to providing rest and stress myocardial perfusion, maintenance of left ventricular function and protection against infarction. *Am. J. Cardiol.*, **1982**, *50*, 130–238.

Kotler, M. N.; Tabatznik, B.; Mower, M. M.; and Tominaga, S. Prognostic significance of ventricular ectopic beats with respect to sudden death in the late postinfarction period. *Circulation*, **1973**, *47*, 959.

Lee, S. J. K.; Sung, Y. K.; and Zaragoza, A. J. Effects of nitroglycerin on left ventricular volumes and wall tension in patients with ischemic heart disease. *Br. Heart J.*, **1970**, *32*, 790.

LeJemtal, T. H.; Keung, E.; Frishman, W. H.; *et al.* Hemodynamic effects of captopril in patients with severe chronic heart failure. *Am. J. Cardiol.*, **1982**, *49*, 1484–1488.

Lesperance, J.; Saltiel, J.; Petitcherc, R.; and Bourassa, M. G. Angulated views in the sagittal plane for improved accuracy of cine-coronary angiography. *Am. J. Roentgenol.*, **1974**, *121*, 565.

Levy, R. I., and Rifkind, B. M. Lipid lowering drugs and hyperlipidaemia. In, Avery, G. S. (ed.) *Cardiovascular Drugs*, Vol. I: *Antiarrhythmic, Antihypertensive and Lipid Lowering Drugs.* ADIS Press Australia Pty., Ltd., Sydney, Australia, **1977**, p. 1.

Levy, W.; Cannon, D. S.; and Cohen, L. S. The nontransmural myocardial infarction in perspective. *Cardiovasc. Rev. Rep.* **1981**, *12*, 1285–1294.

Lie, J. T., and Titus, J. L. Pathology of the myocardium and the conduction system in sudden coronary death. *Circulation*, **1975**, *51*, (Suppl. III), 41–52.

Lloyd-Mostyn, R. H., and Oram, S. Modification by propranolol of cardiovascular effects of induced hypoglycaemia. *Lancet*, **1975**, *2*, 1213.

Longhurst, J. C., and Kraus, W. Exercise-induced ST elevation in patients without myocardial infarction. *Circulation*, **1979**, *60*, 616.

Malinow, M. R. Regression of atherosclerosis in humans: Fact or myth? *Circulation*, **1981**, *64*, 1–3.

Markis, J. E.; Jaffe, C. D.; Cohn, P. F.; *et al.* Clinical significance of coronary arterial ectasia. *Am. J. Cardiol.*, **1976**, *37*, 217.

Maseri, A.; Severi, S.; De Nes, M.; *et al.* "Variant" angina: One aspect of a continuous spectrum of vasospastic myocardial ischemia. *Am. J. Cardiol.*, **1978**, *42*, 1019–1035.

Mason, D. T., and Braunwald, E. The effects of nitroglycerin and amylnitrite on arteriolar and venous tone in the human forearm. *Circulation*, **1965**, *32*, 755.

Master, A. M. The two step test of myocardial function. *Am. Heart J.*, **1935**, *10*, 495.

Mathey, D. G.; Kuch, K. H.; Tilsner, V.; *et al.* Nonsurgical coronary artery recanalization in acute transmural myocardial infarction. *Circulation*, **1981**, *63*, 489.

Mattingly, T. W. The postexercise electrocardiogram. Its value in the diagnosis and prognosis of coronary arterial lesions. *Am. J. Cardiol.*, **1962**, *9*, 935–409.

McHenry, P. L.; Morris, S. N.; and Jordan, J. W. Stress testing in coronary heart disease. *Heart Lung*, **1974**, *3*, 83.

McKeena, W. J.; Chew, C. Y. C.; Oakley, C. M.; *et al.* Myocardial infarction with normal coronary angiogram: Possible mechanism of smoking risk in coronary artery disease. *Br. Heart J.*, **1980**, *43*, 493–498.

McNeer, J. C.; Margolis, J. R.; Lee, K. L.; *et al.* The role of the exercise test in the evaluation of patients for ischemic heart disease. *Circulation*, **1978**, *57*, 64–70.

Merx, W.; Dorr, R.; Rentrop, P.; *et al.* Evaluation of the effectiveness of intracoronary streptokinase infusion in myocardial infarction: Post procedure management and hospital course in 204 patients. *Am. Heart J.*, **1981**, *102*, 1181.

Mikolich, J. R.; Nicoloff, N.; Robinson, P. H.; *et al.* Relief of refractory angina with continuous intravenous infusion of nitroglycerin. *Chest*, **1980**, *77*, 375–379.

Milvy, P., and Siegel, A. J. Physical activity levels and altered mortality from coronary heart disease with an emphasis on marathon running: A critical review. *Cardiovasc. Rev. Rep.* **1981**, *2*, 233–236.

Mock, M. B.; Ringqvist, I.; Fisher, L. D.; *et al.* Survival of medically treated patients in the coronary artery surgery study (CASS) registry. *Circulation*, **1982**, *66*, 562–568.

Morris, S. N.; Phillips, J. C.; Jordan, J. W.; and McHenry, P. L. Incidence and significance of decreases in systolic blood pressure during graded treadmill exercise testing. *Am. J. Cardiol.*, **1978**, *41*, 221.

Moskowitz, R. M.; Piccini, P. A.; Nacarelli, G. V.; and Zelis, R. Nifedipine therapy for stable angina pectoris: Preliminary results of effects on angina frequency and treadmill exercise response. *Am. J. Cardiol.*, **1979**, *44*, 811–816.

Moss, A. J.; Davis, H. T.; DeCamilla, J.; and Bayer, L. W. Ventricular ectopic beats and their relation to sudden and nonsudden death after myocardial infarction. *Circulation*, **1979**, *60*, 998.

Mueller, H., and Chahine, R. A. Interim report of multi-center double-blind, placebo controlled studies of nifedipine in chronic stable angina pectoris. *Am. J. Med.*, **1981**, *71*, 645.

Multicenter International Study. Improvement in prognosis of myocardial infarction by long-term beta-adrenoreceptor blockade using practolol. *Br. Med. J.*, **1975**, *3*, 735.

Multiple Risk Factor Intervention Trial. Risk factor changes and mortality results. *JAMA,* **1982,** *248,* 1465–1502.

Nattel, S.; Ragno, R. E.; and Van Loon, G. Mechanism of propranolol withdrawal phenomena. *Circulation,* **1979,** *59,* 1158–1164.

Norwegian Multicenter Study Group. Timolol-induced reduction in mortality and reinfarction in patients surviving acute myocardial infarction. *N. Engl. J. Med.,* **1981,** *304,* 801–807.

Oliver, M. F. Cholesterol, coronaries, clofibrate and death. *N. Engl. J. Med.,* **1978,** *299,* 1360–1362.

Olvia, P. B. Pathophysiology of acute myocardial infarction. *Ann. Intern. Med.,* **1981,** *94,* 236–250.

Ornish, D.; Scherwitz, L. W.; Doody, R. S.; *et al.* Effects of stress management training and dietary changes in treating ischemic heart disease. *JAMA,* **1983,** *149,* 54–59.

Orzan, F.; Garcia, E.; Mathur, V. S.; and Hall, R. J. Is the treadmill exercise test useful for evaluating coronary artery disease in patients with complete left bundle branch block? *Am. J. Cardiol.,* **1978,** *42,* 35–40.

Perper, J. A.; Kuller, L. H.; and Cooper, M. Arteriosclerosis of coronary arteries in sudden unexpected deaths. *Circulation,* **1975,** *51* (Suppl. III), 27–33.

Pickering, M. B. Exercise and the prevention of coronary heart disease. *Cardiovasc. Rev. Rep.* **1981,** *2,* 227–229.

Popp, R. L. M-mode echocardiographic assessment of left ventricular function. *Am. J. Cardiol.,* **1982,** *49,* 1312–1318.

Prinzmetal, M.; Kennamer, R.; Merliss, R.; Wada, T.; and Bor, N. A variant form of angina pectoris. *Am. J. Med.,* **1959,** *27,* 375.

Profstfield, J. L., and Gotto, A. M., Jr. Lipoproteins in health and disease: Diagnosis and management. *Baylor College of Medicine Cardiology Series,* **1982,** *5,* 1–31.

Proudfit, W. L.; Bruschke, A. V. T.; and Sones, F. M., Jr. Natural history of obstructive coronary artery disease: Ten year study of 601 nonsurgical cases. *Prog. Cardiovasc. Dis.,* **1978,** *21,* 53.

Reeves, T. J.; Oberman, A.; Jones, W. B.; and Sheffield, L. T. Natural history of angina pectoris. *Am. J. Cardiol.,* **1974,** *33,* 423.

Rentrop, P.; Blanke, H.; Karsch, R.; *et al.* Selective intracoronary thrombolysis in acute myocardial infarction and unstable angina pectoris. *Circulation,* **1981,** *63,* 307–317.

Ritchie, M. L. Myocardial perfusion imaging. Bethesda Conference. *Am. J. Cardiol.,* **1982,** *49,* 1341–1347.

Robb, G. P., and Marks, H. H. Postexercise electrocardiogram in arteriosclerotic heart disease. *JAMA,* **1967,** *200,* 110–118.

Robin, E., Cowans, C.; and Puri, P. A comparative study of nitroglycerin and propranolol. *Circulation,* **1967,** *36,* 175–186.

Robinson, B. F. Mode of action of nitroglycerin in angina pectoris. *Br. Heart J.,* **1968,** *30,* 295–301.

Robson, R. H., and Vishwanath, M. D. Nifedipine and beta-blockade as a cause of cardiac failure. *Br. Med. J.,* **1981,** *284,* 104.

Rochmis, P., and Blackburn, H. Exercise tests. A survey of procedures, safety and litigation experience in approximately 170,000 tests. *JAMA,* **1971,** *217,* 1061.

Rodger, J. C.; Sheldon, C. D.; Lerski, R. A.; and Living-ston, W. R. Intermittent claudication complicating beta-blockade. *Br. Med. J.,* **1976,** *1,* 1125.

Rosenman, R. H.; Brand, R. J.; Sholtz, M. S.; and Jenkins, C. D. Relation of corneal arcus to cardiovascular risk factors and the incidence of coronary disease. *N. Engl. J. Med.,* **1974,** *291,* 1321–1323.

Rosing, D. R.; Kent, K. M.; Maron, B.; *et al.* Verapamil therapy: A new approach to the pharmacologic treatment of hypertrophic cardiomyopathy: I. Effects on exercise capacity and symptomatic status. *Circulation,* **1979,** *60,* 1209.

Rowe, D. W.; Oquendo, I.; DePuey, E. G.; *et al.* The noninvasive diagnosis of coronary artery disease in patients with left bundle-branch block. *Tex. Heart Inst. J.,* **1982,** *9,* 397–406.

Rubenson, D. S.; Tucker, C. R.; London, E.; Miller, D. C.; Stinson, E. B.; and Popp, R. R. Two-dimensional echocardiographic analysis of segmental left ventricular wall motion before and after coronary artery bypass surgery. *Circulation,* **1982,** *66,* 1025–1033.

Ruberman, W.; Weinblatt, E.; Goldberg, J. D.; *et al.* Ventricular premature complexes and sudden death after myocardial infarction. *Circulation,* **1981,** *64,* 297–305.

Salem, B. I.; Terasawa, M.; Mathur, V. S.; *et al.* Left main coronary artery ostial stenosis: Clinical markers, angiographic recognition and distinction from left main disease. *Cathet. Cardiovasc. Diagn.,* **1979,** *5,* 125–134.

Sanz, G.; Castaner, A.; Betriu, A.; *et al.* Determinants of prognosis of survivors of myocardial infarction. *N. Engl. J. Med.,* **1982,** *306,* 1065–1070.

Savage, R. M.; Wagner, G. S.; Ideker, R. E.; *et al.* Correlation of postmortem anatomic findings with electrocardiographic changes in patients with myocardial infarction. *Circulation,* **1977,** *55,* 279.

Schroeder, J. S.; Lamb, I. H.; and Hu, M. Do patients in whom myocardial infarction has been ruled out have a better prognosis after hospitalization than those surviving infarction? *N. Engl. J. Med.,* **1980,** *303,* 1–5.

Schulze, R. A., Jr.; Pitt, B.; Griffith, L. S. C.; *et al.* Coronary angiography and left ventriculography in survivors of transmural and nontransmural myocardial infarction. *Am. J. Med.,* **1978,** *64,* 108–113.

Seldinger, S. I. Catheter replacement of the needle in percutaneous arteriography: A new technique. *Acta Radiol.,* **1953,** *39,* 368.

Sheffield, L. T., and Reeves, T. J. Graded exercise in the diagnosis of angina pectoris. *Mod. Concepts Cardiovasc. Dis.,* **1965,** *34,* 1.

Shekelle, R. B.; Shryock, A. M.; Paul, L.; *et al.* Diet, serum and death from coronary heart disease: The Western Electric Study. *N. Engl. J. Med.,* **1981,** *304,* 65–70.

Singh, B. N.; Collett, J.; and Chew, C. Y. C. New perspectives in the pharmacologic therapy of cardiac arrhythmias. *Prog. Cardiovasc. Dis.,* **1980,** *22,* 243.

Skinner, C.; Gaddu, J.; and Palmer, K. N. V. Comparison of effects of metoprolol and propranolol on asthmatic airway obstruction. *Br. Med. J.,* **1976,** *1,* 504.

Slogoff, S.; Keats, A. S.; and Ott, E. Preoperative propranol therapy and aortocoronary bypass operation. *JAMA,* **1978,** *240,* 1487–1490.

Solberg, L. E.; Nissen, R. G.; and Bliestra, R. E. Prinzmetal's variant angina—response to verapamil. · *Mayo Clin. Proc.,* **1978,** *53,* 256–259.

Sones, F. M., Jr. Acquired heart disease: Symposium on present and future of cineangiocardiography. *Am. J. Cardiol.,* **1959,** *3,* 710.

Sones, F. M., Jr., and Shirey, E. K. Cine coronary arteriography. *Mod. Concepts Cardiovasc. Dis.,* **1962,** *31,* 735.

Sos, T. A.; Lee, J. G.; Levin, D. C.; and Baltaxi, H. A. New lordotic projection for improved visualization of the left coronary artery and its branches. *Am. J. Roentgenol.,* **1974,** *121,* 575.

Specchia, G.; de Servi, S.; Falcone, C.; *et al.* Significance of exercise-induced ST segment elevation in patients without myocardial infarction. *Circulation,* **1981,** *63,* 46–53.

Stadel, B. V. Oral contraceptives and cardiovascular disease. *N. Engl. J. Med.,* **1981,** *305,* 612–618.

Stratton, J. R.; Lighty, G. E.; Pearlman, A. S.; and Ritchie, J. L. Detection of left ventricular thrombus by two-dimensional echocardiography: Sensitivity, specificity, and causes of uncertainity. *Circulation,* **1982,** *66,* 156–166.

Strauss, H. W., and Boucher, C. A. Radionuclide angiography. Bethesda Conference RNA. *Am. J. Cardiol.,* **1982,** *49,* 1337–1341.

Subramanian, B.; Bowles, M. J.; Davies, A. B.; and Raftery, E. B. Combined therapy with verapamil and propranolol in chronic stable angina. *Am. J. Cardiol.,* **1982,** *49,* 125–132.

Swan, H. J. C. Editorial: Thrombolysis in acute myocardial infarction: Treatment of the underlying coronary artery disease. *Circulation,* **1982,** *66,* 914–916.

Taylor, W. R.; Forrester, J. S.; Magnusson, P.; *et al.* Hemodynamic effects of nitroglycerin ointment in congestive heart failure. *Am. J. Cardiol.,* **1976,** *38,* 469–473.

Thadani, U.; Davidson, C.; Chir, B.; Singleton, W.; and Taylor, S. H. Comparison of the immediate effects of five β-adrenoreceptor-blocking drugs with different ancillary properties in angina pectoris. *N. Engl. J. Med.,* **1979,** *300,* 750–755.

Thadani, U.; Fung, H.; Kdrke, A. C.; and Parker, J. O. Oral isosorbide dinitrate in the treatment of angina pectoris. *Circulation,* **1980,** *62,* 491–502.

Thompson, P. D., and Kelemen, M. H. Hypotension accompanying the onset of exertional angina. *Circulation,* **1975,** *52,* 28.

University Group Diabetes Program. A study of the effects of hypoglycemic agents on vascular complications in patients with adult-onset diabetes. I. Mortality results. *Diabetes,* **1979,** *19* (Suppl. 2), 785.

Vaughan-Williams, E. M.; Baywell, E. E.; and Singh, B. N. Cardiospecificity of beta-receptor blockade. A comparison of the relative potencies on cardiac and peripheral vascular beta-adrenoceptors of propranolol, of practolol and its ortho-substituted isomer. *Cardiovasc. Res.,* **1973,** *7,* 226.

Visser, C. A.; Kan, G.; David, G. K.; *et al.* Two-dimensional echocardiography in the diagnosis of left ventricular thrombus: A prospective study of 67 patients with anatomic validation. *Chest,* **1983,** *83,* 228.

Waal, H. Propranolol-induced depression. *Br. Med. J.,* **1967,** *2,* 50.

Waal-Manning, H. Problems with practolol. *Drugs,* **1975,** *10,* 336.

Waters, D. D.; Szlachcic, J.; Bourassa, M. G.; *et al.* Exercise testing in patients with variant angina: Results, correlation with clinical angiographic features and prognostic significance. *Circulation,* **1982,** *65,* 265–274.

Weaver, W. D.; Lorch, G. S.; Alvarez, H. A.; and Cobb, L. A. Angiographic findings and prognostic indicators in patients resuscitated from sudden cardiac death. *Circulation,* **1976,** *54,* 895.

Williams, D. O.; Bommer, W. J.; Miller, R. R.; Amsterdam, E. A.; and Mason, D. T. Hemodynamic assessment of oral peripheral vasodilator therapy in chronic congestive heart failure: Prolonged effectiveness of isosorbide dinitrate. *Am. J. Cardiol.,* **1977,** *39,* 84–90.

Wright, P. Untoward effect associated with practolol administration. Occulomucocutaneous syndrome. *Br. Med. J.,* **1975,** *1,* 595.

Zir, L. M.; Miller, J. E.; Dinsmore, R. E.; *et al.* Interobserver variability in coronary arteriography. *Circulation,* **1976,** *53,* 627.

Chapter 12
SURGICAL TREATMENT OF PATIENTS WITH CORONARY ARTERY DISEASE

Robert J. Hall

HISTORY

The earliest operative treatment proposed for patients with refractory symptoms of coronary artery disease (CAD) was thoracic sympathetic ganglionectomy, usually T_1 to T_4 or T_5. Attempts to increase myocardial collateral blood flow through epicardial connections included procedures such as suturing the omentum to the epicardium (O'Shaughnessy, 1937), as well as the application of talc, asbestos, or other irritants to the epicardial surface (Harken et al., 1955; Thompson and Plachta, 1957). Coronary venous obstruction also was combined with arterial anastomosis to the great cardiac vein in an attempt to retroperfuse the ischemic myocardium via the venous circulation (McAllister et al., 1948). None of these procedures achieved any widespread use. Subsequent attempts to increase myocardial blood flow included direct implantation of the internal mammary artery into the myocardium of the left ventricle (Vineberg, 1946; Vineberg and Walker, 1964; Effler et al., 1965; Gorlin and Taylor, 1966; Effler, 1976). Anastomoses developed between the implanted systemic artery and the coronary arterial bed in a number of patients with beneficial clinical results (Vineberg and Walker, 1964; Effler, 1976). Ligation

of the internal mammary artery became popular temporarily in the late 1950s. This procedure was effective presumably by increasing flow through pericardial branches after occlusion of the major internal mammary artery channel. The procedure fell into disrepute and was abandoned when it was demonstrated that "sham" ligation of the internal mammary arteries was equally effective in reducing angina (Diamond et al., 1960).

Direct operation in patients with obstructed epicardial coronary arteries evolved after angiographic visualization of the coronary arteries was developed in the early 1960s (Sones and Shirey, 1962). Early procedures included coronary endarterectomy, pericardial patch angioplasty, and resection of a diseased portion of the coronary artery with interposition of a saphenous venous graft (Mundth and Austen, 1975; Effler, 1976). The earliest reported use of a Dacron tube graft, or of a reversed segment of autologous saphenous vein as a conduit from the aorta to the coronary artery, was in 1963 in a child with coronary-to-right-ventricle fistula (Hallman et al., 1965), and in 1965 in children with anomalous origin of the left coronary from the pulmonary artery (Cooley et al., 1966). The late follow-up of the first patient with atherosclerotic CAD who received an aorticocoronary saphenous vein graft in 1964, was reported in 1973 (Garrett *et al.,* 1973). The technique of myocardial revascularization in patients with coronary disease by means of saphenous vein bypass graft from the aorta to the coronary artery was first reported in 1969 from two separate clinics (Favaloro, 1969; Johnson *et al.,* 1969). Presently, more than 3,000 patients in our institution and 100,000 patients annually in the United States undergo myocardial revascularization by aortocoronary bypass (ACB). The frequency and popularity of this modality for the treatment of patients with CAD require the practitioner to have a clear understanding of the management of patients through the period of bypass surgery and follow-up, and of the short- and long-term results. Current indications are best considered after these factors are studied.

CORONARY ARTERY BYPASS

Coronary artery bypass became widely accepted before scientific and statistical proof of its effectiveness. Widespread experience has now shown that before patients can be properly selected for ACB, and the benefits of revascularization over medical treatment ascertained, a thorough assessment of all aspects of the procedure is essential. An understanding of these details, including patient management, surgical considerations, complications, results, rehabilitation, and long-term survival, is essential if the physician is to make an effective decision.

Presurgical Management

Patients admitted to the hospital for ACB are continued on a regimen of antianginal medication, and the dosage is further optimized if required. The patient and family members have a high level of anxiety during this period, and this can be alleviated if all aspects of the hospitalization are conducted in an efficient, relaxed, and reassuring manner. Clinical evaluation of the patient for evidence of other significant disease processes, which may affect the patient during open heart surgery, has usually been performed before this admission. If not, certain considerations are important at this time.

A history of symptoms of cerebrovascular insufficiency, prior cerebrovascular accident, or the finding of cervical carotid bruits indicates the need for careful neurological evaluation. Results of noninvasive carotid artery echo flow studies may aid in excluding significant

extracranial common or internal carotid artery occlusive disease. If the patient's condition is questioned further, contrast carotid, and at times vertebral, angiography is required. Significant extracranial carotid occlusive disease (75% or greater diameter narrowing), in even asymptomatic patients, poses a risk of cerebrovascular accident with open heart surgery. Patients with these lesions are managed best by appropriate carotid endarterectomy, one side at a time if bilateral disease is present, four to seven days before ACB. Such staging of surgery appears to yield better results than concomitant carotid endarterectomy and ACB (Loop *et al.,* 1982).

Attention is also directed to the patient's respiratory system. Symptoms or physical findings of significant chronic obstructive or bronchospastic lung disease necessitate careful pulmonary evaluation—blood gas analysis and pulmonary function testing. If required, presurgical bronchodilator therapy is initiated, and at times operation is delayed temporarily while the pulmonary status is optimized. At a minimum, certain patients are identified for closer postoperative respiratory attention because of the potential for increased difficulties.

A history of renal insufficiency or the finding of azotemia increases the risk of open heart surgery. If secondary to a diuretic-induced volume contraction, this condition should be corrected before operation. In patients with parenchymal renal disease, added precautions toward preventing further renal impairment are required, and volume contraction is avoided insofar as possible. Preoperative and intraoperative administration of mannitol intravenously is advocated in this setting by some nephrologists.

Prothrombin-inhibiting drugs (*Coumadin,* and so on) are discontinued five to seven days before surgery, and although some physicians recommend discontinuing antiplatelet agents for two or more weeks before open heart surgery, this may not always be practical and is probably unnecessary. A recent report indicates that saphenous vein bypass patency is enhanced when prophylaxis with dipyridamole (*Persantine*) is initiated before operation and continued postoperatively with the agent administered via nasogastric tube the first 24 hours after operation (Chesebro *et al.,* 1982).

Surgical Considerations in ACB

The heart is approached for ACB through a median sternotomy. The operation requires a quiet, nonbeating heart, necessitating the support of circulation by temporary cardiopulmonary bypass. Blood is routed from the right atrium to the ascending aorta through a heart-lung machine which assumes the pumping function of the heart and oxygenates the venous blood. In the early years of coronary bypass surgery, asystole was produced by intermittent cross-clamping of the aorta, producing temporary ischemic arrest. Since 1976 to 1977, preservation of the myocardium has been improved by chemical and hypothermic cardioplegia. The heart is cooled externally by placing iced saline into the pericardial sling, and chilled cardioplegic solution (see Table 12-1 for composition) is injected into the cross-clamped ascending aorta and gains access to the myocardium via the coronary arteries. Cardiac hypothermia and standstill reduce myocardial oxygen requirements and protect the myocardium during the period the bypasses are constructed. Segments of the saphenous vein from the lower extremity are the conduits most frequently used to bypass from the proximal aorta to the distal portion of each of the narrowed or occluded coronary arteries. The vein is reversed to disable venous valves present in the peripheral veins.

The saphenous vein grafts are sutured end-to-side to the opened distal coronary artery and to the proximal aorta using a running suture of 6-0 *Prolene*. (Figures 12-1 and 12-2). The technique of these delicate anastomoses is facilitated by the use of 3-diopter magnifying loupes and narrowly focused high-intensity "cold" light on the immediate surgical field. A single saphenous vein may be used to perform two or more distal anastomoses in sequence by side-to-side anastomosis to one (or several) coronary artery(ies) and by end-to-side anastomosis to an adjacent coronary artery or to the distal segment of the same coronary artery if multiple obstructions are present in one vessel. The trend toward complete revascularization has resulted in more bypasses being placed; at present a patient may commonly undergo by-

pass to three to five coronary artery branches (average, 3.2 bypasses per patient) (Hall *et al.,* 1983) (Figure 12-3).

The internal mammary artery also has been used as a bypass conduit, usually to bypass the left anterior descending or diagonal coronary arteries. Excellent patency rates have been reported with use of internal mammary grafts (Kay *et al.,* 1974; Loop *et al.,* 1977); however, the size of the artery, lower rate of flow achieved relative to that possible with saphenous vein grafts, and the additional time required to dissect the internal mammary artery have limited their use to conduits.

Endarterectomy. One of the original procedures attempted in coronary revascularization was mechanical removal of the atherosclerotic plaque within the lumen of the coronary artery (Sawyer *et al.,* 1967; Mundth and Austen, 1975). Inadequacies of the method led to the development of, and replacement by, ACB. During the years, patients with severely diseased vessels have been managed by blunt removal of the atherosclerotic plaque from the coronary artery at and distal to the site of anastomosis, together with ACB. In our institution the combined use of endarterectomy has resulted in a somewhat higher early mortality and greater frequency of perioperative infarction and is avoided whenever possible. Severe diffuse atherosclerotic disease, unfortunately, dictates the necessity of endarterectomy in some patients (Hall *et al.,* 1983).

Aneurysmectomy and Operation for Ventricular Tachyarrhythmias. A discrete, large left ventricular aneurysm requires resection and concomitant ACB if indicated (Elayda *et al.,* 1982). Various surgical techniques have been used to treat patients who have aneurysmal formation, or severe thinning of the interventricular septum, and generally involve either plication or support with an onlay patch of Dacron cloth. At times, patients with large akinetic areas of the free wall of the left ventricle, without a discrete aneurysm, are managed by plication rather than resection.

The salutary, though nonpredictable, effect of left ventricular aneurysm resection in patients with recurrent life-threatening ventricular tachyarrhythmias has been reported (Sami, et al., 1978). Recent advances in intracardiac electrophysiologic studies have led to development of surgical techniques which attempt to isolate, resect or interrupt reentry pathways that contribute to the genesis of reentry ventricular tachycardia (Fontaine *et al.,* 1982). These

Table 12-1. CARDIOPLEGIA SOLUTION (per 500 ml 5% Dextrose and 0.45% NaCl)*

Potassium chloride	20.0 mM	(1492.0 mg)
Magnesium chloride	7.5 mM	(1527.03 mg)
Sodium bicarbonate	2.5 mM	(210.0 mg)
Calcium chloride	0.0 mM	(147.147 mg)

* From the Texas Heart Institute, Houston, Texas.

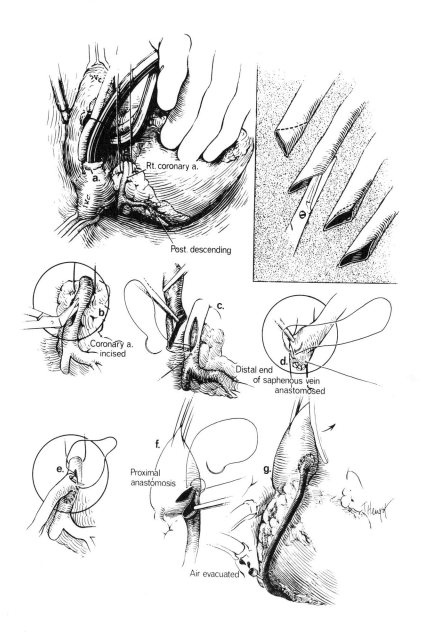

Figure 12-1. Drawing showing aortocoronary saphenous vein bypass to the right coronary artery using temporary cardiopulmonary bypass with caval cannulation for venous outflow and ascending aortic cannulation for arterial return. *a.* The caval clamps are applied, and the ascending aorta is cross-clamped. A traction suture is placed around the artery proximal to the anticipated site of anastomosis. *b.* The proposed distal end of the reversed saphenous vein graft is beveled slightly (inset). *c.* The distal anastomosis is performed using a 6-0 monofilament double-armed polypropylene suture, starting at the distal end of the arteriotomy. *d.* The right side of the anastomosis is done first, using a simple continuous suture. *e.* If the vessel is unusually sclerotic, the sutures are inserted in the artery from inside to outside to prevent lifting a plaque. The left side of the anastomosis is performed using the other needle, and the two ends are tied together. *f.* The proximal anastomosis to the ascending aorta may be performed with the aorta cross-clamped or with a partial occlusion clamp on the ascending aorta after the aortic cross-clamp is released. We prefer a transverse or oblique aortotomy just above the origin of the right coronary artery. *g.* A small ellipse of aortic tissue is removed. A 5-0 monofilament double-armed continuous suture is preferred. Air is evacuated from the saphenous vein through a 25-gauge needle, as the clamp is released from the ascending aorta. (From Cooley, D. A., and Norman, J. C. *Techniques in Cardiac Surgery.* Texas Medical Press, Houston, **1975,** pp. 156–157.)

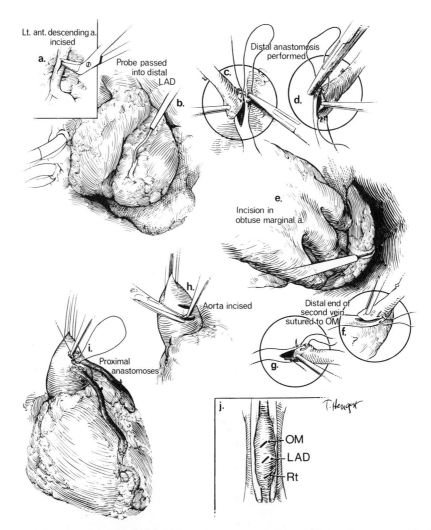

Figure 12-2 labels:

Lt. ant. descending a. incised

a.

Probe passed into distal LAD

b.

Distal anastomosis performed

c.

d.

e.
Incision in obtuse marginal a.

h.
Aorta incised

Distal end of second vein sutured to OM

f.

g.

i.
Proximal anastomoses

j.
OM
LAD
Rt

T. Heugot

Figure 12-2. Drawing showing double aortocoronary bypass with anastomoses to the left anterior descending coronary artery and the obtuse marginal branch of the circumflex artery. In general, the technique of anastomosis is the same as for the right coronary artery, using temporary cardiopulmonary bypass and topical cardiac hypothermia (Fig. 12-1). *a.* The first anastomosis performed is to the left anterior descending coronary artery. *b.* After an arteriotomy is made, distal patency of the artery is verified by the use of a coronary probe. *c.* The anastomosis is performed from the upper or proximal angle of the incision toward the distal end. *d.* The right side of the anastomosis is then completed. *e.* To expose the circumflex branches, the heart must be completely elevated from the pericardium and rotated toward the right. A second assistant standing on the patient's right side provides exposure by retracting the heart with a hand over the wet gauze pack. The obtuse marginal branch of the circumflex is incised longitudinally using a scalpel and fine scissors. *f* and *g.* Acutely angled scissors are useful to enlarge the arteriotomy in a retrograde direction toward the cardiac apex. The anastomosis is performed using a 6-0 monofilament simple continuous suture. *h.* The apex of the heart is returned to the pericardial sac. The aortotomy incisions are made in a transverse direction. *i.* The surgeon must estimate the appropriate length of the veins before making the anastomoses, being careful not to make the grafts too short. Ellipses of aortic wall are then excised, and the anastomoses are completed with 5-0 monofilament sutures. *j.* The aortic anastomoses are made using a partial-occlusion clamp. The optimum position of the aortotomy incisions is shown in the drawing. (From Cooley, D. A., and Norman, J. C. *Techniques in Cardiac Surgery.* Texas Medical Press, Houston, **1975,** pp. 158–159.)

204

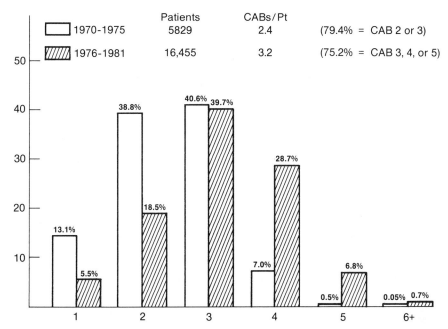

Figure 12-3. Number of coronary arteries bypassed per patient. Texas Heart Institute experience—1970 through 1975 compared with 1976 through 1981 (From Hall, R. J., Elayda, M. A., Gray, A., *et al.* Coronary artery bypass: Long-term follow-up of 22,284 consecutive patients. *Circulation,* **1983,** *68*(Suppl. II):II20-26. By permission of the American Heart Association, Inc.)

pathways are in the endocardium and frequently encircle the base of a ventricular aneurysm or adjacent zone of an infarct scar. After the ventricle is opened, these areas can be isolated electrically from the remainder of the heart by an encircling endocardial ventriculotomy (Guiraudon *et al.,* 1978). Electrophysiologic identification of other sites of micro reentry, usually in areas of dense endocardial scarring, has permitted surgical resection of these endocardial plaques or destruction of focal endocardial areas with cryosurgical techniques (Josephson *et al.,* 1979; Horowitz *et al.,* 1980). These surgical methods, directed at treating patients with life-threatening ventricular tachyarrhythmic complications of CAD, are currently developmental and require further experience for validation of their efficacy.

Pacemakers. A small number of patients who undergo ACB experience temporary suppression of sinoatrial impulse formation or of atrioventricular conduction, and pacing wires are sewn loosely into the ventricular myocardium. The wires are guided out of the mediastinum through a separate anterior tract and permit temporary electronic pacing of the ventricle with an external pulse generator. Pacing is usually required for only several hours

(usually no longer than 12 to 24 hours) and can be discontinued when normal sinoatrial or atrioventricular function resumes. The temporary pacing wires can be easily extracted externally four to eight days after operation. When poor ventricular function is present, pacing electrodes placed on both the atrium and the ventricle permit temporary external atrioventricular sequential pacing, preserving the atrial contribution to ventricular filling and enhancing left ventricular function. Rarely, the preexistence of a serious abnormality of sinoatrial impulse formation or of atrioventricular conduction is identified before ACB, and a permanent epicardial pacemaker is implanted.

Weaning from Cardiopulmonary Bypass. After the bypasses are completed and any residual intracavitary air is vented from the ascending aorta and the left ventricle, the patient is taken off cardiopulmonary bypass in a decremental fashion. Normal sinus rhythm usually resumes spontaneously, although direct-current countershock may be required to terminate ventricular fibrillation. The need for cardiotonic agents to support myocardial contractility as the patient is weaned from cardiopulmonary bypass presently is infrequent, unless the patient has had severe preoperative left ventricular depression or has sustained severe perioperative myocardial injury. Under these circumstances, temporary intra-aortic balloon-assisted circulation is implemented so the duration and amount of circulatory support provided by inotropic agents can be limited. The current, infrequent need for postcardiopulmonary inotropic support has resulted from improved protection of the myocardium during surgery, due in large part to the effectiveness of cold and potassium cardioplegia employed during ACB (Sturm et al., 1981).

After cardiopulmonary bypass is terminated, the chest is closed and a mediastinal tube and, if needed, pleural drainage tubes are placed to vacate and quantitate residual bleeding.

POSTOPERATIVE MANAGEMENT

Postoperative management is optimally conducted by close coordination among members of the surgical, anesthesia, and cardiological staffs. A skilled, experienced recovery room nursing staff is essential in the management of patients during the first 24 to 48 hours after ACB. These nurses follow the clinical status of the patient closely, observe vital signs continuously, and monitor the cardiac rhythm, ventilation, blood loss, and urinary output. Frequent arterial blood gas determinations are made to guide ventilator adjustments. Although complex monitoring systems are used by some centers, we have found that display of the interarterial pressure and the electrocardiographic recording at each bedside, with appropriate high and low audible alarm signals, is adequate. The central venous pressure is monitored hourly by a saline manometer via a catheter in the superior vena cava. Body temperature is monitored by means of a rectal probe. Flow of urine and loss of mediastinal and pleural blood are measured hourly. Frequent blood gas and pH determinations, and electrolyte measurements are made; and, if abnormal, the mechanism is identified and corrected. Hypokalemia is particularly common in the period after cardiopulmonary bypass and is corrected by infusion of 10 mEq of potassium chloride added hourly to the intravenous solution. Patients with hyperglycemia, glycosuria, and resultant polyuria are treated with insulin as required. Occasional inordinate hypertension necessitates temporary treatment with trimethaphan camsylate (Arfonad) or nitroprusside drip with close attention paid to careful monitoring of blood pressure. Hypovolemia may be the cause of an intense sympathetic

discharge, peripheral vasoconstriction, and central hypertension and is corrected by volume expansion. Reoperation for continued bleeding in the postoperative period has become relatively infrequent in recent years (Loop et al., 1981). If the postoperative course is complicated, serial measurement of the pulmonary artery and pulmonary capillary wedge pressures and of the cardiac output, using a balloon flotation catheter, is required to successfully manage the patient's cardiac, pulmonary, and fluid volume status.

Low Cardiac Output States

Postoperative myocardial insufficiency and low cardiac output may be the consequence of either severe preoperative ventricular dysfunction or, more often, perioperative myocardial damage. Patients with low cardiac output are managed with inotropic and vasodilator therapy and require a pulmonary artery catheter for appropriate monitoring of pressure and cardiac output. Severe depression of myocardial function requires hemodynamic support with intra-aortic balloon pumping. From 1972 to 1979 at our institution, intra-aortic balloon pumping was required for management of slightly more than 2% of the patients who had postoperative low output syndromes (Sturm et al., 1980). Of these, 82% had initiation of intra-aortic balloon assistance in conjunction with weaning from cardiopulmonary bypass. Management also included simultaneous manipulation of intravascular volume, myocardial stimulation with inotropic agents, and control of afterload with vasodilator therapy, titrated to reduce peripheral resistance to less than 1,800/dynes/sec/cm^{-5}. Among patients who require intra-aortic balloon assistance, a 60% survival can be expected (Sturm et al., 1980; McGee et al., 1980).

Perioperative Myocardial Infarction

The incidence of perioperative infarction has declined over the last decade and ranges from 4 to 10%. Incidence as low as 2.4% (Kouchoukos et al., 1980) and 1.2% (Loop et al., 1981) has been reported. The reduced frequency of perioperative infarction is related to myocardial preservation techniques utilizing cold potassium cardioplegia. It is of interest that most perioperative infarctions occur in the distribution of a patent graft (Loop et al., 1981).

Perioperative infarction is diagnosed by means of electrocardiographic changes, elevated serum cardiac enzyme levels, and radionuclide techniques such as ^{99m}Tc-pyrophosphate (PYP) scintigraphy and gated blood pool ventriculography. We routinely record a 12-lead electrocardiogram shortly after operation and on postoperative days one and two. The serum level of cardiac enzymes is measured on the first (16 to 20 hours postoperative) and second days after operation.

Moderate elevation of the levels of the standard cardiac enzymes is attributable to thoracotomy and cardiac surgery alone, although elevation of SGOT levels above 100 and LDH levels above 500 have been most suggestive of new myocardial necrosis (Dawson et al., 1972). In our laboratory, elevation of the creatine kinase-MB, measured by immunoradiometric assay, to levels above 8.5 units has been highly specific for new myocardial necrosis (DePuey et al., 1983).

Electrocardiographic Changes

Perioperative myocardial infarction may produce the classic evolutionary ST-T and Q-wave changes, or may be manifested by abrupt appearance of new Q waves on the first postoperative ECG recording. Most perioperative infarctions are evident from the initial ECG record, with a smaller number becoming evident only on the first or second postoperative day or, rarely, later during the recovery period. In the presence of a QRS deformity such as that produced by prior myocardial infarction, by left bundle branch block, or ventricular paced rhythms, the diagnosis of infarction by ECG is not possible, and the occurrence of a perioperative infarction must be judged by enzyme changes or by results of technetium pyrophosphate myocardial imaging.

Nonspecific ST- and T-wave changes are common after surgery. Most patients demonstrate some generalized ST-segment elevation caused by injury to the epicardium resulting from trauma at surgery. The ST-segment vector of diffuse surgical epicardial trauma usually is directed between 0 and 60 degrees in the frontal plane and oriented slightly anteriorly. Subsequent generalized moderate T inversion, occurring after several days and lasting several weeks, is a continuation of this same process and should not be misconstrued as the consequence of myocardial damage. Axis shift to the left, probably the consequence of thoracotomy and pericardotomy, is common and results in reduced inferior R forces and, at times, development of a new Q wave in leads III and, occasionally, AVF. In our experience, this is usually not the consequence of new inferior infarction but represents a frequent source of ECG misinterpretation in the postoperative period.

The extent of a perioperative infarction can be assessed early in the postoperative period by recording at bedside an equilibrium gated blood pool radionuclide ventriculogram which provides information on the ejection fraction of the left ventricle as well as the location and magnitude of new wall motion abnormalities (DePuey et al., 1980). Occasionally, the differential diagnosis of abnormal hemodynamics, consistent with either right heart failure or pericardial tamponade, is resolved when the features of extensive right ventricular infarction are elicited by radionuclide angiography.

The recovery of patients who experience a perioperative myocardial infarction is handled at a slower rate than those who have an uncomplicated course. Management in an intensive care area and a step-down unit is used to provide appropriate monitoring and a more gradual convalescence. Some patients with evidence of perioperative infarction by electrocardiographic criteria will have little or no new ventricular wall motion abnormality by radionuclide angiography (DePuey et al., 1980), and can be progressed at a normal rate.

Progression of Recovery of the Uncomplicated Patient

Most patients can be transferred to a standard hospital room on the second postoperative day after the chest tubes are removed and an x-ray of the chest is reviewed to exclude an unintentional pneumothorax. Low-dosage therapy with a beta-blocker is reinstituted orally on the first or second postoperative day, usually 40 to 80 mg per day of propranolol, to prevent the manifestations of beta-blockade withdrawal. This practice has also reduced by nearly 50% the incidence of postoperative atrial flutter and fibrillation, a common occurrence between the first and seventh postoperative day. Deep-breathing exercises and use of an incentive inspirometer facilitate clearing of postoperative atelectasis. From this time forward, patients are ambulated progressively, assisted at first and then progressively on their own as strength resumes. Progressive ambulation is encouraged, and most patients are walking about the ward a total of 1 or more miles daily by the seventh to ninth postoperative day. The electrolyte levels and a complete blood count are checked on the fourth postoperative day, and anemia is corrected with infusion of packed red blood cells or by oral iron and folate therapy, as indicated. The BUN and creatinine levels are checked at this time to detect the occasional occurrence of renal insufficiency. Results of chest roentgenography on the fourth postoperative day provide guidance for further management of postoperative atelectasis or pleural effusion.

Anticoagulation is not employed routinely after ACB, since lower extremity phlebitis is uncommon and pulmonary emboli are rare, probably as a consequence of early postoperative ambulation. Under certain conditions such as advanced age or obesity which may delay ambulation, or when there has been simultaneous implantation of a prosthetic valve, anticoagulation is desirable. It has been our policy for the past decade to initiate antiplatelet therapy with dipyridamole (PERSANTINE), 100 to 150 mg daily, and buffered acetylsalicylic acid, 300 to 600 mg per day, on the second postoperative day, after chest tubes are removed. If no contraindication or intolerance is exhibited, the agents are continued indefinitely. Dipyridamole (PERSANTINE), initiated prior to ACB and continued in the early postoperative period via nasogastric tube and thereafter orally, along with aspirin, for long-term therapy, recently has been shown to enhance saphenous vein graft patency significantly (Chesebro et al., 1982).

OTHER COMPLICATIONS

Wound Infection

Among more than 9,000 consecutive procedures, 0.66% of patients developed significant sternal complications and 0.39%, sternal infections. Of these patients, 95% survived (Ott et al., 1980). Predisposing factors are chronic obstructive lung disease, diabetes mellitus, obesity, closed-chest cardiac massage, prolonged assisted ventilation, and excessive postoperative bleeding. Proper management includes early diagnosis, surgical debridement, rewiring, and primary closure with substernal drainage and appropriate antibiotic therapy.

Neurological Complications

A neurological deficit occurs in a small number of patients after ACB, either as the result of air or particulate embolization from the heart or the aorta at the time of surgery (Slogoff et al., 1982), or due to concomitant intrinsic cerebrovascular disease. The complication occurs in 1 to 3% of all patients and is more frequent in the elderly—6.5% of patients over 69 years of age in one series (Loop et al., 1981). Although the neurological deficit is transient in many, permanent residual symptoms persist in some patients. The frequency of minor neurological deficits may be much higher if careful psychometric testing were to be done before and after operation.

Renal Insufficiency

Renal insufficiency is uncommon following ACB and usually is related to, and a complication of, decreased renal blood flow secondary to conditions of extensive blood loss or low cardiac output. A considerable number of these patients recover with meticulous management and dialysis.

Pulmonary Insufficiency

Pulmonary insufficiency most often is observed in patients with preexisting chronic pulmonary disease. Unexpected severe respiratory failure due to the "adult respiratory distress syndrome" which usually follows major hemorrhage or cardiogenic shock is observed infrequently. Recovery is unpredictable and requires intense management of the patient's pulmonary status and fluid balance.

Postpericardiotomy Syndrome

This inflammatory process of both the pericardial and pleural mesothelial surfaces occurs, in varying degrees of severity, in from 5 to 20% of patients. The syndrome consists of pleuritic-like pain, fever of moderate degree, pericardial (and often pleural) friction rub, and effusion into the pericardial (and often pleural) space. Although the syndrome often occurs after discharge of the patient, it may occur during the convalescent period in the hospital. The course is usually benign, limited to three to four days, and the patient is best treated with analgesics and nonsteroidal anti-inflammatory agents. Rarely, the brief and nonsustained use of steroids is required for more severe manifestations of the syndrome. Patients who experience recurrence of the syndrome at intervals of several weeks or months are again managed with a repeat course of nonsteroidal anti-inflammatory agents, followed by an increased dosage of acetylsalicylic acid suppression. Multiple recurrences during long periods are rare and appear to occur more often in patients who have been managed more extensively and for prolonged periods with corticosteroids. The unusual occurrence of renal insufficiency concomitant with the use of the nonsteroidal anti-inflammatory agents must be kept in mind and renal function checked when these agents are used (Bennett *et al.,* 1980).

DISCHARGE

Predischarge counseling includes instructions directed toward modification of coronary risk factors. Dietary instructions are designed to achieve normal body weight and to correct observed abnormalities in lipids. A low-sodium diet, routine during the recovery period in the hospital, is continued somewhat less stringently for several more weeks. The importance of continued abstinence from cigarette smoking is stressed again at this time. Antihypertensive therapy is continued if required, although the blood pressure may have normalized during hospital confinement. If so, reevaluation of the need for antihypertensive therapy must be made at subsequent office visits as blood pressure usually becomes elevated upon return to normal daily activity and stresses. Low-dose beta-blocker therapy is continued four to six weeks after operation when it can be terminated gradually, unless necessary for control of blood pressure or arrhythmia. The possible beneficial role of long-term administration of a beta-blocker after ACB has not been established.

At discharge, usually eight to nine days after operation, the patient is instructed to increase the daily walking routine in a progressive fashion along with the progressive resumption of activities of everyday living. Lifting, in excess of 10 to 15 lb, and more strenuous exercises are not permitted until the median sternotomy is well healed, usually six weeks after surgery. Many patients with sedentary employment will return to work three to four weeks after surgery, usually limiting their time to one half a day's work for the first week or two. Return to light manual labor is usually delayed for six weeks, and heavy labor is not resumed for eight to twelve weeks after operation.

Office visits at intervals of several weeks after discharge permit evaluation of the patient's progress. Exercise stress testing is usually accomplished at eight to twelve weeks after operation and before resumption of heavy manual labor or more strenuous physical activities. Such testing serves to assess the success of myocardial revascularization and also serves as a baseline for yearly postsurgical follow-up and evaluation. Exercise testing is also psychologically reassuring to patients and an important step in their rehabilitation process.

Formal Rehabilitation Program

After ACB, most patients are capable of progressive rehabilitation and return to gainful employment without entering a formal program of rehabilitation. This is especially true of patients who have been gainfully employed up to the period before ACB or who have not had prolonged periods of medical disability prior to operation. Daily exercise programs such as walking can be accomplished easily and the distance or speed advanced in a progressive manner. In similar fashion, patients gradually resume household chores, occupational duties, and recreational and athletic activity, delaying arduous activity until the sternotomy is healed, about six weeks after operation. More strenuous activities are delayed until the postoperative exercise testing has been accomplished.

Patients who have had long periods of disability secondary to symptomatic CAD, or have abided by prolonged restrictions of activity, following a prior infarction (often inappropriately prescribed), may present a more difficult rehabilitation problem. Such individuals have often lost confidence in themselves and frequently have experienced long periods of unemployment before operation. A formal, highly disciplined rehabilitation program has the most to offer this group of patients. Programs, employing progressive and monitored exercise, permit patients to gain confidence in their ability along with the added advantage of peer psychology as they perform with groups of patients who have similar problems. Return to gainful employment, however, often continues to be a difficult problem. There is ample evidence that return to full employment is related to many factors (Oberman, *et al.,* 1982; Smith *et al.,* 1982). One adverse factor is a long period of unemployment before ACB. Another factor is the type of employment. Those in unskilled and semiskilled jobs return to work less frequently than the more skilled employees and professionals. The age of the patient also plays a role, with the older patient more often choosing early retirement rather than return to full-time employment. Although the level of nonwork physical activity generally is increased after ACB, this has no relationship to return to gainful employment. The attitudes of industry vary, with some employers less desirous of permitting the return of a previously disabled employee following ACB. Although these attitudes are changing gradually, they still persist to varying degrees. Other factors include non-work income, attitude of the family, and the patient's psychological perception of his health. In our own experience with patients 60 years of age or younger who underwent ACB between 1976 and 1981, 64% have returned to full-time, and 11% to part-time, employment; of patients 50 years of age or younger, 72% and 10% have returned to full- and part-time employment, respectively (Hall, 1982).

Long-Term Follow-up

Periodic follow-up of patients after ACB allows reevaluation, and reinforcement, of measures directed toward controlling coronary risk factors. After ACB, exercise testing is performed yearly in each patient. Excellent exercise performance and absence of an ischemic response provide evidence of continued adequate myocardial perfusion. Recurrence of symptoms and deterioration of exercise tolerance, along with the return of an ischemic response to exercise testing, have been correlated

with graft occlusion or, more frequently, significant progression of the native atherosclerotic coronary occlusive disease.

ASSESSING THE RESULTS OF CORONARY ARTERY BYPASS

Early Mortality

During the last decade the early (30-day) mortality has decreased in all major centers and presently ranges from 1 to 4% (Rahimtoola, 1982; Hall et al., 1983) (Figure 12-4). This reduction is due to gains in surgical, anesthetic, and cardiologic experience as well as improved techniques of myocardial preservation. During a 12-year period (1970–1981) the early mortality among 22,284 patients undergoing ACB without other procedures in our institution was 2.9%, and in 1981 was 1.9% (Hall et al., 1983). The decline in early mortality has occurred even though the patients selected for ACB have more extensive disease, have worse myocardial function, are older, and receive more bypasses per patient, resulting in

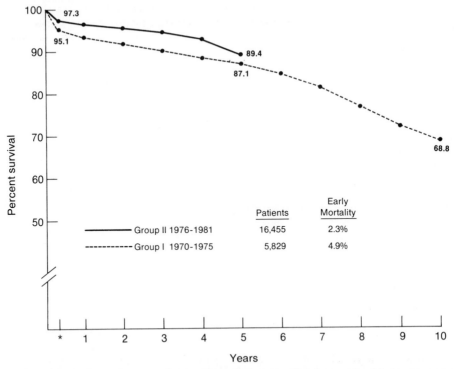

Figure 12-4. Early mortality and actuarial survival curves of patients undergoing aortocoronary bypass alone, 1976 through 1981, compared with 1970 through 1975; Texas Heart Institute experience. (From Hall, R. J., Elayda, M. A., Gray, A., et al. Coronary artery bypass: Long-term follow-up of 22,284 consecutive patients. *Circulation,* **1983**, *68*(Suppl. II):II20-26. By permission of the American Heart Association, Inc.)

more complete myocardial revascularization. Early mortality in women undergoing ACB has been consistently higher than in men (Boloöki *et al.*, 1975; Kennedy *et al.*, 1981; Hall *et al.*, 1983) (Figure 12-5). Early mortality also increases progressively with the age of the patient; after the age of 60, the risk to male and female patients becomes more identical (Table 12-2). Eighty per cent of the early deaths following ACB are secondary to cardiac causes (Hall *et al.*, 1983).

Relief of Angina

Angina decreases in more than 90% of patients who undergo ACB, with complete relief in approximately 70% (King and Hurst, 1980). The degree of improvement is related to patency of the vein graft and to completeness of revascularization (Assad-Morrell *et al.*, 1975), with both factors having improved in patients operated on in more recent years. Relief of

Table 12-2. EARLY MORTALITY (PER CENT) ACCORDING TO AGE AND SEX IN ALL PATIENTS WHO HAD CORONARY ARTERY BYPASS*

| | EARLY MORTALITY | | | |
| | MEN | | WOMEN | |
AGE (YR)	NO. OF PTS.	(%)	NO. OF PTS.	(%)
10–19	5	(20.0)	—	—
20–29	32	—	8	(12.5)
30–39	776	(1.2)	62	(6.5)
40–49	4,333	(1.5)	424	(5.7)
50–59	8,036	(2.1)	1,094	(4.8)
60–69	5,059	(3.8)	1,180	(5.0)
70–79	916	(5.3)	330	(7.0)
80–89	17	(5.9)	11	(9.1)
90–99	1	—	—	—
Total	19,175	(2.6)	3,109	(5.3)

* From Hall, R. J., *et al.* Coronary artery bypass: long-term follow-up of 22,284 consecutive patients. *Circulation,* **1983,** *68* (Suppl. II), II 20–26. By permission of the American Heart Association, Inc.

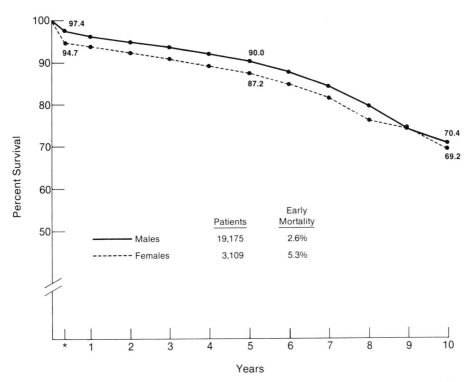

Figure 12-5. Early mortality and actuarial survival curves contrasting male and female patients undergoing aortocoronary bypass alone; Texas Heart Institute experience. (From Hall, R. J., Elayda, M. A., Gray A., *et al.* Coronary artery bypass: Long-term follow-up of 22,284 consecutive patients. *Circulation,* **1983,** *68*(Suppl. II):II20-26. By permission of the American Heart Association, Inc.)

angina persists for a number of years, although symptoms have returned in some patients after a variable period of complete relief. Return of symptoms has occurred at a rate of 2 to 4% per year (Cameron *et al.,* 1979; Campeau *et al.,* 1979), and more often has been related to progression of native disease than to vein graft occlusion (Campeau *et al.,* 1978b).

Graft Patency

Saphenous vein graft patency of 80 to 90% at one year has been reported (Bourassa *et al.,* 1977; Fitzgibbon *et al.,* 1979; Loop *et al.,* 1981). Approximately one half of the grafts occluded at one year had become occluded during the first month after ACB. After the first year, the average annual rate of graft occlusion was 2 to 3% per year (Campeau *et al.,* 1978c; Loop *et al.,* 1981); and in patients operated in the later years of the last decade, graft occlusion may be less than 1% per year (Campeau *et al.,* 1978c). Early postoperative graft occlusion appears to be a function of the size of, and flow into, the recipient artery and the technical efficacy of the anastomosis itself. Late occlusion is the result of fibrous proliferation of the wall of the vein graft and atheromatous changes (Rimm *et al.,* 1976; Barborick *et al.,* 1977). Atherosclerotic changes occur in 9% of vein grafts within the first five years (Campeau *et al.,* 1978c).

Patency of an internal mammary artery graft, used most often for bypass of the left anterior descending coronary artery, has been reported to be 95% (Green, 1972) or higher and superior to saphenous vein grafts (Loop *et al.,* 1981).

Progression of native coronary disease is reported to be no different in the proximal segments of grafted and nongrafted vessels by the sixth year after operation, and little if any progress was observed in the distal arteries (Bourassa *et al.,* 1978). Patency in sequential grafts reportedly is high (Loop *et al.,* 1981) and facilitates achieving more complete revascularization since relatively smaller adjacent vessels can be bypassed. Adequate long-term observations in patients who have received sequential grafts are not yet available.

Improved Exercise Capacity

Unlike treatment with vasodilator or beta-blockade therapy, after which exercise capacity improves but does not increase above the pretreatment pulse and blood pressure double-product level, the increase in exercise capacity following ACB is achieved at a higher double product. Patients are able to exercise longer, at higher work loads, and to greater maximum heart rate/blood pressure product without symptoms. Preoperative positive "ischemic" treadmill test results revert to a normal response, even at greater work levels, in 75 to 90% of patients after ACB. The degree of improved exercise capacity, freedom from symptoms, and persistently negative treadmill test results, likewise, are related to the completeness of revascularization and vein graft patency, with a gradual and small deterioration of these benefits occurring with the passage of time (Busch *et al.,* 1977).

Improved Myocardial Perfusion

The decrease of symptoms, increase of exercise capacity, and reversion of a positive "ischemic" treadmill test result to negative are all consistent with improved myocardial blood flow after ACB. Large flows in the grafted vessel have been documented by flow-meter studies at the time of surgery, and a smaller flow, a function of inadequate distal run-off as well as the quality of the anastomosis, has resulted in lower levels of graft patency at one week and one year (Marco, 1980). Restoration of flow to areas of myocardium beyond subtotal and total occlusion is also observed at postoperative angiography. Clinical improvement is related to the completeness of revascularization, also supporting improved myocardial perfusion (Peduzzi and Hultgren, 1979). The decrease of left ventricular ejection fraction that occurs with exercise in patients with CAD is also reversed following successful ACB (Kent *et al.,* 1978). Exercise-induced abnormalities detected by means of thallium-201 perfusion in patients with CAD are likewise eliminated after successful ACB. Resting thallium-201 perfusion defects also have been eliminated after ACB which supports the concept of resting myocardial ischemia in some patients (Berger *et al.,* 1979; Beller *et al.,* 1980). Exertional hypotension during treadmill testing, believed to be due to severe exercise-induced ischemia of the left ventricle, is reversed following ACB (Li *et al.,* 1979). The evidence that coronary bypass surgery increases myocardial perfusion in patients with CAD is compelling and is based upon a variety of observations.

Improved Myocardial Function

One of the most impressive responses to a significant myocardial perfusion deficit secondary to coronary artery narrowing is regional and, at times, global deterioration of contractility during exercise. This has been documented angiographically (Sharm *et al.*, 1976) and serves as the basis for exercise stress testing using radionuclide gated blood pool ventriculographic imaging (Kent *et al.*, 1978). These exercise-induced segmental and global wall motion abnormalities are reversed after successful ACB (Kent *et al.*, 1978; Ott *et al.*, 1980). Myocardial dysfunction present at rest may manifest as regional wall motion abnormalities, global abnormalities, reduced overall ejection fraction of the left ventricle, or in altered ventricular hemodynamics with increased left ventricular end-diastolic, pulmonary venous, and pulmonary artery pressures. Myocardial dysfunction at rest may be the result of either myocardial scarring from prior infarction or resting myocardial ischemia. Although patients with the former will not benefit from reperfusion, ventricular dysfunction secondary to ischemia should be reversed after ACB and has been reported in a number of studies (Helfant *et al.*, 1974; Chesebro *et al.*, 1979; Stadius *et al.*, 1980). Identification of these subsets of patients is not uniformly possible, but among those whose resting abnormalities are more likely to be due to ischemia are the patients with severe left main disease, severe triple-vessel disease, and with an unstable anginal pattern; and patients with an area of asynergy without prior history of infarction, especially if electrocardiographic evidence of infarction is not present in the asynergic area. Improved myocardial contractility by contrast ventriculography following administration of nitroglycerin (Helfant *et al.*, 1974; Chesebro *et al.*, 1979; Stadius *et al.*, 1980), in the potentiated beat after a premature ventricular contraction (Klausner *et al.*, 1976; Banka *et al.*, 1979), or decrease of a resting segmental radionuclide ventriculographic abnormality in the postexercise recovery period (DePuey *et al.*, 1981a; Rozanski *et al.*, 1982) are all predictive of ventricular dysfunction secondary to resting ischemia and are correlated with improved left ventricular function after ACB (Massin *et al.*, 1978).

Protection Against Myocardial Infarction and Sudden Death

Although none of the prospective multicenter studies has shown a reduced rate of late myocardial infarction in patients treated surgically, in a study done at the Veterans' Administration Hospital in Houston a lower incidence of reinfarction was demonstrated by patients treated surgically (Mathur and Guinn, 1979). As the rate of perioperative infarction decreases and more complete revascularization is accomplished with current surgical techniques, the reduction of late infarction may become more evident. Other data, using historical control patients, are suggestive of a threefold reduction of late infarction (Mason *et al.*, 1980). Data supporting a decrease in the incidence of sudden death have also been reported (Hammermeister *et al.*, 1977; Vismara *et al.*, 1977).

Increased Longevity

Natural history studies of patients with CAD reveal disparate late survival between patients at low risk and patients at high risk, either by the number of vessels involved (one-, two-, and three-vessel disease) or by the degree of left ventricular myocardial dysfunction. Although current medical management was not available during older historical studies (Proudfit *et al.*, 1978), these same trends are still strongly evident in life-survival studies of patients treated medically, including use of the beta-blocking drugs, during the 1970s (Harris *et al.*, 1979; Mock *et al.*, 1982a; Mock *et al.*, 1982b). After ACB, the difference in late survival between patients in low- and in high-risk subsets has been abolished (Anderson *et al.*, 1974; Campeau *et al.*, 1978; Anderson *et al.*, 1979; Kirklin *et al.*, 1979; Stone and Goldschlager, 1979; Hall *et al.*, 1980; Detre *et al.*, in press), with surprisingly excellent late survival of all subgroups, even among those with the most severe disease (Figure 12-6). The five-year survival of patients with three-vessel disease (including patients with both near-normal and abnormal ventricular function) of 91 to 94% (Figure 12-7) (Mathur *et al.*, 1980) is sufficiently close to the expected survival of the "normal" United States population (Hurst *et al.*, 1978; Lawrie *et al.*, 1978), that it can be clearly concluded that late survival following ACB is enhanced. The outcome of studies which randomly assigned patients to medical or surgical therapy, while at first controversial (Murphy *et al.*, 1977), now appears to confirm this conclusion, especially in certain subsets of patients whose prognosis on medical therapy is poor (Loeb *et al.*, 1979; European Cooperative Surgery Study Group, 1979; Gunnar *et al.*, 1980; Detre *et al.*, in press).

Patients with Poor Left Ventricular Function

Patients who have already suffered one or several prior myocardial infarctions, and who

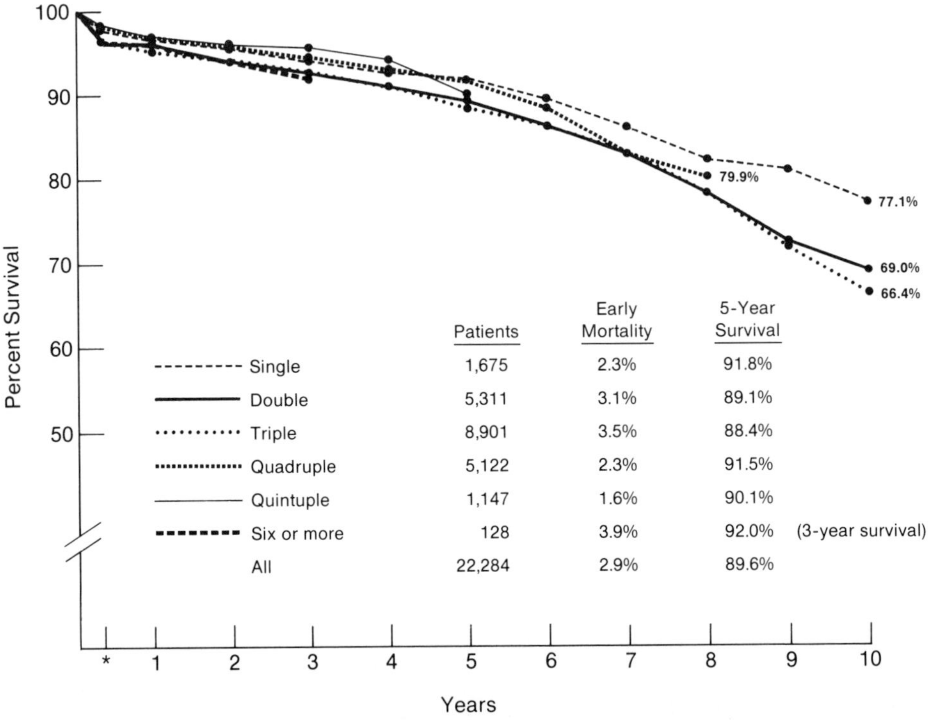
100
90
80
70
60
50
Percent Survival
79.9%
77.1%
69.0%
66.4%
Patients
Early Mortality
5-Year Survival
Single 1,675 2.3% 91.8%
Double 5,311 3.1% 89.1%
Triple 8,901 3.5% 88.4%
Quadruple 5,122 2.3% 91.5%
Quintuple 1,147 1.6% 90.1%
Six or more 128 3.9% 92.0% (3-year survival)
All 22,284 2.9% 89.6%
* 1 2 3 4 5 6 7 8 9 10
Years

Figure 12-6. Life survival curves of 22,284 patients undergoing aortocoronary bypass alone, comprising the Texas Heart Institute experience from 1970 through 1981. The similarity of long-term survival of patients with diverse degrees of severity of coronary artery disease is evident. Note that the survival curve for patients with 6 or more coronary arteries bypassed is projected for only three years. (From Hall, R. J., Elayda, M. A., Gray, A., *et al.* Coronary artery bypass: Long-term follow-up of 22,284 consecutive patients. *Circulation,* **1983,** *68*(Suppl. II):II20-26. By permission of the American Heart Association, Inc.)

demonstrate electrocardiographic evidence of infarction, frequently have severely depressed ejection fractions. The natural history of these patients on medical treatment alone is poor with five-year survival rates of 33% (Mock *et al.,* 1982a,b). Results of bypass surgery in patients with significant depression of myocardial function has been variable (Spencer *et al.,* 1971; Yatteau *et al.,* 1974), although some investigators have reported satisfactory early survival and improved long-term survival among patients who undergo bypass surgery (Manly *et al.,* 1976; Zubiate, *et al.,* 1977). Proper selection of patients for operation from the subsets with a major reduction of ejection fraction continues to be difficult. Even in the presence of quite depressed ventricular function with the ejection fraction below 30%, if angina is a significant clinical symptomatic marker of myocardial ischemia and residual contractile areas of myocardium are in the distribution of severely narrowed coronary arteries, ACB can be performed with considerable confidence of a good result (Faulkner *et al.,* 1977; Jones *et al.,* 1978; Hellman *et al.,* 1980). The decision-making process is much more difficult when more severe degrees of depression of global function exist, with ejection fractions in the range of 20% or less. In the presence of overt congestive failure, surgical revascularization is unlikely to be beneficial. There remain some patients in this category, however, who have residual angina and in whom all coronary vessels are completely or subtotally occluded. On the premise that total occlusion of the last remaining vessel(s) would be fatal, we have performed ACB on patients in this category who have adequate distal vessels, with surprisingly low surgical mortality and satisfactory late results. Although the ejection fraction may remain unchanged, angina has disappeared, and the management of these patients with congestive failure has been facilitated. At times, the ejection fraction improves to a considerable de-

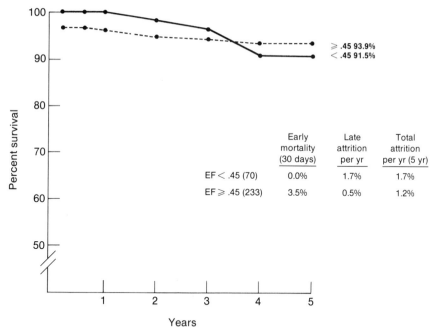

Figure 12-7. Life survival curves of patients with triple vessel disease undergoing aortocoronary bypass. There is no significant difference in the 5-year survival between patients with ejection fraction above and below 45%. (From Mathur, V. S., Hall, R. J., Garcia E., *et al.* Prolonging life with coronary artery bypass surgery in patients with three-vessel disease. *Circulation,* **1980,** *62*(Suppl. I), 90–98. By permission of the American Heart Association, Inc.)

gree, but at the present there are no decisive indicators that consistently predict improvement in ventricular function in this subgroup of patients. Response of the ejection fraction to an acute intervention, when measured in these low ranges, is difficult to evaluate. Exercise-induced thallium-201 defects have been cited (Akins *et al.,* 1980) as a method of detecting silent and reversible ischemia, but such studies are frequently difficult to interpret in the patients with advanced three-vessel disease. We have relied upon a number of clinical criteria in selecting patients for ACB who have markedly depressed left ventricular function. These include persistent exertional angina and the discovery of total or severe high-grade occlusive disease of all proximal vessels, especially the severe occlusive disease that jeopardizes residual contractile segments of myocardium. Asynergy in an area of myocardium that does not show ECG changes of infarction, especially if the proximal coronary artery is severely occluded, is also favorable. Decisions regarding these patients must be made on an individual basis, weighing all available factors. Additionally, patients with poor left ventricular function

will frequently require assisted circulation with intra-aortic balloon pumping and careful pharmacological support during the postoperative period (Golding *et al.,* 1980; Sturm *et al.,* 1980).

Poor Distal Vessels

Small distal vessels frequently indicate diffuse disease and increase the likelihood of technically inadequate graft placement, poor run-off, increased potential for vein graft occlusion, and incomplete revascularization. Visualization of vessels beyond total occlusion depends upon delayed collateral filling which may come from either or both the ipsilateral and/or the contralateral major coronary artery. A coronary artery that is totally occluded proximally and appears small, or is only faintly visualized by retrograde collateral flow, is usually adequate for bypass when the myocardium in its distribution is free of infarction evident by electrocardiography, especially if that segment shows reasonable contractility by means of ventriculography. Excellent angiography and delayed imaging are required to best visualize these "ghost" vessels and to ascertain that continuity exists between segments that collateralize from different coronary artery sources. Even with the best imaging techniques, "ghost" vessels that appear inadequate for bypass angiographically are often found to be of adequate size at the time of operation and as visualized through the vein graft at the time of postoperative angiography (Levin *et al.,* 1982; Rahimtoola, 1982). At times, diffuse distal vessel disease has so multifragmented the coronary circulation that any degree of complete revascularization with ACB is impossible. Each of these cases requires careful individual consideration, including estimating the severity of symptomatic incapacity and the potential risk-benefit ratio, before arriving at a therapeutic decision.

SELECTION OF PATIENTS FOR AORTOCORONARY BYPASS

Surgical bypass of proximal high-grade coronary occlusive lesions provides the immediate benefit of restoring direct aortocoronary blood flow to an underperfused area of myocardium. The limitations of ACB include the morbidity and mortality of open heart surgery, reliance upon the technical skill of the surgeon in establishing functioning anastomoses and in bypassing all major significant coronary lesions, and the natural history of intimal and atherosclerotic changes in the graft as well as progression of atherosclerosis in the native coronary vessels. The indications for ACB continue to evolve and undergo refinement as our understanding of CAD—the natural course and risk in various subsets for subsequent morbid and fatal events—continues to improve.

During the decade of the 1960s, the early period of coronary angiography, our understanding of CAD was vastly expanded and paved the way for surgical treatment. Similarly, the decade of the 1970s served to develop our understanding of short- and long-term effects of ACB and to further define subsets of patients who were at low and high natural risk of coronary disease. During this decade, surgical techniques and skills have evolved, methods of myocardial protection during anesthesia and bypass surgery have been developed (Kouchoukos *et al.,* 1979; Kouchoukos *et al.,* 1980), acute surgical mortality (Kennedy *et al.,* 1981; Loop *et al.,* 1981; Cooley *et al.,* 1982; Hall *et al.,* 1983) and perioperative infarction rates have been reduced to a remarkably low level (Kouchoukos *et al.,* 1980; Stadius *et al.,* 1980; Loop *et al.,* 1981), and we have developed knowledge of the clinical improvement and

late survival that can be expected from ACB (Rahimtoola *et al.,* 1981). We have increasing evidence that not only has early mortality diminished, but late survival has improved after surgery in patients during the latter half of the past decade, probably as the consequence of both better myocardial protection and more complete revascularization (Kouchoukos *et al.,* 1980; Stadius *et al.,* 1980; Hall, 1982). With better knowledge of the predictors of subsequent events in CAD and the results that can be achieved with surgical treatment, we can properly select patients for ACB based upon assessment of a risk-benefit ratio according to the clinical and angiographic characteristics that are present (Hall, 1982).

Clinical Indications

Angina pectoris, either incapacitating to the patient on medical therapy or unacceptable to the patient because of interference with a desired life-style, is an indication for bypass, if suitable coronary anatomy is present. It can be anticipated with a high level of confidence that an improved life-style and freedom from symptoms will be achieved. Additionally, patients who fall into clinical subsets that are known to be at higher natural risk of CAD (Table 12-3) should undergo coronary angiographic studies to further characterize the extent and distribution of disease.

Asymptomatic individuals who have been found to have serious, reversible ischemia, either on routine exercise testing or during the

---

Table 12-3. CLINICAL AND FUNCTIONAL FEATURES OF PATIENT SUBSETS AT INCREASED NATURAL RISK

Unstable angina, accelerating angina, or angina recurring at rest

Continued postinfarction angina

Episode(s) of prolonged coronary insufficiency without infarction

Exercise-induced fall of blood pressure or decline of pulse rate

Exercise test positive at Bruce stage I or II

Major area of ischemia with thallium-201 exercise testing, especially at low level of exercise

Major exercise-induced decrease of ejection fraction or major exercise-induced wall motion abnormality with gated blood pool radionuclide study, especially at low level of exercise

An ischemic response on modified treadmill testing early after transmural or nontransmural myocardial infarction

Recovery from out-of-hospital cardiac arrest

Recurrent ventricular tachycardia or high-grade ventricular ectopy course of evaluation for an unrelated problem, also should undergo coronary angiography and ACB if the coronary anatomy indicates the patient to be in high natural jeopardy (Thurer et al., 1979; Loop et al., 1981). The surgical mortality in a subgroup of 33 asymptomatic patients with severe CAD who underwent ACB was 0% and the five-year survival was 97% (Hall et al., 1980).

Angiographic Indications for ACB

Coronary angiography usually is performed in individuals with known CAD whose clinical characteristics are suggestive that surgical consideration is indicated. In other patients angiography is performed when the diagnosis of a chest pain syndrome or of an electrocardiographic abnormality is unclear. In these circumstances, the finding of normal coronary arteries or of minimal CAD can be of great benefit to a patient who may have been incapacitated by the diagnosis of CAD. In the cooperative national study of unstable angina, 5 to 10% of patients who underwent angiography demonstrated normal coronary arteries (National Cooperative Study Group, 1978).

In the patient with CAD, angiography will characterize the location, extent, and degree of coronary narrowing, characterize coronary collateral circulation, and define the degree of left ventricular contraction abnormalities. In the final analysis from an anatomical standpoint, the indications for operation stem from the estimated amount of left ventricular myocardium in significant jeopardy.

Major narrowing of the left main coronary artery ($\geqslant$ 50% diameter narrowing) places enough of the left ventricular myocardium in jeopardy that the superiority of surgical bypass over medical management became evident early in the Veterans' Administration studies (Takaro et al., 1976) and is evident in other randomized studies (European Coronary Surgery Study Group, 1982). Patients with proximal occlusive disease ($\geqslant$ 50% diameter narrowing) of all three coronary arteries, and subsets of patients with two-vessel disease that includes involvement of the proximal left anterior descending artery, demonstrate sufficiently better late survival after bypass that surgery appears preferable to medical treatment (European Coronary Surgery Study Group, 1982). Patients with single-vessel disease on medical therapy experience such favorable late survival that statistical differences between medical and surgical therapy are difficult to demonstrate. When it progresses to total occlusion, a high-grade proximal lesion in the left anterior descending artery usually produces a large area of myocardial infarction. Individuals with this lesion appear to be treated better by ACB. Patients with single lesions of the right or circumflex arteries apparently fare well on medical management. However, when these vessels have unusually large areas of myocardial distribution, surgery may be preferable. Examples include a very dominant right coronary artery with a cascade of several additional large posterior left ventricular branches beyond the posterior descending coronary artery, or a dominant left system with a circumflex artery giving rise to a number of marginal branches as well as to the posterior descending coronary artery (Table 12-4).

Table 12-4

Anatomical Subsets That Have Better Life Survival After ACB

Left main CAD, $\geqslant$ 50% diameter narrowing
Three-vessel disease, $\geqslant$ 50% diameter narrowing
Two-vessel disease, $\geqslant$ 50% diameter narrowing; subset including LAD

Subsets That May Have Better Life Survival After ACB

High-grade two-vessel disease, 75% diameter
High-grade proximal LAD disease
High-grade proximal LCX single-vessel disease, with dominant LCX supplying multiple marginal branches and PD
High-grade proximal RCA single-vessel disease with several posterior LV branches in addition to the PD
High-grade proximal LCX single lesions with a number of marginal branches, but RCA gives off the PD

ACB, aortocoronary bypass; CAD, coronary artery disease; LAD, left anterior descending; LCX, left circumflex; LV, left ventricular; PD, posterior descending coronary artery; RCA, right coronary artery

When considering any patient for ACB, the clinician will usually assess both anatomical and clinical characteristics. If there are clinical or exercise-testing features indicative of significant reversible ischemia, especially when a major amount of myocardium is in jeopardy, surgical bypass is favored, even when only single-vessel disease is present. Currently, transluminal coronary balloon angioplasty is an alternative to surgical bypass in these latter patients (see below). Conversely, when the clinical characteristics place the patient in a low-risk subset, especially if the degree of coronary artery narrowing is less severe, continued medical management and serial follow-up are warranted. This takes into consideration the fact that bypass surgery does not cure patients with CAD; additionally, there is natural progression of both native coronary disease and occlusive changes in the vein grafts as well. Serial follow-up consists of periodic reevaluation of the patient's symptomatic status and interval (usually yearly) stress testing. With this strategy, bypass surgery can be delayed successfully in many patients for a number of years. The patient and his primary physician must participate in this plan fully, and a change in the symptomatic status of the patient should precipitate prompt reassessment.

Classification of CAD into one-, two-, and three-vessel disease, unfortunately, is an oversimplification. Narrowing of a single marginal branch of the circumflex, especially when it is one of several, does not jeopardize the amount of myocardium that would be involved by an equivalent lesion of the proximal circumflex trunk. Similar anatomical conditions producing less jeopardy include narrowing of the left anterior descending artery beyond the first large diagonal branch and several major septal perforating branches; or isolated posterior descending artery narrowing, especially if there is an additional right coronary artery branch beyond the crux. The mass of left ventricular myocardium in jeopardy is an important factor when deciding about surgical treatment.

Also of importance is the distinction between total occlusion and subtotal or near occlusion of a coronary vessel. In the former, the vessel cannot become more narrow, and the condition of the patient is usually stable. A coronary vessel with subtotal high-grade narrowing is at risk of becoming totally occluded; and the patient (and the distal myocardium) is in considerable jeopardy of an acute event — infarction or death. Variable circumstances

prevail even when different conditions accompany a totally occluded coronary artery. Patients with a single totally occluded vessel usually have a major transmural infarction in the distribution of this vessel, with the infarction evident both clinically and electrocardiographically. Such patients represent the fortunate survivors of this particular subset. They are usually asymptomatic, perform well on exercise stress testing, and, when managed medically, have exceptionally fine late survival rates. Conversely, an occasional patient with total occlusion of a proximal vessel may present with little or no evidence of myocardial infarction and manifest continued angina or recurrent episodes of coronary insufficiency with ST- and/or T-wave abnormalities. In these latter patients, the major myocardium in the distribution of this vessel is still in jeopardy. Ventricular wall function in this distribution may be near normal or variably depressed; yet, if depressed, the wall function usually demonstrates the markers of reversible myocardial ischemia cited earlier. These include wall motion potentiation following an induced premature ventricular contraction, following nitroglycerin administration, or in the recovery phase of radionuclide exercise testing. Such a patient with total occlusion will profit from bypass surgery, and the wall motion abnormality can be expected to improve. These examples contrast total occlusion (resulting in a completed scar) with no additional viable myocardium in jeopardy and total occlusion resulting in severe ischemia with major myocardial jeopardy. The underlying coronary anatomy that distinguishes these two diverse consequences of total occlusion must be the adequacy, although marginal, of collateral flow which retains myocardial viability in the latter condition.

Other clinical features also determine the choice of medical or surgical treatment. In patients of advanced age, the risk of immediate mortality of bypass surgery is increased (Table 12-2), and there is also increased perioperative morbidity, especially due to complications of the central nervous system. Accordingly, one is prone to intensify medical treatment in the older patient, especially in those beyond age 70, and reserve operation for patients who are refractory to vigorous medical management (Figure 12-8). When making this decision, one should bear in mind that overall physiological age — physical and mental — is more important than the actual chronological age of the

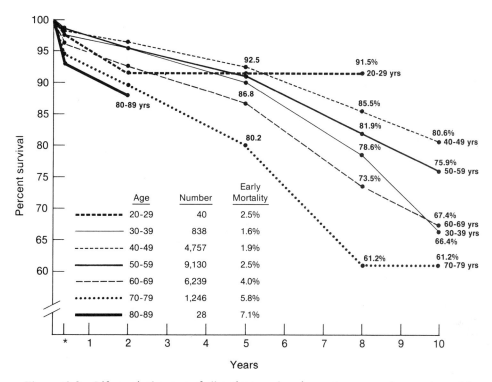

Figure 12-8. Life survival curves of all patients undergoing aortocoronary bypass alone at the Texas Heart Institute from 1970 through 1981, demonstrating the patient's age at the time of aortocoronary bypass. The accelerated attrition of those patients between 30 to 39 years at the time of aortocoronary bypass possibly reflects the gravity of the premature atherosclerotic process in these individuals; Texas Heart Institute experience. (From Hall, R. J., Elayda, M. A., Gray, A., *et al.* Coronary artery bypass: Long-term follow-up of 22,284 consecutive patients. *Circulation,* **1983,** *68*(Suppl. II):II20-26. By permission of the American Heart Association, Inc.)

patient. Similar overall consideration of the risk-benefit ratio must prevail when disease of other major organ systems is present. The separate risks to longevity posed by each process must be weighed separately when making a therapeutic decision. Individual, careful analysis of each patient is essential.

The concept in the lay mind that surgery is "curative" also must be refuted. This attitude makes it "easier" to choose surgical therapy, even when less severe disease is identified angiographically. Neither medical therapy nor surgical bypass is "curative." Even after successful ACB, there are progression of the native disease at a variable and difficultly defined rate, an annual identifiable risk of graft closure, and, to varying degrees, a slow deterioration of the benefits achieved from even the most successful bypass surgery. Stated another way, ACB does not "assure immortality" but merely sets back the "clock of time" a variable number of

years. The atherosclerotic processes progress relentlessly. There are many patients whose disease is of such severity that they are at high natural risk. Undeniably, surgery adds years to their lives. To deny such a patient surgery is inappropriate. Conversely, to recommend surgery for a patient with milder degrees of occlusive disease, who is at low natural risk, is to operate prematurely. Such individuals may have to return for a second operation when they, more appropriately, might be undergoing a first operation. When less severe degrees of disease are identified, a medical regimen should be initiated and a careful plan designed for serial clinical and functional testing followup. If clinical or functional indicators change during the course of follow-up, such patients would undergo repeat angiography; and it would not be unreasonable, even without clinical indicators, to perform a "second-look" angiogram after four to six years.

In summary, the choice of treatment of patients with CAD is made on an individual, patient-to-patient basis which takes into consideration the total clinical and angiographic risk factors; the mode of therapy chosen best fits the conditions at that time.

Repeat ACB

Patients who return after ACB with recurrence of symptoms usually require reassessment, both functionally with stress testing and anatomically with angiography. In general, consideration for repeat surgery will follow the thoughts outlined in the previous section. The risk of repeat ACB is considerably higher than a first bypass operation, and the results are not as favorable consistently. This is not unexpected since the characteristics, single or multiple, that caused failure of the first bypass surgery usually persist, e.g., poor recipient coronary vessels for bypass, inadequate run-off, or associated biological risk ractors, which accelerate the natural progress of the atherosclerotic process. As a consequence, repeat ACB is elected with greater reservation, demanding a more rigorous application of the principles set forth previously.

NONOPERATIVE DILATION OF CORONARY ARTERY STENOSIS (TRANSLUMINAL CORONARY BALLOON ANGIOPLASTY)

A method of transluminal dilation of atherosclerotic femoral artery disease in humans was first reported in 1964 (Dotter and Judkins). This technique subsequently was adapted in Europe to more extensive use in patients with peripheral vascular disease, and ultimately, in 1977, to patients with stenosis of the coronary arteries (Gruntzig et al., 1979). Observations of the results in a large number of patients accumulated in the National Heart, Lung and Blood Institute registry have been reported (Kent et al., 1982), and guidelines for use have been identified (Williams et al., 1982). The procedure is applicable in patients with discrete subtotal coronary occlusive disease, usually confined to a single coronary vessel, although investigation of this procedure in patients with multivessel disease is progressing. Early experience indicated successful immediate dilation of the coronary artery lumen in 59 to 66% of patients, with the stenosis reduced from an average of 85% narrowing of the lumen diameter to 30 to 35% narrowing (Gruntzig et al., 1979; Kent et al., 1982). Improvements in

catheter and balloon design and increased operator experience have further aided in improving these results. Similarly, nonfatal complications, including myocardial infarction and necessary emergency surgery, which occurred in 18% of patients in the early registry report (Kent et al., 1982), should now occur in only 10% or less of the patients when the procedure is performed by experienced operators (Williams et al., 1982). The mortality has been 1% or less.

One-year follow-up of patients who had initially successful angioplasty has revealed clinical improvement in 83%. Ten per cent have required repeat angioplasty or coronary bypass surgery (Kent et al., 1982). In our experience, early restenosis has occurred in 8% of the patients and later restenosis in 3%. Among patients in whom balloon angioplasty has been successful, 85% are free of symptoms. Results of exercise testing by means of treadmill or radionuclide ventriculography have corroborated effective myocardial revascularization (Mathur, 1982).

Transluminal balloon coronary angioplasty requires a skilled operative team, angiographic equipment capable of high resolution and multiangular projections, and the immediate availability of a skilled surgical team (Williams et al., 1982). The beneficial effects of balloon angioplasty reside not only in compression of the atherosclerotic plaque but also controlled disruption of the media of the coronary artery, with enlargement of the vessel itself. Angioplasty allows the patient the advantage of avoiding surgical bypass and thoracotomy but, presently, is applicable to only approximately 5% of patients who are surgical candidates. The role of balloon angioplasty in the treatment of patients with multivessel disease has not, as yet, been established firmly.

Patients selected for coronary balloon angioplasty, in general, should be surgical candidates, have significant narrowing of the lumen of the coronary artery, and demonstrate clinical or functional evidence of significant reversible ischemia. Transluminal coronary angioplasty has also been performed in some patients with acute myocardial infarction following partial recanalization with intracoronary infusion of streptokinase (Meyer et al., 1982).

Aortocoronary bypass and transluminal coronary angioplasty are both extremely effective in reestablishing prograde coronary flow to the myocardium beyond a serious coronary artery narrowing. Neither method of treatment is curative and, at this time, the short- and long-term effects of ACB are better defined than those of transluminal coronary angioplasty. The advantages of angioplasty—ease of performance and avoidance of a major surgical procedure—are balanced by the relatively small number of patients with CAD in whom this procedure is suitable. Increasing experience with transluminal angioplasty in patients with multiple-vessel disease may broaden the applicability of this technique. Decision to use either form of therapy must always incorporate consideration of the long-term needs and benefits of the patient. Invasive treatment, whether surgical or angioplasty, is not competitive with medical management of patients with coronary artery disease but, rather, is complementary. The clinician must constantly strive to select the form of treatment that is in the best interest of the patient at that particular time. Coronary artery disease is a progressive process, and any decision regarding therapy must be reassessed regularly as the patient is followed clinically.

REFERENCES

Akins, C. W.; Pohost, G. M.; Desanctis, R. W.; and Block, P. C. Selection of angina-free patients with severe left ventricular dysfunction for myocardial revascularization. *Am. J. Cardiol.,* 1980, *46,* 695–700.

Anderson, R. P.; Li, W.; Balfour, R. I.; and Horton, W. B. Surgical management of left main coronary artery stenosis and ischemic left ventricular dysfunction. *J. Thorac. Cardiovasc. Surg.,* 1979, *77,* 369.

Anderson, R. P.; Rahimtoola, S. H.; Bonchek, L. I.; and Starr, A. The prognosis of patients with coronary artery disease after coronary bypass operations. Time-related progress of 532 patients with disabling angina pectoris. *Circulation,* 1974, *50,* 274.

Assad-Morrell, J. L.; Frye, R. L.; Connolly, D. C.; *et al.* Aorto-coronary artery saphenous vein bypass surgery. Clinical and angiographic results. *Mayo Clin. Proc.,* 1975, *50,* 379.

Banka, V. S.; Bodenheimer, M. M.; Shah, R.; and Helfant, R. H. Intervention ventriculography: Comparative values of nitroglycerin, post-extrasystolic potentiation and nitroglycerin plus post-extrasystolic potentiation. *Circulation,* 1979, *53,* 632.

Barborick, J. J.; Batayias, G. E.; Pintar, K.; *et al.* Late lesions in aortocoronary artery vein grafts. *J. Thorac. Cardiovasc. Surg.,* 1977, *73,* 596.

Beller, G. A.; Watson, D. D.; Ackell, P.; and Pohost, G. M. Time course of thallium-201 redistribution after transient myocardial ischemia. *Circulation,* 1980, *61,* 791.

Bennett, W. M.; Muther, R. S.; Parker, R. A.; Feig, P.; Morrison, G.; Golper, T. A.; and Singer, I. Drug therapy on renal failure: Dosing guidelines for adults. Part II: sedatives, hypnotics, and tranquilizers; cardiovascular antihypertensive, and diuretic agents;

miscellaneous agents. *Ann. Intern. Med.,* 1980, *93,* 286–325.

Berger, B. C.; Watson, D. D.; Burwell, L. R.; Crosby, I. K.; Wellons, H. A.; Teates, C. D.; and Beller, G. A. Redistribution of thallium at rest in patients with stable and unstable angina and the effect of coronary artery bypass surgery. *Circulation,* 1979, *60,* 1114.

Bolooki, H.; Vargas, A.; Green, R.; *et al.* Results of direct coronary surgery in women. *J. Thorac. Cardiovasc. Surg.,* 1975, *69,* 271–277.

Bourassa, M. G.; Campeau, L.; and Lesperance, J. Effects of bypass surgery on the coronary circulation: Incidence and effects of vein graft occlusion. In, Rahimtoola, S. H. (ed.) *Coronary Bypass Surgery.* F. A. Davis, Philadelphia, 1977, p. 107.

Bourassa, M. G.; Lesperance, J.; Corbara, F.; Saltiel, J.; and Campeau, L. Progression of obstructive coronary artery disease 5 to 7 years after aortocoronary bypass surgery. *Circulation,* 1978, *57* and *58* (Suppl. I), 100.

Busch, U.; Garcia, E.; Hall, R. J.; Mathur, V. S.; de Castro, C. M.; Guttin, J.; Dear, W. E.; and Cooley, D. A. Serial graded exercise testing in follow-up of coronary artery bypass: A preliminary report. *Cardiovasc. Dis. Bull Tex. Heart Inst.,* 1977, *4,* 149.

Cameron, A.; Kemp, H. G., Jr.; Shimomura, S.; *et al.* Aortocoronary bypass surgery. A 7-year follow-up. *Circulation,* 1979, *60* (Suppl. I), 9.

Campeau, L.; Corbara, F.; Corchet, D.; and Petitclerc, R. Left main coronary artery stenosis. The influence of aortocoronary bypass surgery on survival. *Circulation,* 1978a, *57,* 1111.

Campeau, L; Hermann, J; Lesperance, J.; *et al.* Loss of the improvement of angina between 1 and 6 years after aortocoronary bypass surgery: Correlations with changes in vein grafts and in coronary arteries. *Circulation,* 1978b, *58* (Suppl. II), 16 (abstr.).

Campeau, L.; Lesperance, J.; Corbara, F.; Hermann, J.; Grondin, C.; and Bourassa, M. D. Patency of aortocoronary saphenous vein bypass grafts 5 to 7 years after surgery. *Can. J. Surg.,* 1978c, *21,* 118.

Campeau, L.; Lesperance, J.; Hermann, J.; *et al.* Loss of improvement of angina between 1 and 7 years after aortocoronary bypass surgery. Correlations with changes in vein grafts and in coronary arteries. *Circulation,* 1979, *50* (Suppl. I), 1.

Chesebro, J. H.; Clements, I. P.; Fuster, B.; *et al.* A platelet-inhibitor-drug trial in coronary artery bypass operations: Benefit of perioperative dipyridamole and aspirin therapy on early postoperative vein graft patency. *N. Engl. J. Med.,* 1982, *307,* 73–78.

Chesebro, J. H.; Ritman, E. L.; Frye, R. L.; *et al.* Regional myocardial wall thickening response to nitroglycerin. A predictor of myocardial response to aortocoronary bypass surgery. *Circulation* 1979, *57,* 592.

Cooley, D. A.; Hall, R. J.; Elayda, M. E.; *et al.* Aortocoronary bypass surgery: Long term follow-up of 21,561 patients over one decade. *Circulation,* 1982, *66* (Suppl. II), 219 (abstr.).

Cooley, D. A.; Hallman, G. L.; and Bloodwell, R. D. Definitive surgical treatment of anomalous origin of left coronary artery from pulmonary artery: Indications and results. *J. Thorac. Cardiovasc. Surg.,* 1966, *52,* 798–808.

Cooley, D. A., and Norman, J. C. *Techniques in Cardiac*

Surgery. Texas Medical Press, Houston, 1975, pp. 158–159.

Dawson, J. T.; Hall, R. J.; Garcia, E.; and Cooley, D. A. Myocardial infarction after coronary artery bypass (CAB) surgery. *Circulation,* 1972, 46 (Suppl. II), 144 (abstr.).

DePuey, E. G.; Aessopos, A. E.; Monroe, L. R.; *et al.* Creatine kinase-MB immunoradiometric assay to diagnose myocardial infarction following aortocoronary bypass surgery. *J. Nucl. Med.,* 1983, 24, 35 (abstr.).

DePuey, G.; Mammen, G.; Sonnemaker, R. E.; *et al.* Identification of myocardial viability by improvement in left ventricular function in the post exercise recovery period. *J. Nucl. Med.,* 1981b, 22, 80–81.

DePuey, E. G.; Mathur, V.; Hall, R. J.; and Burdine, J. A. Infarct-induced wall motion abnormalities in aortocoronary bypass patients: Correlation with electrocardiographic, enzymatic, and scintigraphic diagnostic criteria. *Cardiovasc. Dis. Bull. Tex. Heart Inst.,* 1980, 7, 382–396.

DePuey, E. G.; Rivas, A. H.; Thompson, W. L.; *et al.* Improvement in left ventricular function following bypass surgery assessed by exercise radionuclide ventriculography in the early postoperative period. *Proceedings,* 26th Annual Meeting, Society of Nuclear Medicine, March 26–29, 1981a, New Orleans, La.

Detre, K.; Peduzzi, P.; Murphy, M.; *et al.* Effect of bypass surgery on survival of patients in low- and high-risk subgroups delineated by the use of simple clinical variables. The Veterans Administration Cooperative Study Group for Surgery for Coronary Arterial Occlusive Disease. *Circulation,* 1981, 63, 1329–1338.

Diamond, E. G.; Kittle, C. F.; and Crockett, J. E. Comparison of internal mammary artery ligation and sham operation for angina pectoris. *Am. J. Cardiol.,* 1960, 5, 483–486.

Dotter, C. T., and Judkins, M. Transluminal treatment of arteriosclerotic obstruction: Description of a new technic and a preliminary report of its application. *Circulation,* 1964, 30, 654–670.

Effler, D. B.; Sones, F. M., Jr.; Groves, L. L.; and Suarez, E. Myocardial revascularization by Vineberg's internal mammary artery implant. Evaluation of postoperative results. *J. Thorac. Cardiovasc. Surg.,* 1965, 50, 527–533.

Effler, D. B. Myocardial revascularization surgery since 1945 A.D. *J. Thorac. Cardiovasc. Surg.,* 1976, 72, 823–828.

Elayda, M. A.; Hall, R. J.; Mathur, V. S.; *et al.* Survival in patients with coronary artery bypass and left ventricular aneurysmectomy. *Circulation,* 1982, 66 (Suppl. II), 92 (abstr.).

European Cooperative Surgery Study Group. Coronary artery bypass surgery in stable angina pectoris: Survival at two years. *Lancet,* 1979, 1, 889.

European Coronary Surgery Study Group. Prospective randomized study of coronary artery bypass surgery in stable angina pectoris. A progress report on survival. *Circulation,* 1982, 65 (Suppl. II), 67.

Faulkner, S. L.; Stoney, W. S.; Alford, W. C.; *et al.* Ischemic cardiomyopathy: Medical versus surgical treatment. *J. Thorac. Cardiovasc. Surg.,* 1977, 74, 77–82.

Favaloro, R. G. Saphenous vein graft in the surgical treatment of coronary artery disease. Operative technique. *J. Thorac. Cardiovasc. Surg.,* 1969, 58, 178–185.

Fitzgibbon, G. M.; Burton, J. R.; and Leach, A. J. Coronary bypass graft fate: Angiographic grading of 1400 consecutive grafts early after operation and of 1132 after one year. *Circulation,* 1979, 57, 1070.

Fontaine, G.; Guiraudon, G.; and Frank, R. Stimulation studies and epicardial mapping in ventricular tachycardia: Study of mechanism and selection for surgery. In, Kulbertus, H. E. (ed.) *Re-entrant Arrhythmias.* MTP Press, Lancaster, England, 1977, p. 334.

Garrett, H. E.; Dennis, E. W.; and DeBakey, M. E. Aortocoronary bypass with saphenous vein graft. Seven-year follow-up. *JAMA,* 1973, 223, 792–794.

Golding, L. A. R.; Loop, F. D.; Peter, M.; *et al.* Late survival following use of intraaortic balloon pump in revascularization operations. *Ann. Thorac. Surg.,* 1980, 30, 48.

Gorlin, R., and Taylor, W. J. Selective revascularization of the myocardium by internal-mammary-artery implant. *N. Engl. J. Med.,* 1966, 275, 283–290.

Green, G. E. Internal mammary artery-to-coronary artery anastomosis. Three-year experience with 165 patients. *Ann. Thorac. Surg.,* 1972, 14, 160.

Gruntzig, A. R.; Senning, A.; and Siegenthaler, W. E. Nonoperative dilatation of coronary-artery stenosis: Percutaneous transluminal coronary angioplasty. *N. Engl. J. Med.,* 1979, 301, 61–68.

Guiraudon, G.; Fontaine, G.; Frank, R.; *et al.* Encircling endocardial ventriculotomy: A new surgical treatment for life-threatening ventricular tachycardias resistant to medical treatment following myocardial infarction. *Ann. Thorac. Surg.,* 1978, 26, 438.

Gunnar, R. M.; Loeb, H. S.; Palac, R.; and Figarre, R. Improved survival in patients with chronic angina pectoris treated surgically: Report of a randomized prospective study of aortocoronary bypass from Hines, Illinois. In, Update II. *The Heart,* edited by Hurst, J. W., New York, McGraw-Hill, 1980, p. 205.

Hall, R. J. Coronary artery bypass: Facts and figures. *Tex. Heart Inst. J.,* 1982, 9, 478–482.

Hall, R. J.; Elayda, M. A.; Gray, A.; *et al.* Coronary artery bypass: Long-term follow-up of 22,284 consecutive patients. *Circulation,* 1983, 68 (Suppl. II), II 20–26.

Hall, R. J.; Mathur, V. S.; Garcia, E.; and de Castro, C. M. The prolongation of life by coronary bypass surgery. In, Hurst, J. W. (ed.) *Update II, The Heart.* McGraw-Hill, New York, 1980, pp. 175–204.

Hallman, G. L.; Cooley, D. A.; McNamara, D. G.; and Latson, J. R. Single left coronary artery with fistula to right ventricle: Reconstruction of two-coronary system with Dacron graft. *Circulation,* 1965, 32, 293.

Hammermeister, K. E.; DeRoyen, T. A.; Murray, J. A.; and Dodge, H. T. Effect of aortocoronary saphenous vein bypass grafting on death and sudden death. Comparison of nonrandomized medically and surgically treated cohorts with comparable coronary disease and left ventricular function. *Am. J. Cardiol.,* 1977, 39, 925.

Harken, D. E.; Black, H.; Dickson, J. F., III; and Wilson, H. E., III. De-epicardialization: A simple, effective surgical treatment for angina pectoris. *Circulation,* **1955,** *12,* 955.

Harris, P. J.; Harrell, P. E., Jr.; Lee, K. L.; *et al.* Survival in medically treated coronary artery disease. *Circulation,* **1979,** *60,* 1259.

Helfant, R. H.; Pine, R.; Meister, S. G.; *et al.* Nitroglycerin to unmask reversible asynergy. Correlation with post-coronary bypass ventriculography. *Circulation,* **1974,** *50,* 108.

Hellman, C.; Schmidt, D. H.; Kamath, M. L.; *et al.* Bypass graft surgery in severe left ventricular dysfunction. *Circulation,* **1980,** *62* (Suppl. I), 103.

Horowitz, L. N.; Harken, A. H.; Kastor, J. A.; and Josephson, M. E. Ventricular resection guided by epicardial and endocardial mapping for the treatment of recurrent ventricular tachycardia. *N. Engl. J. Med.,* **1980,** *302,* 589.

Hurst, J. W.; King, S. B.; Logue, R. B.; *et al.* Value of coronary artery bypass surgery. *Am. J. Cardiol.,* **1982,** *42,* 308–329.

Johnson, W. D.; Flemma, R. J.; Lepley, D., Jr.; and Ellison, E. H. Extended treatment of severe coronary artery disease: A total surgical approach. *Ann. Surg.,* **1969,** *170,* 460–470.

Jones, E. L.; Craver, J. M.; Kaplan, J. A.; *et al.* Criteria for operability and reduction of surgical mortality in patients with severe left ventricular ischemia and dysfunction. *Ann. Thorac. Surg.,* **1978,** *25,* 413.

Josephson, M. E.; Harken, A. H.; and Horowitz, L. N. Endocardial excision: A new surgical technique for the treatment of recurrent ventricular tachycardia. *Circulation,* **1979,** *60,* 1430.

Kay, E. B.; Naraghipour, H.; Beg, R. A.; *et al.* Internal mammary artery bypass graft. Long-term patency rate and follow-up. *Ann. Thorac. Surg.,* **1974,** *18,* 269.

Kennedy, J. W.; Kaiser, G. C.; Fiser, L. D.; *et al.* Clinical and angiographic predictors of operative mortality from the collaborative study in coronary artery surgery. *Circulation,* **1981,** *63,* 793.

Kent, K. M.; Bentivoglio, L. G.; Block, P. G.; *et al.* Percutaneous transluminal coronary angioplasty: Report from the registry of NHLBI. *Am. J. Cardiol.,* **1982,** *49,* 2011.

Kent, K. M.; Borer, J. S.; Green, M. V.; *et al.* Effects of coronary artery bypass on global and regional left ventricular function during exercise. *N. Engl. J. Med.,* **1978,** *298,* 1434–1439.

King, S. B., III, and Hurst, J. W. The relief of angina pectoris by coronary bypass surgery. In, Hurst, J. W. (ed.) *Update II, The Heart.* McGraw-Hill, New York, **1980,** pp. 71–83.

Kirklin, J. W.; Kouchoukos, N. T.; Blackstone, E. H.; and Berman, A. Research related to surgical treatment of coronary artery disease. *Circulation,* **1979,** *60,* 1613.

Klausner, S. C.; Ratshin, R. A.; Tybert, J. V.; *et al.* The similarity of changes in segmental contraction patterns induced by post-extrasystolic potentiation and nitroglycerin. *Circulation,* **1976,** *54,* 615.

Kouchoukos, N. T.; Oberman, A.; Kirklin, J. W.; *et al.* Coronary bypass surgery: Analysis of factors affecting hospital mortality. *Circulation,* **1979,** *60* (Suppl. II), 58 (abstr.).

————. Coronary bypass surgery: Analysis of factors affecting hospital mortality. *Circulation,* **1980,** *62* (Suppl. I), 84.

Lawrie, G. M.; Morris, G. C., Jr.; Tidwell, J. F.; *et al.* Improved survival after 5 years in 1,144 patients after coronary artery bypass surgery. *Am. J. Cardiol.,* **1978,** *42,* 709–715.

Levin, D. C.; Cohn, L. H.; Koster, J. K., Jr., and Collins, J. J., Jr. Accuracy of angiography in predicting quality and caliber of the distal coronary artery lumen in preparation for bypass surgery. *Circulation,* **1982,** *66* (Suppl. II), 93.

Li, W.; Riggins, R. C. K.; and Anderson, R. P. Reversal of exertional hypotension after coronary bypass grafting. *Am. J. Cardiol.,* **1979,** *44,* 607.

Loeb, H. S.; Pifarre, R.; Sullivan, J.; *et al.* Improved survival after surgical therapy for chronic angina pectoris. One hospital's experience in a randomized trial. *Circulation,* **1979,** *60* (Suppl. I), 22.

Loop, F. D.; Hertzer, N. R.; Beven, E. G.; *et al.* Intermediate-term results of combined (simultaneous) carotid endarterectomy and coronary artery surgery. *Circulation,* **1982,** *66* (Suppl. II), 91.

Loop, F. D.; Irarrazaval, M. J.; Bredee, J. H.; *et al.* Internal mammary artery graft for ischemic heart disease. Effect of revascularization on clinical status and survival. *Am. J. Cardiol.,* **1977,** *39,* 516.

Loop, F. D.; Sheldon, W. C.; Lytle., B. W.; *et al.* The efficacy of coronary artery surgery. *Am. Heart J.,* **1981,** *101,* 86–96.

Manly, J. C.; King, J. C.; Zeft, H. J.; and Johnson, W. D. The "bad" left ventricle. *J. Thorac. Cardiovasc. Surg.,* **1976,** *72,* 841–848.

Marco, J. D. Myocardial perfusion by coronary artery bypass. In, Hurst, J. W. (ed.) *Update II, The Heart.* McGraw-Hill, New York, **1980,** pp. 13–31.

Mason, D. T.; Amsterdam, E. A.; De Maria, A. N.; *et al.* The prevention of myocardial infarction by coronary bypass surgery. In, Hurst, J. W. (ed.) *Update II, The Heart.* McGraw-Hill, New York, **1980,** p. 103.

Massin, B. M.; Botvinick, E. H.; Brundage, B. H.; *et al.* Relationship of regional myocardial perfusion to segmental wall motion. A physiologic basis for understanding the presence and reversibility of asynergy. *Circulation,* **1978,** *58,* 1154–1163.

Mathur, V. S. Functional results of revascularization with percutaneous transluminal coronary angiography. *Tex. Heart Inst. J.,* **1982,** *9,* 477 (abstr.).

Mathur, V. S., and Guinn, G. A. Chronic stable angina: Prospective randomized study with 4–7 year follow-up to evaluate surgical vs. medical treatment. *Chest,* **1979,** *76,* 359 (abstr.).

Mathur, V. S.; Hall, R. J.; Garcia, E.; *et al.* Prolonging life with coronary artery bypass surgery in patients with three-vessel disease. *Circulation,* **1980,** *62* (Suppl. I), 90–98.

McAllister, F. F.; Leighninger, D.; and Beck, C. S. Revascularization of the heart by graft of systemic artery into coronary sinus. *JAMA,* **1948,** *137,* 436.

McGee, M. G.; Szycher, M.; Turner, S. A.; *et al.* Use of composite biomer/butyl rubber/biomer material to prevent transdiaphragmatic water permeation during long-term, electrically-actuated left ventricular assist device (LVAS) pumping. *Cardiovasc. Dis. Bull. Tex. Heart Inst.,* **1980,** *3,* 278.

Meyer, J.; Merx, W.; Schmitz, H.; *et al.* Percutaneous

transluminal coronary angioplasty immediately after intracoronary streptolysis of transmural myocardial infarction. *Circulation,* **1982,** *66,* 905.

Mock, M. M.; Ringqvist, I.; Fisher, L.; Davis, K.; *et al.* The survival of nonoperated patients with ischemic heart disease: The Coronary Artery Surgery Study (CASS) registry. *Am. J. Cardiol.,* **1982a,** *49,* 1007 (abstr.).

————. Survival of medically treated patients in the Coronary Artery Surgery Study (CASS) registry. *Circulation,* **1982b,** *66,* 562–568 (abstr.).

Mundth, E. D., and Austen, W. G. Surgical measures for coronary heart disease (first of three parts). *N. Engl. J. Med.,* **1975,** *193,* 13–19.

Murphy, M. L.; Hultgren, H. N.; Detre, K.; *et al.* Treatment of chronic stable angina. A preliminary report of survival data of the randomized Veterans Administration Cooperative Study, *N. Engl. J. Med.,* **1977,** *297,* 621–627.

National Cooperative Study Group to Compare Medical and Surgical Therapy. I. Report of protocol—Patient population. Unstable angina pectoris. *Am. J. Cardiol.,* **1978,** *42,* 839.

Oberman, A.; Wayne, J. B.; Kouchoukos, N. T.; *et al.* Employment status after coronary artery bypass surgery. *Circulation,* **1982,** *65* (Suppl. II), 115–119.

O'Shaughnessy, L. Surgical treatment of cardiac ischemia, *Lancet,* **1937,** *1,* 185.

Ott, D. A.; Cooley, D. A.; Solis, R. T.; and Harrison, C. B., III. Wound complications after median sternotomy: A study of 61 patients from a consecutive series of 9,279. *Cardiovasc. Dis. Bull. Tex. Heart Inst.,* **1980,** *7,* 104–111.

Peduzzi, O., and Hultgren, H. N. Effect of medical vs. surgical treatment on symptoms in stable angina pectoris. The Veterans Administration Cooperative Study of Surgery for Coronary Arterial Occlusive Disease. *Circulation,* **1979,** *60,* 888.

Proudfit, W. L.; Bruschke, A. V. G.; and Sones, F. M., Jr. Natural history of obstructive coronary artery disease. Ten-year study of 601 nonsurgical cases. *Prog. Cardiovasc. Dis.,* **1978,** *21,* 53.

Rahimtoola, S. H. Coronary bypass surgery for chronic angina—1981: A perspective. *Circulation,* **1982,** *65,* 225–241.

Rahimtoola, S. H.; Grunkemeier, G.; Tepley, J.; *et al.* Changes in coronary bypass surgery leading to improved survival. *JAMA,* **1981,** *246,* 1912.

Rimm, A. A.; Blumlein, S.; Barboriak, J. J.; *et al.* The probability of closure in aortocoronary vein bypass grafts. *JAMA,* **1976,** *236,* 2637.

Rozanski, A.; Berman, D.; Grary, R.; *et al.* Preoperative prediction of reversible myocardial asynergy by postexercise radionuclide ventriculography. *N. Engl. J. Med.,* **1982,** *307,* 212–216.

Sami, M.; Chaitman, B. R.; Bourassa, M. D.; *et al.* Long term follow-up of aneurysmectomy for recurrent ventricular tachycardia or fibrillation. *Am. Heart J.,* **1978,** *96,* 303–308.

Sawyer, P. N.; Kaplitt, M. J.; Sobel, S.; and DiMaio, D. Application of gas endarterectomy to atherosclerotic peripheral vessels and coronary arteries. Clinical and experimental results. *Circulation,* **1967,** *35–36* (Suppl. I), 163.

Sharma, B.; Goodwin, J. F.; Raphael, M. J.; *et al.* Left ventricular angiography on exercise: A new method of assessing left ventricular function in ischemic heart disease. *Br. Heart J.,* **1976,** *38,* 59–70.

Slogoff, S. Anesthetic considerations for the patient with ischemic heart disease. *American Society of Anesth. Refresher Course in Anesthesiology,* **1980,** *8,* 179–188.

Slogoff, S.; Girgis, K. Z.; and Keats, A. S. Etiologic factors in neuropsychiatric complications associated with cardiopulmonary bypass. *Anesth. Analg.* (*Cleve.*), **1982,** *61,* No. 11.

Smith, H. C.; Hammes, L. N.; Gupta, S.; *et al.* Employment status after coronary artery bypass surgery. *Circulation,* **1982,** *65* (Suppl. II), 120–125.

Sones, F. M., Jr., and Shirey, E. K. Cine coronary arteriography. *Mod. Concepts Cardiovasc. Dis.,* **1962,** *31,* 735–738.

Spencer, F. C.; Green, G. F.; Tice, D. Z.; *et al.* Coronary artery bypass grafts for congestive heart failure: A report of experience with 40 patients. *Cardiovasc. Surg.,* **1971,** *62,* 529–542.

Stadius, M.; McAnulty, J. H.; Cutler, J.; *et al.* Specificity, sensitivity and accuracy of the nitroglycerin ventriculogram as predictor of surgically reversible wall motion abnormalities. *Am. J. Cardiol.,* **1980,** *45,* 399 (abstr.).

Stone, P. H., and Goldschlager, N. Left main coronary artery disease: Review and appraisal. *Cardiovasc. Med.,* **1979,** *4,* 165.

Sturm, J. T.; Fuhrman, T. M.; Sterling, R.; *et al.* Combined use of dopamine and nitroprusside therapy in conjunction with intraaortic balloon pumping for the treatment of postcardiotomy low-output syndrome. *J. Thorac. Cardiovasc. Surg.,* **1981,** *82,* 13–17.

Sturm, J. T.; McGee, M. G.; Fuhrman, T. M.; *et al.* Treatment of postoperative low output syndrome with intraaortic balloon pumping: Experience with 419 patients. *Am. J. Cardiol.,* **1980,** *45,* 1033–1036.

Takaro, T.; Hultgren, H. N.; Lipton, M. J.; Detre, K. M.; and participants in the study group. The Veterans Administration Cooperative Randomized Study of Surgery for Coronary Arterial Occlusive Disease. II. Subgroup with significant left main lesions. *Circulation,* **1976,** *54* (Suppl. II), 107.

Thompson, S. A., and Plachta, A. Fourteen years' experience with cardiopexy in treatment of coronary artery disease. *J. Thorac. Cardiovasc. Surg.,* **1957,** *27,* 64.

Thurer, R. L.; Lytle, B. W.; Cosgrove, D. M.; and Loop, F. D. Asymptomatic coronary artery disease managed by myocardial revascularization: Results at five years. *Circulation,* **1979,** 59–60 (Suppl. I), 14.

Vineberg, A. M. Development of anastomosis between coronary vessels and transplanted internal mammary artery. *Can. Med. Assoc. J.,* **1946,** *55,* 117.

Vineberg, A. M., and Walker, J. The surgical treatment of coronary artery heart disease by internal mammary artery implantation. Report of 140 cases followed up to thirteen years. *Prog. Cardiovasc. Dis.,* **1964,** *45,* 190–206.

Vismara, L. A.; Miller, R. R.; Price, J. E.; *et al.* Improved longevity due to reduction of sudden death by aortocoronary bypass in coronary atherosclerosis.

Prospective evaluation of medical versus surgical therapy in matched patients with multivessel disease. *Am. J. Cardiol.,* **1977,** *39,* 919.

Williams, D. O.; Gruntzig, A.; Kent, K. M.; Myler, R. K., *et al.* Guidelines for the performance of percutaneous transluminal coronary angioplasty. *Circulation,* **1982,** *66,* 693.

Yatteau, R. R.; Peter, R. H.; Behar, V. S.; *et al.* Ischemic cardiomyopathy: The myopathy of coronary artery disease. *Am. J. Cardiol.,* **1974,** *34,* 520–525.

Zubiate, P.; Kay, J. H.; and Mendez, A. M. Myocardial revascularization for the patient with drastic impairment of function of the left ventricle. *J. Thorac. Cardiovasc. Surg.,* **1977,** *73,* 84–86.

Chapter 13

CARDIOVASCULAR NUCLEAR MEDICINE: APPLICATIONS IN PATIENTS WITH CORONARY ARTERY DISEASE

E. Gordon DePuey and John A. Burdine

The technological revolution of today has brought with it improvements in the noninvasive diagnosis of disease, with one example being the evolution of nuclear medicine cardiovascular techniques. A combination of advances in computer science and electronics has made it possible to evaluate many of the parameters of cardiac function utilizing radiopharmaceuticals and current imaging instrumentation. Within the past few years, nuclear medicine testing has made a major impact on clinical cardiology, and the testing a patient receives today is vastly different from that of just five years ago. Most of the newer techniques are primarily adjunctive to the traditional cardiologic testing. Radionuclide ventriculography, for example, has created a shift in emphasis on the data derived from cardiac catheterization and coronary angiography, but has not affected the invasive procedures where anatomical rather than physiological information is desired. With the advent of mobile scintillation cameras, important clinical information can be collected at the patient's bedside in the intensive care or coronary care units, in some instances providing critical information that could only be obtained previously by an invasive technique not routinely available in this setting. *In vitro* radioimmunoassay tests for

the presence of abnormal levels of cardiac proteins in blood constitute additional nuclear medicine procedures which have recently been introduced and are growing rapidly in application. The total spectrum of current nuclear medicine testing involves the diagnosis of myocardial infarction, including that associated with aortocoronary bypass surgery, the localization and sizing of infarcts, determination of the presence and extent of coronary artery disease, intervention testing related to drug administration, and assessment of the physiological effects of measures directed toward cardiac rehabilitation.

RADIONUCLIDE PROCEDURES TO DIAGNOSE MYOCARDIAL INFARCTION

^{99m}Tc-Pyrophosphate Imaging

Based upon the observation that hydroxyapatite crystals were formed within mitochondria in the peripheral zones of an acute infarct, ^{99m}Tc-pyrophosphate, a calcium chelate that was being used for bone imaging, was discovered to also collect at the periphery of irreversibly damaged myocardial tissue (Buja *et al.*, 1977). Following infarction, uptake of this radiopharmaceutical usually begins with 12 to 24

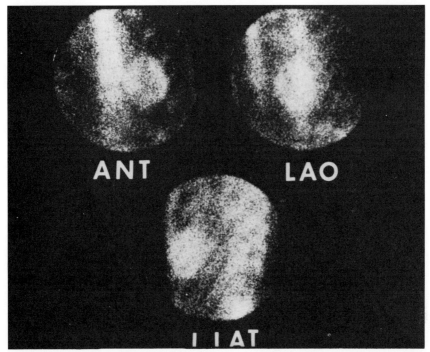

Figure 13-1. Acute anterior transmural myocardial infarction. There is intense ^{99m}Tc-pyrophosphate accumulation in the region of the entire anterior and lateral aspect of the left ventricle. In the anterior view a central area of less intense tracer concentration is present, indicating a central necrotic area within the infarct receiving relatively less tracer than the tissue at its periphery.

hours, reaching a maximum concentration in most instances by 48 hours. The time at which detectable tracer accumulation is present in an acute infarct is also, in part, dependent on the residual blood flow to the zone of infarction (Bruno *et al.*, 1976). If the infarct is very large, central areas may receive no residual blood flow and thus will appear as areas of decreased tracer concentration. This "doughnut pattern" is frequently associated with subsequent aneurysm and poor patient prognosis (Figure 13-1) (Rude *et al.*, 1979). In contrast, infarcts that are due to transient coronary occlusion, i.e., spasm, reperfuse quickly and thus accumulate tracer as soon as two to three hours following the acute event (Bruno *et al.*, 1976; Long *et al.*, 1980; Parkey *et al.*, 1981). Thus, the timing of identifiable tracer accumulation in an infarct may yield valuable information regarding the pathophysiology of the infarct and patient prognosis. In uncomplicated infarction tracer avidity declines fairly rapidly so that by 7 to 10 days many patients will have little if any localization remaining. In some instances, concentration persists, raising the question of reinfarc-

tion or aneurysm formation (Olson *et al.*, 1979). The sensitivity of the technique is quite good, with studies in dogs suggesting that infarcts involving as little as 3 g of myocardial tissue are consistently detected (Willerson *et al.*, 1977). ^{99m}Tc-PYP imaging is not as useful in detecting acute subendocardial infarcts in comparison with transmural, since tracer uptake is generally more diffuse and of less intensity (Figure 13-2) (Massie *et al.*, 1979). Patients with unstable angina pectoris also may have low-grade scan abnormalities, and whether such patients, in fact, have patchy myocardial necrosis is a possibility under current investigation (Perez *et al.*, 1975; Prasquier *et al.*, 1977; Jaffe *et al.*, 1979; Olson *et al.*, 1981).

It is also possible to utilize the distribution of pyrophosphate as an indicator of infarct size. Anterior and lateral infarcts can be accurately sized, but due to geometric considerations, measurement of those involving the inferior or posterior aspect of the left ventricle may be inaccurate (Botvinick *et al.*, 1975; Holman *et al.*, 1978). Recently tomographic radionuclide procedures have increased the accuracy in

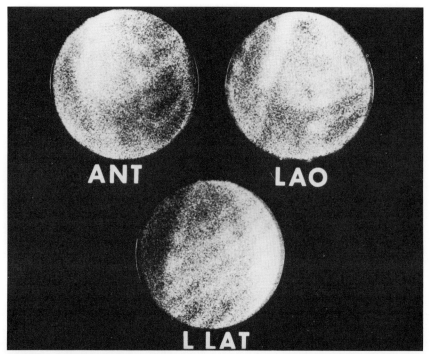

Figure 13-2. Diffuse subendocardial infarction. There is a moderate diffuse increase in tracer accumulation in the region of the entire left ventricle, seen best in the left anterior oblique view. In this patient a subendocardial infarct was documented, although a similar image pattern may be present in patients with unstable angina or myopericarditis. Occasionally residual tracer accumulation in the blood pool may present a similar image pattern.

infarct size estimation with pyrophosphate imaging (Keyes *et al.,* 1978). It should be emphasized, however, that the distribution of pyrophosphate in some patients tends to overestimate infarct size. Studies in animals have shown that pyrophosphate also localizes within tissue immediately adjacent to the zone of necrosis (Marcus *et al.,* 1976; Zaret *et al.,* 1976).

A major application of this imaging technique is in the evaluation of patients for perioperative myocardial infarction. Serum enzyme levels are routinely elevated following open heart surgery due to skeletal muscle trauma, hypothermia, and hemolysis associated with cardiopulmonary bypass. Electrocardiographic abnormalities frequently occur due to pericardial and epicardial trauma and cardiac axis shift, allowing only the larger areas of necrosis to be accurately diagnosed. In contrast to the electrocardiogram and serial enzyme studies, PYP imaging proved to be the most accurate testing modality since it is unaffected by these noninfarct perioperative changes (Klein *et al.,* 1976; Platt *et al.,* 1976;

Klausner *et al.,* 1977; Burdine *et al.,* 1979). The test is also useful in suspected right ventricular infarction, or in any circumstance where there is clinical suspicion and other tests are equivocal or negative (Wackers *et al.,* 1978; Kronenberg *et al.,* 1979).

^{201}Tl *Imaging*

The first radioisotope utilized to image regional myocardial perfusion was ^{43}K, but it had undesirable imaging characteristics that precluded satisfactory results with a standard scintillation camera. The potassium analogue, ^{201}Tl, soon replaced ^{43}K, and has been used extensively in recent years. Its rate of clearance from the myocardium is less rapid than ^{43}K resulting in more available imaging time (Nishiyama *et al.,* 1976). As an indicator, its biochemical distribution within the myocardium is similar to that of potassium, so that the concentration of thallium decreases or is absent in ischemic or dead tissue. Comparative studies using radiolabeled microspheres injected into the left atrium have demonstrated that thallium distribution is directly proportional to coronary blood flow at normal and reduced levels (Figure 13-3) (Strauss *et al.,* 1975; Mueller *et al.,* 1976; Nielsen *et al.,* 1980; Grunwald *et al.,* 1981). This circumstance makes it potentially useful in selected patients during the first 18 hours following myocardial infarction wherein other clinical studies are negative or equivocal, and a pyrophosphate study would be unsatisfactory in most cases due to inadequate concentration of the radiopharmaceutical (Figure 13-4) (Pitt and Thrall, 1980). A 97% sensitivity in detecting acute transmural myocardial infarction during the first 12 hours has been reported using thallium (Berger *et al.,* 1978). Some authors have indicated that a thallium abnormality is usually more consistent with true infarct size than the information gained from a pyrophosphate image (Berger *et al.,* 1978; Keyes *et al.,* 1981). However, this is a subject of controversy since thallium also is deficient in the zone of ischemia which may surround dying and dead myocardial tissue (Wackers *et al.,* 1976; Fletcher *et al.,* 1980). Thus, as in the case of pyrophosphate imaging,

thallium scan abnormalities should be looked to only as a rough estimate of infarct size.

Whereas pyrophosphate abnormalities frequently disappear after two weeks, thallium abnormalities with infarction persist indefinitely and thus may be helpful in following evolutionary changes. As agents for detecting the presence of infarction, thallium and pyrophosphate are comparable. However, the fact that thallium imaging may be abnormal due to resting ischemia alone, whereas pyrophosphate usually is not, makes it more difficult to interpret the thallium image in some instances. In addition, thallium image abnormalities which may be indistinguishable from those caused by acute infarction may result from old scars or aneurysms, coronary spasm, mitral valve prolapse, or congestive cardiomyopathy (Gutgesell *et al.,* 1980). The inability of thallium imaging to differentiate acute infarction from areas of scar is a severe limitation to the use of this imaging modality in diagnosing acute myocardial infarction (MI) in patients with a prior history of MI, unless of course a previous baseline scan is available for comparison.

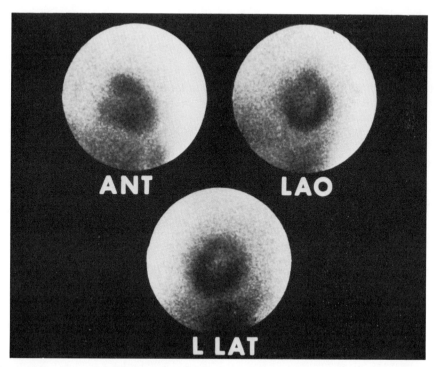

Figure 13-3. Normal thallium myocardial perfusion images. Homogeneous tracer distribution is noted throughout the myocardium. Diminished-to-absent tracer concentration is present in the location of the valve planes, and a central area of absent tracer concentration is noted in the location of the left ventricular cavity.

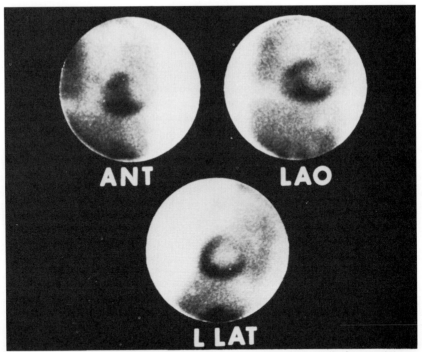

Figure 13-4. T1-201 myocardial perfusion images demonstrating a large lateral myocardial infarction. There is a well-localized area of absent tracer concentration in the region of the anterolateral wall of the left ventricle noted in the anterior view, and in the left anterior oblique view a well-defined absolute defect is present in the posterolateral region.

Cardiac Protein Radioassay

Developments in laboratory *in vitro* methods during the past decade have resulted in steady improvement in the accuracy of serum enzyme assays for the diagnosis of acute myocardial infarction. This approach now centers around the enzyme creatine kinase (CK) and its three isoenzymes: MM, MB, and BB. Skeletal muscle contains large quantities of CK-MM which is released following any form of muscle trauma including intramuscular injections of drugs such as those commonly given to patients presenting with chest pain. Approximately 80% of CK contained within the myocardium is also in the MM form, and the remainder is in the MB form. The CK-BB isoenzyme is primarily located in brain tissue. Because of its nonspecificity, at least 15% of patients with chest pain but without myocardial infarction have an elevation in total CK (Goldberg and Winfield, 1972).

The isoenzyme CK-MB is contained primarily within the myocardium with trace amounts present in the prostate and the mucosa of the small intestine. For practical purposes, a significant elevation of CK-MB is virtually diagnostic of myocardial cell necrosis in a consistent clinical setting (Roberts and Sobel, 1978). The first technique utilized to measure CK-MB on a clinical basis was serum electrophoresis. Because of the negative charge on the B-subunit, the MB isoenzyme has an intermediate electrophoretic mobility as compared to BB and MM, the latter of which does not migrate. This technique produced a significant advantage over conventional total CK assays, and a diagnostic accuracy of 95% has been reported (Wagner *et al.*, 1973; Blomberg *et al.*, 1975). Using fluorometric analysis with column chromatography, some further improvement in sensitivity and specificity was obtained, and using sequential blood samples, animal experimentation has demonstrated that the area under a CK-MB curve plot is proportional to infarct size (Sobel *et al.*, 1972; Fiolet *et al.*, 1977; Yasmineh *et al.*, 1977; Shell *et al.*, 1981).

Recent advances in radioimmunoassay have added substantial improvement in sensitivity compared to the electrophoretic and fluorometric techniques, resulting in the detection of CK-MB in the range of 0.01 IU/L (Roberts *et al.,* 1977; Willerson *et al.,* 1977; Rothkopf *et al.,* 1979; Yazaki and Nagai, 1979). This hundredfold improvement theoretically permits the identification of extremely small areas of myocardial necrosis which fall beneath the threshold for electrocardiographic and scintigraphic detection. However, the initial radioimmunoassay antibodies were specific for the B-subunit, and therefore small quantities of CK-BB product significant interference in patients with coexistent cerebral effects such as those produced by general anesthesia or concurrent cerebrovascular accidents. We have recently been involved in testing a new radioassay which has been bioengineered to be specific for the MB fraction. A solid phase anti-CK-B antibody separates CK-MB and CK-BB from the patient's serum. ^{125}I-labeled anti-CK-M is then added to bind to the immobilized CK-MB, and the bound radioactivity is compared to that obtained using purified human CK-MB standards. In initial clinical trials, results have been excellent in the diagnosis of acute myocardial infarction including that sustained in the perioperative setting of aortocoronary artery bypass surgery (DePuey *et al.,* 1982b; DePuey *et al.,* 1983).

Another recently introduced radioassay pertains to the determination of serum myoglobin levels. Myoglobin is an oxygen-binding compound present in myocardial tissue which is released into the serum and urine following acute myocardial infarction. Abnormal serum levels of myoglobin can be detected by this technique very early in the course of infarction (Kagen *et al.,* 1975; Stone *et al.,* 1977; Sonnemaker *et al.,* 1979; Witherspoon *et al.,* 1979). However, like CK, high levels of myoglobin are also contained in skeletal muscle which renders the test nonspecific in patients with intramuscular injections, trauma, DC cardioversion, and so forth. For the same reasons, the assay is unreliable in the diagnosis of perioperative myocardial infarction.

EVALUATION OF VENTRICULAR FUNCTION

In parallel with the development of static myocardial imaging with infarct-avid radiopharmaceuticals such as ^{99m}Tc-pyrophosphate and perfusion-related potassium analogues such as ^{201}Tl, assessment of global and segmental changes in the ventricular myocardium became possible using specialized electronics and radiopharmaceuticals that localize within the intravascular space. With the electrocardiographic signal from the patient triggering an electronic device called a "gate," it became possible to collect image data from the patient's beating heart during intervals confined to endsystole and end-diastole. Radioactive counts from multiple cardiac cycles were summed in a computer until a satisfactory data base for an image was present. This information was then displayed as composite end-systolic and end-diastolic images. By alternating the display of these composite images in a "flip-flop" fashion, an appreciation of the changes in configuration of the intraventricular blood pools could be obtained with the scintillation camera aimed at the heart from a variety of angles, including the right anterior oblique and left anterior oblique. In the next stage of development, the gating mechanism divided the R-R ECG interval into multiple segments, and sequential frames were collected beginning with the first portion of ventricular contraction and ending at end-diastole. These frames were then processed by the computer to construct a ventricular volume curve and a frame-mode display of the beating heart. Continuing refinements including image filtering and contrast enhancement techniques have resulted in excellent quality images that approach the contrast levels obtained in cineangiograms (Figure 13-5). Evaluation of segmental wall motion for most of the ventricular segments can be done with a high level of precision and accuracy (Harris *et al.,* 1981). Since the radiotracer is distributed uniformly throughout the blood pool, the radioactive count rate measured externally is proportional to LV volume. By monitoring changes in the count rate over the LV throughout the cardiac cycle, an LV volume curve may be obtained. Quantitative indices obtained from the ventricular volume curve such as the ejection fraction and systolic emptying rates have proven to be equally accurate and reproducible in assessing global function (Figure 13-6) (Links *et al.,* 1980; Swain *et al.,* 1981; Bonow *et al.,* 1981; Dehmer *et al.,* Denenberg *et al.,* 1981.) The application of these dynamic techniques has encompassed much of clinical cardiology including screening of patients with symptoms such as dyspnea or edema for the presence of cardiac dysfunction, evaluation of patients with myocardial infarction during critical phases of management, in the determination of complications such as ventricular aneurysm,

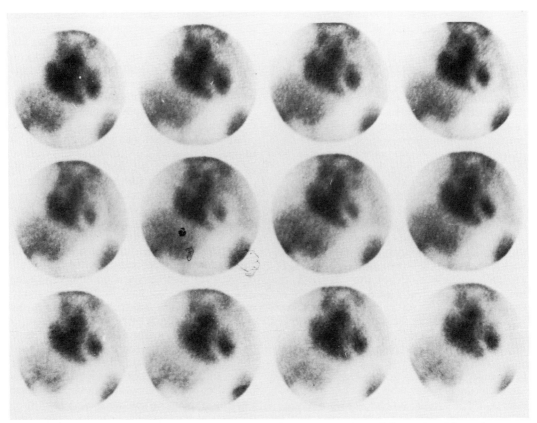

Figure 13-5. A series of gated cardiac images obtained in the 45-degree left anterior oblique view progressing horizontally from end-diastole (upper left corner) to end-systole (second or third image in the second row) and throughout the diastolic filling phase again to end-diastole (lower right corner).

and in the selection and follow-up of patients for aortocoronary artery bypass surgery (Nichols *et al.*, 1978; Winzelberg *et al.*, 1979; DePuey *et al.*, 1980; Boucher *et al.*, 1980; Preston, 1980; Boucher *et al.*, 1981; Freeman *et al.*, 1981; Kelly *et al.*, 1981).[201] Tl may also be used to obtain information about regional myocardial perfusion in these same circumstances. Assessment of right ventricular function is also possible, providing information regarding RV function in patients with congenital heart disease, COPD, pulmonary hypertension, and RV infarction (Maddahi et al., 1980.)

EXERCISE TESTING WITH RADIONUCLIDES

In considering patients who present with chest pain or those undergoing rehabilitation following myocardial infarction, the most important testing modalities are those that pro-

vide information concerning ventricular response to exercise. The technique which we use employs a bicycle ergometer and a computerized scintillation camera with continuous ECG monitoring. A basic understanding of physiological changes in response to exercise is necessary for satisfactory interpretation of the nuclear medicine studies. In the normal individual during strenuous bicycle exercise there is a dramatic redistribution of blood flow to the working musculature and myocardium resulting from the local effects of metabolites such as adenosine and carbon dioxide. Sympathetic stimulation causes vasoconstriction in the non-working musculature and splanchnic bed with the resultant collapse of the venous capacitance vessels in these areas. This phenomenon, coupled with the rhythmic muscular pumping of blood out of the legs during exercise and the enhancement of the negative intrathoracic

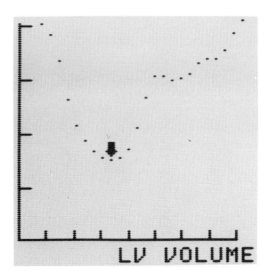

LV VOLUME

Figure 13-6. Count-rate-determined 24-point left ventricular volume curve obtained from a region surrounding the left ventricle in left anterior oblique gated images. The preejection period, rapid systolic emptying phase, slower phase of systolic emptying, rapid diastolic filling phase, period of diastasis, and the final atrial kick are well defined. The *arrow* indicates the point of end-systole used for ejection fraction calculation.

pressure during deep breathing, markedly increases the venous return to the heart. In the healthy individual the heart readily accommodates this increased venous return by increasing cardiac output through an increase in heart rate and myocardial contractility, thus supplying the increased demand for oxygen and nutrients and removing accumulated metabolites with greater efficiency. During maximal exercise, the velocity of left ventricular contraction increases, as well as the rate of development of myocardial wall tension and intracavitary pressure within the left ventricle. The enhanced contractility produces a significant decrease in end-systolic volume and therefore ejection fraction (Clausen, 1976; Smith *et al.*, 1976; Vatner and Pagani, 1976). With the patient in the supine position at rest, the left ventricle is maximally dilated during diastole, and the diastolic dimensions change little if any during exercise (McCallister *et al.*, 1968; Dehmer *et al.*, 1981c). (In the upright position, there is an increase in left ventricular end-diastolic volume during exercise, which also contributes to the increase in ejection fraction) (Rerych *et al.*, 1978). Similarly, the right ven-

tricle increases its contractility during exercise. Little change in pulmonary blood volume occurs in the normal individual in response to added workload (Nichols *et al.*, 1979; Okada *et al.*, 1979). Following the cessation of exercise, there is an abrupt termination of the pumping mechanisms described previously with a consequent sudden pooling of venous blood in the dilated peripheral vasculature. In contrast to normal individuals, patients with cardiac disease are frequently exercise-limited by symptoms related to coronary ischemia or insufficient cardiac output. In the normal subject, coronary blood flow may increase by a factor of six during exercise. However, in areas of coronary stenosis (defined by us as intraluminal narrowing equal to or greater than 70%), flow may not be able to increase to meet myocardial oxygen demands, particularly as a patient approaches maximum work load. In addition, some patients with fixed coronary lesions may have associated spasm, which further limits regional blood flow to the myocardium (Fuller *et al.*, 1980). When myocardial oxygen demand exceeds supply during exercise, deterioration of regional wall motion occurs. If this process worsens as the oxygen deficit rises, global dysfunction may result. Several abnormalities in ventricular function have been associated with coronary artery lesions. The most specific indicator is a regional motion abnormality including hypokinesis, akinesis, or dyskinesis. The image quality of radioisotope ventriculography has improved substantially as computer processing techniques continue to be refined. Not only have better resolution and contrast resulted, but image derivations are now possible including functional images of regional volume changes, regional ejection fraction, and, more recently, images of regional ventricular function expressed as phase for the study of the systolic wave form and identification of tardykinesis (Figure 13-7). The most important parameter of global function has been measurement of the ejection fraction. In our experience, a decrease in ejection fraction during exercise or a failure to increase by approximately five points strongly suggests ischemic changes or other abnormalities such as valvular heart disease, cardiomyopathy, and some forms of congenital heart disease. It has recently been noted that patients who decrease their ejection fractions by more than five points during exercise frequently have critical single-vessel disease or severe multivessel disease, thus substantially jeopardizing their prognosis. An increase

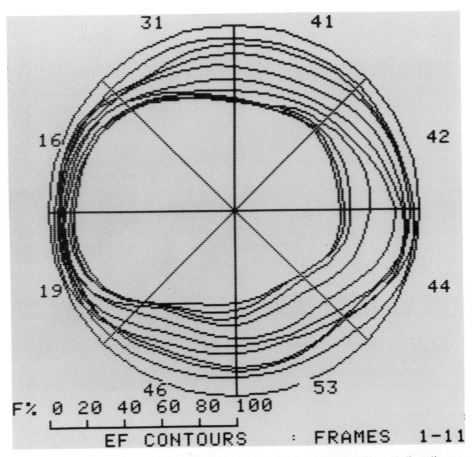

Figure 13-7. Left ventricular isocontours obtained throughout systole. The end-diastolic contour of the left ventricle is normalized to a circle, and the outline of the left ventricle during systole is plotted by isocontour mapping. There is obvious marked hypokinesis of the intraventricular septum (9 o'clock) and tardykinesis of the inferoposterior wall (3 to 4 o'clock). The circle is divided into eight octants, and the regional ejection fraction for each octant is indicated.

in end-systolic volume by 5% or greater over the resting volume is also considered abnormal and may in fact be a more sensitive indicator of cardiac dysfunction than the ejection fraction change described above. A marked increase in end-diastolic volume during supine exercise is likewise considered abnormal (McCallister *el al.*, 1968; Dehmer *et al.*, 1981c). In the upright position diastolic volume is relatively lower at rest due to blood pooling in the lower extremities and may normally increase by 20% due to enhanced venous return to the heart.

Following the cessation of exercise, there is an abrupt termination of the venous pumping mechanism described above with a consequent sudden pooling of venous blood in the dilated peripheral vasculature. Blood shifts to the pe-

ripheral structures with a resultant decrease in left ventricular end-diastolic and end-systolic volumes, but the increase in left ventricular contractility and ejection fraction usually persists for some time due to persistently elevated tissue and circulatory catecholamine levels (DePuey *et al.*, 1982b).

^{201}Tl EXERCISE TESTING

The noninvasive assessment of regional myocardial perfusion with ^{201}Tl was the first nuclear cardiology procedure to have a major clinical impact in the diagnosis of coronary artery disease. The ECG-monitored treadmill test had contributed substantially to the diagnosis of stress-induced myocardial ischemia, but there was a growing recognition of the technique limitations, including low sensitivity in detecting single-vessel disease and a relatively high number of false-positive results. Consequently, interest began to focus on the use of radioactive potassium and potassium analogues in an attempt to develop an image of the myocardium that was equivalent to regional perfusion.

For exercise testing, a standard treadmill or a bicycle ergometer may be used. It is most important for a patient to achieve a fairly high work load to obtain satisfactory imaging results, and the criteria for normalcy include achievement of 80 to 90% of maximum predicted heart rate, as well as a maximum heart rate systolic blood pressure product of 20,000 to 25,000 (Brady et $al.$, 1980). In the final minute or so of the exercise period, the patient is injected with ^{201}Tl and then imaged immediately following the cessation of exercise in several positions, usually including anterior, 45-degree LAO, and 60-degree LAO projections. The initial distribution of thallium monitored

in these images is directly proportional to regional myocardial blood flow. Thus, areas of myocardium supplied by normal coronary arteries where blood flow dramatically increases with exercise will have more tracer concentration than areas supplied by stenotic arteries in which blood flow cannot increase or may actually decrease due to superimposed spasm (Figure 13-8). Since thallium rapidly redistributes into ischemic areas, it is important that all images be completed within 20 to 30 minutes following cessation of exercise (Beller et $al.$, 1980; Grunwald et $al.$, 1981).

The interpretation of ^{201}Tl myocardial images requires a knowledge of the physiology of potassium and potassium analogues. Approximately 90% of ^{201}Tl is extracted by the myocardium on the first transit through the coronary arteries (Grunwald et $al.$, 1981). The total activity level of the myocardium and skeletal muscle rises markedly during exercise as cardiac output is augmented to these areas. Images taken immediately following exercise

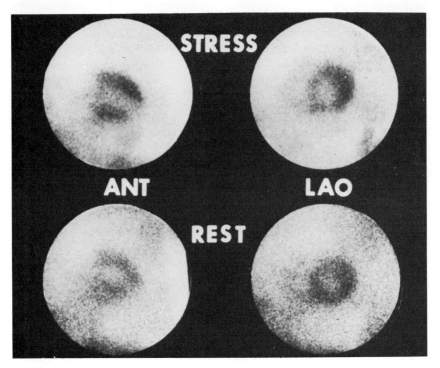

Figure 13-8. Thallium myocardial perfusion images obtained immediately following peak treadmill exercise (above) and at a four-hour delayed interval (below). In the initial stress images, there is a localized area of absent tracer concentration at the left ventricular apex in the anterior view and moderately diminished concentration throughout the intraventricular septum in the left anterior oblique view. In the delayed redistribution images tracer concentration has returned to normal. These scan findings are consistent with exercise-induced ischemia of the apex and septum.

demonstrate decreased activity in the watershed of a stenotic vessel and in areas of scarring as well. In severe ischemia, decreased activity, in fact, may occur at rest (Gibson et al., 1980).

Following exercise, redistribution of ^{201}Tl occurs into ischemic areas so that images obtained four to five hours following tracer injection permit separation of ischemic areas from those that are scarred, since the latter do not have a restoration of normal activity levels during the resting interval. Thus, ischemic areas will frequently have a normal concentration of tracer in the delayed images, whereas the activity level in areas of scarring will continue to be decreased.

Other changes in the distribution of thallium may be helpful in interpretation of the study. For example, during exercise, thallium activity in the liver progressively decreases to a negligible level at peak work load (Cook et al., 1976). Therefore, the absence of significant thallium activity in the liver is a good indicator of adequate stress. It has also been observed that many patients with significant ischemia have increased lung activity following exercise even if they are unable to achieve maximum work loads (Bingham et al., 1978; Bingham et al., 1980). In terms of lesion recognition, it is estimated that a minimum of 5.0 g of contiguous ischemic tissue with a decrease in activity at least 25% in comparison to the surrounding area is necessary for the imaging technique to demonstrate an abnormality (Mueller et al., 1976). Technical changes such as the introduction of the 7- to 10-hole pinhole collimator and the rotating slant-hole collimator have not at this point made major improvements in imaging accuracy (Mullani et al., 1981; Ritchie et al., 1981). Current efforts toward improved imaging of ^{201}Tl include oblique reconstructions of the ventricular myocardium utilizing emission-computed tomography (Holman et al., 1979; Keyes et al., 1981; Mullani et al., 1981; Tamaki et al., 1981).

The major current application of the procedure is in patients in whom the results of stress electrocardiography are equivocal or difficult to interpret (Iskandrian et al., 1980; Ong et al., 1980; Iskandrian and Segal, 1981; Melin et al.,1981). If significant coronary artery stenosis is considered to be a 50% or greater narrowing of the diameter of the lumen of a vessel, most reports indicate a sensitivity for ^{201}Tl stress imaging between 80 and 90%, and a specificity between 70 and 80% (Ritchie et al., 1978; Massie et al., 1979; Rigo et al., 1981). The sensitivity for stress electrocardiography in those studies ranges between 50 and 70% with a comparably low specificity. The low specificity for the ECG technique is frequently attributed to drug effects, bundle branch block, previous infarction, and metabolic and electrolyte changes. False-positive thallium studies have been reported in patients with mitral valve prolapse and mitral stenosis, but perhaps the greatest source of false-positive interpretations is due to scan artifacts produced by overlying soft tissue structures which attenuate the low-energy thallium emissions (Dunn et al., 1981).

GATED RADIONUCLIDE VENTRICULOGRAPHY

Using the scintillation camera with a special purpose computer, high-resolution and high-contrast movie-mode images can now be obtained of the intracardiac blood pool during exercise. This technique has proven to be an optimal method for measuring ventricular response to exercise and is an excellent testing modality to follow patients during cardiac rehabilitation. Ejection fractions, rates of systolic emptying and diastolic filling, absolute or relative left ventricular volumes, and mathematically derived left ventricular pressure changes may be measured from the same data collection interval. The exercise protocol currently used is as follows:

1. The patient is NPO at least four hours prior to exercise testing. This is very important for several reasons. Patients are considerably less comfortable when exercising with a full stomach, and if an arrhythmia with cardiac arrest occurs, there is a much greater chance of aspiration of gastric contents. Also, the presence of food in the stomach produces visceral dilatation and shunts blood away from the central circulation and working musculature to the gut, theoretically decreasing the patient's exercise capacity. Furthermore, ECG changes unrelated to ischemia have been identified in the postprandial state, and there is a consistent increase in the resting left ventricular ejection fraction (Brown et al., 1981).

2. The procedure is thoroughly explained to the patient and written informed consent is obtained. Although there are no known risks from the radiopharmaceuticals administered or the radiation dose, there is a small, but definite, risk of exercise-induced problems in patients with known or suspected cardiovascular disease.

3. Following radiopharmaceutical adminis-

tration, resting images are obtained in the 30-degree right anterior oblique and 45-degree left anterior oblique views.

4. The patient is then requested to begin exercising using a bicycle ergometer and continuous data collection is performed with the camera in the 45-degree left anterior oblique view. An initial work load of 300 kpm at 50 revolutions per minute is used, with the workload being incremented by 100 kpm every three minutes as tolerated by the patient. In patients who are poorly conditioned or who have arthritis or peripheral vascular disease, the study is generally initiated with a lower work load, and the incremental additions may be less.

5. The heart rate and blood pressure are continuously monitored, and the patient is encouraged to continue exercise to the point of leg fatigue, exhaustion, appearance of electrocardiographic abnormalities, or chest pain. Exercise, of course, is immediately terminated if there is an untoward drop in blood pressure or heart rate.

6. With the camera remaining in the 45-degree LAO projection, images are obtained at three to six minutes postexercise.

Although ejection fraction calculations from the various data collection intervals may be performed by several automated, operator-independent techniques, our experience suggests that in a significant number of patients careful manual selection of the left ventricular edges is necessary to best separate the left ventricle from the aortic outflow tract and left atrium.

For interpretation, the resting, exercise, and postexercise images are viewed simultaneously by the physician in order to achieve satisfactory comparison of regional wall motion between the various studies.

Other abnormalities, which are not specific for coronary artery disease, include a decrease in the rate of systolic emptying and the rate of diastolic filling, both of which may be determined from the computer-constructed ventricular volume curve. Pulmonary blood volume may be estimated with this technique, but is much more accurately measured by positron-emission tomography. A significant increase in pulmonary blood volume during exercise is considered to be a sensitive indicator of cardiac dysfunction (Nichols et al., 1979; Okada et al., 1979).

Utilizing these criteria, particularly the ejection fraction and regional wall motion changes, it is generally reported that 85 to 90% of pa-

tients with coronary artery disease may be identified with exercise radionuclide ventriculography (Borer et al., 1977; Bodenheimer et al., 1979; Borer et al., 1979; Jengo et al., 1980). The specificity of the study varies with the patient population. Some of the parameters of left ventricular function are nonspecific for coronary disease, as previously indicated, and are consistent with cardiac dysfunction of any variety. Several influences that diminish the sensitivity and specificity of the test should be kept in mind. The most important of these is failure of the patient to achieve a satisfactory work load, creating an inadequate myocardial oxygen demand (Brady et al., 1980). This may occur because of fatigue, leg pain, or more important circumstances such as cardiac arrhythmia. A linear relationship between the so-called "double product" (heart rate times systolic blood pressure) and myocardial oxygen demand has been demonstrated. Therefore, any factors that limit the rate pressure product also limit myocardial oxygen demand, and thus diminish the sensitivity of the test. Propranolol, a common medication given to patients with coronary artery disease, also acts to restrict the rate pressure product and is a common cause of false-negative tests (Marshall et al., 1981). Patients taking short- and long-acting nitrates may experience increased coronary blood flow with a concomitant reduction in left ventricular end-diastolic pressure (Slutsky et al., 1980). This circumstance alters the myocardial supply/demand relationship and may interfere with the test results.

In patients whose resting ventricular function is abnormal, such as those having previous myocardial infarction, the sensitivity and specificity of the test are considerably lower than in patients with normal resting left ventricular function. In our series, only 26% of patients with prior infarcts and significant coronary disease outside of the infarct distribution had associated wall motion abnormalities (DePuey et al., 1980b). There are several possible explanations for this finding. First, it is often difficult to determine additional segmental motion abnormalities in patients with previous extensive infarcts, particularly if they involve the apex and anterior wall. Also, patients with prior infarction frequently are exercise limited.

Other helpful applications of the test include the evaluation of resting wall motion abnormalities in the consideration of scarring versus ischemia. In the postexercise period when there is decreased ventricular preload due to peripheral pooling of blood, left ventricular end-diastolic pressure is reduced. Circulating catecholamines also remain significantly elevated (150% of resting values). These combined factors result in increased myocardial contractility. Areas of myocardium that are ischemic at rest, but not significantly scarred, frequently potentiate their motion during the postexercise period as opposed to areas of scarring that remain unchanged (DePuey et al., 1982a).

Dramatic improvement in both exercise tolerance and global and regional left ventricular response is routinely observed following aortocoronary bypass surgery and percutaneous transluminal coronary angioplasty (DePuey et al., 1981). A failure to improve left ventricular response to exercise serves as a sensitive indicator of bypass graft occlusion, unsuccessful dilatation, or restenosis of the coronary artery.

Also, in patients following cardiac surgery, chest pain may be difficult to evaluate due to poststernotomy syndromes.

In patients under consideration for valvular surgery, the point of decision is frequently difficult to reach since premature replacement of a valve subjects the patient to unnecessary risk of systemic emboli, lifetime anticoagulant therapy, infection, and so forth. By contrast, irreversible deterioration of left ventricular function may occur if surgery is inappropriately delayed. A fall in left ventricular ejection fraction during exercise has been reported to indicate irreversible myocardial damage, and utilizing this criterion, the sequential evaluation of patients with aortic valve disease in particular using exercise radionuclide ventriculography may be a very helpful tool in determining the appropriate time for surgery (Borer et al.,

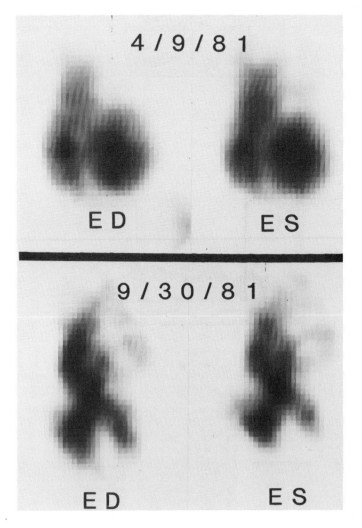

Figure 13-9. End-diastolic *(ED)* and end-systolic *(ES)* left anterior oblique gated blood pool images obtained at rest and during exercise before *(Top)* and after *(Bottom)* percutaneous transluminal angioplasty of the left anterior descending coronary.

Table 13-1. CASE STUDY

	9/17/79	12/8/80
Duration of exercise	8 min, 24 sec	11 min, 27 sec
Double product (HR × SBP)	14,000	17,340
Total work (kpm)	3,600	5,224
Resting ejection fraction	0.44	0.52
Exercise ejection fraction	0.46	0.58

* This 61-year-old man sustained an acute myocardial infarction in 1977 and underwent aortocoronary bypass surgery for incapacitating angina in 1978. In January, 1979, he noted recurrent chest pain and syncope. He was hospitalized and found to have intermittent ventricular arrhythmias. Cardiac catheterization and coronary angiography demonstrated that two of four bypass grafts were occluded. A course of medical management was decided upon, including antiarrhythmic agents, platelet antagonists, and propranolol.

The patient entered a cardiac rehabilitation program on 9/17/79. In Table 13-1, the parameters of exercise tolerance and left ventricular performance are listed upon entrance into the program and after 15 months, at which time the patient was asymptomatic. Improvement in exercise tolerance, as well as resting and exercise left ventricular function, are demonstrated.

1978; Bonow *et al.*, 1980; Sorenson *et al.*, 1980; Mirsky *et al.*, 1981).

Finally, exercise radionuclide ventriculography is very useful in establishing a baseline for cardiac rehabilitation of patients who have sustained myocardial infarction or undergone coronary artery bypass procedures. Based on sequential studies, specific improvement in segmental and global function is observed in such patients which correlates extremely well with the results of other tests and the patient's general clinical status (Figure 13-9) (Table 13-1) (Jensen *et al.*, 1980; Verani *et al.*, 1981). Following revascularization procedures, the technique can also provide evidence of graft occlusion, and in patients with myopathy and/or valvular disease, exercise radionuclide ventriculography is very useful in determining optimal surgical and medical management (Kent *et al.*, Urquhart *et al.*, 1981).

REFERENCES

Beller, G. A.; Watson, D. D.; Ackell, P.; and Pohost, G. M. Time course of thallium-201 redistribution after transient myocardial ischemia. *Circulation,* **1980,** *61,* 791–797.

Berger, H. J.; Gottschalk, A.; and Zaret, B. L. Dual radionuclide study of acute myocardial infarction. Comparison of thallium-201 and technetium-99m stannous pyrophosphate imaging in man. *Ann. Intern. Med.,* **1978,** *88,* 145–154.

Bingham, J. B.; McKusick, K. A.; Strauss, H. W.; *et al.* Influence of coronary artery disease on pulmonary uptake of thallium-201. *Am. J. Cardiol.,* **1980,** *46,* 821-826.

Bingham, J. B.; Strauss, H. W.; Pohost, G. M.; and McKusick, K. A. Mechanisms of lung uptake of T1-201. *Circulation,* **1978,** *58,* II-62.

Blomberg, D. J.; Kimber, W. D.; and Burke, M. D. Creatine kinase isoenzymes. Predictive value in the early diagnosis of acute myocardial infarction. *Am. J. Med.,* **1975,** *59,* 464–469.

Bodenheimer, M. M.; Banka, V. S.; Fooshee, C. M.; and Helfant, R. H. Comparative sensitivity of the exercise electrocardiogram, thallium imaging and stress radionuclide angiography to detect the presence and severity of coronary heart disease. *Circulation,* **1979,** *60,* 1270–1278.

Bonow, R. O.; Bacharach, S. L.; Green, M. V.; *et al.* Impaired left ventricular diastolic filling in patients with coronary artery disease: Assessment with radionuclide angiography. *Circulation,* **1981,** *64,* 315–323.

Bonow, R. O.; Borer, J. S.; Rosing, D. R.; *et al.* Preoperative exercise capacity in symptomatic patients with aortic regurgitation as a predictor of postoperative left ventricular function and longer-term prognosis. *Circulation,* **1980,** *62,* 1280–1290.

Borer, J. S.; Bacharach, S. L.; Green, M. V.; *et al.* Real-time radionuclide cineangiography in the noninvasive evaluation of global and regional left ventricular function at rest and during exercise in patients with coronary-artery disease. *N. Engl. J. Med.,* **1977,** *296,* 839–844.

———. Exercise-induced left ventricular dysfunction in symptomatic and asymptomatic patients with aortic regurgitation: Assessment with radionuclide cineangiography. *Am. J. Cardiol.,* **1978,** *42,* 351–357.

Borer, J. S.; Kent, K. M.; Bacharach, S. L.; *et al.* Sensitivity, specificity and predictive accuracy of radionuclide cineangiography during exercise in patients with coronary artery disease. Comparison with exercise electrocardiography. *Circulation,* **1979,** *60,* 572–580.

Botvinick, E. H.; Shames, D.; Lappin, H.; *et al.* Noninvasive quantitation of myocardial infarction with technetium-99m pyrophosphate. *Circulation,* **1975,** *52,* 909–915.

Boucher, C. A.; Bingham, J. B.; Osbakken, M. D.; *et al.* Early changes in left ventricular size and function after correction of left ventricular volume overload. *Am. J. Cardiol.,* **1981,** *47,* 991–1004.

Brady, T. J.; Thrall, J. H.; and Pitt, B. The importance of adequate exercise in the detection of coronary heart disease by radionuclide ventriculography. *J. Nucl. Med.,* **1980,** *21,* 1125–1130.

Brown, J. M.; White, C. J.; Sobol, S. M.; and Lull, R. J. Increased left ventricular ejection fraction after a meal: Potential source of error in performance of radionuclide angiography. *Am. J. Cardiol.,* **1983,** *51,* 1709–1711.

Bruno, F. P.; Cobb, F. F.; Rivas, F.; and Goodrich, J. K. Evaluation of ^{99m}technetium stannous pyrophosphate as an imaging agent in acute myocardial infarction. *Circulation,* **1976,** *54,* 71–78.

Buja, L. M.; Tofe, A. J.; Kulkarni, P. V.; *et al.* Sites and mechanisms of localization of technetium-99m phosphorus radiopharmaceuticals in acute myocardial infarcts and other tissues. *J. Clin. Invest.,* **1977,** *60,* 724–740.

Burdine, J. A.; DePuey, E. G.; Orzan, F.; *et al.* Scintigraphic, electrocardiographic, and enzymatic diagnosis of perioperative myocardial infarction in patients undergoing myocardial revascularization. *J. Nucl. Med.,* **1979,** *20,* 711–714.

Clausen, J. P. Circulatory adjustments to dynamic exercise and effect of physical training in normal subjects and in patients with coronary artery disease. *Prog. Cardiovasc. Dis.,* **1976,** *18,* 459–495.

Cook, D. J.; Bailey, I.; Strauss, H. W.; *et al.* Thallium-201 for myocardial imaging: Appearance of the normal heart. *J. Nucl. Med.,* **1976,** *17,* 583–589.

Dehmer, G. J.; Firth, B. G.; Lewis, S. E.; *et al.* Direct measurement of cardiac output by gated equilibrium blood pool scintigraphy: Validation of scintigraphic volume measurements by a nongeometric technique. *Am. J. Cardiol.,* **1981,** *47a,* 1061–1067.

Dehmer, G. J.; Firth, B. G.; Hillis, L. D.; *et al.* Alterations in left ventricular volumes and ejection fraction at rest and during exercise in patients with aortic regurgitation. *Am. J. Cardiol.,* **1981b,** *48,* 17–27.

Dehmer, G. J.; Lewis, S. E.; Hillis, L. D.; *et al.* Exercise-induced alterations in left ventricular volumes and the pressure-volume relationship: A sensitive indicator of left ventricular dysfunction in patients with coronary artery disease. *Circulation,* **1981c,** *63,* 1008–1018.

Denenberg, B. S.; Makler, P. T.; Bove, A. A.; and Spann, J. F. Normal left ventricular emptying in coronary artery disease at rest: Analysis by radiographic and equilibrium radionuclide ventriculography. *Am. J. Cardiol.,* **1981,** *48,* 311–315.

DePuey, E. G.; Krajcer, Z.; Boskovik, D.; *et al.* Exercise radionuclide ventriculography in evaluating successful transluminal coronary angioplasty. *Circulation,* **1981,** *64,* IV-261 (abstr.).

DePuey, E. G.; Mammen, G. P.; Rivas, A. H.; *et al.* Post-exercise potentiation of wall motion to identify myocardial viability. *Cardiovasc. Dis. Bull. Tex. Heart Inst.* **1982a,** *9,* 127–134.

DePuey, E. G.; Mathur, V.; Hall, R. J.; and Burdine, J. A. Infarct-induced wall motion abnormalities in aortocoronary bypass patients: Correlation with electrocardiographic, enzymatic, and scintigraphic diagnostic criteria. *Cardiovasc. Dis., Bull. Tex. Heart Inst.,* **1980a,** *7,* 382–396.

DePuey, E. G.; Monroe, L. R.; Sonnemaker, R. E.; *et al.* A new creatine kinase-MB specific radioassay to diagnose myocardial infarction. *J. Nucl. Med.* **1982b,** *23,* P6 (abstr.).

DePuey, E. G.; Sonnemaker, R. E.; Garcia, E.; and Burdine, J. A. Exercise radionuclide ventriculography in patients with prior myocardial infarction. *J. Nucl. Med.,* **1980b,** *21,* 5 (abstr.).

DePuey, E. G.; Aessopos, A.; Monroe, L. R., *et al.* Clinical utility of a two-site immunoradiometric assay for creatine kinase-MB in the detection of perioperative myocardial infarction. *J. Nucl. Med.,* **1983,** *8,* 703–709.

Dunn, R. F.; Wolff, L.; Wagner, S.; and Botvinick, E. H. The inconsistent pattern of thallium defects: A clue to the false positive perfusion scintigram. *Am. J. Cardiol.,* **1981,** *48,* 224–232.

Fiolet, J. W. T.; Willebrands, A. F.; Lie, K. I.; and Ter Welle, H. F. Determination of creatine kinase isoenzyme MB (CK-MB): Comparison of methods and clinical evaluation. *Clinica Chim. Acta,* **1977,** *80,* 23–35.

Fletcher, J. W.; Mueller, H. S.; and Rao, P. S. Sequential thallium-201 myocardial scintigraphy after acute infarction in man. Comparison to creatine kinase-MB release pattern. *Radiology,* **1980,** *136,* 191–195.

Freeman, M. R.; Gray, R. J.; Berman, D. S.; *et al.* Improvement in global and segmental left ventricular function after coronary bypass surgery. *Circulation,* **1981,** *64,* II-34–II-39.

Fuller, C. M.; Raizner, A. E.; Chahine, R. A.; *et al.* Exercise-induced coronary arterial spasm: Angiographic demonstration, documentation of ischemia by myocardial scintigraphy and results of pharmacologic intervention. *Am. J. Cardiol.,* **1980,** *46,* 500–506.

Gibson, R. S.; Taylor, G. J.; Watson, D. D.; *et al.* Prognostic significance of resting anterior thallium-201 defects in patients with inferior myocardial infarction. *J. Nucl. Med.,* **1980,** *21,* 1015–1021.

Goldberg, D. M., and Winfield, D. A. Diagnostic accuracy of serum enzyme assays from myocardial infarction in general hospital population. *Br. Heart J.,* **1972,** *34,* 597–604.

Goldman, M. R., and Boucher C. A. Value of radionuclide imaging techniques in assessing cardiomyopathy. *Am. J. Cardiol.,* **1980,** *46,* 1232–1236.

Grunwald, A. M.; Watson, D. D.; Holzgrefe, H. H.; *et al.* Myocardial thallium-201 kinetics in normal and ischemic myocardium. *Circulation,* **1981,** *64,* 610–618.

Gutgesell, H. P.; Pinsky, W. W.; and DePuey, E. G. Thallium-201 myocardial perfusion imaging in infants and children. Value in distinguishing anomalous left coronary artery from congestive cardiomyopathy. *Circulation,* **1980,** *61,* 596–599.

Harris, D. N. F.; Taylor, D. N.; Ogilivie, B. C.; *et al.* Left ventricular segmental wall motion—a comparison between equilibrium radionuclide angiography and contrast angiography. *Br. J. Radiol.,* **1981,** *54,* 296–301.

Holman, B. L.; Chisholm, R. J.; and Braunwald, E. The prognostic implications of acute myocardial infarct scintigraphy with ^{99m}Tc-pyrophosphate. *Circulation,* **1978,** *57,* 320–326.

Holman, B. L.; Hill, T. C.; Wynne, J.; *et al.* Single-photon transaxial emission computed tomography of the heart in normal subjects and in patients with infarction. *J. Nucl. Med.,* **1979**, *20,* 736–740.

Iskandrian, A. S., and Segal, B. L. Value of exercise thallium-201 imaging in patients with diagnostic and nondiagnostic exercise electrocardiograms. *Am. J. Cardiol.,* **1981**, *48,* 233–238.

Iskandrian, A. S.; Wasserman, L. A.; Anderson, G. S.; *et al.* Merits of stress thallium-201 myocardial perfusion imaging in patients with inconclusive exercise electrocardiograms: Correlation with coronary arteriograms. *Am. J. Cardiol.,* **1980**, *46,* 553–558.

Jaffe, A. S.; Klein, M. S.; Patel, B. R.; *et al.* Abnormal technetium-99m pyrophosphate images in unstable angina: Ischemia versus infarction? *Am. J. Cardiol.,* **1979**, *44,* 1035–1039.

Jengo, J. A.; Freeman, R.; Brizendine, M.; and Mena, I. Detection of coronary artery disease: Comparison of exercise stress radionuclide angiocardiography and thallium stress perfusion scanning. *Am. J. Cardiol.,* **1980**, *45,* 535–541.

Jensen, D.; Atwood, J. E.; Froelicher, V.; *et al.* Improvement in ventricular function during exercise studied with radionuclide ventriculography after cardiac rehabilitation. *Am. J. Cardiol.,* **1980**, *46,* 770–777.

Kagen, L.; Scheidt, S.; Roberts, L.; Porter, A.; and Paul, H. Myoglobinemia following acute myocardial infarction. *Am. J. Med.,* **1975**, *58,* 177–182.

Kelly, M. J.; Giles, R. W.; Simon, T. R.; *et al.* Multigated equilibrium radionuclide angiocardiography: Improved detection of left ventricular wall motion abnormalities and aneurysms by the addition of the left lateral view. *Radiology,* **1981**, *139,* 167–173.

Kent, K. M.; Borer, J. S.; Green, M. V.; *et al.* Effects of coronary-artery bypass on global and regional left ventricular function during exercise. *N. Engl. J. Med.,* **1978**, *298,* 1434–1439.

Keyes, J. W.; Brady, T. J.; Leonard, P. F.; *et al.* Calculation of viable and infarcted myocardial mass from thallium-201 tomograms. *J. Nucl. Med.,* **1981**, *22,* 339–343.

Keyes, J. W.; Leonard, P. F.; Brody, S. L.; *et al.* Myocardial infarct quantification in the dog by single photon emission computed tomography. *Circulation,* **1978**, *58,* 227–232.

Klausner, S. C.; Botvinick, E. H.; Shames, D.; *et al.* The application of radionuclide infarct scintigraphy to diagnose perioperative myocardial infarction following revascularization. *Circulation,* **1977**, *56,* 173–181.

Klein, M. S.; Coleman, E.; Weldon, C. S.; *et al.* Concordance of electrocardiographic and scintigraphic criteria of myocardial injury after cardiac surgery. *J. Thorac. Cardiovasc. Surg.,* **1976**, *71,* 934–937.

Kronenberg, M. W.; Wooten, N. E.; Friesinger, G. C.; *et al.* Scintigraphic characteristics of experimental myocardial infarct extension. *Circulation,* **1979**, *60,* 1130–1140.

Links, J. M.; Douglass, K. H.; and Wagner, H. N., Jr. Patterns of ventricular emptying by Fourier analysis of gated blood-pool studies. *J. Nucl. Med.,* **1980**, *21,* 978–982.

Long, R.; Smyes, J.; Allard, J.; *et al.* Differentiation between reperfusion and occlusion myocardial necrosis with technetium-99m pyrophosphate scans. *Am. J. Cardiol.,* **1980**, *46,* 413–418.

Maddahi, J.; Berman, D. S.; Matsuoka, D. T.; *et al.* Right ventricular ejection fraction during exercise in normal subjects and in coronary artery disease patients: Assessment by multiple-gated equilibrium scintigraphy. *Circulation,* **1980**, *62,* 133–140.

Marcus, M. L.; Tomanek, R. J.; Ehrhardt, J. C., *et al.* Relationships between myocardial perfusion, myocardial necrosis, and technetium-99m pyrophosphate uptake in dogs subjected to sudden coronary occlusion. *Circulation,* **1976**, *54,* 647–653.

Marshall, R. C.; Wisenberg, G.; Schelbert, H. R.; and Henze, E. Effect of oral propranolol on rest, exercise and post exercise left ventricular performance in normal subjects and patients with coronary artery disease. *Circulation,* **1981**, *63,* 572–583.

Massie, B. M.; Botvinick, E. H.; and Brundage, B. H. Correlation of thallium-201 scintigrams with coronary anatomy: Factors affecting region by region sensitivity. *Am. J. Cardiol.,* **1979**, *44,* 616–622.

Massie, B. M.; Botvinick, E. H.; Werner, J. A.; *et al.* Myocardial scintigraphy with technetium-99m stannous pyrophosphate: An insensitive test for nontransmural myocardial infarction, *Am. J. Cardiol.,* **1979**, *43,* 186–192.

McCallister, B. D.; Yipintsoi, T.; Hallermann, F. J.; *et al.* Left ventricular performance during mild supine leg exercise in coronary artery disease. *Circulation,* **1968**, *37,* 922–931.

Melin, J. A.; Piret, L. J.; Vanbutsele, R. J. M.; *et al.* Diagnostic value of exercise electrocardiography and thallium myocardial scintigraphy in patients without previous myocardial infarction: A Bayesian approach. *Circulation,* **1981**, *63,* 1019–1024.

Mirsky, I.; Henschke, C.; Hess, O. M.; and Krayenbuehl, H. P. Prediction of postoperative performance in aortic valve disease. *Am. J. Cardiol.,* **1981**, *48,* 295–303.

Mueller, T. M.; Marcus, M. L.; Ehrhardt, J. C.; *et al.* Limitations of thallium-201 myocardial perfusion scintigrams. *Circulation,* **1976**, *54,* 640–653.

Mullani, N. A.; Gould, K. L.; and Gacta, J. M. Tomographic imaging of the heart with thallium-201: Seven-pinhole or rotating gamma camera? *J. Nucl. Med.,* **1981**, *22,* 925–926.

Nichols, A. B.; McKusick, K. A.; Strauss, H. W.; *et al.* Clinical utility of gated cardiac blood pool imaging in congestive left heart failure. *Am. J. Med.,* **1978**, *65,* 785–793.

Nichols, A. B.; Strauss, H. W.; Moore, R. H.; *et al.* Acute changes in cardiopulmonary blood volume during upright exercise stress testing in patients with coronary heart disease. *Circulation,* **1979**, *60,* 520–530.

Nielsen, A. P.; Morris, K. G.; Murdock, R.; *et al.* Linear relationship between the distribution of thallium-201 and blood flow in ischemic and nonischemic myocardium during exercise. *Circulation,* **1980**, *61,* 797–801.

Nishiyama, H.; Sodd, V. J.; Adolph, R. J.; *et al.* Intercomparison of myocardial imaging agents: ^{201}Tl, ^{129}Cs, ^{43}K, and ^{81}Rb. *J. Nucl. Med.,* **1976**, *17,* 880–889.

Okada, R. D.; Pohost, G. M.; Kirshenbaum, H. D.; *et al.* Radionuclide-determined change in pulmonary blood volume with exercise. *N. Engl. J. Med.,* **1979**, *301,* 569–576.

Olson, H. G.; Lyons, K. P.; Aronow, W. S.; *et al.* Prognostic value of a persistently positive technetium-99m stannous pyrophosphate myocardial scintigram after myocardial infarction. *Am. J. Cardiol.,* **1979,** *43,* 889–898.

Olson, H. G.; Lyons, K. P.; Aronow, W. S.; *et al.* The high-risk angina patient. Identification by clinical features, hospital course, electrocardiography and technetium-99m stannous pyrophosphate scintigraphy. *Circulation,* **1981,** *64,* 674–684.

Ong, S. S.; Quaife, M. A.; Dzindzio, L. S.; *et al.* Clinical decision-making with treadmill testing and thallium-201. *Am. J. Med.,* **1980,** *69,* 31–38.

Parkey, R. W.; Kulkarni, P. V.; Lewis, S. E.; *et al.* Effect of coronary blood flow and site of injection on Tc-99m PPi detection of early canine myocardial infarcts. *J. Nucl. Med.,* **1981,** *22,* 133–137.

Perez, L. A.; Hayt, D. B.; and Freeman, L. M. Localization of myocardial disorders other than infarction with ⁹⁹ᵐTc-labeled phosphate agents. *J. Nucl. Med.,* **1975,** *17,* 241–246.

Pitt, B., and Thrall, J. H. Thallium-201 versus technetium-99m pyrophosphate myocardial imaging in detection and evaluation of patients with acute myocardial infarction. *Am. J. Cardiol.,* **1980,** *46,* 1215–1223.

Platt, M. R.; Mills, L. J.; Parkey, R. W.; *et al.* Perioperative myocardial infarction diagnosed by technetium-99m stannous pyrophosphate myocardial scintigrams. *Circulation,* **1976,** *54* (Suppl. III), III-24–III-27.

Prasquier, R.; Taradash, M. R.; Botvinick, E. H.; *et al.* The specificity of the diffuse pattern of cardiac uptake in myocardial infarction imaging with technetium-99m stannous pyrophosphate. *Circulation,* **1977,** *55,* 61–66.

Preston, T. A. Measuring ventricular function after coronary bypass surgery. *Am. Heart J.,* **1980,** *99,* 270–271.

Rerych, S. K.; Scholz, P. M.; Newman, G. E.; *et al.* Cardiac function at rest and during exercise in normals and in patients with coronary heart disease. *Ann. Surg.,* **1978,** *187,* 449–464.

Rigo, P.; Bailey, I. K.; Griffith, L. S. C.; *et al.* Stress thallium-201 myocardial scintigraphy for the detection of individual coronary arterial lesions in patients with and without previous myocardial infarction. *Am. J. Cardiol.,* **1981,** *48,* 209–216.

Ritchie, J. L.; Williams, D. L.; Caldwell, J. H.; *et al.* Seven-pinhole emission tomography with thallium-201 in patients with prior myocardial infarction. *J. Nucl. Med.,* **1981,** *22,* 107–112.

Ritchie, J. L.; Zaret, B. L.; Strauss, H. W.; *et al.* Myocardial imaging with thallium-201: A multicenter study in patients with angina pectoris or acute myocardial infarction. *Am. J. Cardiol.,* **1978,** *42,* 345–350.

Roberts, R.; Parker, C. W.; and Sobel, B. E. Detection of acute myocardial infarction by radioimmunoassay for creatine kinase MB. *Lancet,* **1977,** *2,* 319–321.

Roberts, R., and Sobel, B. E. Creatine kinase isoenzymes in the assessment of heart disease. *Am. Heart J.,* **1978,** *95,* 521–528.

Rothkopf, M.; Boerner, J.; Stone, M. J.; *et al.* Detection of myocardial infarct extension by CK-B radioimmunoassay. *Circulation,* **1979,** *59,* 268–274.

Rude, R. E.; Parkey, R. W.; Bonte, F. J.; *et al.* Clinical implications of the technetium-99m stannous pyrophosphate myocardial scintigraphic "doughnut" pattern in patients with acute myocardial infarcts. *Circulation,* **1979,** *59,* 721–730.

Shell, W. E.; DeWood, M. A.; Kligerman, M.; *et al.* Early appearance of MB-creatine kinase activity in nontransmural myocardial infarction detected by a sensitive assay for the isoenzyme. *Am. J. Med.,* **1981,** *71,* 254–262.

Slutsky, R.; Bartler, A.; Gerber, K.; *et al.* Effect of nitrates on left ventricular size and function during exercise: Comparison of sublingual nitroglycerin and nitroglycerin paste. *Am. J. Cardiol.,* **1980,** *45,* 831–840.

Smith, E. E.; Guyton, A. C.; Manning, R. D.; and White, R. J. Integrated mechanisms of cardiovascular response and control during exercise in the normal human. *Prog. Cardiovasc. Dis.,* **1976,** *18,* 421–443.

Sobel, B. E.; Bresnahan, G. F.; Shell, W. E.; and Yoder, R. D. Estimation of infarct size in man and its relation to prognosis. *Circulation,* **1972,** *46,* 640–648.

Sonnemaker, R. E.; Daniels, D. L.; Craig, W. E.; Floyd, J. L.; and Bode, R. F. Serum myoglobin determination: Laboratory and clinical evaluation. *J. Nucl. Med.,* **1979,** *20,* 120–124.

Sorenson, S. G.; O'Rourke, R. A.; and Chaudhuri, T. K. Noninvasive quantitation of valvular regurgitation by gated equilibrium radionuclide angiography. *Circulation,* **1980,** *62,* 1089–1098.

Stone, M. J.; Waterman, M. R.; Harimoto, D.; *et al.* Serum myoglobin level as diagnostic test in patients with acute myocardial infarction. *Br. Heart J.,* **1977,** *39,* 375–380.

Strauss, H. W.; Harrison, K.; Langan, J. K.; *et al.* Thallium-201 for myocardial imaging. Relation of thallium-201 to regional myocardial perfusion. *Circulation,* **1975,** *51,* 641–645.

Swain, J. L.; Morris, K. G.; Bruno, F. P.; and Cobb, F. R. Comparison of multigated radionuclide angiography with ultrasonic sonomicrometry over a wide range of ventricular function in the conscious dog. *Am. J. Cardiol.,* **1980,** *46,* 976–982.

Tamaki, N.; Mukai, T.; Ishii, Y.; *et al.* Clinical evaluation of thallium-201 emission myocardial tomography using a rotating gamma camera: Comparison with seven-pinhole tomography. *J. Nucl. Med.,* **1981,** *22,* 849–855.

Urquhart, J.; Patterson, R. E.; Packer, M.; *et al.* Quantification of valve regurgitation by radionuclide angiography before and after valve replacement surgery. *Am. J. Cardiol.,* **1981,** *47,* 287–291.

Vatner, S. F., and Pagani, M. Cardiovascular adjustments to exercise: Hemodynamics and mechanisms. *Prog. Cardiovasc. Dis.,* **1976,** *19,* 91–108.

Verani, M. S.; Hartung, G. H.; Hoepfel-Harris, J.; *et al.* Effects of exercise training on left ventricular performance and myocardial perfusion in patients with coronary artery disease. *Am. J. Cardiol.,* **1981,** *47,* 797–803.

Wackers, F. J. T.; Lie, K. I.; Sokole, E. B.; *et al.* Prevalence of right ventricular involvement in inferior wall infarction assessed with myocardial imaging with thallium-201 and techetium-99m pyrophosphate. *Am. J. Cardiol.,* **1978,** *42,* 358–362.

Wackers, F. J. T.; Sokole, E. B.; Samson, G.; *et al.* Value and limitations of thallium-201 scintigraphy in the acute phase of myocardial infarction. *N. Engl. J. Med.,* **1976,** *295,* 1–5.

Wagner, G. S.; Roe, C. R.; Limbird, L. L.: *et al.* The importance of identification of the myocardial-specific isoenzyme of creatine phosphokinase (MB form) in the diagnosis of acute myocardial infarction. *Circulation,* **1973,** *43,* 263–269.

Willerson, J. T.; Buja, L. M.; Stokely, E. M.; *et al.* Infarct sizing in awake, unsedated dogs with acute anterior myocardial infarcts. *J. Nucl. Med.,* **1977,** *17,* 534 (abstr.).

Willerson, J. T.; Stone, M. J.; Ting, R.; *et al.* Radioimmunoassay of creatine kinase-B isoenzyme in human sera: Results in patients with acute myocardial infarction. *Proc. Natl. Acad. Sci.,* **1977,** *74,* 1711–1715.

Winzelberg, G. G.; Strauss, H. W.; Bingham, J. B.; and McKusick, K. A. Scintigraphic evaluation of left ventricular aneurysm. *Am. J. Cardiol.,* **1980,** *46,* 1138–1143.

Witherspoon, L. R.; Shuler, S. E.; Garcia, M. M.; and Zollinger, L. A. Assessment of serum myoglobin as a marker for acute myocardial infarction. *J. Nucl. Med.,* **1979,** *20,* 115–119.

Yasmineh, W. G.; Pyle, R. B.; Cohn, J. N.; *et al.* Serial serum creatine phosphokinase MB isoenzyme activity after myocardial infarction. Studies in baboon and man. *Circulation,* **1977,** *55,* 733–738.

Yazaki, Y., and Nagai, R. Serial determinations of serum cardiac myosin light chain II; a new method for estimation of myocardial infarction size. *Circulation,* **1979,** *59, 60,* II-139.

Zaret, B. L.; DiCola, V. C.; Donabedian, R. K.; *et al.* Dual radionuclide study of myocardial infarction. Relationships between myocardial uptake of potassium-43, technetium-99m stannous pyrophosphate, regional myocardial blood flow and creatine phosphokinase depletion. *Circulation,* **1976,** *53,* 422–427.

Chapter 14

INSURANCE AND RISK EVALUATION IN CARDIOVASCULAR DISEASE

Donald W. Bowne

The insurance industry has a vital interest in heart disease because of its importance as a major contributor to death, disability, and health care costs in this nation. More than a third of all of the deaths among adults in this country are due to cardiovascular disease. Ischemic heart disease accounts for most of these. Heart disease not only produces fatal heart attacks, it also causes the greatest amount of permanent disability among workers under age 65 and is responsible for more days of hospitalization than any other single disease. Progress is being made in the prevention and treatment of heart disease, but not as rapidly as most would like. The number of deaths due to ischemic heart disease among the insured population of the United States has only decreased 1.2% in the past five years (U.S. Dept. Health, Education, Welfare, 1979b). A man at age 45 years today has a life expectancy only five years greater than in 1900. By contrast much greater progress has been made in the prevention and treatment of infectious diseases. As a result, the life expectancy for an infant at birth has increased 25 years since the beginning of this century. The number of people over 65 years of age is steadily increasing. This demographic change makes it more imperative that greater progress be made in combating the degenerative diseases.

" Every man desires to live long, but no man would be old." These words from Jonathan Swift's *Thoughts on Various Subjects* express the wish of each of us. Unfortunately this is a desire that cannot be realized. Some of us will live long. Others will grow old prematurely. Some will be even less fortunate and will be victims of the alternative, premature death. The ultimate mortality, however, will be one hundred per cent.

From birth to death we face the hazard of becoming disabled from sickness or injury. One out of six Americans will be hospitalized this year. Acute illness will cause an average of ten days of disability per person. Chronic illness will limit the activities of more than 14% of the population (Health Insurance Institute, 1980). That all will eventually die, and that a percentage of the population will be disabled, are certainties. The uncertainties are the times when these events will occur and who the unfortunate victims will be. Each of these hazards brings with it two great losses, personal losses and financial losses. This chapter will deal with the financial losses and how insurance is used to protect against such losses.

HISTORICAL BACKGROUND

A. H. Maslow (1954), a pioneer research social scientist, in constructing man's hierarchy of needs, has placed in first priority the satisfaction of his basic physiological needs, i.e., food, shelter, and warmth. As soon as these needs have been met, man attends to his second priority, the quest for security from external danger. As civilization developed, the dangers of attack by wild animals and hostile bands were replaced by new dangers. With the development of bartering, trade, and commerce, came the danger of financial loss and the need for financial security. In ancient times, Babylonian caravans and Phoenician ships were pledged as security for loans. In the fourteenth century, Italian merchants began to insure their ships and cargoes. Thus, property insurance came into being. In England the insurers were initially individuals who worked out of coffeehouses where merchants congregated. For a price, they were willing to assume a portion of the risk on a ship or cargo ready to sail. The individual insurer would write his name beneath the contract; thus, he became known as the "underwriter." Edward Lloyd was the owner of one of these coffeehouses in 1690. Shipowners came to Lloyd's to seek out "underwriters." From this meager beginning, Lloyd's of London evolved. Businessmen still come to Lloyd's today seeking out underwriters. Each individual underwriter is liable for paying losses on the risk that he underwrites. Lloyd's itself, does not write insurance.

In the agrarian society, the farm afforded security. The crops, livestock, and game provided food; the forest provided fuel, and the family unit provided for the elderly and sick. As civilization turned from a predominantly agrarian society to an industrial society, there was a migration from the country farms to the cities, and the new urban dweller had left the security of the farm behind. The barter system gave place to a monetary exchange system, and buying financial security became necessary. Life insurance was the product of urbanization and industrialization.

The earliest known life insurance policy was issued in England in 1583 (Brackenridge, 1977). Gradually individual underwriters were replaced by insurance companies. The first life insurance company in the United States was one now known as the Presbyterian Ministers' Fund which was founded in 1759. The industry has grown tremendously in the past century. In 1840, only $4,690,000 worth of life insurance was in force throughout the United States. In 1978, there was $2,870,000,000 in force. Two thirds of all the individuals in this nation own some form of life insurance.

THE NATURE AND PRINCIPLES OF INSURANCE

Definition of Insurance

Insurance is a contract whereby, for a stipulated consideration called the premium, one party (the insurer) agrees to pay the other party (the insured), or his beneficiary, a fixed sum upon the occurrence of death, disability, or some other specified event. In the life insurance contract, the event is death; in the health insurance contract, the event is disability; and in property insurance on your home, the event is fire, wind storm, flood, or theft.

On the surface, insurance might appear to be a form of gambling. For example, a man buys a new home and takes out fire insurance on the house. It might appear that he is betting with the insurance company that his house will burn down. Actually, insurance is the opposite of gambling. Gambling creates risks. Insurance helps to lessen and spread risks, and it is economically advantageous. The odds are highly in favor of his house not burning down. For a small premium charge, the insurance company guarantees, however, that if it does burn down, he will be indemnified for the loss. He joins with a large group of policyholders who have a similar risk to share the loss, should such a loss occur. This same principle is applicable to life and health insurance. It is important to note that you can only insure something that you have. You cannot insure your home against fire once it has started burning. Neither can you take out life insurance when death has occurred or is known to be near at hand, nor health insurance when you are already very ill.

The Nature of the Perils

Although all forms of insurance are alike in that they combine similar risks into groups in order that the costs may be equally shared, the nature of the risks or perils of the various types of insurance are quite different. The peril that your home will burn may never occur, but, relative to life insurance, the peril of death will certainly occur. Death is an uncertainty from year to year, but the probability of death increases each year until it becomes a certainty. It is necessary, therefore, in life insurance to protect the insured during his whole life by accumulating a reserve fund to meet the absolute certain death claim when it does occur.

The risk of disability does not follow as consistent a pattern as the risk of death. Some persons never become disabled. The risk of disability does increase, however, with age. In addition, the cost of health care has been increasing each year, necessitating constant premium adjustment to meet the increased costs of claims.

The Sharing of Losses

The sharing of losses is the function of insurance. The aim is to have the losses of the unfortunate few paid by the contributions of the many who are exposed to the same risk. This, then, is the insurance principle: the transfer of the risk to the insurance company by payment of a premium. The company functions as a mechanism of reimbursement for actual losses that occur within the group.

The Laws of Probability

We stated earlier that insurance was the opposite of gambling. The insurance principle involving large numbers converts an uncertainty into a certainty. The laws of probability upon which insurance is based, did, however, have their origin in gambling. During the seventeenth century, when gambling was a fashionable and popular sport, a gentleman gambler named Chevalier de Mere sought the advice of a famous French mathematician, Blaise Pascal, about various games of chance. It is interesting to note that Pascal laid the groundwork for the theory of probability. It remained for the physicist, Nicolas Bernoulli, to actually develop the theory in 1713. By utilizing the laws of probability, actuaries are able to measure the risk and calculate the premiums required to cover the shared losses of the insureds.

Certainty may be expressed by unity or one. The impossible event is represented by zero. The probability of an event happening is equal to the number of favorable chances divided by the total number of chances, provided that all chances are equally alike. Certainty, or one, equals the sum of all of the separate probabilities. The calculation of probability of events happening, when combined with the law of large numbers, becomes the basis for accurate predictions of mortality and morbidity by insurance companies. The law of large numbers tells us that as the number of trials increases, the variation from the law of probability decreases. It is for this reason that insurance companies must base their predictions of mortality on a very large number of lives to insure that the deviation from the expected mortality loss will be relatively small.

Forecasting Future Events

One can use the knowledge of what has happened to a group in the past to predict what will happen to a group in the future by the use of inductive reasoning, provided that the two groups qualify under similar sets of conditions. The death rate of a sufficiently large group can be used to predict the mortality of another large group under similar circumstances at another time. The accuracy of this prediction depends upon the size of the group and the accuracy of the statistics. To insure one life is a gamble. To insure 100 lives is less of a gamble. If the number of lives is increased to a half million, however, the fluctuation in mortality rate from year to year will vary only a fraction of 1 per cent. The larger the number of risks of like nature that are combined into one group, the

less uncertain will be the amount of loss that will be experienced in a given period. Insurance companies cannot predict what will happen to any specific individual, but they can predict with a great deal of accuracy what will happen within a large group of individuals. From this knowledge, the company can set a premium that will cover the losses incurred within the large insured group. Just as the insurance company cannot predict what will happen to any given individual, neither can the individual predict when he will die, or when he will be disabled. The prudent man lessens the risk of the attendant economic loss by transferring the risk to an insurance company through the purchase of an insurance policy.

LIFE INSURANCE

Mortality Tables and Rate Making

History. The earliest known compilations of death registration were the weekly bills of mortality posted by order of the Council of London as early as 1532. It is not surprising to find that the use of inductive reasoning to predict future events by using past happenings had its embryonic application in mortality studies shortly after Francis Bacon had formulated his new approach to scientific studies. In 1662, John Graunt, the son of a London draper, analyzed these records of posted mortality and published his findings in a book. In this publication he constructed a Table of Survivors which was a forerunner of future life tables. His efforts, though crude, were commendable because he had no special training for this task. This was a time, however, of brilliant analytical minds, the time of Wren, Boyle, and Descartes. Graunt's findings of the effect of age upon mortality made it possible for Edmund Halley, the English astronomer, to compile a series of mortality tables. These life tables were contained in an essay published in 1693, titled "An Estimate of the Degrees of Mortality of Mankind Drawn from Curious Tables of the Birth and Funerals at the City of Breslaw." Records of births and deaths had been regularly kept in this city in Silesia since 1584. Halley had calculated the probable expectancy of life at any given age and thus laid the basic foundation for scientific life insurance.

Mortality Tables. Mortality tables are compact models of mortality and survival experience describing rates of death and survival among a given collection of persons in a specific period of time. The business of life insurance is concerned with the probability of death. Estimating this probability is accomplished by analyzing past mortality experience. This requires observation of what happened to a large number of people for a specified length of time. The number of people who die during that period and the number who survive are recorded.

As a matter of convenience, the probability of death is usually measured over a period of one year. The term "mortality rate" is the probability that an individual will die within one year. The annual mortality rate of any group is determined by dividing the number of deaths during the year by the number of people alive at the beginning of the year in that specific group. For example, if, during the year, ten people died in a group originally numbering 1,000, the annual mortality rate for that year would be $10 \div 1,000$, or 0.01. A mortality rate of 0.01 means that in a group of 100 one person will die, or in a group of 1,000 ten people will die during the year. This is a gross oversimplification of mortality since many factors can affect the determination. Persons who enter or leave the group during the year must be counted as fractions. Age, sex, occupation, state of health, and many other factors also affect the probability of death.

Mortality tables based on census canvasses of the population and death certificate registration contain significant elements of error. Census data, collected by a multitude of different interviewers, are subject to many errors of inaccuracy, misclassification, and misunderstanding. Death certificate registers are often incomplete and inaccurate. Because of these errors, mortality tables based on population and death registration only approximate the true mortality. The mortality experience on insured lives has proved more accurate. It is for this reason that virtually all mortality tables used today by life insurance companies are based on the experience of insured lives. These tables, however, will show a lower mortality than the population as a whole. They are derived from a select group of people who have purchased life insurance. They are generally in a higher economic and social class, receive better medical care, and are in some state of reasonable health at entry to be eligible for acceptance.

A mortality table usually shows the mortality rate for each age. Each mortality rate represents the probability that a person at that exact age will die during the following year. Two additional columns are usually added to the table, the "number living" and "the number dying." Table 14-1 shows a small portion of the 1958 Commissioners Standard Ordinary Mortality Table for males.

Table 14-1. 1958 COMMISSIONERS STANDARD ORDINARY MORTALITY TABLE (MALE LIVES)

AGE	NUMBER LIVING AT BEGINNING OF DESIGNATED YEAR	NUMBER DYING DURING DESIGNATED YEAR	MORTALITY RATE PER 1,000
0	10,000,000	70,800	7.08
1	9,929,200	17,475	1.76
2	9,911,725	15,066	1.52
3	9,896,659	14,449	1.46
4	9,882,210	13,835	1.40
5	9,868,375	13,322	1.35
6	9,855,053	12,812	1.30
7	9,842,241	12,401	1.26
8	9,829,840	12,091	1.23
9	9,817,749	11,879	1.21
10	9,805,870	11,865	1.21

Methods of Rate Making. Insurance companies often use the 1958 Commissioners Standard Ordinary Mortality Table for determining how much money to keep in reserve for future payment of liabilities. They use tables based on their own most recent experience, however, to establish premium rates. Computation of rates depends upon many factors in addition to mortality rates. One of these is the manner in which the premium is to be paid. If the premium is paid in a single cash sum annually, semiannually, or at shorter intervals, the company has use of the premium dollars to produce investment income for varying lengths of time. These options determine, in part, the amount of overhead that will be generated by bookkeeping expenses. The age and sex of the insured, the acquisition costs, the benefits to be provided, the rate of interest received on company investments, and other company expenses, all figure into the computation of rates in addition to the mortality costs.

The Life Insurance Contract

Characteristics of the Contract. The life insurance contract must meet the same legal requirements as any other contract. (1) There must be an agreement based on an *offer* made by one of the parties, and an acceptance of that offer in the same terms without modification by the other party. (2) The parties to the contract must be *legally capable* of making a valid contract. (3) There must be a *valuable consideration.* (4) The *purpose* of the agreement must be lawful. In addition, as an insuring agreement, it becomes a contract of *utmost good faith* and as such is governed by legal principles that relate specifically to insurance contracts. Each party is entitled to rely upon the representations of the other, without attempt to deceive, misrepresent, or withhold material information.

Parties to the Contract. Everyone is presumed to be capable of making a valid contract. There are, however, certain classes of people who have limited contractual powers. These include insane persons, intoxicated persons, and minors. The contract with a minor is not void, but is voidable. The adult is bound by the contract, the minor ordinarily is not.

Mutual Assent. Every contract must have an offer and an acceptance. Traditionally, the life insurance application is the offer if the initial premium accompanies it. The company may issue a conditional receipt for the initial premium, conditional upon the applicant's insurability. The issuance of the policy as applied for, by the insurance company, becomes the acceptance. If the policy is issued other than as applied for, the company is considered to have rejected the original offer and to have made a counteroffer. The counteroffer must then be accepted by the applicant before a contract has been completed. The insurance becomes effective at the time of the medical examination, provided the applicant is found insurable.

If the initial premium does not accompany the application, and the company approves the application, issues the policy, and delivers it to the applicant while he is in good health, this becomes the offer. The acceptance comes with the payment of the first premium.

Valuable Consideration. The consideration is the price given or asked in exchange for a promise. The initial premium becomes adequate consideration for the promises made by the insurance company, and this puts the insurance into effect.

Purpose Must Be Lawful. For a contract to be valid, it must be for a legal purpose and not contrary to public policy. Each party to a life insurance contract is aware that the other party may receive far more in equivalent value under the contract than the other, depending on how long the insured lives. It is, therefore, called an aleatory agreement rather than a communative agreement where approximate worth is expected and received.

Insurable Interest. The requirement that there be an insurable interest is basic to the insurance contract and takes the agreement out of the gambling category. Certain insurable interest requirements must be met to make the contract valid. The insurable interest arises from the relationship of the party taking out the insurance and the insured. There must be an expectation of advantage or benefit from the continuance of life in the insured, as opposed to an advantage in his death. The advantage may arise from one of natural affection or be purely a monetary one from a business relationship. The interest may arise from affection through blood relationship or marriage, on the one hand, or from being a creditor, or as surety for the insured. In the absence of insurable interest, the policy contract is unenforceable.

Concealment, Misrepresentation, and Fraud. Insurance is a contract of highest faith and the rule of *caveat emptor* (let the buyer beware) does not apply. The insurer is entitled to rely upon information submitted to him and expects full disclosure of all facts material to a consideration of the risk. Statements made by the applicant are considered representations and not warranties. The company cannot technically void the contract because of misstatements unless they are material to the risk or were made with fraudulent intent. The application and medical history forms are designed to provide full disclosure. These documents become a permanent part of the contract, and their execution by the agent and the examining physician, therefore, should be done with all due care. Concealment of material facts is ground for recision of the contract. The claim may be denied if the declarations were fraudulent or made with the intent to deceive. A sympathetic agent or physician who fails to record a significant history or impairment really does the applicant a great disfavor. If death were to occur within the contestable period, in all likelihood, a thorough investigation of the claim would be made. If it were found that material information had been withheld, the claim would be denied, and the beneficiaries would not receive the

financial security originally planned. A policy may be reformed to carry out the intention of the parties to the contract, if a mutual error has been made. The incontestable clause does not prevent reformation. In some cases, fraud can vitiate a contract even after the contestable period has elapsed.

It has been estimated that losses due to fraud cost the entire insurance industry in the United States currently over four billion dollars annually. This continues to grow each year. In 1974, the National Chamber of Commerce estimated the loss to be one half the present amount. The indirect costs are probably five times the direct costs and are paid for by the public through increased taxes for police, firemen, and other social services. Arson is a prime example of fraud in the property and casualty insurance field. In life insurance, fraud may vary from nondisclosure of material information to murder made to look like an accident. Insurance fraud traditionally has been easy to commit, time consuming to prove, difficult to prosecute, and punishable by light sentences.

Standard Provisions of the Contract. INCONTESTABLE CLAUSE. This clause was introduced into the contract to provide greater assurance to the public that they would not have relatively unimportant misstatements used at a later date to deny liability. The interpretation has been liberalized by the courts far beyond the original intention. It now often prevents an insurance company from voiding a life insurance contract even on grounds of material misrepresentation or fraud after the contestable period, which is usually two years.

OTHER CLAUSES. The grace period usually provides for thirty days of grace after the premium is due before the policy is considered lapsed. A reinstatement provision usually allows a policyholder who has allowed his policy to lapse by nonpayment of premium to reinstate it within a three-year period. He must, however, furnish evidence of insurability satisfactory to the company. Other standard provisions deal with cash value and policy loans.

Special Provisions of the Contract. SUICIDE CLAUSE. The typical suicide clause provides that if, within two years of the date of issue of the policy, and while the policy is still in force, the insured, whether sane or insane, shall die by his own hand or act, the company will be liable only for the amount of the premiums paid. This amount will be paid in one sum to the beneficiary.

AVIATION EXCLUSION. Coverage in case of death from aviation, except as a passenger on a scheduled airline, is usually excluded in all double-indemnity provisions. At present, most companies accept within their standard classifications all commercial airline passengers.

WAR EXCLUSION. War clauses are used to control adverse selection against the company by those going into military service in time of war. The clauses provide for a return of premiums with interest in the event that death occurs under conditions excluded by the clause.

DOUBLE INDEMNITY. This clause or rider provides that double the face amount of the insurance policy is payable if the death of the insured is caused by accidental means. Deaths due to natural causes are sometimes claimed to be accidental, and this leads to litigation.

Risk Selection

Purpose of Selection. If every person in the country were to be issued the same amount of life insurance, under the same plan, and if one could be certain that all policies would remain in force, there would be much less need for selection. This, however, is not the case. Some applicants are young, some are old, some healthy, some near death, some will purchase a small amount of insurance, others a large amount, some will buy term insurance, others will purchase an endowment. As soon as an individual is given a choice, antiselection against the interest of the company will occur. The healthy will be less anxious to buy insurance; while those near death will rush at the opportunity. In addition, they will buy larger amounts at the lowest possible premium. This would result in the healthy paying excessive premiums to cover the losses of the unwell. Insurance strives for equity. It is for this reason that the company must determine the risk of each applicant in order that he may be classified into groups that can be assessed a fair premium charge. Groups with expected higher mortality rates pay a higher premium.

Factors Affecting Risk. AGE. The probability of death increases as a person grows older; degenerative diseases are more likely to appear as age increases. For this reason, insurers tend to exercise greater precaution in underwriting older age groups. Medical examinations, electrocardiograms, and chest x-rays are more frequently required, if the amount of insurance applied for justifies the added expense. Most companies will not insure persons over 70 years of age.

SEX. Mortality rates for women are now lower at all ages than for men. Most companies reflect this difference by charging women lower premiums or paying higher dividends, which is really a return of premium.

BUILD. This includes the applicant's height, weight, and distribution of the weight. Overweight, even in a moderate degree, brings with it extra mortality with the highest mortality experienced in the middle and older age groups. Underweight is not considered as significant today as it was a generation ago when tuberculosis was common. However, it does alert the underwriter to look for chronic disease or other impairment of health.

PHYSICAL CONDITION. The probability that the company will require an examination by a physician increases as the age of the applicant and the amount at risk increase. Special emphasis is placed on blood pressure, build, heart findings, and urinalysis. The company is more likely to be satisfied with a para-medical screening examination, or a medical history alone, for the younger applicant and for the lower amounts at risk. The paramedical examination develops the medical history; measures height, weight, pulse rate, blood pressure; and includes a urinalysis.

PERSONAL HISTORY. The health record is usually the most important of the personal history factors. The underwriter looks for significant history of illness or injury in the past that might adversely affect future life expectancy. Medical statements usually are obtained from attending physicians and hospitals to fully investigate past history.

FAMILY HISTORY. If the history shows that mother, father, and siblings have not died prematurely, and the parents lived beyond age 60, credits against other impairments may be given. A history of several members in the family with diabetes mellitus, coronary artery disease, or cancer may be cause for assessing an increased mortality ratio. Certain serious illnesses with dominant inheritance may be a cause for rejection.

OCCUPATION. The type of work that an applicant does may affect the risk. The increased peril may be from accident or health conditions related to environmental hazards. Steeplejacks, bartenders, and asbestos workers are examples of individuals with hazardous employment.

HABITS. The underwriter is particularly concerned about the applicant's use of alcohol or drugs. Those who drink socially in moderation are considered at no appreciable increase in risk. If alcohol is consumed in large amounts, the applicant may be rejected or offered insurance at substandard rates, depending on the degree of abuse. Drug addicts are not insurable. A history of drug and alcohol abuse in the past requires careful underwriting to determine whether permanent damage has occurred and what the probability of relapse may be.

MORAL HAZARDS. Moral codes change with each generation. Insurance companies today are less concerned about sexual morality than they were in the past. If the relationship between two persons appears to be a stable one with a low risk for violent acts, an insurable interest would be recognized. The applicant's reputation in personal activities and in meeting business obligations has a bearing on the moral risk involved. The risk of a gangster or thief dying prematurely is so great that he would be considered uninsurable.

AVIATION. The safety of air travel improves each year. Travel as a passenger on a commercial airline is considered as not increasing the mortality risk. Private pilots with good safety records, who are mature, experienced, and fly more than 150 hours per year, generally qualify as standard risks.

HOBBIES AND AVOCATIONS. Increased leisure time and a rising standard of living have made hobbies and avocations important considerations in underwriting of life and health insurance risks. Hang gliding, sky diving, mountain climbing, scuba diving, auto and motorcycle racing, all involve a significant hazard that must be considered in underwriting risks for life insurance.

Information Sources

The Application. This primary source of information is usually completed by the insurance agent. It contains personal information about the applicant such as age, sex, marital status, past and present occupations, home and business addresses, amount and kind of insurance applied for, other insurance in force, and designated beneficiaries.

Medical Examination. The medical examination consists of two parts. Part I is the medical history furnished by the applicant in response to specific questions asked by the medical examiner. The questions relate to past and present medical history, family history, and a systemic review. Specific emphasis is placed on recent medical history. The names and addresses of all physicians seen within the last five years are requested, along with reasons for the consultations. A question about habituating drugs and treatment for alcoholism is also included. The applicant signs at the bottom of the declarations attesting to the truthfulness of the statements and gives authorization to the company to obtain additional information from attending physicians and hospitals if necessary. The medical examiner dates and signs the declarations as a witness. This document becomes a permanent and integral part of the insurance contract.

Part II consists of the physical examination. Here, the examiner records measured height and weight; blood pressure; pulse rate; and the results of his examination of the heart, lungs, abdomen, skin, extremities, and the nervous system. A check of the urine for albumin and sugar is also included. The examiner should record exact blood pressure and pulse readings and should not round off these figures.

Additional studies such as electrocardiogram, chest x-ray, blood screening tests, and a home office urine specimen may be requested if the age of the applicant, and the amount of insurance at risk, warrant the expenditures. Other ancillary tests may be required at a later date, if a suspicious history requires clarification. These age and amount rules are determined on an actuarial basis. The test in a certain age group must pick up additional impairments that would otherwise go unrecognized. In addition, the generated savings in mortality costs resulting from the test must exceed the cost of obtaining the test in all individuals in that group. If these criteria are met, then that test will be a requirement since it is cost effective. Frequent reevaluation of age and amount rules are required in this time of rapidly escalating medical costs. Insurance companies have found it necessary to accept ever larger amounts of life insurance risks on a nonmedical basis, or only with a paramedical screening examination.

In recording the history and performing the physical examination, the physician becomes legally a special agent of the insurance company, with limited authority to act for the company. Even though the examining physician's authority is narrowly restricted within this special area, he has the power to bind the company by his acts and his knowledge concerning the most important factor in insurability, the physical condition of the applicant. Knowledge of the medical examiner about prior illnesses and impairments of the applicant, which are not disclosed on the application, is often imputed to the company and may effectively prevent the company, by estoppel, from asserting an otherwise valid defense based on misrepresentation of material facts. It is for this reason that insurance companies must place great reliance on the integrity and thoroughness of the medical examiner. The physician has the legal responsibility to ask all of the questions on the application form and record all pertinent facts, as well as convey any knowledge he has about the health of the applicant. Additional information that might be contradictory to the applicant's declarations can be recorded on Part II of the medical examination. This portion does not become part of the contract, thus it is not seen by the applicant. In this way confidentiality can be preserved. If an attending physician completes an insurance medical examination on one of his own patients, he becomes a special agent for the insurance company. If he knows that the patient/applicant has a significant illness, but fails to reveal this information, he places the company at great risk. The company, on discovery of this fact, could conceivably seek recourse from the physician for this omission. If all physicians were aware of this agency responsibility, more complete and careful examinations would be performed.

Inspection Reports. The medical examination is not all inclusive, nor is it a foolproof safeguard against adverse selection. The applicant may not disclose significant health history either deliberately or unintentionally. Additional investigation is required for the larger amount policies. Inspection agencies and credit bureaus are called upon for supplementary information about health, finances, business reputation, habits, and motor vehicle violations. The larger the amount of insurance at risk, the more thorough will be the inspection.

Intercompany Data. Insurance companies require as many relevant facts as possible to make a fair and equitable underwriting decision. Their position of trust requires that other policyholders who share the risk be protected from dishonesty and fraud. One means of assuring this is an exchange of intercompany data. Codes for medical findings, both favorable and unfavorable, are reported to a central collecting agency. When an application for insurance is received, participating companies may obtain these codes to serve as an alert to possible important impairments. Each applicant is informed that disclosure will be made to, and information received from, such a data center.

Classification of the Risk. Mention has been made of the insurance philosophy which seeks equity among policyholders sharing risks. From this arose the need to further classify applicants of the same age into groups who would generate approximately the same mortality experience. Per cent increase in mortality is used for this classification. Those who fall within the group not expected to experience an added mortality ratio greater than 25% are considered standard risks. Those with an expected added mortality ratio greater than 25% are considered substandard. The substandard risks are further classified into classes or tables representing increasing degrees of expected mortality. The additional assessment is added to the 100% mortality that all of us will eventually experience and is called the expected mortality ratio.

Some insurance companies will only insure standard or slightly substandard risks; others may accept applicants with mortality ratios up to 500%; and a few will even accept risks with ratios over 500%. Some companies specialize in substandard risks. Smaller companies often limit the amount of risk that they will assume, placing the excess amount with a reinsurance company. A 200% mortality ratio is less ominous than it sounds. It means that if, at age 50 years, 8 persons are normally expected to die during the year out of 1,000 standard lives at the beginning of the year, 16 deaths could be expected. A 300% mortality ratio would mean there would be 24 expected deaths.

Those persons expected to generate a mortality experience higher than that acceptable to the company or the reinsurer are rejected. Those falling within the group expected to have a better than standard expectancy may be offered life insurance as a preferred risk with lower premium rates. In order to qualify for preferred rates, the applicant will have to show evidence of exceptionally good health. Some companies require the applicant to be a nonsmoker.

The standard group classification is broad enough to include approximately 91% of the applicants for ordinary life insurance. About 3% of applicants are rejected as uninsurable risks, and the remaining 6% are offered coverage at substandard rates. Of those who are considered substandard, 20% are by reason of their occupation or other hazards, and 80% are for medical reasons. Cardiovascular-renal disease accounts for 31% of the medical ratings, with obesity accounting for 19% *(1979 Life Insurance Fact Book).*

Originally, insurance companies had to rely almost entirely on judgment as a method of classifying and rating applicants for insurance. Gradually, as experience developed, quantitative evaluation of specific hazards and impairments was possible. Initially companies relied only on their own mortality statistics. Then companies began to pool their respective studies. From this has come, for example, the recent updating of the 1959 *Build and Blood Pressure Study* (Society of Actuaries). Recently, the *Combined Study on Atrial Fibrillation* (Gajewski, 1981) was completed. Tens of thousands to millions of lives entered into these studies.

New developments in medical treatment, with changing mortality in specific diseases, require constant re-evaluation of various impairments. Compa-

nies supplement their own actuarial experience with published clinical studies, if they are based on sound scientific methods. In this way, much progress has been made in insuring ever-increasing numbers of persons. In the final analysis, all data must be interpreted in the light of experience and judgment.

Risk Selection in Cardiovascular Disease

Different Perspectives of Clinical and Insurance Medicine. A private physician may tell a patient that he is in excellent health only to find out that on application for life insurance, the person is considered a substandard risk. This is due to the difference in the nature of clinical and insurance medicine. Clinicians talk in terms of survival rates, while life actuaries are more apt to talk in terms of mortality rates. They may be looking at the same problem but from different points of view. The clinician is dealing with one individual. The insurance company is evaluating a large group. If the diagnosis is obscure, the clinician can often await further developments and defer his final clinical opinion. The insurance company, however, must make its decision at the moment, either to accept or reject. If future events show the company to have been too conservative and to have overestimated the risk, the applicant can apply for a reduction in, or removal of, the rating with a resultant decrease in premium. The reverse, however, is not possible. Once the company has made its decision, even though the risk may have been underestimated, it must live with its decision and cannot terminate the insurance or increase the premium.

Occasionally misunderstandings arise from slightly elevated blood pressure, systolic murmurs, and rapid pulse rates. The clinician may conclude that these slight impairments are not significant to his patient's health. The insurance statistics, however, show that if a large group of persons with only slight elevation of blood pressure is followed over the years, some of these will progress into significant hypertension, and the group as a whole will experience a higher mortality. The company has to deal with the future, and since it is not able to pinpoint who among the group will show progressive disease, it must assess a slightly higher premium for all within the group to cover the increased mortality costs. The same holds true for systolic heart murmurs of low intensity and for mild tachycardias. If the attending physician has additional evidence which proves, for example, that the systolic murmur is functional, the company will welcome an appeal of its decision.

Cardiovascular Disease

Heart disease is the leading cause of death and disability in the United States and accounts for 35% of deaths due to all causes. Ischemic heart disease, or coronary artery disease, causes nearly 90% of the cardiovascular deaths; of these myocardial infarctions claim 650,000 deaths each year. About 25,000 babies are born in this country annually with congenital heart lesions. Thus, cardiovascular disease is of great importance to insurance companies as well as to the clinician and the nation.

Death rates from heart disease increased rapidly after 1940, but then began to level off in the early 1960s. Between 1962 and 1967, the decrease in mortality in white males was 2.7%, and in white females 6.8%. Between 1969 and 1973, the rate of decrease became even greater, with the decrease in mortality in white males at 4.9%, and white females 8.8%. In 1973, the overall death rate from heart disease was lowest in white males 20 to 24 years of age (3.7 per 100,000), and highest among males 75 years and over (5,503.9 per 100,000). Women in these respective age groups showed rates of 2.0 and 4,146.3 per 100,000 (Singer and Levinson, 1976). Between 1968 and 1977, the death rate from heart disease declined by about 22%.

The mortality from cardiovascular disease in the United States in the black population is much higher than among the white. This results, in part, from the high prevalence of hypertension and hypertensive heart disease in the nonwhites. In 1977, nonwhite males between the ages of 35 and 74 years experienced 25% more deaths from cardiovascular disease than did their white counterparts. Black females had almost twice the rate of white females.

The Eighth Revision of the *International Classification of Diseases* in 1968 (U.S.D. H.E.W., 1978) changed classification and coding and, as a result, caused a significant break in the continuity of mortality statistics for certain categories of heart disease, especially hypertensive and to a lesser extent rheumatic and ischemic heart disease. These changes offset one another so that this revision seems not to have produced a significant break in the overall mortality of all heart disease. This welcomed decline in heart disease mortality promises to continue into the future. Factors contributing to the decline are increased detection

and more effective treatment of hypertension, decreased dietary consumption of saturated fats, improved medical care, and health education directed toward a healthier life-style to include smoking cessation, regular vigorous exercise, and a prudent optimal caloric diet.

Hypertension. An abnormally elevated blood pressure is estimated to be present in 23 million Americans. One out of every seven adults suffers from hypertension. It is the most important contributor to cerebrovascular accidents which annually account for about 200,000 deaths and disable another 250,000 persons under age 65 years. Hypertension is also an important contributor to the more than 1,250,000 heart attacks which cause in excess of 650,000 deaths in this country each year. The prevalence of hypertension and its profound effect on mortality and morbidity make it a concern of high priority to the life underwriter. Even mild elevations of systolic and diastolic pressures are accompanied by a significant rise in mortality ratio, even though such an elevation might not be considered important to the clinician.

The definition of elevated blood pressure as proposed by the New York Heart Association has wide acceptance. Any blood pressure up to and including 139/89 is regarded as *normotensive.* Any systolic pressure of 160 or over, or any diastolic pressure of 95 or over, will be classified as *definitely hypertensive.* Readings between the limits of normotensive and definitely hypertensive will be considered *borderline hypertensive* (New York Heart Association, 1955).

The 1960–1962 National Health Survey on a sample United States population, age 18 to 79 years, numbering 6,672 persons, both male and female, showed the prevalence of normotensives to be 70%, borderline hypertensives to be 15%, and definite hypertensives also 15%. The prevalence of systolic hypertension increased markedly with age up to at least 75 years in males and 65 years in females. The prevalence of diastolic hypertension, however, leveled off or decreased at about 45 years of age in males, and 55 years in females. Under the age of 35 years, the prevalence of borderline hypertension is much higher in males than females, but this differential disappears at older ages. The prevalence of definite hypertension is less in females than males under age 55 years, but the reverse is true at age 55 years and up (U.S. Department of Health, Education, and Welfare, 1964).

It is estimated that there are 23 million definite hypertensives in this country today. The number with borderline hypertension exceeds 20 million. Stamler (1973), in a study of high blood pressure in the United States, estimated that only one half of all hypertensives are aware of their problem. For this reason, it has been called the "silent disease." Of the one half who are aware of their disease, only one half come under treatment. Thus, there is great need for widespread screening for hypertension, along with programs to educate the public and physicians of the dangers of this disease and the need for effective early treatment.

The prevalence of hypertension among blacks is substantially higher than among whites in every age group. The proportion of black men, aged 45 to 64 years, with definitely elevated systolic and diastolic blood pressure appears to be twice that among white men. In black women, aged 45 to 54, the proportion with elevated blood pressure is two and one half times that of white women. However, at ages 55 to 64, black women with hypertension number only one third higher than white women at that age. This difference does not appear to be related to any difference in socioeconomic status. It may be due to a genetic factor.

By far the largest body of data relating to mortality in hypertensives is that developed in the *Build and Blood Pressure Study 1959*. This endeavor combined the experience of 26 large insurance companies on some 4,000,000 policies issued between 1935 and 1953. Included in this group were 200,000 persons with mild to moderate hypertension ranging from 140 to 170 mm Hg systolic, and 90 to 115 mm Hg diastolic. From this study came some significant findings: (1) The mortality was lowest among the group with a systolic pressure of 98 to 127, and diastolic pressure of 48 to 67. (2) Even relatively small increases above average blood pressure represent substantial departure from optimal blood pressure and are associated with an increase in mortality. (3) Progressive elevation in blood pressure is accompanied by a progressive increase in mortality.

Other findings were that the prevalence and incidence of hypertension are highly correlated with overweight. Weight control should be considered an integral part of blood pressure control. Cardiac enlargement and left ventricular hypertrophy and strain as shown by the electrocardiogram are adverse prognostic indicators.

Prior to the late 1950s, treatment of hypertension was not very effective. With the continued progress in the development of the antihypertensive drugs, there has been a steady decrease in mortality from hypertension. It has been estimated that there has been a reduction of at least 30% in the mortality of "benign" hypertension, with an increasingly greater reduction in severe hypertension. A large life insurance study on policies issued from 1960–1971, which were rated for hypertension, found that the mortality in those persons under treatment was 127%, compared to 183% for those without a history of treatment. Untreated malignant hypertension has a first-year mortality ratio in the range of 900 to 1,000%, with a low survival rate of 0.05. When treated, the survival rate rose to 0.36 (Pilgrim, 1974). Many companies disregard elevated readings that were not recorded in the last five years. Such an underwriting practice indicates that if the blood pressure of the hypertensive is controlled at normal levels by treatment for five years, the mortality experience will be the same as for normotensive persons. Mortality studies indicate that treatment should be given early, even for those with borderline hypertension. Those persons in this borderline group may respond to weight reduction, sodium restriction, exercise, and relaxation therapy, without having to resort to chemotherapeutic agents.

The National High Blood Pressure Program was initiated in 1973 (National Conference on High Blood Pressure Education, 1973) to alert the public to the high frequency and significance of blood pressure elevation. The age-adjusted death rate from all cardiovascular disease has declined about 15% since that time. Stroke mortality fell by 25% between 1972 and 1976. Awareness, discovery, education, and more effective treatment of hypertension have all played a part in this improvement.

Smoking History. Personal habits play a critical role in the development of many serious diseases. Cigarette smoking is clearly the largest single preventable cause of illness and premature death in this nation today. Since the Surgeon General's first warning in 1964 (Report of the Advisory Committee), 34,000,000 men and women have been wise enough to stop smoking. A larger group of 54,000,000, however, continue this self-destructive habit. Those who choose to smoke join a club that has an increased mortality ratio of at least 70%. An excellent recent insurance study suggests that this increased ratio is close to 85% (Cowelland Hirst, 1980). Tobacco is associated with 346,000 premature deaths a year. A person 30 years of age, who smokes two packs a day, shortens his life-span by eight or nine years. Of the 650,000 deaths due to coronary artery disease each year, 25% are attributed to smoking-related illnesses. The incidence of myocardial infarction is about three and one half times greater in smokers than in nonsmokers. The chance of a heart attack being fatal is 21 times greater in a smoker.

Many insurance companies are still hesitant to assess the increased mortality to the cigarette smoker that is warranted. Instead, they have granted credits to nonsmokers. The amount of credit has gradually increased and is presently about 40%, which is still underevaluated. Some companies will not issue preferred insurance to cigarette smokers. Smoking cessation is an investment in a healthier and significantly longer life.

Serum Cholesterol and Triglycerides. The level of serum cholesterol has been tied to the pathogenesis of coronary atherosclerosis by the correlation between the level of blood cholesterol and the incidence of coronary heart disease. Studies have frequently shown that the higher the level of cholesterol, the higher the subsequent attack rate of ischemic heart disease. The Framingham Study showed that the risk of coronary artery disease in young men was six times greater in those who had a serum cholesterol level of more than 260 mg % than in those with a level less than 220 mg %. Between the ages of 50 to 59 years, the difference was threefold. The comparative ten-year experience for men in the National Cooperative Pooling Project showed no increase in the cumulative mortality when the serum cholesterol level was under 250 mg %. The group with a level of 250 mg % or above did show an excess mortality with a ratio of 124 to 140%.

If the phenotype is type I or V, any elevation of the lipids is usually disregarded by the life underwriter. In phenotypes II, III, and IV, if known, or in cases where the phenotype is not known, an increased mortality ratio is assessed, depending upon the age of the applicant and the level of the elevation. For example, ten debits are assessed for those under 29 years of age if their level exceeds 225 mg %. At age 50 years and up, the level would have to exceed 325 mg % to generate a debit. Levels in excess of 500 mg % require an extra mortality ratio of 80% for all ages.

Elevated serum triglycerides, present in the fasting state, also are associated with an increased incidence of premature atherosclerosis, and some studies have shown even a greater correlation than the cholesterol level. Values in excess of 250 mg % warrant an assessment of an extra mortality ratio of about 55% to age 29 years and 20% at age 50 years. Levels in excess of 750 mg % are considered at 125 to 55% extra mortality, depending on the age of the applicant.

Suspicious Chest Pain. The evaluation of chest pain is difficult and requires a great deal of judgment. The underwriter is primarily concerned about chest pain that might be a manifestation of coronary artery disease. Insurance companies would like to have a complete and exact diagnosis on every applicant for insurance. This, however, is neither practical nor possible. It is often necessary to make an evaluation of a history of chest pain without the benefit of an extensive diagnostic investigation. The amount of insurance at risk may not warrant the expenditure of large sums of money for additional information and tests. The company does not wish to inconvenience its clients with added procedures, nor does it wish to assume liability for any adverse reactions that might arise from invasive techniques. Considerable weight, therefore, must be given to the attending physician's opinion. However, the description of the pain as given by the applicant and the examining physician must also be evaluated. The rating applied must be based on an index of suspicion. When the individual is a male over 40 years of age, and where serial electrocardiograms were taken during a relatively long period of hospital stay, the index of suspicion becomes higher. The evaluation assigned, therefore, may vary from a standard risk to one close to angina pectoris.

Angina Pectoris. Just as the greater recognition and improved treatment have reduced the mortality and liberalized the underwriting of hypertension, so too has there been an equally dramatic change in the underwriting of coronary artery disease in the past decade. In 1945, some companies would not knowingly insure persons with coronary artery disease. Only a few years ago, it was not unusual to assess an extra mortality ratio of 150% to 250% for suspicious chest pain. If a diagnosis of definite angina pectoris were established, a temporary extra premium of $5.00 to $7.50 per $1,000 of insurance would be added each year for the first five years of the policy. Today, angina pectoris diagnosed by classical symptoms is assessed only an extra mortality ratio of 100%. If the diagnosis has been confirmed by a positive exercise test or a coronary angiogram, this will be increased to 125% with a small temporary extra of $2.50 per $1,000 until age 40 years. After this age is reached, no temporary extra is required. The purpose of the temporary extra is to collect the additional premium on the front end in those diseases where the first five-year mortality is high. These recent changes reflect the improved mortality experience in angina at all ages, but especially after age 40 years.

Although angina pectoris can be associated with other diseases such as luetic coronary ostial disease, periarteritis, congenital anomalies of the coronary arteries, and aortic valve disease, coronary atherosclerosis is by far the principal cause of this entity. Most studies that have evaluated the mortality experience associated with coronary artery disease other than myocardial infarction have shown the mortality for angina pectoris to be slightly less than that resulting from myocardial infarction. The trends by age and duration are not as clearly defined however. Stable angina carries a better prognosis than does unstable angina. Patients who have angina pectoris as a new complaint will succumb at an average rate of 4% per year. Associated hypertension increases the mortality significantly. In one life insurance study, the mortality was four times greater in angina pectoris with hypertension than it was in those with normotension. The Framingham Study, at the end of nine years, showed the cumulative survival ratios for males and females in the angina pectoris group to be 86 and 89.2%, respectively. In the myocardial infarction group, they were only 37.8 and 58.9%.

Myocardial Infarction. Heart attacks claim about 650,000 deaths each year in the United States. They are the ultimate expression of the coronary atherosclerotic process and are caused, in most cases, by coronary thrombosis. Myocardial infarctions account for about 90% of all heart disease deaths and 35% of deaths due to all causes. Ischemic heart disease takes its greatest toll during the most productive years of life when there is the greatest family responsibility. Between the ages of 35 and 64 years, it accounts for nearly 88% of the deaths from heart disease.

The incidence of coronary artery disease is much more common among males than fe-males. Under age 45 years, ten times more males than females are afflicted. The sex preference for males falls off rapidly between 45 and 60 years, during which period males have twice as many heart attacks as females. In the very elderly, the incidence is about the same. Mortality is related to the extent of coronary artery disease, as shown on angiography, and the degree of impairment of left ventricular function. A single significant lesion in the descending coronary artery carries with it a probability of 90% five-year survival. Significant three-vessel disease, on the other hand, has only a 50% probability of five-year survival. When the myocardium is so impaired in its function, as the result of a myocardial infarction, that congestive heart failure results, there is a 25 to 33% probability that the patient will die within one year (Singer and Levinson, 1976).

Of the 650,000 deaths from heart attacks in this country per year, 350,000 of these deaths occur within the first hour, often before the patient reaches the hospital. This mortality can only be decreased by early monitoring, with adequate and effective treatment of arrhythmias, bradycardia, and shock. There is some evidence that suppression of ectopy does reduce the very early mortality. The greatest incidence of death in the first 24 hours occurs in males in their 20s. It then tends to decrease with age through the 40s and then increases again with age. The highest mortality is in the 55- to 64-year age group. After the first 24 hours, the mortality tapers off. Myocardial infarction survival after the first year is similar to that of angina pectoris. The risk of death in the first year is 8 to 13% and falls thereafter to an average of 4% per year.

Factors that add to the mortality from myocardial infarction are hypertension, history of angina pectoris of more than one month's duration, shock, congestive heart failure, and conduction defects. It is estimated that about 50% of those who suffer a heart attack have one or more of the three most important risk factors: elevated blood pressure, continued history of cigarette smoking, and an elevated serum cholesterol.

An international comparison (Brackenridge, 1977) of age-adjusted death rates from coronary artery disease in the United States, Canada, and Western European countries shows males in each of these countries to have a mortality of from 2.6 to 3.5 times greater than that in the female population. Males in Finland and the United States have the highest rates, with the lowest mortality in males occurring in the Southern European countries.

Most insurance companies will consider applicants who have had a myocardial infarction only after they have returned to their normal activities and are back to work. This eliminates the group with the very early high mortality as well as those left with severe impairments. Ratings are based on the age at the time of application for insurance and the seriousness of the disease as indicated by the findings after recovery.

For underwriting purposes, applicants who have had a myocardial infarction can be classified into three groups of expected increasing mortality. The group expected to generate the lowest mortality have the following characteristics: (1) a history of only one infarction, (2) resumed normal duties within three months of the attack, (3) no subsequent anginal pain, (4) normal or stable electrocardiograms in the postinfarction period, (5) taking no medication for the heart disease except prophylactically, and (6) no other cardiovascular-renal impairments. This group is assessed a permanent rating appropriate for an added expected mortality ratio of 125%, plus a temporary extra of $5.00 per $1,000 until the age of 40 years, when this temporary extra is reduced to $2.50 per $1,000 until age 50 years, at which time the temporary extra will no longer be required. These ratings reflect the improved survival expected in those over 40 and 50 years of age. It is possible for a person over 50 years in this category, with a good family history, and who does not smoke cigarettes, to be offered life insurance at only a slight substandard premium.

The second group with a higher expected mortality would have the following characteristics: (1) a history of one or more infarctions, (2) resumed normal activities within six months after the attack, (3) may have an occasional nondisabling episode of anginal pain, (4) show electrocardiographic residual of the infarction with only moderate deterioration, (5) taking no medication for heart disease except prophylactically, and (6) may have some expected increase in mortality from other cardiovascular-renal impairment. This category would be assigned an expected increased mortality ratio of 225%, with a $10.00 temporary extra per $1,000 until age 40 years, and then $5.00 temporary extra to age 50 years.

The third and highest acceptable risk category would have the same characteristics as the second group, with the exception that the applicant may have (1) fairly frequent episodes of anginal pain, and (2) more extreme electrocardiographic changes. This group would be assessed an expected increased mortality ratio of 325%, with the temporary extras increased to $15.00 per $1,000 to age 40 years and then $7.50 per $1,000 to age 50 years.

Coronary Artery Bypass Surgery. The past two decades have seen spectacular advances in the operative approach toward correcting congenital and acquired lesions of the heart. Ischemic heart disease has shared these advances. Coronary artery bypass surgery has become one of the most common procedures performed by cardiac surgeons. Pioneer efforts in this type of arterial surgery began in the early 1960s. Recent surveys have shown that more than 100,000 bypass operations were performed in this country in 1979, and it is estimated that 125,000 were done in 1980.

Early mortality after surgery has been decreasing from year to year. In the Texas Heart Institute Study (Hall, 1973) of 1,105 patients who underwent coronary artery bypass surgery alone or with endarterectomy, the early mortality fell to 3.2% in 1972. A group of 1,000 patients at the Cleveland Clinic (Sheldon, 1973) experienced an early mortality of 1.2% in 1971. The University of Oregon Study (Anderson, 1974) showed a survival ratio of 96.4% at four years. Excess mortality was the greatest in the first year with a mortality ratio of 240%, with 14 extra deaths per 1,000 per year. Over the next three years, the mortality was only slightly above the expected level with a mortality ratio of 125%. The overall mortality for four years was 124% for single-vessel disease, 158% for two-vessel disease, and 215% for three-vessel disease. These results must be interpreted with caution because of the small number of deaths (17) in the series.

Most studies indicate that the quality of life can be improved by the operation because of relief of chest pain and increased ability to work. There is also growing evidence that improved mortality can be expected in the early postoperative years. Individuals with good left ventricular function have the better prognosis. Time and more randomized studies are needed to establish the long-term prognosis of the operation.

Initially, insurance companies required that one year elapse between the date of surgery and the consideration for life insurance. This time period has gradually shortened until now, when many companies will consider the person for life insurance when complete recovery from the operation has occurred, and the patient has returned to normal activities. Some companies are now willing to offer policies at an extra mortality ratio of 100% plus a temporary extra of $2.50 per $1,000 to age 40 years, provided that there is no residual anginal pain.

Electrocardiography. The electrocardiogram is almost as important in the selection of risks for life insurance as is the sphygmomanometer. The incidence of heart disease increases with age, and the electrocardiogram provides an additional aid in detecting unknown or undeclared myocardial disease. This is especially true in males past 40 and females past 55 years of age. For this reason, the larger the amount at risk, and the older the applicant, the more likely it is that this test will be required.

T-WAVE CHANGES. The most common nonspecific electrocardiographic abnormalities found are those affecting the T waves. T waves that are flat or disproportionately low in amplitude in relation to that of the QRS complex are referred to as minor T-wave changes. Those that are inverted or diphasic, where one would normally expect an upright T wave, are considered major changes. A significant difference in opinion in the electrocardiographic evaluation can arise between the clinician and the insurance medical director in this particular area of T-wave changes. The clinician, in examining a patient, may find everything normal on the physical, except for minor T-wave changes. The chances are that he will consider the changes insignificant and interpret the tracing as normal and reassure the patient that he is in excellent health. The insurance physician, in all probability, will view this tracing in a different light, particularly if the applicant is a male over 40 years of age. We all know that T-wave changes can be transient and vary with position, food intake, and electrolyte loss associated with diarrhea. The medical director, however, views the applicant as one of a large group of individuals who have minor T-wave changes. He knows that this large group will generate mortality experience greater than standard. Within this group with minor T-wave changes will be some individuals who owe their changes to early myocardial disease. Since the director cannot identify which ones within the group will die prematurely from their heart disease, he must assess each one within the group a slight extra mortality ratio to maintain

equity. Isolated minor T-wave changes in males over 40 years are significant. They are much less significant in females and in males under 40 years.

The fact that even minor T-wave abnormalities, unaccompanied by any other electrocardiographic or clinical abnormality, demonstrate a significant increase in coronary occlusions and mortality ratio is based on pioneer work done by Kiessling, Schaaf, and Lyle in 1951 and reaffirmed in 1961. A file of 30,000 electrocardiograms on approximately 11,000 home office employees of Prudential Insurance Company provided the data on a group of males 40 to 69 years of age. The first study showed a mortality ratio of 166% in those males who were normal in all other respects except for the presence of minor T-wave changes. A control group without minor T-wave changes showed a mortality ratio of 78%. The second study showed a mortality ratio of 147%. It becomes apparent that, although electrocardiograms showing minor T-wave changes may be of little prognostic value in evaluating an individual patient, such changes generate significant increased mortality within a large group.

It is much less common to find isolated major T-wave changes in normal healthy people, although it can occur. Usually such changes are associated with significant and obvious organic disease. The more pronounced the T-wave inversion, the greater the possibility of cardiovascular disease. Isolated major T-wave changes in a female warrant a bit more liberal underwriting. Males with such isolated changes would be evaluated at 55 to 100% increased mortality ratio, while females would warrant 55% additional mortality.

EXERCISE ELECTROCARDIOGRAMS. Master and his associates introduced the Master's two-step test in 1942. It was soon discovered that many false negatives resulted from failure of the test to produce a sufficient increase in heart rate (Master, 1968). The single test gave way to the double Master's test which was later modified by increasing the number of trips by 15%. Bicycle ergometry and treadmill exercise stress tests have now made the double Master's test obsolete. Patients can now be monitored while exercising and can be taken to the desired target heart rate. False-positive and false-negative tests do occur, and final evaluation must be spiced with judgment. A negative exercise test will usually persuade the insurance underwriter to erase the debits required for minor T-wave changes and reduce the debits for suspicious chest-pain history. A negative coronary angiogram, if available, is even more reassuring. A positive test, on the other hand, will bring with it an assessment of an extra mortality ratio of 100%. A study by Robb and Marks (1967) showed that a group of persons who developed isolated T-wave inversion with exercise experienced a mortality ratio of 166%. In the group with ischemic ST segment depression, there was a mortality ratio of 285%. Those with a downward sloping, depressed ST segment showed a higher mortality than those with a depressed flat segment. Mortality increased with the increase in depth of the depression.

BUNDLE BRANCH BLOCKS. Studies (Singer, 1968) have shown that, in the absence of associated cardiovascular abnormality, incomplete right bundle branch block and indeterminate intraventricular conduction delay carry with them no increase in mortality risk. A complete right bundle branch block does have an associated higher mortality ratio in the older age groups of 155 to 180%. The presence of a complete left bundle branch block is much more significant, with a greater chance of being a manifestation of serious heart disease. This warrants the assessment of 155 to 275% mortality ratio, depending upon the age of the applicant, with the higher ratio being assessed to those over 50 years of age. Of the two divisions of the left bundle branch, the anterosuperior is more susceptible to interruption because of its longer and thinner structure and because of a single blood supply. A posteroinferior block is rare and, when present, is very apt to be overlooked. Left anterior hemiblock in a person over age 60 years carries with it a slight increase in mortality in a high percentage of cases due to its association with significant myocardial disease in this age group. When the left anterior hemiblock is combined with a complete right bundle branch block, to give a bifascicular block, the risk of complete atrioventricular block becomes greater. Waich (1974) and his colleagues in Venezuela found only about 19% of bifascicular blocks associated with healthy hearts. Lenegre's disease, involving a sclerodegenerative processs of the conducting system, is one of the most common causes of right bundle branch block and left anterior hemiblock.

ATRIOVENTRICULAR BLOCK. A PR interval prolonged beyond the accepted limits of normal may be just a physiological variant or may be caused by a number of causes including nonspecific fibrosis of the bundle of His, congenital anomalies, digitalis toxicity, rheumatic carditis, and ischemic heart disease.

In first-degree AV block, the conduction time is prolonged, but all impulses are conducted to the ventricles. Averill and Lamb (1960) reviewed the electrocardiograms on over 67,000 apparently healthy asymptomatic men in the U.S. Air Force and found an incidence of first-degree AV block of 5.2 per 1,000. On further investigation of 139 of these men, only 3.6% were found to have evidence of organic heart disease. If this conduction defect is associated with known heart disease, the risk is classified, for insurance purposes, in accordance with that disease. Where the prolonged PR interval is the only abnormality present, no debits are assessed under 40 years of age, with 20 to 55% extra mortality ratio assessed for the older age groups.

Second-degree AV block can be divided into two categories: Mobitz type I and Mobitz type II. In the type I block, the Wenckebach phenomenon is seen. Here there is a progressive deterioration in the capacity of the His bundle to transmit atrial impulses, with progressive prolongation of the PR interval until one impulse completely fails to be conducted to the ventricles. Averill and Lamb (1960), found three in their group of 67,000. Although this type block can occur in normal hearts, or on occasion in anxiety, the probability of organic disease becomes greater when it is present. A slightly higher mortality is expected than in first-degree AV block. In type II block, beats are dropped without preceding lengthening of the PR intervals, and in this type of block the PR interval of the conducted beats may be either normal or prolonged. An occasional dropped beat will receive less concern than will a constant block where the ventricles respond to every second, third, or fourth atrial beat. The concern stems from the frequently found progression into a complete heart block.

A third-degree, or complete AV block, shows a complete dissociation between atrial and ventricular rhythms. Congenital malformation of the heart may cause such a block. The most common cause is ischemic heart disease. Primary disease of the specialized conducting tissue may also be responsible. A third-degree block may produce a great variety of symptoms from lightheadedness to fatal Adams-Stokes attacks. At younger ages an extra mortality ratio of 125% is added. The risk increases with age until at age 50 years and above a 275% extra mortality is added. The ratings for second- and third-degree blocks are probably high in view of recent advances in pacemaker design and usage.

WOLFF-PARKINSON-WHITE SYNDROME. This entity shows a preexcitation pattern of the right ventricle on the electrocardiogram. The PR interval is shortened, the QRS complex is widened, and characteristic delta waves slur the upstroke of the R waves. This syndrome is of importance to the underwriter as much for the confusion and misdiagnosis it causes as for the associated increase in mortality. This syndrome often simulates, somewhat, the pattern of a myocardial infarction, and when the QRS complexes are wide and in association with a tachycardia, it can be confused with ventricular tachycardia. Because of frequent misinterpretation of electrocardiograms, insurance companies prefer to review all tracings in their home office.

An Air Force study (Averill and Lamb, 1960) found the incidence of this preexcitation syndrome to be 1.5 per 1,000. The syndrome is important because of its frequent association with tachycardias and arrhythmias. The most common arrhythmias are paroxysmal supraventricular tachycardia (70%), atrial fibrillation (16%), and atrial flutter (4%). Wolff-Parkinson-White without a history of tachycardia will require the assessment of a slight increase in mortality ratio for those over 30 years of age. If there is a history of of tachycardia, extra mortality debits of 30 to 80% will be assessed. Those over 40 years of age will receive the higher number of debits.

Cardiac Arrhythmias

Ectopic Beats. Ectopic beats may arise from any locus outside the normal sinus pacemaker. They may be supraventricular or ventricular in origin. Premature atrial beats occur at all ages, and most often are seen in the absence of heart disease. Averill and Lamb (1960) found an incidence of 0.4% in the Air Force Study on healthy males. Atrial disease may be the cause, and here the ectopy predisposes to atrial tachycardia, flutter, and fibrillation. As an isolated finding, however, they are of little significance to the life underwriter.

Ventricular extrasystoles are the most common form of rhythm disturbance. They may occur in healthy persons or may result from some form of heart disease, electrolyte imbalance, or they may be drug induced. Hypoxia is a potent cause of ventricular extrasystoles. A study of Rodstein et al. (1971) found that when ventricular ectopy occurred in persons over 45 years, and at a rate of ten or more per minute, the group showed a mortality ratio of 148%. When the origin of the ectopic beats was multifocal or they occurred in a bigeminy or trigeminy pattern, their significance increased. Extrasystoles associated with cardiac abnormalities or hypertension resulted in a significant mortality hazard. The presence of premature ventricular contractions may require the assessment of an increased mortality ratio up to 80%, depending on the age, frequency, and pattern.

Supraventricular Tachycardia. This entity is common in both normal and diseased hearts. In healthy hearts supraventricular tachycardia is usually tolerated well, but can on occasion, when rates are very rapid, precipitate shock and heart failure.

SINUS TACHYCARDIA. Here the impulses arise from the SA node, and the rapid rate may be caused by vagal depression or sympathetic accelerator stimulation. It may occur as the result of emotion, exercise, digestion, or stimulating drugs. When the increased rate is persistent, there may be an underlying cause of hyperthyroidism, chronic anxiety, anemia, or failing myocardium. Any large group of individuals with sinus tachycardia will contain some persons with undiagnosed organic disease as the causative factor. The group as a whole will experience some increase in mortality. For this reason, a persistent rapid pulse rate above 90 per minute will cause the life underwriter to assess an increased mortality ratio. The debits assessed will increase as the average pulse rate increases. A persistent pulse over 120 per minute might be cause for rejection.

PAROXYSMAL ATRIAL TACHYCARDIA (PAT). It is often difficult or impossible to distinguish between atrial and AV nodal tachycardia. Since the prognosis is essentially the same, they are considered together. Paroxysmal atrial tachycardia is seen in normal and diseased hearts and can occur at any age. In most cases, PAT is of no clinical importance. Occasionally the frequency and the duration of the attacks may interfere with normal activity. Prolonged, severe attacks can lead to congestive heart failure and increase the risk of myocardial infarction. The probability of associated organic heart disease increases when the first attack occurs at older ages. Those individuals with the onset of PAT after age 40 or 50 years, or those who experience frequent and prolonged attacks, warrant the assessment of an extra mortality ratio of 30 to 55%.

Atrial Fibrillation and Flutter. Atrial flutter is manifested by the atria beating regularly at a rate of 250 to 350 per minute. The flutter usually occurs in paroxysms that last longer than those of PAT. It is generally believed that atrial flutter almost always occurs in diseased hearts, with the greatest frequency occurring in rheumatic heart disease with mitral stenosis.

Atrial fibrillation is characterized by extremely rapid, irregular, atrial impulses and ineffectual atrial contractions, accompanied by irregular ventricular response. It is one of the more common disorders of the heart beat. The fibrillation may occur in paroxysms or may become established as a chronic, permanent condition. This arrhythmia is commonly associated with mitral stenosis of rheumatic heart disease, hyperthyroidism, and coronary heart disease with failure.

A recent cooperative study (Gajewski, 1981) of atrial fibrillation in an insured population pooled the experience of 393 life insurance companies. There were 46,058 policyholders with atrial fibrillation identified. Follow-up study was restricted to 3,099 individual cases with 71 observed deaths over an average duration of 3.3 years. This study revealed that there was a great difference in the mortality rate of those with paroxysmal atrial fibrillation as compared to those with chronic fibrillation. The paroxysmal group, with no other identifiable cardiovascular impairment, had a normal mortality. Those associated with mitral stenosis or coronary heart disease had a significant increased mortality (199%). Patients with chronic atrial fibrillation, with or without other cardiac impairment, experienced a much higher risk than the paroxysmal group. This varied from a mortality ratio of 379% to a high of 1,737%, the latter occurring with mitral stenosis. Atrial fibrillation, when associated with mitral stenosis, is cause for rejection for life insurance coverage. Paroxysmal atrial fibrillation, not associated with known organic heart disease, might well be considered insignificant. Between these two extremes, appropriately graded ratings would be imposed.

Cardiac Hypertrophy and Enlargement

The identification of ventricular hypertrophy from electrocardiograms is not a simple process. The intelligent interpretation must use multiple criteria such as proposed by Sokolow and Lyon (1949) and should be correlated with the clinical history and physical findings. The presence of electrocardiographic evidence of ventricular hypertrophy or strain alerts the medical underwriter to look for causes of pressure or volume overload. Left ventricular hypertrophy is commonly associated with hypertensive cardiovascular disease or aortic valve disease. Right ventricular hypertrophy in the young suggests possible congenital heart disease, and in the older applicant, mitral stenosis, chronic lung disease or pickwickian syndrome. When present, electrocardiographic evidence of ventricular hypertrophy or strain will affect considerably the insurability of the applicant.

Heart size determination in insurance medicine is more of a problem than in clinical medicine. Additional studies cannot be conveniently made, and the decision cannot be postponed to await future developments. Two measurements of heart size are commonly used, utilizing the PA view of the chest x-ray. The cardiothoracic ratio compares the transverse diameter of the heart to the internal diameter of thorax at its widest point. If it exceeds 50%, it is assumed that there is cardiac enlargement. The second measurement, the Clark–Ungerleider scale, expresses the transverse diameter of the heart as a ratio to the predicted diameter for height and weight. It is considered enlarged if it exceeds the predicted by 10%. It is rare for cardiac enlargement to exist as an isolated abnormality. It is usually secondary to organic disease. If there is slight enlargement without known cardiac disease, a small extra mortality ratio might be assessed. Definite enlargement associated with other evidence of heart disease could be cause for rejection.

Congenital Heart Disease

The incidence of congenital cardiac abnormalities is difficult to ascertain. Estimates vary from 1 to 8% of newborns. Major anomalies probably occur in about 0.3 to 0.6% of livebirths. One half of the children born with congenital malformations of the heart and great vessels die during the first year. This early mortality occurs despite an estimate that 90% of these defects can be corrected or palliated. Among adults it is estimated that congenital heart disease constitutes less than 1% of all clinical heart disease.

Insurance companies are still reluctant to insure children under 15 years of age with congenital heart lesions. Postponing coverage avoids the early mortality risks. For example, only 60% of those with transposition of the great vessels are alive at one year. In addition, this practice also avoids antiselection in a group of young people where there is little economic need for life insurance. The majority of uncorrected cardiac anomalies are uninsurable. This is particularly true in the severe forms of congenital lesions showing cyanosis or heart failure.

Ventricular septal defects, atrial septal defects, and cases of patent ductus arteriosus comprise more than one half of the clinically diagnosed congenital lesions (MacMahon *et al.,* 1953). Fortunately these most common defects are amenable to surgical correction. The prognosis for ventricular septal defects depends somewhat on the size of the defect as well as the extent of pulmonary or systemic vascular resistance. Small defects with minimal left-to-right flow are usually associated with normal pulmonary artery pressure and are well tolerated. Those with low pulmonary flow and low pulmonary vascular resistance show no excess mortality. Those with a high pulmonary blood flow or a right-to-left shunt are found to have a poor prognosis.

Atrial septal defects may be primum, secundum, or complete AV canal defects and can vary in size and significance. Individuals with primum or complete AV canal defects are more apt to develop symptoms of failure or arrhythmias early and are thus more apt to have an early surgical correction. Secundum-type defects tend to develop symptoms later in life, thus this lesion is the usual type seen in adulthood. The average age of death for those persons with unoperated atrial septal defects of the secundum type is 40 years. The larger defects, repaired with patch grafts, have an increased incidence of embolism and arrhythmias. Correction of the defect will not reverse established pulmonary hypertension, and those with elevated pulmonary pressures before the operation do poorly postoperatively. Operative mortality is estimated to be about 9% without pulmonary hypertension, and 50% in those with pulmonary hypertension.

Congenital aortic stenosis accounts for about 5% of all cases of congenital defects of the heart and great vessels. About 80% are valvular or subvalvular; the remainder are idiopathic hypertrophic subaortic stenosis and left ventricular outflow obstruction due to abnormal mitral valve attachment.

Most insurance companies will consider applicants with uncorrected atrial septal defects, ventricular septal defects, pulmonary stenosis, and aortic and subaortic stenosis only after they have reached age 15 years. Higher mortality ratios are assessed at the younger age groups and gradually decrease with age as time proves the lesions to be of lesser hemodynamic significance. At age 15 years an extra mortality of about 300% would be expected. This would gradually decrease to 125% at age 50 years and over. If there is evidence that a good evaluation revealed little or no hemodynamic changes, and that no surgical correction was advised, a more favorable underwriting evaluation would be made. A normal chest x-ray would warrant further reduction. The presence of pulmonary hypertension would be considered very unfavorable.

Surgical advances in the correction of congenital defects have made it possible to offer insurance coverage to an increasing number because of improved mortality experience. Not too many years ago, no cases were accepted. Surgically corrected septal defects in the better cases warrant the assessment of a small increase in mortality ratio over the first two or three postoperative years. After that period, they may be considered standard in the absence of a high pulmonary resistance. Surgically corrected coarctation of the aorta now receives favorable treatment after the passage of several years. Repair by end-to-end anastomosis receives slightly more favorable treatment than repair with a graft. When surgical treatment is carried out early in life, the individual is considered a slightly better risk. Patent ductus arteriosus after surgical correction and return to normal activities without residual murmurs is considered a standard risk. Dextrocardia without other associated anomalies is also accepted as standard.

Heart Murmurs and Valvular Heart Disease

The life underwriter's interest in heart murmurs is essentially whether or not the murmur is a sign of some organic lesion that will shorten the applicant's life-span. If the exact cause of the murmur has definitely been established, this becomes a welcome bonus to the underwriter. Usually the precise diagnosis has not been established. The medical director must often evaluate the risk on the description of the murmur as supplied by the examining physician or the attending physician. Full and accurate appraisal is not always possible. It is neither practical nor economically prudent to have every applicant with a heart murmur examined by a cardiologist. The evaluation is often based on the location, intensity, timing, and radiation of the murmur, in determining whether the murmur is innocent or organic.

Systolic Murmurs. Innocent intracardiac murmurs are almost always systolic in timing. They can be found at all ages, but are most common in children, tend to be less common during middle age, and then increase in frequency over age 50 years. The intensity of the murmur parallels the ejection velocity of blood from the ventricular chambers and has a crescendo-decrescendo quality. Since most of the blood is ejected during the first half of systole, the murmurs are short, peak early, and are primarily in the first half of systole. In children they are more apt to occur in the pulmonary area but can occur in all areas. In the elderly, they are more apt to radiate to the aortic area and occasionally can be maximal at the apex. Dilation and elongation of the aorta most probably set up eddy currents to cause many of these murmurs in the elderly. Innocent murmurs are usually softer than grade III in intensity. They tend to decrease or disappear in the upright position. The presence of a pansystolic murmur rules against its being innocent.

If the underwriter is convinced that a murmur is an innocent one, no extra mortality debits will be assessed. If he is not certain, the murmur will be classified into one of several categories depending upon its location, intensity, timing, and radiation. Despite the diagnostic uncertainties involved, insurance studies have shown the value of such a classification in predicting the mortality, hence aiding in the risk classification. A large group of insured lives (Singer and Levinson, 1976), with inconstant, localized, apical, systolic murmurs of grade I or II intensity, with no evidence of cardiac enlargement, and with normal blood pressure, produced a mortality ratio of 107%. These can be insured at standard risk. A similar group, with the exception that the murmur was constant, experienced a mortality ratio of 124%. These, also, can be issued insurance at a standard rate. When "slight heart enlargement" was added, the mortality ratio jumped to 296%, requiring the assessment of a significant substandard premium.

When the apical murmur is constant and also transmitted to the left, or when a specific diagnosis of mitral regurgitation is made, the mortality ratio sharply increases to 220%. This further climbs to 267% with a positive history for rheumatic fever or chorea. If mitral stenosis is present, and there is x-ray evidence of cardiac enlargement, the applicant would either be rejected or offered life insurance at a very high rate.

Basal systolic murmurs of slight intensity, localized to the pulmonary area, not transmitted, and with the characteristics of an innocent murmur, will be accepted at standard risk. Basal systolic murmurs at the aortic area, even though not transmitted, are treated with greater concern for they alert the underwriter to the possibility of narrowing of the left ventricular outflow tract. When the murmur is transmitted into the great vessels of the neck, the probability of a significant lesion becomes greater. In a large group of insured lives, where the systolic aortic murmur was faint and considered functional, the mortality ratio proved to be 176%. This is considerably higher than the expected mortality. When the murmur was not localized, or was considered organic, the mortality ratio jumped to 400% (Singer and Levinson, 1976).

Aortic stenosis is the most common lesion of the aortic valve. If rheumatic in origin, it is often combined with mitral stenosis. Other causes are congenital, idiopathic, and calcific. The obstruction to the outflow tract may be valvular, subvalvular, or supravalvular. The majority of valvular lesions are congenital in origin. In applicants under 30 years of age without a history of rheumatic fever, the chances are great that it is congenital in origin. Beyond 50 years of age, the probability increases that calcific aortic stenosis exists which may have its primary cause as rheumatic, idiopathic, or a congenital bicuspid aortic valve. Sudden death occurs in 5 to 15% in most series. This may be due to coronary occlusion, ventricular fibrillation, cardiac standstill, or cerebral ischemia. Occasionally the lesion is associated with a "pulsus tardus et parvus" and a small pulse pressure. The electrocardiogram may show left ventricular hypertrophy. When the obstruction is one third or more of the orifice, symptoms develop. The increased mortality justifies the life underwriter's serious concern about aortic murmurs.

Diastolic Murmurs.   MITRAL STENOSIS. Diastolic murmurs are considered much more serious by the life underwriter. When heard at the apex, mitral stenosis is highly suspect. The three hallmarks on auscultation are (1) a loud and snapping first heart sound, (2) an early diastolic opening snap, and (3) a rumbling diastolic murmur beginning after the opening snap. The rumble is characteristically low pitched, often localized at the apex, heard best with the bell stethoscope held with a light touch, and the patient in the left lateral recumbent position.

The basic hemodynamic problem in a tight mitral valve is the blocking of the outflow of blood from the left atrium into the left ventricle. The pressure increases in the left atrium and is transmitted to the pulmonary veins to cause congestion. Dyspnea becomes an early sign. Chronic pulmonary congestion, pulmonary thrombosis and emboli, respiratory infections, and episodes of pulmonary edema contribute to a precipitous decline. In a tight mitral valve, the average period of time between the onset of symptoms to complete incapacity is about seven years. Atrial fibrillation is an additional risk factor. The mortality ratio is a minimum of 400%.

AORTIC INSUFFICIENCY. The principal cause of aortic insufficiency is rheumatic fever, with syphilis and bacterial endocarditis much less common as a cause. Although mitral stenosis occurs with greater frequency in females, aortic regurgitation is more common in males. Even a slightly incompetent valve results in a significant reflux of blood back into the left ventricle each minute. This occurs because of the large diastolic pressure gradient across the valve. The resultant increase in diastolic volume of the left ventricle causes a more forceful contraction with a prolonged period of systolic ejection. The left ventricle enlarges, first by dilation, and then by hypertrophy, as a compensatory mechanism. If the lesion is pure regurgitation, the ability of the heart to compensate is great, and the life expectancy is much better than in mitral stenosis. The severity of the regurgitation influences the period of time it takes for the left ventricle to fail. When failure does occur, it may be quite sudden. When the dilation causes a functional mitral regurgitation, the decline is hastened by pulmonary congestion and associated right heart failure.

The characteristic murmur of aortic insufficiency is a soft, high-pitched, blowing diastolic murmur, with its intensity diminishing progressively in a decrescendo fashion. Usually the duration of the murmur is directly related to the severity of the regurgitation. It is best heard in the second right interspace, or along the left border of the sternum, with the patient leaning forward in the standing or sitting position. The murmur is one of the more difficult ones to hear. Other characteristic findings are a wide pulse pressure, Corrigan's pulse, visible pulsations in the neck vessels, capillary pulse, and pistol-shot femorals. A mortality ratio of 285 to 300% must be applied to the best cases. Additional debits are added for cardiac enlargement noted on x-ray.

Prolapse of the Mitral Valve (Barlow's Syndrome). With the development of sophisticated techniques in recent years, such as intracardiac phonocardiography, cineangiography, and echocardiography, there has developed an increasing interest in prolapse of the mitral valve. The click coincides with leaflet prolapse. The posterior leaflet is more prone to prolapse because it comprises two thirds of the circumference of the mitral orifice. The prolapse results from an exaggerated inflation or ballooning of the prolapsed leaflet, and typically occurs in mid- to late systole. The murmur, when present, is produced by mitral regurgitation, which is usually of minimal hemodynamic significance. However, in a few individuals, the insufficiency may progress to a degree where it does become significant. The click moves toward the first sound with interventions that decrease left ventricular volume, as with the Valsalva maneuver, and toward the second sound when left ventricular volume is increased by squatting or release of the Valsalva maneuver. This syndrome is rather common with a surprisingly high incidence in otherwise healthy young females. The entity is associated with certain distinct complications: (1) ventricular arrhythmias, (2) sudden death, (3) ruptured chordae tendineae, (4) bacterial endocarditis, and (5) calcification of the valvular tissue. The relatively recent recognition of the syndrome has precluded the development of any large mortality study of mitral prolapse. Because of the complications, we feel there is an increased mortality, and we arbitrarily assess an extra mortality ratio of 55% for life insurance.

Myocarditis

Myocarditis implies inflammation of the myocardium. It has been found in association with bacterial, viral, rickettsial, mycotic, and parasitic diseases. Usually the myocardial manifestations are minimal in comparison to the other clinical manifestations, thus often remain hidden. Alcohol and toxic chemicals also can cause myocardial inflammation. On occasion, the etiological agent may remain obscure. The clinical picture may be characterized by fatigue, tachycardia disproportionate to the degree of fever, cardiac arrhythmias, cardiac enlargement, electrocardiographic changes, and occasionally pericarditis, as with the Coxsackie B virus. In some infectious illnesses the myocarditis develops during the convalescent period, suggesting a hypersensitivity response. Most patients recover spontaneously; diphtheritic and Chagas' myocarditis are the major exceptions.

Diphtheria can be associated with a severe myocarditis which occurs in 10 to 25% of those with the disease. Fortunately, the prevalence of the disease has been markedly reduced through immunization. Most of the acute cases of bacterial and viral myocarditis are self-limiting. If episodes leave no clinical or electrocardiographic evidence of residual damage, there is no appreciable increase in mortality risk and the individual would be considered a standard risk for life insurance after full recovery.

Rheumatic fever is the predominant cause of clinically significant myocarditis and is of concern to the life underwriter. Fortunately, both the incidence and severity of the disease have decreased over the past several decades. Improved standards of living, along with proper antibiotic therapy for streptococcal infections, are responsible for this favorable change. Mortality studies of the insured population with a history of a single episode of rheumatic fever demonstrate that there is only a slight increase in expected mortality. These persons can be considered standard risks after two years have elapsed if there are no residual murmurs. When the history is recent, or when there has been more than one attack, the increased mortality is such that a slight substandard rate is indicated. A history of rheumatic fever in an applicant with a heart murmur requires the assessment of an additional mortality ratio, with higher debits imposed in the younger age groups.

Cardiomyopathies

Much confusion has arisen in the classification of cardiomyopathies. Generally, the term is reserved for those disorders of the heart muscle not secondary to the common etiological forms of heart disease. Often the cause may be unknown. This group can be subdivided into four principal types: hypertrophic, congestive, constrictive, and obliterative. The first two are the most common, with the latter two quite rare. This descriptive and functional classification is further complicated by the fact that one type may evolve into one or more of the other types.

Hypertrophic Cardiomyopathy. This group can be further divided into two subtypes: idiopathic hypertrophic subaortic stenosis (IHSS) and idiopathic concentric hypertrophy. IHSS is characterized by marked hypertrophy of the left ventricle, particularly the interventricular septum at its uppermost part, causing an obstruction of the outflow tract of the left ventricle during systole. About one third of the cases have a familial history of the disease. A systolic murmur at the apex and along the left sternal border and electrocardiographic changes of left ventricular hypertrophy are common. In addition, 25% have two of the electrocardiographic findings seen in Wolff-Parkinson-White syndrome: a short PR interval and delta waves. Deep septal Q waves may be seen in the posterior and left lateral leads. Chest x-ray shows an enlarged heart in approximately 50% of the cases, predominantly left ventricular enlargement. In two series of IHSS studied (Reynolds and VanderArk, 1974), there was an excess death rate of 29 per 1,000. Sudden death occurred in more than 50% in another series (Brackenridge, 1977). The expected mortality with IHSS is 3 to 4% a year. The best cases will require a mortality ratio of 540%, and this will increase as the work capacity decreases.

Congestive Cardiomyopathy. This type is characterized by congestive heart failure, arrhythmias, embolic phenomena, and murmurs of mitral or tricuspid insufficiency. Some cases may start with hypertrophy, but eventually marked dilation occurs. Repeated bouts of heart failure, increasing heart size, and intraventricular blocks are signs of grave prognosis. When these occur, about half of the patients are dead within one year, and two thirds within two years.

There are some congestive cardiomyopathies which have a more favorable outcome. Alcoholic cardiomyopathy may develop after excessive abuse of alcohol over a long period of time. The excess death rate is about 101 per 1,000. If total abstinence is adhered to in the early stages of this disease, the changes are reversible. With evidence of regression, normal heart size, and abstinence for at least two or three years, the risk might be considered for life insurance.

Postpartum cardiomyopathy is also of the congestive type. The mechanism for its development is still obscure. Those cases where the cardiomyopathy develops within three months of parturition have a more favorable prognosis than those with a more delayed onset. Those who still show cardiomegaly after six months probably will not regress, and the mortality is high. The overall excess death rate for this entity is 56 per 1,000 according to one series (Reynolds and VanderArk, 1974) that was studied.

Other Related Diseases

Cerebrovascular Accidents. It is difficult to overemphasize the magnitude of the burden imposed on society by cardiovascular disease. The entire arterial system shares in the aging process of the arteries, albeit in varying degrees. The cerebral circulation is no exception. Cerebrovascular accidents contribute more than their fair share to the medical, social, and economic problems related to vascular disease. Stroke is the third leading cause of death in the United States, accounting for 11% of all deaths. Approximately two million people in this nation have neurological manifestations of cerebrovascular disease of all varieties. One half million new acute CVAs occur each year, causing 200,000 deaths (Brackenridge, 1977). For the survivors, disability and dependency are often their residual plight. One out of six survivors will require permanent care in an institution, and three out of four will have a reduced work capacity. Rehabilitation efforts to restore some function in stroke victims occupy a significant portion of every hospital and rehabilitation center.

ISCHEMIC CEREBRAL INFARCTS. Under this heading can be included cerebral thrombosis, embolism, and transient ischemic attacks (TIAs). These three encompass about 88% of all CVAs. Approximately 20 to 25% of the victims will die with their first attack. Recurrent episodes are common. The probability of suffering a recurrence lessens with increasing elapsed time from the first attack. The incidence of strokes, however, has declined appreciably during the past 30 years, mainly as the result of more effective and aggressive treatment of hypertension.

TRANSIENT ISCHEMIC ATTACKS. These episodes may serve as a warning of impending ischemic stroke. A patient presenting with a TIA has a 37% chance of developing a stroke during the subsequent five years if no treatment is given. Although surgery is not the answer to completed strokes, extracranial arterial surgery to prevent further ischemia can

improve the long-term outlook. The procedure of choice is endarterectomy if the carotids are involved. Improvement in symptoms and the quality of life usually results. There is still some question as to whether surgical intervention increases longevity. Carotid arterial angiography carries with it a small, but real, danger of serious side effects, including strokes and death. The rate is about 1% in major medical centers. Surgical removal of stenotic lesions of the internal carotid has about 4% surgical mortality. Although arterial angiography is still the most accurate diagnostic test, noninvasive studies such as oculoplethysmography, Doppler ultrasonography, and ultrasound imaging are safer. The added mortality experience in persons suffering a TIA or ischemic infarct is covered by applying an increased mortality ratio of 100% and, in addition, collecting mortality costs on the front end by assessing a temporary extra premium of about $10 per $1,000 for the first eight years following the stroke.

INTRACRANIAL HEMORRHAGE. This category accounts for about 12% of cerebrovascular accidents. When the hemorrhage is due to hypertensive vascular disease, the mortality is over 50%. The initial mortality rises with the age of the patient; it is approximately 40% in the 40-to-60-year age group, 50% in the 60-to-70-year group, and 80% in those over 70 years of age.

A subarachnoid or other intracranial hemorrhage occurring in a young individual is most likely to be caused either by trauma or the rupture of a berry aneurysm. Approximately 5% of adult Americans have one or more small intracranial saccular aneurysms. The incidence of subarachnoid hemorrhage is, however, only about 11 per 100,000 persons, with approximately 26,000 persons suffering such an attack each year. Unlike other forms of cerebrovascular disease, the incidence of subarachnoid hemorrhage from ruptured aneurysms has not declined appreciably in the last decade. The overall mortality and morbidity remain high; more than one third are fatal, and an additional 18% experience serious neurological sequelae. Techniques for improved early recognition, before the aneurysm ruptures, are necessary in order to reduce the high rates of death and disability. Operative intervention to clip or ligate the aneurysmal neck carries an operative mortality of 5 to 8%. Early operation may prove to be the treatment of choice. There is a gradual decrease in the mortality ratio over the first six years. Those treated surgically warrant more favorable consideration by the life underwriter.

Peripheral Arterial Occlusive Disease. Intermittent claudication is the usual clinical manifestation of occlusive arterial disease involving the lower extremities and is of significant importance to both the life and health underwriter. The ischemia produced in the leg muscles during exercise is analogous to the myocardial ischemia that causes angina pectoris. It indicates that the blood supply to the muscles is inadequate during exercise, and this symptom usually develops before complete occlusive disease occurs. Atherosclerosis obliterans, as this process is called, involves the large- and medium-size arteries. It is the most common cause of arterial disease in the extremities after age 30 years. The superficial femoral arteries are most commonly involved (90%), with aortoiliac and popliteal areas next most common. The incidence is higher in males than in females, and it increases with advancing age.

THROMBOANGIITIS OBLITERANS. Buerger's disease can also cause intermittent claudication. This inflammatory type of obstruction affects chiefly the peripheral arteries and veins. The incidence appears to have decreased markedly in the United States. The prevalence in males is 75 times greater than in females and occurs most frequently between the ages of 20 to 45 years. The exact etiology is unknown. However, it appears to be closely associated with smoking which aggravates the disease. Many insurance companies will not issue life insurance on a person who has Buerger's disease and continues to smoke.

The presence of intermittent claudication increases the mortality ratio of actual-to-expected deaths. In the Framingham Study, over a nine-year interval, the mortality ratio in those who had developed intermittent claudication since their first biennial examination was 200% in males and 300% in females. Excess death rates were 20 and 24 per 1,000 per year. However, other manifestations of arterial disease involving other organs were also often present (Schiffman, 1970).

RAYNAUD'S PHENOMENON OR DISEASE. This syndrome is characterized by paroxysmal bilateral ischemia of the digits induced by cold or emotional stimuli and relieved by heat. Intimal thickening and hypertrophic changes in the muscular coats can develop in those with a severe and prolonged history. Thrombosis of small arteries may occur causing focal gangrene of the digital tips. Mild cases

are merely an inconvenience with very little disability. The progressive form becomes increasingly painful and disabling. Additional risk arises from the fact that Raynaud's phenomenon may be secondary to a systemic disease, such as scleroderma, rheumatoid arthritis, or disseminated lupus.

Diabetes Mellitus. Any discussion of arterial occlusive disease should include diabetes mellitus. Persons with this disease develop atherosclerosis and arteriosclerosis at an earlier age, and the degenerative process progresses more rapidly in these individuals. There is an increased risk of atherosclerotic heart disease, myocardial infarction, of cerebrovascular disease, peripheral vascular disease, kidney disease, and, for that matter, disease of any organ with an arterial blood supply. Coronary insufficiency in the premenopausal diabetic female is 20 times more common than in the nondiabetic female. A myocardial infarction in a male under 40 years should prompt the physician to look for diabetes mellitus or a familial lipid disorder. Fifty per cent of all diabetics die prematurely of myocardial infarction. The five-year survival is one half that of the nondiabetic (30 versus 60%).

Peripheral arteries share in the premature aging process of diabetics; thus, the degree of involvement is often more severe. Gangrene of the feet due to ischemia is 70 times more frequent in diabetics. One of the reasons for the accelerated atherosclerosis is a defective lipoprotein metabolism. Twenty per cent of diabetics have an elevated serum triglyceride level involving the pre-beta fraction with a type IV hyperlipoproteinemia. Low levels of HDL are found in poorly controlled diabetics. In addition, basement membrane defects exist.

Diabetes mellitus is a complex of abnormalities that include a disturbance in glucose metabolism, which is secondary to a deficiency in beta cells of the pancreas. It is protean in its manifestations. During the last 40 years, the prevalence of diabetes seems to have increased 6½-fold, from 0.4% in 1936 to 2.4% in 1978. At present, there are approximately 5,000,000 Americans with known diabetes mellitus, and it is presumed that an equal number exists undiagnosed. The mortality from diabetes mellitus, however, has been decreasing over the past decade by approximately 24%. This parallels the decrease in cardiovascular disease in the general population. The prognosis is dependent, to a large degree, on the patient's willingness and ability to follow a regimen of good control. One mortality study (Goodkin, *et al.,*

1974) showed that those under poor control had an excess mortality two and one half times those under satisfactory control. Mild disease controlled by diet alone has a better prognosis than insulin-dependent or juvenile-onset diabetes. Those requiring larger amounts of insulin experience a greater increase in mortality. Excess mortality tends to increase with the duration of the disease. Proteinuria, signaling renal involvement, has an extremely unfavorable impact on mortality. Most of the excess mortality is accounted for by cardiovascular-renal disease.

Respiratory Disorders. In 1970, respiratory diseases were reported as causing 6.1% of all deaths in the United States. Mortality from acute respiratory diseases, including tuberculosis, has declined significantly in recent years. This is due in great part to improved antibiotics and effective tuberculosis chemotherapy. Tuberculosis was a principal cause of death at the turn of the century, when the rate in the general population was 194 per 100,000. Today, that rate has decreased to 3 per 100,000.

Pneumonia in all forms accounted for 50% of all respiratory deaths in 1970. Usually, however, this occurs as a terminal event in the elderly and debilitated patients suffering from other chronic diseases. Acute upper respiratory tract disease causes more disability days than any other acute illness.

Pulmonary embolism is the most common form of acute pulmonary disease and probably is the most frequent immediate cause of death in the adult hospital population. Pulmonary emboli are found in approximately 10% of all autopsies. In those patients dying in congestive heart failure, the incidence is three to five times more frequent. The most common origin for the emboli is thrombosis occurring in the veins of the legs and pelvis. Acute cor pulmonale is caused by sudden massive obstruction of the pulmonary arteries by a large pulmonary embolus. The chance for recurrent emboli is greatest during the first six months after the original event. Such a history of embolism would require the assessment of a temporary extra premium for life insurance during the first year. Repeated episodes of pulmonary embolism may lead to sustained pulmonary hypertension, right ventricular hypertrophy, and chronic right ventricular failure.

The principal chronic respiratory diseases today, other than cancer, are emphysema, bronchitis, and asthma. Chronic bronchitis means different things to different physicians, thus, the diagnosis is often inexact. Most will agree that cigarette smoking invites this disease. The prevalence appears higher in Great Britain than in the United States. When the diagnosis is made in connection with life insurance, the disease is more apt to be severe than mild. Thus, mortality experience on insured lives usually shows an excess death rate from 6.5 to 11 per 1,000. This increases with age and the presence of emphysema.

Asthma is associated with widespread airway constriction and obstruction. Extrinsic, or seasonal, allergic asthma has a more favorable prognosis for both morbidity and mortality than does intrinsic, or perennial, asthma. The latter has an onset that is more apt to occur in later life, with infection as its precipitating cause. The frequency and severity of the attacks, the degree of disability experienced, and the amount of reduction in pulmonary function all play an important role in the underwriting decision. Emphysema and evidence of chronic obstructive pulmonary disease begin to make their appearance after years of asthmatic attacks.

Chronic respiratory disease has continued as an important cause of mortality and morbidity. It accounts for 10% of the awards for disability under Social Security. Chronic obstructive pulmonary disease (COPD), with its associated decrease in ventilation and perfusion, causes most of this disability. More accurate diagnosis and reporting may be responsible for the continued high prevalence. Where obstruction of the airways is the predominant lesion, with little reduction in the oxygen saturation, congestive heart failure is less likely to occur. Those cases that have a reduction in blood oxygen saturation are more prone to develop heart failure with pulmonary edema and early death. Cor pulmonale is difficult to reverse. It is an ominous sign in COPD. A markedly reduced FEV_1 is also an indicator of poor prognosis. Emphysema may be secondary to obstructive disease. Primary emphysema has been linked with a genetic deficiency or absence of an antienzyme, alpha-antitrypsin. The life underwriter evaluates the severity of the clinical manifestations and the degree of reduced pulmonary function when making his assessment of increased mortality risk.

Improvement in Life Expectancy

The average length of a person's life in the United States has increased by more than 50% in this century. This fact justifies the assumption that through the years we must have been doing something right. However, before we claim too much credit for this improvement, we should analyze when and where the gains were made. Most of the improved life expectancy occurred during the first half of this century. Little change has occurred since the mid-1950s. Between 1900 and 1950, life expentancy increased by 27.3 years, from 47.3 to 68.8 years. From 1950 to 1977, however, life expectancy increased only 4.4 years to 73.2 years. The longevity gains for women have been greater than those for men. Since 1900, life expectancy for females has increased 28.8 years, while that for males only increased 23.0 years (U.S. Department of Health, Education, and Welfare, 1979).

Much of the improved life expectancy has come from advances in public health, sanitation, standard of living, and safety. By far the greatest increase has occurred among newborns as the result of sharp reductions in mortality of infants and young children. Immunization against infectious diseases and the advent of antibiotics deserve much of the credit. Our efforts in combating the degenerative diseases have been less successful. The wellness approach, encouraging the adoption of healthy life-styles, holds promise for improvement in the near future. The need for continued research and efforts in this field becomes more urgent when one considers the shift toward an older population that is occurring in this country. In 1900 there were about 3,000,000 people, or 4% of the population, over age 65 years. In 1978 there were 24,000,000 or 11% of the population. It is projected that by the year 2030 there will be 50,000,000 persons over age 65 years, or 17% of the population.

Cardiovascular-renal disease accounted for 49.3% of deaths among insured lives in 1945. In 1978 this category still accounted for 48.8% of deaths. Progress has been made in the treatment of hypertension. Indications are that some progress has been made in the treatment of coronary artery disease in the last few years. Prudential Insurance Company recently completed a mortality study (unpublished) on coronary artery disease with 15,000 years of exposure with 200 deaths. The overall experience was clearly better than expected. It confirmed that mortality was higher among those who suffered their coronary occlusion at the younger ages. The mortality was fairly level regardless of the number of years elapsed after the attack. As a result, many postcoronary patients previously considered uninsurable are not being insured. The better cases, those past 50 years of age who do not smoke and have a good family history, can be insured at only slightly substandard rates.

HEALTH INSURANCE

The most frequent hazard that an individual faces today is the risk of disability resulting from sickness or accident. Illness causes 4 out of 5 persons to be disabled at least one day a year, while accidental injury disables 1 out of 18 annually. Illness and injury combined are responsible, on an average, for 17.4 days of restricted activity per person each year. More than 74 million accidental injuries occur each year, with an average of almost 10 days of restricted activity per injury. Some other interesting statistics relating to health care are (1) 570 million visits are made to physicians' offices each year, for an average of 4.8 visits per person; (2) 262 million patient days are spent in hospitals each year, with an average stay of 7.3 days; (3) 21 million operations are performed annually, for an average of 1 operation for every 10 people (Health Insurance Institute, 1980).

Although the hazard of becoming disabled is a potential threat to everyone, the incidence and severity of the disability are variable. It is influenced by age, occupation, sex, socioeconomic status, temperament, and motivation. It can vary from severe total disability to a minor annoying irritation. The cost of disability is borne both by the individual and the whole of society. These costs are measured in loss of productivity, loss of earned income, and the expense of medical care.

Some people enjoy poor health; others cannot afford to be sick. In reality, few people can afford the costs associated with sickness today. Most need the security of adequate health insurance to protect against financially devastating illness. Health insurance permits an individual to guarantee for himself and his family, that, in case of disability, he will be compensated for his loss of income and will be reimbursed, in great part, for the expenses associated with receiving adequate treatment for his illness. The majority of people in the United States turn to private health insurance for this security. At the end of 1978, more than 181,000,000 Americans were protected by one or more forms of private health coverage. This is slightly more than 8 out of 10 in the civilian, noninstitutionalized population. Of these, 167,000,000 were under 65 years of age, or 9 out of 10. An additional 15,000,000 adults, 65 years or older, were covered by supplemental private insurance in addition to Medicare. This supplemental coverage is carried by 6 out of 10 senior citizens. The number of persons in this country without private or public protection against health care expenses is estimated to be about 25,000,000, or 13% of the population. Since health insurance is involved in almost every patient seen by a physician, it is appropriate to include in this text some discussion of health insurance.

The major forms of health insurance include Hospital Expense, Surgical Expense, Physician's Expense, Major Medical Expense, Dental Expense, and Disability Income Protection. Such insurance may be provided by a private insurance carrier or some governmental agency. It may be issued on an individual contract basis or be part of a large or small group.

Risk Selection

The general purposes of risk selection in health insurance in some ways are very similar to those in life insurance. Classification of applicants according to the risk of disability strives for equity by establishing large, broad groups of individuals who will generate the same degree of expense and thus be charged a similar appropriate premium. The underwriting process also attempts to eliminate selection against the company. Examples of antiselection would be withholding of information by the applicant, e.g., a history of poor health pending surgery, or recent close exposure to some contagious disease. Careful selection tries to avoid overinsurance where the disability income benefits would exceed the insured's take-home pay.

There are significant differences, however, in underwriting life and health insurance. The task of the health underwriter is more difficult than that of the life underwriter. Although both engage in a process of risk selection and classification, the risks are different. Life insurance has a very well-defined end-point — death. In contrast, there are many multiple subjective variables that enter into health insurance. It is much more difficult to place applicants for health insurance in well-defined, homogenous groups. There is greater opportunity to select against the company. Rating the applicant and charging a higher premium often offer little protection for the insurer. A patient is told by a physician that a cholecystectomy is indicated. She has no major medical insurance at that time, but goes out and purchases a policy and pays her first premium of $100. Four weeks later the operation is performed, and bills for $3,000 are presented to the insurance company, paid, and the policy is then dropped. The issuing company has experienced an appreciable loss. For this and other reasons, it becomes necessary to waiver certain impairments or organs by an exclusion clause or rider in the contract.

The likelihood of injury or sickness is closely associated with age, sex, and occupation. Therefore, these factors often enter into the assessment of the morbidity risk and the premiums charged. Although over 90% of the applicants for life insurance can be included in the standard risk category, only approximately 80% of all applicants for individual health insurance are accepted as standard risks. In addition, the number rejected for health insurance is much greater than for life. The dollars at risk in health insurance underwriting are as great as or greater than life insurance. A man who has $4,000 per month of disability income protection to age 65, and who becomes totally and permanently disabled at age 30, may collect $1,680,000 by the time he reaches age 65

years. An insured, covered by major medical insurance, who suffers extensive burns over a large portion of his body, might well have bills for care of over a million dollars. It is for these reasons that the health underwriter must be more skeptical, inquisitive, and questioning than the life underwriter. Impending operations, chronic disabling diseases, neuroses and psychoses, hazardous occupations and avocations, and seasonal employment must all receive serious scrutiny and may well be cause for rejection. Malingering is another hazard faced in health insurance which is nonexistent in life insurance.

More than 80% of health insurance applications are underwritten on the basis of the applicant's declared history, along with statements from attending physicians and hospitals. Medical examinations are used much less frequently than in life insurance underwriting. Since great reliance is placed on declared history, discovery of significant misstatements or withholding of material information will usually be cause for rejection of the application. Such discovery after issue will bring attempts to have the contract declared invalid. Inspection reports are usually obtained on applicants for disability income protection, if the amount at risk warrants the cost of the report.

Private Health Insurance

It was not until the Great Depression years of the 1930s that insurance was marketed specifically to cover the cost of hospital and medical expenses. Prior to that time such insurance had been linked to income protection plans. Improvements in coverage and rising health care costs served as an impetus for rapid expansion starting in 1950, when only 76 million persons were insured. By 1978, more than 181 million Americans were covered by some form of private health insurance which paid out benefits in excess of $50.8 billion. This amount was an increase of 17.8% over the previous year and four times the amount paid ten years earlier. The increase was primarily due to the rising cost of medical care, expansion of benefits, and higher utilization.

Private health insurance coverage is available through various types of insurers. There are more than 1,200 private insurance companies in this country providing individual and group health insurance. Security from this source was provided to 103 million persons in 1978. These policies provide for payment directly to the insured or, if assigned by the insured, to the provider of the services rendered as reimbursement for charges incurred.

Blue Cross and Blue Shield associations are nonprofit, health care, membership groups which are organized on a geographic basis. They offer coverage both to individuals and to groups. Blue Cross provides for hospital care usually on a "service type" basis. Here, the association enters into a separate contract with member hospitals for reimbursement for covered services rendered. Often this is at a preferred rate, allowing them to pay less than fully billed charges, and less then defined costs. This can result in hospital costs shifting, where the deficit is made up by patients with or without other types of insurance coverage. Blue Shield plans provide coverage for surgical and medical services performed by a physician. At the end of 1978, there were 69 Blue Cross and 69 Blue Shield plans in the United States, with 24 of these being joint plans.

Health Maintenance Organizations (HMOs) provide comprehensive health coverage in return for fixed periodic payments. From 1971 to mid-1978, the number of HMOs increased from 33 to 215, and the number of individuals covered by such groups increased from 3.6 million to 8.2 million. HMOs provide an alternate delivery system to compete with other providers in the private sector. There is an incentive to minimize health care costs, particularly by reducing in-hospital costs. One criticism offered of such plans is that there also may be an incentive to offer the cheapest medical care rather than the best medical care.

Certain types of health insurance coverage are also available from plans that are administered by employers or labor unions, fraternal societies, communities, or rural consumer health cooperatives. Many corporations have established self-funded group health plans. Such companies contract with an insurance carrier or private organization to process claims and do the administrative paperwork and insure only against a certain level of large unpredictable claims. In 1975 only 5% of total insurance company group coverage had this type of arrangement; by 1977 it had grown to 15%.

Hospital Expense Insurance. This type of medical expense insurance is the most widely held health insurance in this country, with over 181 million persons enrolled at the end of 1978. The benefits payable under this contract are of two kinds: (1) the daily hospital benefit which pays for room, board, and general nursing care, and (2) the miscellaneous hospital expense benefit which covers charges for hospital services and supplies not included in the per diem charge.

The room and board benefits may reimburse for the actual charge up to a specific maximum per day, or the maximum payment may be stated to be the usual charge for a semiprivate room. Some plans pay a fixed defined benefit for each day of hospitalization without regard to the actual charge. Usually there is a limit on the maximum number of days for which the benefit is payable. The recent trend has been toward liberal extension of these limits.

The miscellaneous expense benefit is always on an expense-incurred basis. This would include use of the operating room, laboratory services, anesthetics, drugs, and other supplies. Again, the maximum benefit is usually defined.

Surgical Expense Insurance. This coverage pays for surgical procedures performed for the correction of an impairment resulting from sickness or accident. Most policies exclude reconstructive surgery performed for cosmetic reasons. Coverage under surgical expense insurance has grown 20% in the past

decade. At the end of 1978, there were 172 million persons in this country with this type of protection. The two most common plans are the fixed-surgical-fee schedule and the "reasonable and customary" fee schedule. Under the fixed fee schedule, a maximum amount is set for each operation. Usually about 100 of the most common operations are listed with the maximum benefits payable. Operations not included in the list are equated to comparable procedures. The great deficiency of the fixed-fee plan is that it does not keep pace with rising costs and inflation. The schedules are often five to ten years out of date.

As an attempt to remain more current, many insurance companies offer a policy that pays a "reasonable and customary" benefit. A much better terminology would be "usual and prevailing." If the fee is reduced because of the limits of the policy as not being "reasonable and customary," it implies that the surgeon's fee was "unreasonable," which may not necessarily be so. This plan of payment takes into consideration the attending surgeon's "usual" charge for that particular operation and the "prevailing" charges of his peers in that particular geographic area for the same operation. Usual and prevailing fees are determined on a percentile basis. Many pay the 90th percentile. This means that, if the profile contains ten fees for an appendectomy, the 90th percentile payment would be the ninth highest fee. Although this plan of payment keeps pace with changing prices, it does little to help contain runaway inflation.

The expense benefit paid for a particular surgical procedure under the usual and prevailing method includes postoperative care. When the services of an assistant surgeon are deemed necessary, the allowable fee for this service is usually calculated at 20% of the fee allowed for the principal surgeon. When the expertise of two different surgical specialists is required, e.g., an orthopedic surgeon and a neurosurgeon, usually an additional 25 to 50% is allowed, and the total calculated allowable expense is divided equally between the two cosurgeons. When there is a team approach involved, as in cardiac surgery, the total professional fee is often paid to the chief surgeon for the entire team.

Physician Expense Insurance. This type of coverage is sometimes known as Regular Medical Expense Insurance. It pays for charges by physicians for services other than those in connection with surgical procedures and postoperative care. Most such policies cover only in-hospital treatment, although a few may provide for care at home or in the doctor's office. There are usually maximum limits on daily charges and on the number of days of coverage. At the end of 1978, more than 164 million persons had some form of physician expense insurance.

Major Medical Expense Insurance. This type of coverage was first introduced nationally in 1951, and its growth since then has been quite rapid. In 1978 there were 142 million persons with this type of coverage in the United States. Major Medical coverage provides broad and substantial protection for large, unpredictable, medical expenses and supplements basic hospital, surgical, and medical expense benefits. Its purpose is to provide protection against very large bills and catastrophic medical expenses that result from serious accident or prolonged sickness.

The Major Medical Expense benefit is usually subject to a deductible, typically varying from $100 to $1,000. This means that no benefits will be paid until the expenses incurred exceed the deductible. Such a provision eliminates from coverage those sicknesses and injuries that require only relatively minor medical treatment for which medical expenses could be budgeted without hardship. Such a provision reduces the cost of claims settlement and thus increases the proportion of premium payments that can be utilized for policy benefits. It also generates a savings by preventing unnecessary hospitalization for routine diagnostic testing that could be obtained on an outpatient basis.

The total benefits under a Major Medical policy usually have a maximum amount payable which may range from $10,000 per person to an unlimited amount. A recent survey of newly issued group Major Medical benefits revealed that 92% of the surveyed employees had a maximum benefit of more than $100,000, compared with only 23% in 1973. Maximum benefits of $1 million or over were held by 54%, and 30% had unlimited benefits.

Many policies further guard against abuse by incorporating a coinsurance policy provision. Here, both the insured person and the insurer share in a specific ratio, often 20% paid by the insured and 80% paid by the insurer, of the covered losses under the policy.

Disability Income Protection. The earning power of every worker, which is the principal asset in a great majority of families, is constantly at risk of being reduced, or lost completely, by reason of disabling injury or illness. Disability income insurance benefits in health and accident policies provide for the partial replacement of this lost income. The disability may be total or partial. Most policies issued today define total disability as being unable to perform the duties of the insured's usual occupation for the first two years. After that period, the definition changes to the inability to engage in any gainful occupation for which the insured is reasonably fitted by education, training, and experience. The amount of weekly or monthly benefits is defined by the specifications of the policy. Partial disability coverage usually provides for payment of income at a reduced rate, such as 40 to 50% of the full rate for a limited period, often six months.

Tremendous losses were suffered by insurance companies during the Great Depression of 1929 when unemployed insured workers claimed disability to obtain some income. This experience forced insurance carriers to place more stringent limitations on the length of the indemnity period. Short-term disability, with benefits payable for one or two years, is more apt to motivate the patient to strive for recovery and rehabilitation. His motivation may be very different from that of the person who is insured under a lifetime disability contract. As the monthly benefits payable for disability approach the salary earned, the greater becomes the urge for the insured to cling to his disability status. He may resist efforts to have him take advantage of the modern techniques of rehabilitation, which have enabled many severely impaired people to become self supporting.

Heart disease is the greatest cause of permanent disability claims among workers under 65 years in this nation. It is the principal cause of limited activity for some 2.5 million Americans in this age group and is responsible for more days of hospitalization than any other single disorder. Heart attacks cause industry to lose about 132 million workdays per year. The great prevalence of heart disease and the resultant disability that occurs make cardiac rehabilitation a prime concern in the treatment of this disease.

The physician plays a most important role in determining the length of disability for each patient he treats for any disease, whether real or imagined. Every sensible patient confronted with cardiac symptoms has a justified concern about the severity of his condition. This concern generates considerable anxiety in most patients, outwardly expressed to varying degrees. A good cardiac workup may include many tests that are completely foreign to the patient. Early patient education becomes an important element in the care of every patient if superimposed iatrogenic disease is to be avoided. The physician should explain every part of the workup, as well as the final diagnosis. Care must be taken not to misinterpret symptoms, signs, and laboratory data. This is particularly true of faulty interpretation of the electrocardiogram. The tendency is to overread. The medical director of every insurance company sees frequent cases of erroneous diagnosis of coronary artery disease based solely on misinterpretation of normal electrocardiograms. The conscientious physician must be aware of the suffering and the unnecessary disability that may result from inaccurate diagnosis. The manner in which a physician conveys his opinion, and the assessment of the problem, to the patient can have a profound influence on the emotionally susceptible patient and on his progress in the rehabilitative process. As soon as the cardiac patient's condition has stabilized, thoughts and language directed toward a return to a productive life are appropriate to early rehabilitation. The heart lends itself to the somatic expression of thoughts and fears of death. A cardiac neurosis can be difficult to cure. It can contribute to a great loss of productivity through unnecessary disability.

Disability rates vary by the social and economic characteristics of the group in question. The higher the educational attainment, the fewer are the days of disability experienced in most cases. The same occurs as the average family income increases. Blue-collar workers averaged 6.6 work-loss days, while white-collar workers averaged 4.2 days in 1978. There are also geographical differences in average work-loss days due to disability. The West has the highest level of restricted activity days, as well as the highest frequency of physician visits.

Chronic illness has great impact on people by causing a change in their life-styles which prevents them from resuming their major activity or occupation. In 1978, 30.3 million (14.2%) persons in this country suffered a limitation of activity due to one or more chronic conditions. Acute illness caused a loss of 351 million workdays in that same year, with an average loss of 3.8 days per worker. Work-related injuries added another 38.2 million workdays lost from 5.7 million injuries. The loss in earnings to the American worker was in excess of $29 billion. Insurance benefits paid for disability in 1977 amounted to $10.3 billion (Health Insurance Institute, 1980). The need for measures to prevent injuries and chronic illness cannot be stressed enough as a means of reducing this great loss in earnings and productivity.

Government Health Care Programs

Medical and health care services are provided to certain segments of the population in the United States through a variety of public programs at all levels of government, from city to federal. As the number of programs funded by public monies has increased over the years, there has been an increase in the percentage of health care expenditures paid for by public funds. In 1968 governmental outlay for health care amounted to 37.3% of the total national disbursement, compared to 49.6% in 1978. Prior to 1967, state and local allocations exceeded federal expenditures, which accounted for less than 5% of all federal spending. Today, federal spending for health care is more than double the state and local expenditures and accounts for 13% of all federal spending.

Federal health care programs are directed mainly toward six major groups: low income individuals through Medicaid, those over 65 years of age through Medicare, military personnel and their dependents, veterans, federal civilian employees, and Native Americans.

Social Security

The Social Security Act of 1935 became effective in 1937. It inaugurated the Old Age, Survivors, and Disability Insurance under federal sponsorship in the United States. This law has been amended from time to time and currently is subject to further modification to assure the solvency of the program.

Virtually all gainfully employed persons are covered under the program. The principal exceptions are certain government employees and a few very low-income, self-employed, farm, and domestic workers with irregular employment. The basic principles governing the OASDI system is that benefits are (1) based upon the presumption of need occasioned by retirement, (2) need for a floor of protection, and (3) payment related to earnings. In addition, there is a balance between social adequacy and individual equity. The financing is on a self-supporting contribution basis, with no general revenue funds used.

The original act passed in 1935 provided only retirement benefits and a lump-sum death benefit. To this was added, through the years, survivor's benefits and disability benefits. In 1965, the Medicare program was added, and shortly thereafter in 1972, the chronic renal dialysis program was included. Coverage was gradually extended to cover most of the population. Every few years, the benefits have been increased by well-meaning politicians, without great regard for the fiscal integrity and stability of the program. Social Security benefits now represent 25% of federal expenditures. As the result of inflation and high unemployment, the system faces some grave financial problems in the not-too-distant future.

In 1982, the Social Security retirement fund will face a cash shortage, and by 1985, the annual shortfall will reach $30 billion. The immediate problem centers on the huge trust funds for retirement and disability insurance. These are being depleted by a shortfall of revenues and may be in serious deficit by the beginning of 1982. The disability fund should move into a healthy surplus in 1983. The $100 billion retirement fund will be in trouble through 1986, when it will face an annual shortfall of some $30 billion in funds needed to insure continuous payment of benefits. The third Social Security Trust Fund, which covers hospital insurance under Medicare, is expected to start disbursing more funds than it takes in by 1988 and be completely exhausted by the early 1990s. The long-term problem will occur around 2010, when the baby-boom generation begins to enter the ranks of the retired, pushing the fund into a further deficit. Currently, for every 100 workers, there are 31 receiving benefits. By the year 2000, for every 100 workers, there will be 70 receiving benefits. This will require an increase in the Social Security tax of 40%. The solutions to these fiscal problems will require interfund borrowing as a temporary measure, with eventual reduction in benefits and a raise in the age of retirement.

Medicaid. Title XIX of the Social Security Act provides for a program of medical assistance for certain low-income individuals and families. This program, which is known as Medicaid, was created by federal law in 1965. It is administered by each state with certain federal requirements and guidelines. Financing is accomplished through joint contributions from both state and federal funds. Medicaid is designed to help with the payment of medical expenses for those persons who are eligible to receive payments under one of the existing cash-assistance programs. This includes those receiving Aid to Families with Dependent Children and Supplemental Social Security Income. Most states add to these groups other persons who are medically indigent.

Many persons receiving Medicaid are aged and disabled and are also covered under Medicare. Where dual coverage is involved, many states pay for the Medicare premiums and then also pay the deductibles, copayments, and for services not covered by Medicare. In order to qualify for federal matching funds, state programs must provide comprehensive services to include outpatient care, in-hospital services, laboratory and x-ray coverage, skilled nursing and home care for those 21 years or over, family planning, periodic screening examinations, diagnosis and treatment for children under 21 years of age, and physician services whether in or out of the hospital. In 1978, the Medicaid program paid out $17.8 billion in benefits. The average number of recipients per month was nine million. States participate in the program at their option. All states except Arizona have Medicaid programs.

Medicare. This program became effective on July 1, 1966. It is federally administered and provides hospital and medical insurance protection for those 65 years of age and over. In addition, persons under 65 years are also covered if they have been receiving cash benefits under Social Security or Railroad Retirement programs because of disability or are receiving dialysis for chronic renal failure. Medicare consists of two parts. Part A covers hospital insurance and is mandatory. Part B is a supplementary, voluntary plan which helps pay for physician's services and some medical services and supplies not covered under Part A. Social Security taxes finance Part A with contributions shared by employers and employees. The voluntary Part B is financed by monthly premiums paid by those who choose to enroll and by the federal government. Part A contains a deductible which, as of January 1, 1982, increased from $228 to $256 for the first 60 days of care and $65 per day for the next 30 days of hospitalization. The deductible for Part B increased from $60 to $75, with benefits being paid for 80% of the charges over this deductible amount. The premium for Part B was raised to $8.70 per month on July 1, 1980.

Since 1973, certain aliens and some federal civil service employees have been eligible to participate in Part A by paying a premium that was $78 per month as of July 1, 1980. This group has always been eligible to enroll in Part B. Medicare has shared in the escalation of health care costs. In 1967, total benefits paid were $4.5 billion. By 1978, a 448% increase had occurred with the total reaching $24.9 billion. Part of this increase was due to the addition in 1972 of the chronic renal dialysis program to the list of eligible services. Approximately 13% of the total benefits paid are for the care of persons under 65 years of age. In 1978, the cost of Part A was $17.7 billion and Part B, $7.2 billion. A number of insurance companies serve as fiscal intermediaries for the federal government in processing claims and paying benefits.

Military Personnel and Dependents. All active and retired military personnel and their families are eligible for medical care at any Department of Defense medical facility. In addition, the Civilian Health and Medical Program (CHAMPUS) provides payment for care of those unable to use government medical facilities for reason of distance, overcrowding, or unavailability of appropriate treatment at military medical centers. There is a deductible provision for covered medical care rendered in civilian facilities to wives and children of active military personnel, to retired military personnel and their dependents, and to dependents of deceased personnel unless they are eligible for Part A of Medicare. In the fiscal year of 1978, of the $3.4 billion spent on medical care by the Department of Defense, $527 million was for medical services rendered under the CHAMPUS program.

Federal Civilian Employees. Civilian employees of the federal government have the option of participating in a variety of insurance programs including HMOs. Premiums are shared by the employing agency and the employee. Nearly 3.4 million federal civilian employees and annuitants and 6.5 million dependents were covered under these programs in 1978, when the total expenditure amounted to $1.8 billion.

Veteran's Medical Care. The Veterans Administration operates 172 hospitals and 47 outpatient clinics for the care of veterans who have received an honorable discharge from military service. Priority is given to service-connected disability. Of the $5.2 billion spent by the federal government for VA medical services in 1978, $4.9 billion was for medical care and hospital services. Inpatient care was received by 1.3 million veterans in that year.

Indian Health Services. A total of $467 million in federal funds was spent to provide health services to more than 625,000 American Indians and Alaskan Natives in 1978. The services included hospital care and other medical services; construction of hospitals and sanitation facilities, and housing for health service employees; health manpower training and education; health planning; and research.

Workmen's Compensation. One of the oldest type of governmental programs aimed at replacing, in some part, the personal income lost during disability is Workmen's Compensation. The benefits paid from this source are designed to provide partial coverage against medical care costs and lost income resulting from industrial injury or occupational disease. The statutes, courts, and commissions are established at state level.

The first attempts to initiate employer liability for on-the-job accidents in the United States began in the early 1900s. By 1970, all but six of the states had adopted Workmen's Compensation of some variety. Now all states have statutes covering this area of liability. The principle underlying all of these statutes is that injury or disease incurred in the course of employment is compensable by the employer without regard to the question of fault. Industry is to consider this as one of the labor costs of operation. In return, the employer's liability will be limited and fixed by law. Most statutes exclude self-inflicted injury or injury sustained while intoxicated. Benefits include medical costs, disability income, and lump-sum payment for specific injuries such as loss of sight or limb.

Disability is classified into total or partial, temporary or permanent. Benefits are usually determined as some portion of the worker's weekly wage. One objective of Workmen's Compensation is to assist the injured worker in his attempts to return to work. In some states, rehabilitation has become the principal purpose of the statute. There is, however, wide variation among the states. In many states employers must contribute to a state fund. In others, they are permitted to self-insure or utilize private insurance carriers. Federal employee coverage is funded by Congressional appropriations.

Most of the medico-legal problems involving cardiac disease arise in connection with claims of cardiac disability and death attributed to the victim's work. For this reason, heart disease is of particular importance to any review of Workmen's Compensation. Liability arises from accidental injury or occupational disease. At this point in time, heart disease generally does not qualify as an occupational disease. It is possible that in the future, stress of the workplace may generate claims as an occupational disease. Evidence is accumulating that suggests that a sedentary life-style and emotional stress may increase the risk of coronary artery disease. In some states there are statutes establishing the presumption that heart disease can be related to certain occupations such as policemen and firemen. In most cases, however, cardiac claims are based on a thesis that the worker sustained an occupational accident rather than an occupational disease. Courts have ruled an award of compensation if a preexisting cardiac condition was aggravated by a stress, strain, or trauma at work. The fact that the worker previously suffered one or more heart attacks away from his job has not been cause for denial of compensation. Most courts hold that liability is presumed even if the incident at work merely accelerated the cardiac event and disability.

Marked differences among the courts do exist over what constitutes effort or exertion that is greater than the ordinary wear-and-tear of life. For this reason, there is much disagreement as to how much and what kind of physical strain will be considered causative. In general, the more severe the strain and the closer its proximity to the cardiac event, the stronger will be the argument for a causal relationship and a compensable award. When there is a single identifiable event of severe mental stress associated with a heart attack, courts have considered this mental stress as complying with the doctrine of unusual strain. In any event, the courts reserve the right to determine the causal relationship. Their interpretation is usually more liberal than that of the physician.

Workmen's Compensation decisions as to what constitutes permanent and total disability are usually very liberal. Formulae have been devised to serve as guides in evaluating the permanent impairment. Usually this evaluation is based on the nature of the organic cardiac disease and the presence or development of symptoms. The work classification of the New York Heart Association is often used as a guide in determining the per cent of disability.

REFERENCES

Anderson, R. P.; Rahimtoola, S. H.; Bonchek, L. I.; and Starr, A. The prognosis of patients with coronary artery disease after coronary bypass operations. Time-related progress of 532 patients with disabling angina pectoris. *Circulation,* **1974,** *50,* 274–282.

Averill, K. H., and Lamb, L. E. Electrocardiographic findings in 67,375 asymptomatic subjects. I. Incidence of abnormalities. *Am. J. Cardiol.,* **1960,** *6,* 76–83.

Beeson, P. B.; McDermott, W.; and Wyngaarten, J. B. (eds.) *Cecil—Textbook of Medicine,* 15th ed., W. B. Saunders, Philadelphia, **1979.**

Brackenridge, R. D. C. *Medical Selection of Life Risks.* The Undershaft Press, London, **1977.**

Bruschke, A. V. G.; Proudfit, W. L.; and Sones, F. M., Jr. Clinical course of patients with normal, and slightly or moderately abnormal coronary arteriograms. A follow-up study of 500 patients. *Circulation,* **1973,** *47,* 936–945.

Build and Blood Pressure Study, 1959, Vols. I and II. Society of Actuaries, Chicago, **1960.**

Cowell, M. J., and Hirst, B. L. Mortality differences between smokers and non-smokers. *Trans. Soc. Actuaries,* **1980,** *32,* 185–213.

Expectation of life in United States at new high. *Stat. Bull. Metropol. Life Insur. Co.,* **1980,** Oct.-Dec., 13.

Friedberg, C. K. *Diseases of the Heart,* 3rd ed., W. B. Saunders, Philadelphia, **1966.**

Friedman, H. H. *Diagnostic Electrocardiography and Vectorcardiography,* 2nd ed. McGraw-Hill, New York, **1977.**

Gajewski, J., and Singer, R. B. Mortality in an insured population with atrial fibrillation. *J. Am. Med. Assoc.,* **1981,** *245,* 1540–1544.

Goodkin, G.; Wolloch, L.; Gottcent, R. A.; and Reich, F. Diabetes—a twenty year mortality study. *Trans. Assoc. Life Insur. Med. Dir. Am.,* **1974,** *58,* 217–269.

Gregg, D. W. *Life and Health Insurance Handbook,* 2nd ed. Richard D. Irwin, Inc., Homewood, Ill., **1964.**

Greider, J. E., and Beadles, W. T. *Law and the Life Insurance Contract.* Richard D. Irwin, Inc., Homewood, Ill., **1968.**

Haas, K. Occlusive cerebrovascular disease. *Med. Clin. North Am.,* **1972,** *56,* 1281–1297.

Hall, M. F. *Public Health Statistics.* Paul B. Hoeber, New York, **1942.**

Hall, R. J.; Dawson, J. T.; Cooley, D. A.; Hallman, G. L.; Wukasch, D. C.; and Garcia, E. Coronary artery bypass, *Circulation,* **1973,** *48* (Suppl. III), 146–150.

Health Insurance Institute. *Source Book of Health Insurance Data 1979.* Health Insurance Institute, Washington D.C., **1980.**

Higgins, I. T. T. The epidemiology of chronic respiratory disease. *Prev. Med.,* **1973,** *2,* 14–33.

Huebner, S. S., and Black, K. *Life Insurance,* 7th ed., Appleton-Century-Crofts, New York, **1969.**

Hurst, J. W.; Logue, R. B.; Schlant, R. C.; and Wenger, N. K. *The Heart,* 3rd ed. McGraw-Hill, New York, **1974.**

1951 Impairment Study. Society of Actuaries, Chicago, **1954.**

Kannel, W. B. Role of blood pressure in cardiovascular disease. The Framingham Study. *Angiology,* **1975,** *26,* 1–14.

—— Some lessons in cardiovascular epidemiology from Framingham. *Am. J. Cardiol.,* **1976,** *37,* 269–282.

Kiessling, C. E.; Schaaf, R. S.; and Lyle, A. M. A reevaluation of the T wave changes in the electrocardiograms of otherwise normal people. *Trans. Assoc. Life Insur. Med. Dir. Am.,* **1961,** *45,* 45–70.

1979 Life Insurance Fact Book. American Council of Life Insurance, Washington, D.C., **1980.**

Lyle, A. M. A study of premature beats by electrocardiogram. *Trans. Soc. Actuaries,* **1962,** *14,* 493–508.

MacMahon, B.; McKeown, T.; and Record, R. G. The incidence and life expectation of children with congenital heart disease. *Br. Heart J.,* **1953,** *15,* 121–129.

Maslow, A. H. A theory of human motivation. *Psychol. Rev.,* **1943,** *L,* 370–396.

Master, A. M., The Master's two-step test. *Am. Heart J.,* **1968,** *75,* 809.

Mathewson, F. A. L., and Brereton, D. C. Atrio-ventricular heart block. *Trans. Assoc. Life Insur. Med. Dir. Am.,* **1964,** *48,* 210–234.

Moriyama, I. M.; Krueger, D. E.; and Stamler, J. *Cardiovascular Disease in the United States.* Harvard University Press, Cambridge, **1971.**

National Conference on High Blood Pressure Education, 15 January, 1973. U.S. Government Printing Office, Washington, D.C., DHEW Publication No. (NIH) 73–486, **1973.**

New York Heart Association. *Nomenclature and Criteria for Diagnosis of Diseases of the Heart and Blood Vessels.* New York Heart Association, **1955.**

Pilgrim, J. W. 1973 Connecticut General blood pressure study. *Trans. Assoc. Life Insur. Med. Dir. Am.,* **1974,** *58,* 81–89.

Report of the Advisory Committee to the Surgeon General of the Public Health Service. *Smoking and Health.* Dept. Health, Education, and Welfare, Washington, D.C., P.H.S. No. 1103, **1964.**

Reynolds, E. W., and VanderArk, C. R. Primary cardiomyopathies: a review of clinical features, pathology and mortality. *Trans. Assoc. Life Insur. Med. Dir. Am.,* **1974,** *58,* 146–164.

Robb, G. P., and Marks, H. H. Postexercise electrocardiogram in arteriosclerotic heart disease. Its value in diagnosis and prognosis. *JAMA,* **1967,** *200,* 918–926.

Rodstein, M.; Wolloch, L.; and Gubner, R. S. Mortality study of the significance of extrasystoles in an insured population. *Circulation,* **1971,** *44,* 617–625.

Rotman, M., and Trietwasser, J. H. A clinical and follow-up study of right and left bundle branch block. *Circulation,* **1975,** *51,* 477–484.

Schiffman, J. *The Framingham Study,* sect. 25. *Survival Following Certain Cardiovascular Events.* Government Printing Office, Washington, D.C., **1970.**

Sheldon, W. C.; Rincon, G.; Effler, D. B.; Proudfit, W. L.; and Sones, F. M. Vein graft surgery for coronary artery disease. *Circulation,* **1973,** *48* (Suppl. III), 184–189.

Singer, R. B., Mortality in 966 life insurance applicants with bundle branch block and wide qrs. *Trans. Assoc. Life Ins. Med. Dir. Am.,* **1968,** *52,* 94–114.

Singer, R. B., and Levinson, L. *Medical Risks.* Lexington Books, Lexington, Mass., **1976.**

Smith, J. M.; Stamler, J.; and Miller, R. A. The detection of heart disease in children. *Circulation,* **1965,** *32,* 966–976.

Sokolow, M., and Lyon, T. P. The ventricular complexes in left ventricular hypertrophy as obtained by unipolar precordial and limb leads. *Am. Heart J.,* **1949,** *37,* 16.

Stamler, J. Cardiovascular diseases in the United States. *Am. J. Cardiol.,* **1962,** *10,* 319–340.

—— High blood pressure in the United States—an overview of the problem and the challenge. In *National Conference on High Blood Pressure Education, 15 January 1973.* U.S. Government Printing Office. Washington, D.C., DHEW Publication No. (NIH) 73–486, **1973.**

U.S. Department of Health, Education, and Welfare. *Blood Pressure of Adults by Age and Sex, United States, 1960–62.* U.S. Dept. HEW, Vital and Health Statistics, Series 11, No. 4, National Center for Health Statistics, Rockville, Md., **1964.**

—— *Blood Pressure of Persons 18–74 Years, United States, 1971–72.* U.S. Dept. HEW, Vital and Health Statistics, Series 11, No. (NIH) 73-486, **1973.**

—— *Facts of Life and Death.* U.S. Dept. HEW (PHS) Pub. No. 79-1222, National Center for Health Statistics, Hyattville, Md., **1978.**

—— *Health, United States 1979,* U.S. Dept. HEW (PHS) Pub. No. 80-1232, U.S. Government Printing Office, Washington, D.C., **1979a.**

—— *Healthy People—The Surgeon General's Report on Health Promotion and Disease Prevention,* U.S. Dept. HEW (PHS) Pub. No. 79-55071, U.S. Government Printing Office, Washington, D.C., **1979b.**

—— *Mortality Trends for Leading Causes of Death, United States, 1950–69.* U.S. Dept. HEW, Vital and Health Statistics, Series 20, No. 16, National Center for Health Statistics, Rockville, Md., **1974.**

Waich, T. S.; Reverson, G. R.; Barcelo, J. E.; Pena, I.; Mendez, A.; and Jasso, J. An analysis of 293 hemiblocks. *Ann. Life Ins. Med.,* **1974,** *5,* 77.

Chapter 15
HEALTH CARE COSTS

Donald W. Bowne

THE PROBLEM

Health care costs have been increasing faster than any other major category of personal expense. The cost of medical care has grown at an average annual rate of 12.6% over the past 15 years, with the rate of increase rising to 15.2% in 1980 (*Source Book of Health Insurance Data 1979-1980*). The present rate of growth will cause these costs to double every five years. Society is beginning to pay close attention to these expenditures and may soon decide that it is no longer willing to pay the price. Today, the public place rising health care costs high on their list of concerns. They rank it third in importance, after inflation and the high crime rate, and ahead of government corruption, drug addiction, unemployment, and the problems of the elderly. A crisis in health care costs is here, and this crisis warrants the sober concern of all. "Thrift is too late at the bottom of the purse." We would be wise to heed these words of Seneca, for we are nearing the bottom of the purse. This crisis demands the cooperative efforts of everyone, if we are to forestall the collapse of our present health care delivery system and keep it in the realm of free enterprise.

Cost, Quality, and Accessibility

Oscar Wilde defined a cynic as "an individual who knows the price of everything, and the value of nothing." This chapter will deal principally with the rising price of health care. Lest we be accused of not knowing the value of good medical care, we hasten to point out that *cost* is only one of three measures used to judge a nation's health care industry. The other two parameters are the *quality* of care and the *accessibility* of care. Physicians justifiably place quality of care in first priority. We should never overlook, however, the importance of the other two, cost and accessibility.

Most will agree that Americans today are healthier than ever. The fitness buff, however, will be quick to point out that we have a long way to go to achieve our full potential for good health. Great advances have been made in the field of public health and medicine. There has been a dramatic reduction in mortality rates through improvement of the environment, correction of malnutrition, and control of infectious diseases through immunization and antimicrobial agents. This latter improvement is attested to by the fact that only 1% of the people who die before the age of 75 years in the United States die of infectious disease. In 1900 the leading causes of death were influenza, pneumonia, diphtheria, tuberculosis, and gastrointestinal infections. In that year the death rate from these major acute diseases was 580 per 100,000 people. Today, barely 30 people per 100,000 die each year of these illnesses (U.S.

Department of Health, Education, and Welfare, 1979b). It should be noted, however, that much of this progress occurred in the first half of this century, with a much slower gain after 1950. Some might argue, therefore, that costly technology of the current era had only minimal effect on the rise in life expectancy and the decline in infant mortality. For this reason, the emphasis in medicine should shift from the bioscientific strategy to the ecological strategy for health. Others would not agree.

Medical education has never been better, nor has there been any previous time when we have trained brighter or more competent physicians. The medical profession deserves great praise for maintaining the standard of excellence in our medical schools through careful monitoring and accreditation. The 160 medical schools of variable quality that existed in 1910 were reduced to 76 schools of high academic standing in 1945. Under careful guidance this number has increased to 120 without sacrificing quality.

When one looks back at the progress that has been made in the last 50 years, we can have justified optimism for the eventual control and cure of major diseases, and the possible elimination of premature death from illness. The medical community warrants a good grade for the quality of care. This should not lull us into a feeling of complacency, however, for the list of diseases needing prevention and cure is long. Twelve other countries do a better job in preventing deaths from cancer; 26 have a lower death rate for circulatory diseases; 11 have a better record for infant mortality; 14 have a higher life expectancy for men, and 6 a higher expectancy for women. In addition, the mortality from major chronic diseases, such as heart disease, cancer, and stroke, has increased more than 250% in the past 70 years. These figures from *The Surgeon General's Report on Health Promotion and Disease Prevention* (HEW, 1979b) suggest that our 700-fold increase in health spending over the past 20 years has not yielded the striking improvement that we might have hoped. Much of the expenditures have been directed toward the treatment of disease and disability after their occurrence rather than toward their prevention.

The third measure of medical care is accessibility. More Americans today have access to better care than ever. However, the distribution of physicians and the proportion devoted to primary care leave room for improvement. There is an overabundance of physicians concentrated about tertiary and secondary medical care facilities, with too few in a community setting providing primary care. Remote and rural areas and inner-city communities are underprovided. The problem of maldistribution of medical personnel in the United States has not yet been resolved. Overall, however, most will agree that good quality health care is accessible to the great majority of people. Unfortunately, we cannot look with the same pride at what has happened to the other measure, the cost of health care.

What Constitutes Reasonable Cost?

It is difficult to place a price tag on health. How much is good health worth? To the very wealthy, it might be worth a fortune; to the derelict on skid row, it might not be worth a pint of cheap wine. For the unfortunate many with chronic or incurable disease, good health may not be a commodity that can be purchased for any price.

The idealist and humanitarian may argue that health care is not a commodity, it is a right; that no amount of money or effort should be spared to provide the best possible care to the last breath for all, regardless of their ability to pay, regardless of their potential for a productive life. The pragmatist will point out that health care is a commodity; it is bought and sold; money is involved. As a commodity, it is subject to certain rules of economics. One of these is "The Law of Increasing Relative Costs" that states that when a family is forced to pay an ever-increasing proportion of its income in order to get equal amounts of one good (health care), it must sacrifice ever-increasing amounts of another good (food, shelter, clothing). The poor outnumber the rich. Food and shelter hold a higher priority in their hierarchy of needs than does health care. The poor may be forced to seek inferior care or do without any care at all.

Two economic aphorisms should be acknowledged when dealing with health care costs. The first is that "There is no such thing as a free lunch." Someone has to pay the bill, and eventually it trickles down to the consumer. This includes all of us. We pay this bill through higher taxes, higher cost of living, and less take-home pay. The second maxim is "The man who pays the piper calls the tune." The government pays 50%, industry 35%, and the individual 15% of the direct health care expenditures. Government and industry will be calling the tunes more and more, in the near future.

Health care has a price, and this price has been rising at a frightening pace. All should be keenly aware that this is happening. We should take a good, hard look at where we have been, where we are now, and where we are headed. We need to know the cause, the effect, and the cure. The day is fast approaching when our economy cannot afford this tremendous burden. The people will be unwilling to pay the price.

The Change in Health Care Costs

In 1950, the per capita expenditure for health care in this country was $83. Only three decades later it had climbed to $1,067, and it is predicted to reach $3,000 by 1990. Figure 15-1 graphically shows what has happened to health care costs. This nation's spending for health care in 1950 was $12.7 billion, or 4.2% of the Gross National Product (GNP). By 1980, the total national expenditure had spiraled to $247.2 billion, or 9.4% of the GNP. Of that amount, approximately 41% was spent on hospitals, 19% on physician fees, 9% on nursing homes, and 32% on other services such as den-

tist fees, drugs, and medical supplies. Between 1950 and 1980, the GNP increased by 918.1%, the cost of hospital care by 2,586.3%, and the cost of physician services rose 1,623.6%. The total health care bill for the nation increased by 1,950.7%, more than twice as fast as the GNP (*Source Book of Health Insurance Data 1979-1980*).

Health care costs are now doubling every five years. The Health Care Financing Administration has predicted that by the year 2000, the costs will total $2.1 trillion, and by the year 2005 will reach $4.2 trillion. Even though America is a prosperous nation, many have grave doubts that this country can carry such a burden on its back. In order that these astronomical costs can be seen in proper perspective, it should be noted that the total federal tax receipts for fiscal year 1978 were only $297.5 billion, and that the total national debt, incurred over many years, is approaching $1 trillion. There is good reason to be concerned and alarmed about these predictions. Our survival as a nation can depend on the soundness of our economy. We need to weigh the costs and the

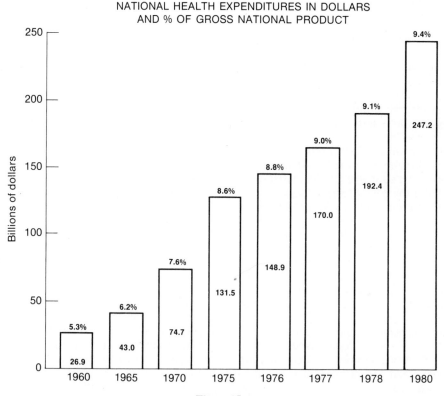

NATIONAL HEALTH EXPENDITURES IN DOLLARS
AND % OF GROSS NATIONAL PRODUCT

Figure 15-1

benefits of our present health care system. We need to restructure some of our priorities and some of our moral values. We need to correct extravagances, overutilization, and waste. We may need to set a course that will take us in a slightly different direction.

Economic burdens of this magnitude affect everyone, and they evoke strong emotional responses that often are not rational. We have a great need to place the blame on someone for our sad plight. We need to point the accusing finger at the guilty party, and usually the direction of the point is away from ourselves. Industry blames labor; labor blames government; government blames the physicians; physicians blame the insurance carriers; the insurance carriers blame the hospitals; the hospitals blame inflation; we all blame the politicians; but none of us blame ourselves! The real truth of the matter is that we all share this blame. It is equally true that the problem is of such magnitude, and such urgency, that it will require the cooperative efforts of all of us who contributed to the problem for its resolution. Only in this way can we avoid becoming the victims of our own preconceptions, prejudices, and special interests.

THE CAUSE

Let us examine what part each of the contributors has played in the causation of this enormous problem and what is their fair share of the guilt.

Price and Quantity

Two factors determine the total cost of producing any goods or service: the unit price and the quantity of the goods produced or the service rendered. This is true of health care. Provide more service, or serve more people, and the total cost rises. Increase the unit price of the component services, and the cost also rises. Price rise has been the primary force behind the huge growth of health care expenditures in the United States. It is estimated that this factor contributed 63% of the rise between 1969 and 1978. Price controls, imposed during the Economic Stabilization Program, were in effect during part of this period, August 1971 through April 1974, and were briefly successful in holding down health care spending. The controls were lifted in 1974, and during the period of 1974 to 1978, prices shot up at an even faster rate and accounted for 80% of the rise in medical costs.

Increased utilization and changes in the health care product caused 25% of the rise in costs for the years 1977 and 1978. The rapid growth of third-party payment removed the economic impediment and made health care more accessible to lower income groups. Insurance encourages increased utilization and creates a greater demand for higher quality care. Utilization increased with age because the elderly have more sickness and experience longer hospital stays. Medicare and Medicaid, which became effective in 1966, provided more health care for the elderly and the poor, who had been previously underserved. In recent years the population has been shifting toward the older age groups. These factors have had significant impact on both the price and the quantity of health care.

Population

It is obvious that a nation growing in population cannot continue to provide the same quality and quantity of health care for each citizen without increasing the total health care bill. During 1980, as the population increased by 1.05%, 2.3 million more people became recipients of medical care in the United States, and the total population reached 228.8 million. In the earlier years, between 1950 and 1965, the population of this country was increasing at a more rapid rate of 1.6% a year, which at that time accounted for about 21% of the increased health care costs for that period. Since 1965, however, there has been a deceleration of the population growth in this nation to an average annual rate of 0.9%. As a result, the population increase has played a less significant role in the rising costs of medical care, accounting for only 6.5% of the increase for the period from 1965 to 1977.

Population growth holds a much greater concern for the world than the increase it causes in health care costs. Scientific advances in medicine and public health have brought about increased fertility, improved infant mortality, and prolongation of human life. Such advances have interfered with pestilence, famine, and war, all previously serving as more significant checks on population growth. As a result, the global population has increased 489% since 1800 to its present 4.89 billion persons, with a promise of reaching 6.09 billion by the turn of the century. If these bioscientific advances which lengthen the life-span are not accompanied by increased productivity, the fear of Malthus takes on new relevance. Overpopulation brings with it limited food supply, crowded living conditions, inadequate medical resources, and rising crimes of violence. The medical profession has a responsibility to share in the solution of these problems which have arisen in part, from their successes.

Shifting Population

Just as scientific advances in medicine and public health have contributed to the population explosion, so too have they caused a shift in the demographic pattern toward the older age groups. This has had significant impact on the increasing health care costs. More Americans live to an older age today than ever. Figure 15-2 shows this change from the middle of the century, as well as the projected change for the near future. Such demographic shifts bring with them both social and biological problems. The proportion of people with sickness and disability increases with age since the elderly are more likely to suffer from multiple, chronic, and disabling diseases.

In 1977, the per capita personal health care expenditure for people over 65 years of age was $1,745.17, or 3.4 times the $514.25 for those under 15 years of age. The elderly account for 28.9% of the total expenditure, although they constitute only 11% of the population. In 1977, the hospital discharge rate per 1,000 population for those 65 years or over was 374.4, while the rate for those under 65 years was only 145.1. The length of hospital stay for this group 65 years and over was almost twice as long, 11.1 days compared to 6.2 days for those under 65 years (U.S. Department of Health and Human Services, 1981). The projected further increase in older citizens in this nation to 50 million, or 17% of the population, by the year 2030 should serve as a stimulus for greater efforts toward the prevention or delay of the chronic diseases of the elderly, both for humanitarian and economic reasons.

Inflation

Prices of almost everything have risen over the past three decades, and health care has not been immune to these changes. The specter of inflation is the most serious problem facing the nation today. Continued high rates over the next decade will pose a serious threat to society

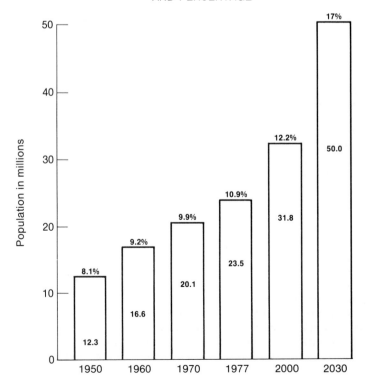

POPULATION 65 YEARS AND OVER BY NUMBERS AND PERCENTAGE

Figure 15-2

as we know it. The rate of inflation has been rising steadily, even as the growth of the real GNP has been slowing. Certainly the easiest culprit to finger as the cause of rising health care costs is inflation. It erodes the buying power of every dollar we earn to a point where our current dollar will buy less than half of what it would ten years ago. As the cost of living increases, so will hospital charges, doctor's fees, and druggist bills. We cannot underestimate the importance of inflation in escalating costs. However, inflation cannot be blamed as the sole cause for our predicament. Actually, its impact on health care costs has declined over the past five years, while the impact of intensity (frequency and quality) of care has doubled. For the twelve-month period ending March, 1974, price increases accounted for 80% of the expenditure growth, while increase in frequency and quality of care was responsible for 14% of the overall growth. Just three years later, in March, 1977, these figures were 66% for inflation and 28% for intensity (Health Care Financing Trends, Fall, 1979).

The causes of inflation are many. Just as the responsibility for rising health care costs must be shared by all, so too must the blame for inflation be allocated to its contributors. We all share a portion of the blame as employers, workers, producers, consumers, and borrowers, albeit to varying degrees. Let us look at some of the major contributors.

Monetary Policy. The monetarists hold that "inflation is at all times and everywhere a monetary phenomenon." They look to the Federal Reserve Board for the source and remedy of inflation. The Board does control the money supply and the credit growth. They decide how much money will be circulated by selling government securities, collecting the money, and placing it in reserve if they wish to decrease the money supply. Conversely, if they choose to buy government securities on the open market, the money payments made decrease the reserve and increase the money supply. In this way their monetary policy determines whether it will be easy or difficult to borrow money. The tighter the money, the higher the interest rates, and this, in turn, lowers the demand and brings down inflation. The Federal Reserve remains the dominant inflation fighter and is, perhaps, the most important determinant of the level of employment, productivity, and purchasing power.

Ideally, money supply should grow at the same rate as the growth of our GNP. Over the past 10 years, the money growth has accelerated to a 9.5% average annual rate, far outstripping the 2.8% growth in the nation's output of goods and services. The money supply has been increased by the Board to fund the federal deficit, providing additional money to pay for programs it could not pay for out of tax revenue. This has diluted the value of the dollar and has shrunk its buying power, until the 1967 dollar is now worth less than 45¢. Any efforts to bring the money supply under control will be insufficient unless federal spending is curtailed to stay within the bounds of the public's willingness to foot the bill through higher taxes. Nonmonetarists would assign less blame to the Federal Reserve Board for inflation.

Fiscal Policy. Annual federal budget deficits have been recorded in 20 of the last 21 years, with an average annual deficit of $61 billion during the last five years. Budget deficits first ballooned as a result of the Vietnam War. The "guns and butter" philosophy of the "Great Society" fostered mounting deficits for war, while expanding social programs, without sufficient increases in taxes to pay for them. This passed the financial burden on to future generations and triggered the inflation spiral. A "psychology of entitlement" developed wherein people feel that society has the responsibility to supply their needs with little regard as to who will pay for them. The big increases in federal outlays came in transfer payments to individuals under Social Security, unemployment insurance, and welfare benefits. Entitlement programs have increased by $270 billion over the past decade and now account for 60% of the federal budget. Some of these programs have been worthy, but they were adopted with little or no thought of future costs. Their adoption was good politics but bad economics. Increased taxes to pay for these increased governmental expenditures can affect the economy by serving as a disincentive to savings and capital investment.

In addition, authorization and appropriation committees in Congress, and agencies within the government, have intentionally exaggerated their requests for money in order to protect themselves against later cuts. There has been budget discipline in appearance only. The budgetary process is a part of any fiscal policy.

The Consumer's Role in Inflation. The consumer has been making ever-increasing demands for more goods and services. These demands have outpaced the supply, and prices have gone up with a resultant wage-price spiral.

The consumer's spending spree has used up money that would have been better saved to provide funds for investment in plants and equipment to increase productivity. The ratio of savings to disposable personal income in the United States is now less than one third of that of other major industrial countries. Much of this consumer-spending spree involved credit cards, time payments, and borrowed money which further fueled inflation. Although the past three decades have brought vast gains in consumer well-being as measured by income, employment, and material possessions, much of the progress may well have only constituted borrowing from the future. The consumer warrants his fair share of the responsibility for inflation.

Productivity. For a 20-year period ending in 1968, productivity in this country grew at a rate of 3% a year. This increase translated into a higher living standard for all of us. Now the United States, once the leader in productivity, has plummeted to ninth place in productivity growth among the leading Western nations. Lagging productivity decreases the supply of goods and services and thus raises prices, which fuels inflation.

Labor becomes more productive if workers become more skilled, have more capital and advanced technology at their disposal, or if the workplace is more efficiently organized. Capital becomes more productive if it eliminates waste and obsolescence, or if it improves its technology through research and development. There have been an influx of young and inexperienced workers into the labor force and a decrease in the work ethic. In addition, restrictive labor rules have lowered production. In 1977 it was estimated that the average hours of work paid for exceeded the hours actually worked by 7.6 hours per week. Capital has not kept pace with obsolescence or the necessary research and development. Both of these factors have contributed to our decreasing productivity.

Although the nation's productivity had grown at a rate of 3.2% annually from 1948 to 1966, it then began to decrease to an annual rate of 2.1% between 1966 and 1973, and to less than 1% since then. At present, it is stationary at 0% increase. Capital, labor, and government all play a vital role in creating goods and services. There has not been the close cooperative effort among these three that is necessary to maximize productivity. The resultant decrease has added significantly to the problem of inflation.

Government Regulations. Excessive government regulation has greatly increased the costs of goods we buy. The buyer pays $600 more for the average automobile, and $2,000 more for the average home, because of government regulations concerning safety, energy, and environment. It is estimated that government regulation cost each man, woman, and child $500 in 1979. These are hidden added costs of government which do not appear in the federal budget, which are not appropriated by Congress, but which are imposed on the private sector by virtue of government rules and regulations. These hidden costs also affect the price tag for health care. It was estimated in the hospitals of New York in 1976 that the costs of coping with government regulations added $24 to the daily bill of each patient, or a total of $1 billion. Virtually every industry has become a regulated industry. The extra work and red tape of compliance have boosted the cost of doing business significantly.

Some of the agencies and government policies that influence our everyday lives and the cost of every product we buy are Occupational Safety and Health Administration (OSHA), Employee Retirement Income Security Act (ERISA), Equal Employment Opportunity (EEO), Internal Revenue Service (IRS), Department of Health and Human Services (H&HS), Social Security (SS), Federal Trade Commission (FTC), Department of Energy (DOE), and the Department of Justice. All of these agencies supposedly have our interests at heart. They promote health and safety, protect us from exploitation, make sure we breathe clean air and drink safe water, and get us more miles per gallon of gasoline. Many of these regulations have merit for they improve the quality of our lives and justify their costs. Others do not. They are the product of bureaucracy with little thought as to whether they are worth the time, effort, and money that they consume. A good example is the recent revision by OSHA of the new antinoise standards, the cost of which is estimated to be $10.5 billion. The cost to engineer the reduction in the level of noise from 90 to 85 decibels in the workplace will be about $20,000 per worker. The same amount of protection could be provided by earmuffs for $10 per worker.

In addition, the various federal agencies often work against each other. The Department of Health and Human Services endorses health care cost containment. When physicians' organizations attempt to take steps to curtail high fees, or institute Peer Review Committees, the

Federal Trade Commission views this as restraint of trade. This Commission obtained a court order that barred the governing board of a state medical society from initiating or participating in health care cost containment in the state's Medicaid Program and with all health insurance carriers. If insurance companies attempt to work with medical associations toward the same end, the Justice Department is apt to consider this conspiracy and collusion. As a result, medical societies have been forced to retreat from activity aimed at reducing price gouging by doctors. Yet, without physician involvement there can be no containment of health care costs. The Department of H&HS wants to cap growth of the physician supply through curtailment of subsidies to medical, dental, and other professional schools, and by restricting the further entry into the United States of foreign-trained physicians. At the same time, the FTC has conducted an investigation to determine whether the medical profession's control over medical school accreditation constitutes a "conspiracy in restraint of trade." The FTC wishes to lift the ban on physician advertising. H&HS forbids hospitals, nursing homes, and home care agencies from engaging in advertising to stimulate use of their facilities.

The list of inconsistencies could be greatly expanded. Regulatory strategies often have had an effect directly opposite to that intended. There is great need for these agencies to coordinate their activities in order to eliminate these conflicting strategies which perpetuate the escalation of inflation and health care costs. This is not to say that government should not be involved in these issues. They pay out about 50% of this nation's expenditures for health care. They have, therefore, both a duty and an obligation to the taxpayers to see that these funds are spent wisely and well. Scrutiny of the cost and quality of health care will require some regulation and monitoring.

Labor

Labor is one of the three contributors to the production of goods, along with capital and natural resources. It deserves great credit for this country's rapid industrial growth. However, labor must also bear its share of responsibility for many of the problems of this nation, including inflation and high health care costs.

Through collective bargaining, organized labor has been responsible for much of the strong steady upward trend in real wages over the past several decades. This has increased the price of goods and contributed to the inflation problem. Some demands of the labor unions have been constructive, while others have interfered with industrial productivity. Explicit union limitation of work loads, such as the number of bricks a mason may lay, the width of the brush that a painter may use, and the requirement of standby workers have all increased the price of labor and have decreased the nation's productivity.

The impact of organized labor on health care costs has been significant. At the bargaining table they have demanded comprehensive health insurance plans with first-dollar coverage with no employee participation through coinsurance. Their aim has been to have union members pay as little out-of-pocket money as possible for medical care. As a result, employers now pay about 85¢ of every dollar for group health insurance. This has removed about 85 million workers from having any responsibility for, or feeling any pain from, excessive medical bills. As a result, patients, hospitals, physicians, and other providers have acted as if medical care had a zero cost without any limits to the amount of funds available for health care.

Industry

Business has become a sizable purchaser of health care services, spending about $60 billion on health care for employees and their dependents in 1981. General Motors, for example, has seen costs of employee health benefits increase from $38 million in 1960 to $1.4 billion in 1979. The cost per employee during that period rose from $84 to $2,285. The added cost for health care per vehicle produced has grown from $10 to $219. This has made General Motors' health insurance provider its largest supplier of services measured in dollars, even larger than U.S. Steel. Health care, next to energy, is industry's biggest cost of doing business. This same costly scenario could be written for thousands of other corporations throughout this nation.

How did industry end up in such a predicament? At the bargaining table they repeatedly acquiesced to labor's demands for more and better health care coverage. They accepted union requests for comprehensive health insurance with first-dollar coverage, with little out-of-pocket cost to labor. Their willingness to do this was increased by the fact that these fringe benefits would be tax free to their employees and tax deductible to them. In 1977, the average annual premium for health insurance per employee was $590, of which the employer paid $501 and the worker $89. This amounted to 82¢ of every health insurance dollar in industry being paid for by the employer. Indeed, corporations have provided a powerful impetus for escalating health care costs by essentially removing the individual from sharing the pain of high medical bills. In essence they have given away the shop by bargaining for the benefit, rather than for a dollar amount, and by so doing, they lost control over the cost of delivery of the service. Health benefits have continued to increase to a point where the average cost per worker is now $1,200 to $1,400. Now companies justifiably want out. They are instituting cost-containment programs, tightening up on disability reviews, and actively participating in business coalitions whose purpose is to lower health care costs. Industry really incurs triple payment when it comes to illness. First, they pay the giant's share of the health insurance premiums; second, they continue to pay salary or disability payments during the illness; and third, they shoulder the indirect costs of disability such as turnover, training, and replacement costs.

Insurance Companies

About 35% of the total health care cost is paid for by insurance carriers. Third-party payers pay 93% of all hospital charges and 66% of all physicians' bills. Over 1,200 private insurance companies provide health coverage for over 103 million persons, with premium income in excess of $61 billion (*Source Book of Health Insurance Data 1979-1980*).

The insurance companies, as paymasters, must join labor and industry as the third member of the triad in sharing their portion of the blame for rising health care costs. The insurance industry has bowed to the demands of the marketplace. Labor asked, industry gave, and insurance companies provided comprehensive coverage with little to no deductibles and no coinsurance. As a result, patients used and overused health services with little concern as to their costs. Insurance companies have anesthetized the consumer to the rising cost of health care. Without direct vested interest in paying the bills, the consumer has failed to recognize the consequences of the escalating costs. Until recently, insurance companies' main concern was with volume sales. Too little emphasis was placed on the quality of business, the economic soundness of the policy provisions, on tight claims control, or the need to bring the patient into the picture with a sizable deduction. As a result, health insurance carriers have lost millions of dollars and now must take drastic action to prevent further losses.

Each year increases in premiums for health insurance have been assessed; and each year health care costs have managed to outpace these best estimates of the actuaries by at least several percentage points. Increases have ranged from 10% to 60%, and yet they still rise. Monthly premiums for comprehensive health insurance for a family of three are in excess of $250 to $300. Few people can afford such coverage. The national averages speak of 12 to 15% increases in cost, yet many carriers are experiencing annual increases in claims costs in excess of 28%. Some companies and plans face serious financial problems; others are withdrawing from the marketplace. If this trend continues, all will suffer. A large uninsured population in any area is not a healthy situation for patients, hospitals, or physicians. Even though some hospitals and physicians have perceived the insurance funds as bottomless wells, these wells are beginning to run dry.

Insurance companies have made other costly mistakes in addition to succumbing to the marketplace. The abandonment of the fixed-fee schedule for operative procedures and the adoption of the "usual, customary, and reasonable" fee in its place have been costly. Young physicians, knowledgeable of the system, submitted high fees from the beginning, thus establishing their "usual" fee at a high level. Many companies use the 80th or 90th percentile to determine the "customary and reasonable" fee. This has skewed the fees to the higher end of the profile or spectrum and has encouraged fees to go even higher. Payment at the 50th percentile would have been a wiser choice.

There is much truth in the observation that "As long as third party payers are willing to pay the bill, no decrease in health care costs will occur." There need to be closer claims reviews, more auditing of hospital bills, and a general tightening of claims payments. Although the percentage of providers who habitually overcharge is relatively small, the total excessive fees they generate is large. For this reason, there is a need for insurance companies to work closely with physician peer review committees, hospital associations, and state licensing boards to deal with those who habitually overcharge. Such cooperative efforts require that the encumbrances which have been imposed by the FTC and the Justice Department be removed.

Health Care Industry

The health care industry is big business from whatever perspective one views it. The industry consumes many dollars—247.2 billion in 1980. Once a cottage industry of individual doctors and charity-supported hospitals, it has become one of the largest and fastest growing industries in the United States, accounting for roughly $1 of every $10 spent in this country. The industry employs many people—6.7 million in 1978. This number has been growing at a rapid rate, 60% between 1970 and 1978, while the total number of employed persons in the nation grew only 20.1%. One out of every seven jobs created during that same period was in the health industry, with 7% of the work force employed in the health field (U.S. Department of Health, Education, and Welfare, 1979). A new medical-industrial complex has been created to take advantage of a lucrative opportunity. Charges for diagnostic tests now amount to $15 billion each year. Prescription drugs manufactured for worldwide sales bring in about $22 billion per year.

We will now turn our attention to some of the individual sectors that work within this large industry and examine what part they have played in the escalation of health care costs. Because more than one half of all persons in the health care industry work in hospitals, this is a good place to start our examination (See Figure 15-3.)

Hospitals. Hospitals have experienced the same operating problems as have other businesses: inflation, high energy costs, federal regulations, declining government funding, increasing public demands for services, and decreasing productivity of labor. Some of their problems, however, are of their own making and arise from the "empire impulse." Each individual and each organization have an inherent urge to build an empire, and hospitals are not immune to this malady. They add more beds that cannot be filled, they acquire new technology which they cannot economically support, and they provide new facilities in excess of community needs. Each hospital covets its own renal dialysis unit, its own heart-lung machine, the latest in radiation equipment, the most modern computer scanner, and the latest imaging equipment. Each tries to keep up with or outdo its neighbor hospital. As a result, hospitals acquire duplicate equipment which is only needed on occasion, but may be used excessively to justify its possession and make it a money-making income producer. This overuse adds greatly to hospital costs. Hospitals are reluctant to decrease their size, their services, or their importance. They suffer from this human frailty. Hospital utilization and costs will now be examined in some detail.

HOSPITAL UTILIZATION. In 1978 about 94,500 people entered community hospitals as patients each day. There were 3.5 million admissions in that year with about one out of every six Americans requiring hospitalization. The daily total hospital census in short-term hospitals is about 718,335 patients (*Source Book of Health Insurance Data 1979-1980*). These figures are large, but it is important to realize that only 2% of all medical care is rendered in a hospital setting. This 2%, however, consumes 55% of the national health expenditures. This imbalance is further accentuated by the estimate that in any given year, half of this nation's hospital resources are spent on only 1.3% of the population. Thirteen per cent of the hospitalized patients account for as much of the hospital billings as do the other 87%. This is a mathematical way of saying that much of the money spent for hospital care goes for chronic and terminal illnesses which require repeated and extended periods of hospitalization.

In 1972, there were 33.3 million discharges from all short-stay hospitals. By 1977, this figure had increased to 36.8 million, an 11% increase. The number of days of care for that same period increased by 6%, from 274.3 to 301.9 million. During this period, the population increase was about 4%. The average hospital stay decreased from 8.2 days to 7.9 days. Actually the increase in hospital utilization is very small when one considers the population increase and the demographic shift to the older age groups during that period. This strongly suggests that the increases in hospital costs stem principally from price increases and an increase in the number of ancillary tests and procedures performed per patient.

Socioeconomic status affects hospital utilization. Persons in the lower income groups have a greater utilization and longer hospital stays. In 1972, the lowest income group had 45% more hospital discharges than the highest income group. By 1977, this had increased to 69% more discharges. In addition, the lowest income group stayed in the hospital 2.4 more days.

The nonmetropolitan areas of the nation had a 15% higher utilization as measured by the discharge rate, but showed 1.8 fewer days of

INFLATION OF THE HEALTH CARE DOLLAR

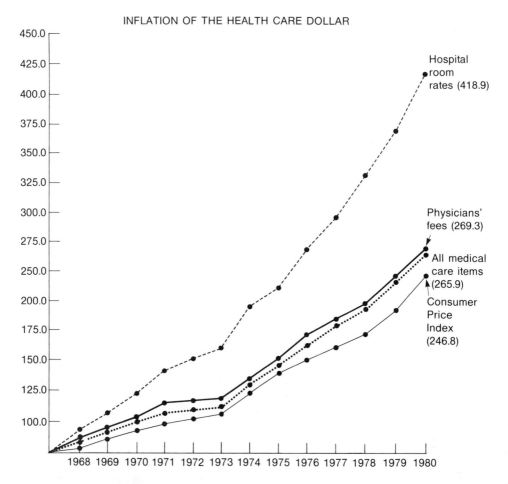

While the **consumer price index** has gone from the 100.0 base in 1967 to 246.8 in 1979, **medical care** has increased to 265.9 in the same time span.

Leading this climb in increased medical expense has been the rise in **hospital room rates** which have increased at a rate more than one and three-fifths times that of the overall C.P.I.

Physicians' fees have followed the trend of rising health care costs but at a rate slightly higher than the overall trend.

Continued increases in consumer price indices for medical care have been the result of higher hospital operating and construction costs, as well as the extensive tests run on inpatient admits.

**CONSUMER PRICE INDICES
FOR MEDICAL CARE ITEMS**
(1967 = 100.0)

Figure 15-3. (Courtesy Group Division, Mutual of Omaha.)

stay in the hospital than the metropolitan group. Older people also have a higher utilization rate as well as a longer average length of stay.

HOSPITAL COSTS. The total operating cost of community hospitals in 1973 was $28.4 billion. By 1978, this had increased by 105% to $58.2 billion, with a 13% increase over the previous year. The escalating costs were gathering momentum. Prior to 1973, the annual rate of increase was less than 11%, by 1978, it was 13%, and for the twelve-month period ending October, 1981, it had zoomed to 15.4%. In 1950, the total hospital care costs for this country were only $3.9 billion, or 30.4% of the total health care bill. By 1978, this figure had climbed to $76 billion, or 39.5% of the total expenditure for health.

The average cost per hospital stay in 1969 was $533. In just nine years this average had climbed to $1,686.40. National averages, however, understate the problem by leveling off the peaks and the valleys. The peaks in hospital bills can be astounding! Burn cases can generate hospital bills in excess of $1 million, neonatal care bills in excess of $100,000, and organ transplants can generate bills to dwarf these. The average costs also vary considerably by state. (See Figure 15-4.) For a one-year period, starting from April, 1980, the costs of running California's 550 acute care hospitals increased 17.7%, occupancy rate increased about 2%, average patient costs on discharge jumped 16.2% to $2,861, the average cost per day rose to $411, and the average cost of an outpatient visit was $82.

A second way to analyze changes in hospital cost is by room rates (Figure 15-5). In 1950, a semiprivate room cost about $30 a day. Since 1965, room rates have increased an average of 12.9% per year. The national average cost per day had grown to $143.85 as of January, 1981. This represented a 36% increase over 1978 (U.S. Department of Health, Education and Welfare, 1979a). The daily rates also vary by geographical area. The West had the highest average at $153, while the lowest per diem rate was in the South at $107. The State of Mississippi ranked the lowest among the states at $78 per day. Alaska had the highest rate, variously estimated to be between $190 and $425, depending on which survey you believe. Again, averages are deceptive. Intensive care beds can generate costs from $500 to $1,000 per day, depending on whether they are for postoperative, coronary, or neonatal care. Studies have shown that the principal reason for admitting a patient to a special care unit was for monitoring rather than for intensive nursing care. Is all of this monitoring necessary and worth the dollars charged? Florida's perinatal care program for newborn intensive care units has experienced costs close to $1,000 per day per infant in level III care beds. An average of $20,000 is spent for the first three weeks of care for a newborn life in their intensive care units.

The rise in hospital costs cannot be blamed on longer periods of hospitalizaion, for this is the only figure that seems to be decreasing. In 1973, the average length of stay in a community hospital was 7.8 days. By 1978, the period of stay had been reduced to 7.6 days. This very modest, yet significant, improvement resulted from more sophisticated medical care and more patients being discharged earlier to convalesce at home. The duration of hospital stay does vary considerably among the states and regions. There seems to be an increasing length of stay as one moves eastward. Utah and Wyoming had the shortest average stay at 5.2 days, while New York State had the longest at 9.7 days. When a comparison was made of the lengths of stay in hospitals in Portland, Oregon, and Baltimore, Maryland, it was found that Portland showed consistently shorter lengths of stays for almost every category of disease: 5.6 days less for uncomplicated acute myocardial infarctions, 4.4 days less for congestive heart failure, 4.5 days less for ischemic heart disease, and 2.5 days less for cataract surgery. Lengths of hospital stays are physician related. A cooperative physician-based effort is absolutely necessary for effective control of hospital overutilization.

EXCESSIVE HOSPITAL BEDS. Another contributing cause for the rise in hospital costs is excessive hospital beds. The national guidelines as set by the Department of Health, Education, and Welfare are slightly less than 4 beds per 1,000 population, with at least 80% occupancy. In 1940, the number of beds in community hospitals in the nation averaged 3.2 per 1,000. The Hill-Burton Act of 1946 was passed to alleviate this shortage. It provided federal funds for the construction of health facilities and stimulated the growth of new and larger community hospitals and increased the total number of hospital beds. By 1977, the number of beds increased 44% and the ratio stood at 4.6 beds per 1,000. The shortage of beds now had turned into the new problem of an excess of beds. Currently, the number of excess beds in this country is variously estimated to be between 68,000 and 83,000 beds, and the occupancy rate is 77%. Washington, D.C., has a marked excess at 7.2 beds per 1,000.

Unoccupied beds cost almost as much (80%) to maintain as occupied beds. The capital investment must be amortized, and the continuing overhead must be paid. This is accomplished by increasing the per diem cost of each occupied bed. The patients pay for the unoccupied beds as well as the beds used. These excess beds add more than $2 billion each year to the nation's hospital bills.

Short-stay hospitals make up about 80% of all beds in this country, with about 90% of these being in community hospitals. These beds can

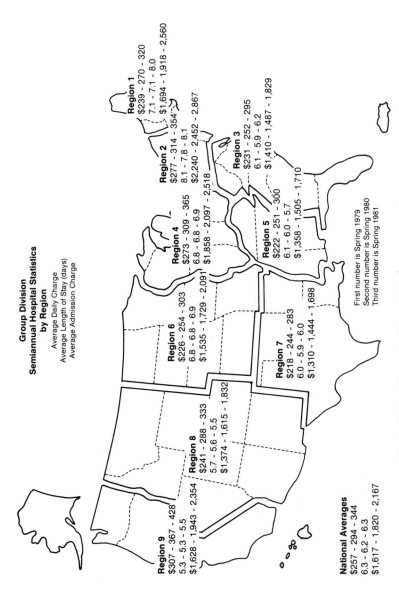

**Group Division
Semiannual Hospital Statistics
by Region**
Average Daily Charge
Average Length of Stay (days)
Average Admission Charge

Region 1
$239 - 270 - 320
7.1 - 7.1 - 8.0
$1,694 - 1,918 - 2,560

Region 2
$277 - 314 - 354
8.1 - 7.8 - 8.1
$2,240 - 2,452 - 2,867

Region 3
$231 - 252 - 295
6.1 - 5.9 - 6.2
$1,410 - 1,487 - 1,829

Region 4
$273 - 309 - 365
6.8 - 6.8 - 6.9
$1,858 - 2,097 - 2,518

Region 5
$222 - 251 - 300
6.1 - 6.0 - 5.7
$1,358 - 1,505 - 1,710

Region 6
$226 - 254 - 303
6.8 - 6.8 - 6.9
$1,535 - 1,729 - 2,091

Region 7
$218 - 244 - 283
6.0 - 5.9 - 6.0
$1,310 - 1,444 - 1,698

Region 8
$241 - 288 - 333
5.7 - 5.6 - 5.5
$1,374 - 1,615 - 1,832

Region 9
$307 - 367 - 428
5.3 - 5.3 - 5.5
$1,628 - 1,943 - 2,354

First number is Spring 1979
Second number is Spring 1980
Third number is Spring 1981

National Averages
$257 - 294 - 344
6.3 - 6.2 - 6.3
$1,617 - 1,820 - 2,167

Figure 15-4. (Courtesy Group Division, Mutual of Omaha.)

288

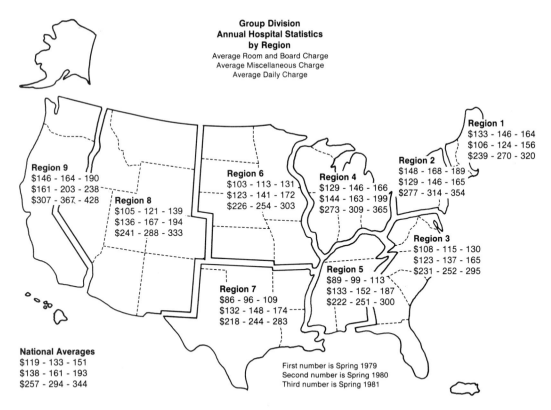

Figure 15-5. (Courtesy Group Division, Mutual of Omaha.)

be further broken down into 56% as community nonprofit, 30% run by state or local government, and 14% proprietary. The number of
these short-stay beds increased at an annual
rate of 1.6% between 1972 and 1977. This
trend needs to be reversed.

The number of long-stay hospitals, principally government-owned psychiatric hospitals,
has actually decreased from 757 in 1972 to 597
in 1977. The cause of this decrease has been the
outpatient treatment of psychiatric patients
made possible by the newer psychotherapeutic
drugs. There are some who feel that this progress may have been a step backward.

Extreme examples of the hospital bed excess
are a government hospital in the South with a
250-bed capacity, which has never had more
than 50 patients, and the metropolitan hospital
in a depressed section of a city that cost $200
million to build, but has never had a single
patient because it would cost $350 a day to stay
there.

LABOR COSTS. A significant portion of
hospital costs go for labor. In 1978, these costs
represented 49.7% of hospital expenditures and

totaled $28.9 billion. However, when expressed
as a percentage of expenditures, payroll costs
have been claiming a smaller share. In 1962,
they constituted 61.9% of total costs. For the
period of 1965 to 1977, labor costs rose at an
annual rate of 11%, while the nonlabor component increased at a faster rate of 15.3%.

It is interesting to note that the ratio of hospital employees to patient has been increasing at
a steady rate. In 1960, the ratio was 1.5 employees per patient. By 1965, this had increased
to 2.24 per patient; and by 1977, it had risen to
3.15 to 1. This increase in employee-to-patient
ratio resulted from the increasing technical
complexity of hospital care. Laboratories required more highly trained technicians and sci-
entists. Intensive care units demanded larger
staffs. These changes in personnel when combined with higher wages, upgrading of workers'
skills, and shortening of the workweek have all
contributed to higher payroll costs. At the same
time, nonpayroll expenses were rising due to
the purchase of more sophisticated equipment,
higher amortization costs, higher service and
maintenance costs.

IMPROVED TECHNOLOGY. One of the most important causes for the rise in hospital and health care costs is the cost of the great scientific advances that have been made in the equipment available for diagnosis and treatment. The past decade has seen tremendous progress in health care technology. These new modalities have added billions of dollars to the cost of medical care for services that never before were available: organ transplants, renal dialysis, laser beams, computerized axial tomography (CAT), echocardiography, fetal monitoring, xerography, isotopic scanning, nuclear magnetic resonance, sophisticated computer systems to name only a few. The average cost of a CAT scanner is about $700,000, and an echocardiograph machine can cost in excess of $100,000. This new and more complicated technology has required more skilled and more highly trained technicians to operate the equipment. This has brought increases to the salary budget.

These technological advances have refined and improved our diagnostic and therapeutic capabilities, and they have prolonged the lives of many. No one would suggest a step backward. It is not the legitimate use of such instruments that requires curtailment. It is the un-necessary proliferation, the duplication of equipment, and the overutilization of these devices that warrant our concern. Health care technology can be overutilized and can become unreasonable both medically and economically when its use is not tempered with judgment.

ANCILLARY HOSPITAL SERVICES. About 29¢ of every health dollar goes for hospital room and board. Rising room rates have high visibility and are easily identified by all who have a concern for hospital costs. Hospitals are aware of this fact and use other billings to mask their charges as they search for alternate ways to meet their expenses. As a result, ancillary or miscellaneous services of hospitals consume 37¢ of every health dollar. (See Figure 15-6.) These high ancillary charges result from overutilization of modern technology and also from high markups for supplies and services.

It is difficult to understand why 50 to 100 blood gas analyses are required during the first day of admission of a newborn or a child on pediatric service, at a charge of $45 per test; why seven spinal taps with stains and cultures are needed in one day; why some drugs are marked up 2500%, or why a cotton ball should cost a dollar. Yet we see such charges all too

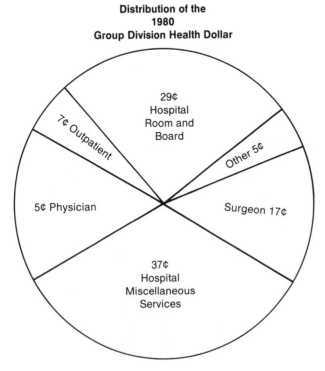

Distribution of the
1980
Group Division Health Dollar

29¢
Hospital
Room and
Board

7¢ Outpatient

Other 5¢

5¢ Physician

Surgeon 17¢

37¢
Hospital
Miscellaneous
Services

Figure 15-6. (Courtesy Group Division, Mutual of Omaha.)

frequently. Such practices do not arise out of medical necessity. One wonders whether or not they represent a philosophy, that borders on the dishonest, of "get ours while we can" as long as the third party will pay for them. Patients and treating physicians are unaware of these charges, for they rarely see the hospital bill. Large bills often contain thousands of dollars of charges for services never performed. One bill for neonatal hospital care of about $80,000 contained charges of $4,500 for services and laboratory procedures never provided (Lewis 1977). Routine audits of hospital charges return $1.83 for every dollar spent on the audit. But surely, it should not be necessary to routinely audit reputable hospitals that we entrust with our lives. It would be good policy perhaps if each attending physician were required to review every tenth hospital bill rendered to his patients. This would serve a dual purpose: make him aware of the high cost of unnecessary laboratory and ancillary services, and alert him to the frequent charges for services never rendered. Charges for diagnostic tests consume an appreciable portion of the health dollar, averaging about $15 billion a year.

HOSPITAL COST SHIFTING. A very serious problem for the health insurance industry has been the practice of "cost shifting." Losses experienced by hospitals from Medicare, Medicaid, and Blue Cross contracts have been made up by raising prices for cash-paying patients and their private insurance carriers.

The Medicare Act, Title XVIII, passed in 1965, provided for payment of hospital bills by the Social Security Administration on a *retrospective* hospital cost reimbursement plan plus 2% allowance as a profit or surplus payment over costs. The original intention was to pay costs in full. However, as the cost of hospital care rose, hospitals found that because of the retrospective plan, they were always falling behind in reimbursement from Medicare. In addition, the Social Security Administration began to disallow an increasing number of defined costs in an attempt to keep expenditures from increasing. The hospitals then began to shift these resultant losses to the private sector.

The Medicaid Program, jointly funded by federal and state funds, produced a similar experience to an even greater degree. They also began by paying regular billed charges. Gradually, some states switched to the retrospective reimbursement system of Medicare, with even more disallowed costs. Medicare and Medicaid

"cost shifting" in 1973 amounted to about $500 million. By 1979, it had increased to $3 billion; in 1981, it is estimated to have been $5 billion. This shortfall cost shifting is an indirect tax being paid by cash-paying patients and their insurance carriers to make up for Medicare and Medicaid deficiencies.

Blue Cross plans in most states have also adopted retrospective defined-cost reimbursement methods and thus pay less than fully billed charges and less than defined costs. Blue Cross plans also receive sizable cash discounts from hospitals in their service areas which adds to the cost-shift burden.

Cost shifting has caused hospital prices for many to escalate out of proportion to actual hospital costs. Although the stated national annual average increase in hospital cost is given as 15%, many insurance carriers are actually finding their hospital charges rising in excess of 28% annually. This growing disparity brought about by cost shifting is forcing major medical insurance carriers either to discontinue this type of coverage or raise the premiums to such a level that they are unaffordable. There should be equity in hospital prices with all paying on the same basis.

PROPRIETARY HOSPITALS. Medicare and Medicaid opened the floodgate of dollars for health care. American business was quick to respond to the opportunities in this lucrative field. As a result, a new complex of profit-seeking medical companies has emerged in the last decade. These corporations have invested in hospital chains, nursing homes, psychiatric clinics, diagnostic laboratories, emergency treatment centers, renal dialysis units, and home health aide providers—all engaged in supplying services once provided by nonprofit hospitals and agencies. There are now over 100 companies listed on the New York and American Stock Exchanges, with dozens more offered over-the-counter. This is now a $12-billion-a-year industry. More than 1,351 hospitals, or 19.3% of all hospitals in the United States, are owned by investors or operated by investor-owned management companies. Six large international corporations dominate the field with annual earnings increasing at a rate of 25 to 30%. It is predicted that by the year 1990, 70% of this nation's hospitals will be under some sort of multifacility management.

These companies insist that they are not adding to the cost of health care, even though they reap a sizable profit. They hold that all hospitals must make a profit if they are to stay in business. These corporations feel that they render quality care through efficient management, striving for cost effectiveness. This is done through labor management, bulk buying, systems control, and "better use of ancillary services which are highly profitable."

Their critics hold that profit making has no place in health care because it leads to cut-rate medicine of reduced quality. These companies "skim" the market and take only the best-paying and best-insured patients and refuse charity cases, which places a burden on the nonprofit hospitals. In addition, they are accused of offering only the profitable services and of leaving the nonprofit hospitals with the losers, such as emergency rooms and obstetrical services. Profit making does not lend itself to educational programs for interns, residents, and nurses. Longer hospital stays will result since they generate greater profits. If these indictments by their critics are true, we should see the development of a two-tiered hospital system: one for the privileged, and one for the underprivileged. It remains for the proprietary hospitals to demonstrate that they are not raising the cost of health care.

Physicians. The relative number of physicians has been increasing at a faster rate than the population of this nation. Between the years 1970 and 1979, the number grew by more than 51% to a total of 454,564. A large percentage of these doctors are in active practice. In 1977, 91% were professionally active. With the population of the country growing at a slower rate than the number of active physicians, the ratio of physicians to population has increased. It grew from 14.2 physicians per 10,000 population in 1950 to 17.9 per 10,000 in 1977. Most of this increase has been since 1960. The ratio continues to grow, and it is estimated that 7 additional physicians per 10,000 will be added by 1990. The projected number of 525,000 physicians in that year would give an estimated surplus of 60,000 (Bureau of Health Manpower, 1979).

DISTRIBUTION. There has been a disproportionate distribution of physicians geographically. The North East region had the highest ratio of 20.4 per 10,000, while the North Central region had the lowest ratio of 14.5. Within each geographical region is a further maldistribution evidenced by the shortage of physicians in the rural and inner-city areas. The number of doctors engaged in primary care has remained fairly constant at about 39% during the past decade. A change did occur within this group, however. There was a 4% decrease in the number of general practitioners, while the number of internists increased 49%, and the number of pediatricians increased 35%. Other medical specialties increased by 15%. This suggests that primary care physicians are becoming more specialized, which tends to bring higher fees for services.

Examination of the trends among the surgical specialties during that same period of the 1970s shows an increase of 18% in the combined surgical specialties. General surgeons, who represent about one third of this group, increased by 10%. The obstetrician-gynecologists, who make up about one quarter of the surgical group, increased by 25%, orthopedists by 29%, anesthesiologists by 29%, pathologists by 21%, psychiatrists by 18%, and radiologists by 16%.

IMPACT ON COSTS. One would logically expect that with the increased ratio of physicians to population, competition, because of the surplus, would cause a drop in fees for services and operations. This has not been the case. In fact, the opposite has occurred. The surplus has caused prices to go up. The forces of supply and demand that normally affect prices and allocation of resources in most markets are not at work in the health care sector. This is equally true of hospitals. There is little competition because the consumer (sick person) does not shop for a doctor or a hospital. The buyer of health care has difficulty in making an informed choice, particularly when his health is at stake and when a third party is picking up the bill. The physician, upon whom the patient relies, becomes both the buyer and the seller of health service. He not only provides the medical services, but he also decides how much medical service the patient is to receive. Here demand and prices can be controlled independent of supply.

It is interesting to note, that as the number of obstetrician-gynecologists was increasing 25%, the birth rate was decreasing. There were one million fewer births in 1977 than there were in 1961, the year when the number of births peaked. The crude birth rate had decreased 36% from 1950. Although this birth rate was decreasing, the rate of cesarean sections doubled between the years 1967 and 1977. The rate of hysterectomies performed on women 15 to 44 years of age increased 22%, and the ligation of fallopian tubes tripled in this age group. Dilation and curettage increased 23% in this same age group, 17% for females 45 to 64 years of age, and 20% for women 65 years and older. Oophorectomies increased 23% for ages 15 to 44, and 48% for the group 45 to 64 years. This increase in surgical operations is not unique to the gynecologists. Although there is no evidence that there was a change in the prevalence of conditions leading to surgical intervention, the surgical rates continued to rise over this period of time. The surgical rate per 1,000 population had climbed from 78.4 in 1967 to 94.5 in 1977. Some of this increase was due to changing criteria for performing surgery, to new surgical techniques, and new protocols for the management of certain conditions. We need to ask ourselves, however, whether dollars available have influenced our medical judgment.

The number of operations grew by 2.2% in 1979 and 2.8% in 1980. Biopsies were the most frequent surgical procedure performed, 5.2 per 1,000 population. In the decade from 1967 to 1977, the number of cardiac catheterizations increased tenfold among men age 45 to 64 years. This procedure became an important study in choosing suitable candidates for coronary artery bypass surgery. The frequency increased with the increase in treadmill stress testing. Prostatectomies increased 41% in males 45 to 64 years and 17% in males 65 years and over. During this same period, some important decreases also occurred. The number of tonsillectomies was cut in half. Appendectomies decreased 20% in people under 45 years. Repair of inguinal hernias declined 5% in males over 65 years.

With the increases in the number of surgical procedures that are being performed has come a growing concern that surgery is perhaps being used excessively in this country. Has the surplus of surgeons and the availability of health coverage encouraged unnecessary surgery?

The increased number of physicians dilutes the number of patients a doctor sees or the number of operations a surgeon performs. The surgeon's malpractice insurance premiums and his office overhead are high and remain fairly constant whether he does 200 or 800 operations a year. If he does relatively few operations a year, he may have to charge considerably more for each operation to meet his expenses and turn a profit. The low patient load increases the unit price. Thus, the surplus of physicians forces the cost of health care up rather than bringing it down through competition. The competitive forces of the marketplace do not operate in setting physician's fees.

The public perceives the physician as having more influence in the daily operation of a hospital than he really does. They see the hospital as the doctor's workshop and are ready to hold him responsible for all of its shortcomings. Usually the administrator and the board of governors have controlling power, set much of the policy, and determine the hospital fees to be charged. Physicians should remember, however, that since they control much of the patient care activity of the hospital, they greatly influence the cost picture. They determine who will be admitted, how long the patient will stay, and what tests will be ordered. Although physicians may not be able to *cause* cost reduction in the hospitals, they can *contribute* to hospital cost reduction. They can run up costs by unnecessary ordering and demands. They can make utilization, tissue, and quality review committees either very effective or allow them to be a sham. The physician does impact greatly on the total health care costs, and his influence is usually understated.

PHYSICIAN'S FEES.   For the twelve-month period ending with June, 1981, charges for physician services rose 10.5%, while the Consumer Price Index rose 9.6%. The cost of physician services represents the second largest share of spending for personal health purposes after hospital care. (See Figure 15-6.) The cost of these services in 1978 was $35.3 billion, or about 46% of the cost of hospital care. This was an increase of 9.5% over the previous year. In 1950, the amount spent on physician services was only $2.7 billion. Although the absolute amount spent has shown substantial increase, the proportion spent on physician services actually decreased from 21.7% in 1950 to 18.3% in 1978.

Surgical charges vary considerably by geographical region and also by whether the area is metropolitan or rural. In 1979, the average surgical charge for a hysterectomy in New York City was $1,259, while in Atlanta it was $736. In nonmetropolitan south-central Pennsylvania it was $649, and in Alabama $549. Physician fees also vary considerably by type of practice and specialty, as well as by region. In that same year the average fee for an initial office visit for the West was $34 for the surgical specialties, while for the general practitioner it was $21. Midwest figures were $25 and $16, respectively. The national average cost of having a baby in 1977 was $888.40 for the hospital and $568 for physician fees, for a total of $1,456.

DEFENSIVE MEDICINE. It is estimated that about $3 billion is spent annually for malpractice insurance. Patients, in their demands for more and better medical care, have set perfectionist standards for physicians and hospitals. They perceive unsatisfactory results as malpractice. Sympathetic jurors' large malpractice awards, and the willingness of lawyers to take cases on a contingency fee basis, have encouraged the dissatisfied patient to sue. We have become a litigious society. This resulted in a malpractice crisis that peaked in 1976. Premiums in California rose 15% in 1975, an astounding 327% in 1976, and another 9% in 1977. In 1981, the physician-owned liability company and a state-run association requested rate increases of 52% and 367.8%, respectively. The insurance commissioner disapproved these requests and granted 26.6% and 27.8% increases. These huge costs of doing business are passed on to the consumer and result in further increases in the unit price of an operation or an office visit.

There is also an indirect increase in costs that results from this malpractice crisis. Physicians and hospitals feel that they must practice defensive medicine almost to the point of paranoia. This has resulted in more laboratory tests; additional treatments, consultations and prescriptions; and extended hospital confinements. An attitude of "leaving no leaf unturned" in the search for disease and abnormalities has developed. This additional cost of defensive medicine is estimated to add another 3%, or $5 billion, annually to health care costs. This is in addition to malpractice premiums.

Nursing Homes. Nursing homes have claimed an increasing share of health expenditures. In 1950, they accounted for only $187 million or 1.5% of the total bill. By 1978, this amount had increased to $15.8 billion, or 8.2% of the total health care costs. The annual rate of increase over this period of time was 17.2% a year (*Source Book of Health Insurance Data 1979–1980*).

The Medicare Program, the increasing number of elderly, and the rising costs of hospital care all served as a stimulus to nursing home expansion. The average monthly charge rose from $186 in 1964 to $689 in 1977, for an annual average increase of 10.6%. Charges for services increase with the size of the home and the age of the patient. Nursing home care is much less expensive, however, than hospital care.

Governmental Expenditures for Health Care

Public expenditures for health care are those made by federal, state, and local governments and include Medicaid, Medicare, programs for veterans and armed forces personnel, crippled children, end-stage renal disease, and workmen's compensation benefits. These public expenditures have increased 1.6 times as fast as private spending.

When Medicaid and Medicare went into effect in 1966, public spending began to grow rapidly. The public expenditure per capita in 1965 was $54.13; by 1978, it had increased 6.5-fold to $350.40. In 1980, governmental spending accounted for about 50% of the total health care costs. In that year, Medicaid and Medicare, combined, paid for 27.8% of all personal health care in this nation (U.S. Department of Health, Education and Welfare, 1979a). It is quite obvious, therefore, that if any health care cost-containment program is to be effective, it must encompass the governmental programs that consume 50% of the health care dollar and have been growing at a rate 1.6 times faster than costs paid by private funding.

Medicaid. Title XIX of the Social Security Act became law in 1965. The program is financed jointly with federal and state funds. It is designed to provide assistance to those groups who have low incomes and are medically needy—the poor, the disabled, the aged, and low-income families receiving Aid for Dependent Children.

Prior to the enactment of this law, physicians were expected to donate a certain portion of their time and expertise, gratis, to care for indigent patients in hospital wards and clinics. The value of this voluntary free physician and hospital service was in the billions of dollars each year. With the enactment of the Medicaid program, physicians and hospitals began to receive payment for these services which had previously been given free of charge. Medicaid also encouraged greater utilization of health services by this previously underserved low-income group. As a result, costs began to grow rapidly. In 1967, the program cost $2.3 billion. By 1977, it had increased sevenfold to $16.3 billion, and by 1980, the cost had grown to $25.3 billion, providing medical services for about 24 million recipients. Payment for physician services made up 9.2% of these expenditures (U.S. Department of Health, Education, and Welfare, 1979). The fees paid for Medicaid patients are considerably below the usual charges for services to other patients and are even more austere than Medicare fees. There have been significant abuses, fraud, and overcharges uncovered among providers of medical sevices for both Medicaid and Medicare patients.

Medicare. The Medicare program, Title XVIII of the Social Security Act, became effective in 1966. It was designed to provide basic health insurance coverage for persons 65 years of age and over. This federally funded program reduces the financial burden of the elderly who have an increased prevalence of chronic disease and disability and usually have a reduced income. It covers a significant portion of the elderly population's health care bill, 44.3% in 1977 (74% for hospitals and 21.7% for physicians).

The program has grown dramatically since its inception. In 1967, the total benefits paid were $4.5 billion. By 1978, these costs had increased 448% to $24.9 billion. By 1980, Medicare covered 29 million persons and cost $36.7 billion. This was an increase of 815% over the first full year of operation.

In 1972 Congress added the End-Stage Renal Disease Program (ESRD) to the Medicare Act. This legislation funded 80% of the cost of hemodialysis through Medicare. The average annual cost per patient is about $25,000 a year, with over 50,000 patients receiving dialysis. About 5% of the total Medicare funds are now being used to aid this 0.2% of the Medicare population. By 1985, the ESRD program will cost Medicare nearly $2.68 billion to serve 83,700 patients. Proprietary dialysis centers have evolved to provide increasing amounts of this service. It is estimated that a reduction of the in-center population for dialysis by 10%, through the use of home dialysis and continuous ambulatory peritoneal dialysis, would save Medicare about $75 million a year.

Veterans Administration. The Veterans Administration operates 172 hospitals and 228 outpatient clinics in this country. It is the nation's largest health care system and controls almost 10% of all the psychiatric beds in the United States. Each year 1.2 million veterans receive inpatient care, and 17.8 million receive outpatient treatment in these facilities.

The cost of running this large complex of veterans centers has risen, as have other health care costs. In 1970, the annual expenditure was $1.8 billion. By 1980, this cost had increased 361% to $6.5 billion. By 1984, these costs are predicted to reach $7.9 billion.

Research and Development. Federal funding for health research and development increased at an annual rate of 12.6% from 1960 to 1978. At the beginning of this period, the amount of federal funds expended for these purposes was $918 million. Over the next 18 years, the amount allocated for research increased 414% to $3.8 billion. The National Institutes of Health accounted for 68.1% of the funds allocated, with the money going to cancer research increasing at the most rapid rate, 20.6% annually.

Cardiovascular Diseases and Their Costs

When one considers that there are more than 40 million persons in this nation afflicted with some form of cardiovascular disease, it is not surprising that the total cost of this category of disease was in excess of $46 billion in 1981. Cardiovascular diseases accounted for almost $26 billion for hospital and nursing home services, over $6 billion in physician and nursing services, $3 billion for medication, and over $11 billion of lost productivity due to disability.

Heart disease accounted for 8% of all hospital discharges and 11% of all hospital patient days between 1972 and 1977. It claimed 28.9 million hospital days in 1978. Heart disease placed higher than cancer, which was responsible for 5% of hospital discharges and 8% of all days of stay. The average length of disability from heart disease is 7.8 weeks and accounts for 8.9% of all disability claim dollars (U.S. Department of Health, Education, and Welfare, 1979a).

There is great need for continued efforts to reduce the prevalence and severity of cardiovascular disease both for economic and humanitarian reasons. Controlling stress responses, prudent diet, smoking cessation, and increased vigorous exercise all hold promise for significant impact on this costly group of diseases.

Cardiac Surgery. The surgical operation that now leads the list in dollar costs in this country is coronary artery bypass surgery for coronary artery disease. At the present time, money spent for the diagnosis and surgical management of coronary artery disease, together, accounts for nearly 2% of the total health care budget.

Nearly 300,000 coronary angiograms were

performed in the United States in 1980, at a total cost of between $600 million and $900 million. It is estimated that 1.5 million cardiac radionuclide scanning procedures were done in 1981, at a cost of another $450 million to $600 million. These two procedures illustrate the marked increase in costs that has resulted from newer, more complicated technology. Coronary arteriography with left ventriculography is the most accurate and informative procedure for diagnosing coronary artery disease and helps discover about 80,000 to 100,000 new candidates for surgery each year. About 40% of patients who receive coronary angiograms go on to have corrective surgery performed.

The first bypass procedure was performed in 1964. It is estimated that since that time more than 700,000 such operations have been done in this country. The number of cases in 1979 was about 100,000, and this increased to 125,000 in 1980. This is predicted to increase to 200,000 annually.

In 1980, the total cost of this one procedure approached $2 billion. If all Americans who could benefit from this operation were to have it done, it would cost in excess of $100 billion. This huge amount would be required for just one specific operation to treat only 0.04% of the population. The question needs to be asked, can we afford it? The hospital costs for coronary bypass surgery range from a low of $11,000 to as high as $25,000. This is exclusive of the surgical fees which can run from $3,500 to $6,000 for the principal surgeon. Complicated cases often generate surgical fees of $9,000 or more. Additional fees for two assistants, a cardiologist, an intensive care physician, and a technician for pump perfusion can add $2,500 to $3,000 more per case. In a three-month period in 1979, Blue Shield of California paid surgeons $709,000 for this operation, which was 20% more than the next most expensive procedure, total hysterectomy.

Most of these coronary bypass operations are performed by about 700 cardiac surgeons. In spite of the new, improved technology with automated routines, and the shared responsibility of the team approach, the fees of the primary surgeons have not dropped. As experience grows, one would expect costly extenuating factors and fees to decrease.

The cost of heart transplants dwarfs the cost of coronary artery surgery. The average cost of a heart transplant at Stanford in 1978 to 1979 was $110,000, exclusive of surgical fees. These patients spent an average of 46 days in an intensive care unit and 27 days additional in a regular care setting. It is estimated that the installation of an artificial mechanical heart will generate bills of about $200,000. As newer and more complicated surgical and medical procedures become common practice, health care costs will escalate at an even greater rate. Someday we will have to pause and make a social decision as to whether society can afford such a rapidly expanding expensive technology.

Disability Costs. Up to this point, we have directed our attention to the *direct* medical costs related to disease and disability. These, as we have seen, are appreciable. Figure 15-7 shows the estimated range of these medical costs for six of the common disabling diseases, including the predisability, the disability, and the postdisability costs.

There are, however, extremely high additional costs borne by industry and society that are generated by disabled workers. These include the costs of salary continuation, long-term disability payments, lost productivity, the costs of replacement and retraining, increased pension payments, increased insurance premiums, and organizational disruption. Many of these costs are difficult to price. The costs that are measurable, however, usually amount to three to six times the direct medical costs.

The number of disabled persons in this country is increasing at a rate 3.5 times that of the population. Heart disease has contributed significantly to this problem, accounting for about 15.5% of the disability due to chronic diseases. Disability costs this nation billions of dollars annually. Many of the disabling events are preventable, and large amounts of money can be saved through efforts aimed at prevention of disability. This can be accomplished by educating and training people to adopt a healthier and safer life-style. Rehabilitation efforts to return the already disabled patient to a productive life as soon as possible can be equally cost effective.

POSSIBLE SOLUTIONS
Alternate Delivery Systems

The great majority of people in this country have been satisfied with the quality of medical care provided and have desired that the rendering of such care continue to be within the free enterprise system. As the dissatisfaction and concern about the rising cost of medical care have grown, however, planners have turned to alternate methods of delivering

Disability Medical Condition	Predisability Medical[a] (Prior 5 Years)	Disabilitating Event—Medical[b] (1 Year)	Post Disability Medical[a] (Next 15 Years)
Heart Attack	0-25,000	26,000	20,000-60,000
Stroke	0-20,000	9,000	5,000-20,000
Alcoholism	0-25,000	11,000	20,000-40,000
Back Injury	0-25,000	21,000	5,000-30,000
Diabetes	1,000-25,000	5,000	5,000-20,000
Cancer	0-20,000	27,000	20,000-40,000

[a]Many respondents did not estimate these costs, so the ranges reported were rounded estimates from only 12 of the 48 respondents.

[b]Only about one third of all respondents (15) provided estimates of the medical cost of the debilitating event. A rounded average is reported.

Figure 15-7. Medical costs of disability. (Reprinted by permission of the publisher from *Human Resource Planning,* Vol. 4, No. 4. Copyright 1981 by the Human Resource Planning Society.)

health care that hold promise of providing more efficient and less costly service.

Health Maintenance Organizations. Health Maintenance Organizations (HMOs) hold considerable promise of lowering health care costs. They offer an alternate delivery system of health care by providing physician and hospital services to their enrollees in exchange for a fixed annual fee. Here, the HMO and the consumer share the financial risk of ill health. A sick person is a financial asset to the fee-for-service or cost-plus health care provider. He becomes a liability, however, to an HMO. Thus, there is a financial advantage to prevent sickness or speed recovery in the HMO setting. The greatest savings come from reduced hospital costs, where the rate of savings varies from 10 to 40%. There is an incentive for the HMO physicians to ration expensive services, eliminate unnecessary laboratory procedures, avoid overutilization, and keep patients out of expensive hospitals where possible.

The concept of such an alternate competitive delivery system is not new. The Kaiser-Permanente Health Plan, one of the oldest in the country, was established in the 1930s. The HMO Act of 1973 provided further impetus for the establishment of HMOs. It required companies to offer employees covered by corporate health insurance the choice of an HMO where one existed. This also made capital funding available by providing $350 million in grants and loans. There have been approximately 235

HMOs established. Of the 148 that have been federally qualified, 19 have failed. In spite of these failures, rising health care costs will serve as a further stimulus for the establishment of more HMOs, which will compete with fee-for-service providers.

Outpatient Surgery. One method of reducing health care costs is to perform the medical or surgical procedure required in the least expensive setting that will still allow the delivery of safe, high-quality care. Certain surgical procedures done in an outpatient facility provide such an opportunity. Many of the commonly performed operations can be done well, safely, and cheaper on an outpatient basis. These include biopsies of easy access, excision of superficial lesions, diagnostic dilatation and curettage, tubal ligation, vasectomy, tonsillectomy and adenoidectomy, repair of hernia, and hemorrhoidectomy. It is estimated that about 30% of the surgical procedures currently being done as in hospital cases could be performed on an outpatient basis at about 30 to 50% of the cost. Ambulatory surgical centers are rapidly being established throughout the country to satisfy this need.

Emergency Medical Treatment Centers. Patients without a regular family physician, or those whose personal physician is not available, frequently travel to hospital emergency rooms for routine treatment. About two thirds of all visits to emergency rooms are nonemergency cases. This is very expensive; the average cost of a hospital emergency room visit in some areas is now $82. Medical entrepreneurs have been quick to seize the opportunity to compete for such business. As a result, many emergency medical treatment centers are springing up as the "convenience stores" of medical care. These centers offer quick service with no appointment required, and at a fee 30 to 50% cheaper than that charged by the hospital emergency rooms. The average cost of a visit ranges from $35 to $45. The patient must pay cash up-front and seek his own reimbursement if covered by insurance. Most of these centers provide quality care.

Second Opinion for Elective Surgery. There has been a growing concern that surgery is being used excessively in this country. Excess utilization may be, in part, the result of the oversupply of surgeons and the ready availability of third-party payment for operative services.

Some insurance companies have attempted to reduce the number of unnecessary operations by the institution of second-opinion elective surgery programs. Any operation for an impairment that is not an emergency, i.e., where a delay of the operative intervention would not be life-threatening, is considered elective surgery. Patients who are to have elective surgery are required to have a second opinion from a consultant, who is a board-certified specialist, to confirm the need for surgery. These programs may be voluntary or mandatory. If mandatory, a second opinion is required to assure full payment for the procedure. Failure to obtain the second opinion would result in the payment of a lesser amount. Voluntary programs have not proved to be as cost effective as the mandatory plans because the participation is much lower. The percentage of decrease in number of operations performed and the resultant savings realized from second-opinion programs vary considerably among the studies done. In general, the savings seem to be in the neighborhood of 5 to 14%. The bottom line as to the true value of second-opinion elective surgical programs has yet to be determined.

Preadmission Testing. Physicians often hospitalize their patients earlier than necessary in order to have certain essential laboratory tests performed in preparation for surgery. In many cases, these tests could be performed on an outpatient basis with a resultant reduction in the length of hospital stay. If every hospital stay could be reduced by just one day about $6 billion could be saved each year in this country. Such a provision covering preadmission testing in health insurance policies is cost effective if the program is publicized to the policyholders.

Home Health Care. This provision in an insurance contract encourages the patient to be discharged from the hospital as soon as possible. The cost for such home care is considerably lower than hospital confinement. Although the hospital may be the most effective place to administer medical care, it is also the most expensive. Early discharge to convalesce at home can often be accomplished if home health care is available.

Rehabilitation Centers. We have seen how large both the direct and indirect costs of disability can be for the individual, for industry, and for society. It is to the benefit of all to return, where possible, the disabled patient to a productive life. Rehabilitation centers start their efforts toward this objective usually on the first visit. Subsequent visits are directed toward this end. The benefits obtained are particularly rewarding in cardiovascular diseases. The positive approach of rehabilitation can prevent disabling cardiac neurosis and iatrogenic disease. These efforts are most productive when instituted early in the recovery state.

Preventive Medicine. It is estimated that life-style is responsible for 70% of cirrhosis, 69% of automobile accidents, 54% of heart disease, and 37% of cancer (U.S. Department of Health, Education, and Welfare, 1979b). Indeed, how we live and what life-style we choose have great influence on our state of health and on our longevity. If we choose to smoke, drink to excess, lead a sedentary life, be a worrywart, and drive carelessly on our highways, we have made the principal causes of sickness and death, to a great extent, diseases of choice.

Good logical reasoning dictates that the most effective way of reducing health care costs is not to get sick. A healthy life-style can help to make this goal a more probable reality. The wellness approach holds great promise of reducing illness and its associated costs. A study done at the Southwestern Home Office of Prudential Insurance Company showed a correlation between the level of cardiorespiratory fitness and the number of days of disability absences as well as the number of dollars spent for medical care. Those employees participating in a physical fitness program averaged 60% fewer disability days than the Home Office as a whole. The turnover rate among the participants was only one fourth of the rate for the other employees.

Within the program, those at a low level of fitness averaged nearly five times more days of disability and six times higher medical costs than those at a high or good level of cardiorespiratory fitness (Bowne *et al;* 1980).

Flexible Insurance Benefits Approach. We have mentioned that labor has demanded comprehensive health insurance with first-dollar coverage, and that industry has been willing to accede to these demands, because they can be written off as a business expense and are nontaxable to the employee. There is considerable sentiment in Congress favoring a cap on the value of insurance benefits allowed each employee. Any excess above the limit would be considered taxable income. Such a restriction would act as an incentive for a flexible or "cafeteria" benefit plan, which allows each employee to select those benefits that meet his individual needs and that he perceives as being the most valuable for him. Such a restriction and plan would decrease the insurance costs for industry and eventually trickle down to the consumer.

Deductibles and Coinsurance. The consumer must be brought back into a position of directly sharing in the cost of health care with out-of-pocket contributions. This is best done by having a $200 to $500 deductible amount for which he is responsible in each health insurance contract. In addition, a coinsurance provision requiring the insured to pay 20% of the costs over a nominal basic amount would be an effective control.

In summary, we have seen that health care has a price, and the price has been escalating at a very rapid rate. We have reached a point where these costs are of such magnitude that society is having a difficult time paying the bill. All of us share the responsibility for this crisis, which is of such greatness and urgency that it warrants the concern of all. Its solution will require the cooperative efforts of government, physicians, hospitals, individuals, industry, labor, and insurance companies. If our combined efforts to contain these costs are not successful, we may succumb to an alternative solution that could bring an end to quality health care as we know it.

REFERENCES

Ankrum, A. D., and List, N. Competitiveness and/or competition—the place for PRSO. Testimony before the House Ways and Means Committee, Washington, D.C., March 25, **1981.**

Barret, C. A. (ed.) Key economic and social issues of the early 1980s. The Conference Board of Canada, Ottawa, October 1979, published **1980.**

Bowne, D. W.; Hellman, E. C.; Richardson, H. E.; and Clarke, A. E. Physical fitness programs for industry—an extravagance or wise investment? *Trans. Assoc. Life Insur. Med. Div. Am.,* **1980,** *64,* 210-222.

Consensus Development Conference. Medical and scientific aspects of coronary artery bypass surgery. National Center for Health Care Technology. JAMA, **1981,** *246,* 1645-1649.

Davis, J. C., and Detmer, D. E. The ambulatory surgical unit. *Ann. Surg.,* **1972,** *175;* 4.

Edwards, M.R. What does permanent disability cost? *Human Resource Planning,* **1981,** *4,* No. 4.

Ellwood, P. M., and Herbert, M. E. Health care: should industry buy it or sell it? *Harvard Bus. Rev. Library* **1973,** 1.071, 5-13.

Fuchs, V. R., and Newhouse, J. P. (eds.) The economics of physician and patient behavior. *J. Human Resources* (Suppl.), **1978,** *13,* 3-262.

Goldsmith, J. C. The health care market: can hospitals survive? *Harvard Bus. Rev.,* **1980,** *58,* 100-112.

——— Outlook for hospitals: systems are the solution. *Harvard Bus. Rev.,* Sept.-Oct. **1981,** *59* (5), 130-141.

Goldstein, K. (ed.) *Statistical Bulletin.* The Conference Board, New York, **1981,** *14,* 2-16.

Government regulations. *Hospitals,* **1978,** *52,* 17.

Griffith, J. R.; Hancock, W. M.; and Munson, F. C. Practical ways to contain hospital costs. *Harvard Bus. Rev. Library* **1973,** 1.071, 61-69.

Guidotti, T. L. What characterizes an ideal health care system? *Pharos,* **1981,** *44,* 20-23.

Hartumian, N. S.; Smart, C. N.; and Tompson, M. S. The incidence and economic costs of cancer, motor vehicle injuries, coronary heart disease and stroke: a comparative analysis. *Am. J. Public Health,* **1980,** *70,* 1249-1260.

Kiefhaber, A.; Weinberg, A.; and Goldbeck, W. *A Survey of Industry Sponsored Health Promotion, Prevention and Education Programs.* Washington Business Group on Health, Washington, D.C., **1979.**

Leone, R. A. The real cost of regulation. *Harvard Bus. Rev.* **1977,** *55,* 57-66.

Lewis, R. California physicians will get refunds from malpractice insurers. *A.M.A. News,* **1979,** *22,* 1.

Lewis, R. F. Financing the nation's health care. An address to Financial Executives Institute, New Orleans, **1977.**

McCarthy, E. G., and Finkel, M. L. Second opinion elective surgery programs: outcome status over time. *Med. Care,* **1978,** *16,* 984-994.

——— Second consultant opinion for elective gynecologic surgery. *Am. J. Obstet. Gynecol.,* **1980,** *56,* 403.

Medicine and profits—Unhealthy Mixture. *U.S. News & World Report,* August 17, **1981,** 50-54.

National Health Education Committee. *The Killers and the Cripplers.* David Mckay Company, New York, **1976.**

Rees, A. Government regulation: a source of higher prices. *Answers to Inflation and Recession: Economic Policies for a Modern Society.* The Conference Board, New York, **1975,** pp. 65-70.

Relman, A. S. The new medical-industrial complex. *N. Engl. J. Med.,* **1980,** *303,* 963-970.

Report of Committee on Stress, Strain and Heart Disease. American Heart Association. *Circulation,* **1977,** *55,* 825A–835A.

Roe, B. B. The UCR boondoggle. A death knell to private practice. *N. Engl. J. Med.,* **1981,** *305,* 41–45.

Samuelson, P. A. *Economics,* 10th ed. McGraw-Hill, New York, **1976.**

Seidman, B., and Binns, W. G. *Labor-Management Group Position Papers on Health Care Costs.* Labor-Management Health Care Task Force, Washington, D.C., **1978.**

Source Book of Health Insurance Data 1979-1980. Health Insurance Institute, Washington, D.C., **1980.**

Statistical Bulletin. Work history following coronary artery bypass surgery. *Stat. Bull. Metropol. Life Insur. Co.,* Oct.-Dec., **1979.**

Tobin, J. Critique of conventional policies: monetary policy and the control of credit. *Answers to Inflation and Recession: Economic Policies for a Modern Society.* The Conference Board, New York, **1975,** 1–19.

U. S. Department of Health, Education, and Welfare. *Facts of Life and Death.* U.S. Dept. HEW (PHS) Pub. No. 79-1222, National Center for Health Statistics, Hyattville, Md., **1978.**

———*Health Care Financing Trends.* Health Care Financing Administration, U.S. Government Printing Office, Washington, D.C., Fall **1979.**

——— *Health United States.* U.S. Dept. HEW (PHS) Pub. No. 80-1232, U.S. Government Printing Office, Washington, D.C., **1979a.**

——— *Healthy People—The Surgeon General's Report on Health Promotion and Disease Prevention.* U.S. Dept. HEW (PHS) Pub. No. 79-55071, U.S. Government Printing Office, Washington, D.C., **1979b.**

U.S. Department of Health and Human Services, *Health Care Financing Review.* HFCA Pub. No. 03146, Health Care Financing Administration, U.S. Government Printing Office, Washington, D.C., Sept., **1981.**

———*Supply and Distribution of Physicians and Physician Extenders.* Graduate Medical Education National Advisory Committee Staff papers. U.S. Dept. HEW Pub. No. (HRA) 78-11. Health Resources Administration, Hyattville, Md., 1978.

Chapter 16
SUMMARY AND CONCLUSIONS

Lysle H. Peterson

As stated in Chapter 1, the term "cardiovascular rehabilitation" means many things to many people. The term has been used to cover an array of practices. To many, its major ingredient is exercise; to others, it includes psychological, nutritional, and related medical management as well. Facilities or centers that have specialized solely in cardiovascular rehabilitation generally have struggled to survive and many have failed. Survival problems are multiple; however, successful establishment of this field, like any other field, ultimately and above all requires that the benefits of cardiovascular rehabilitation are clearly demonstrated, well understood, and accepted broadly, because it is a health care service that should draw its patients by referral; moreover, reimbursement for the services must be approved by the insurance industry, including Medicare. Further, because the start-up costs are substantial, and time is required to develop an adequate referral base, a devoted center must be able to sustain capital and operating debts for relatively long periods, i.e., have adequate "staying power."

The fact that a small proportion of the total patient population with disabilities associated with manifest cardiovascular disorders is referred for rehabilitation is, in itself, evidence that the benefits of rehabilitation have not been adequately demonstrated. Moreover, many of those physicians, who do accept the view that exercise, stress management, and good nutrition together with close medical management are important for their patients, believe that they can offer such services from their offices without specialized facilities.

The major purposes of this book are (1) to demonstrate the benefits that are achievable by the application of sound principles of cardiovascular rehabilitation; (2) to demonstrate that to maximize the achievement of these benefits, a cardiovascular rehabilitation center not only must deal with exercise in an effective manner, but also must combine proper exercise management with concurrent, closely interacting medical, psychological, and nutritional management; thus, cardiovascular rehabilitation should be *comprehensive* in nature; (3) to demonstrate that the maximization of benefits of comprehensive cardiovascular rehabilitation can best be provided in a center or facility devoted to comprehensive cardiovascular rehabilitation, and, conversely, that it would be difficult or impossible to maximize the potential benefits in another way such as from a busy practitioner's desk; (4) to demonstrate the validity of the position taken by the American Medical Association (Council on Scientific

Affairs, 1981), Medicare (1983), and American Heart Association Affiliate Publications (1980–1983) that a cardiovascular rehabilitation program must be directed and closely supervised by an appropriately experienced, licensed physician, i.e., that careful physician monitoring is essential. Indeed, the HCRC is operated similarly to an intensive or critical care facility regarding the role of physicians, nurses, and monitoring and advanced cardiopulmonary life support facilities. These further include the support and cofunctioning of experienced, licensed psychological and nutritional experts.

SUMMARY OF DEMONSTRATED BENEFITS

Åstrand and Rodahl (1977) published a table of documented benefits of exercise. The exercise was, of course, of such a nature as to achieve effective conditioning. Table 16-1 utilizes the Åstrand and Rodahl table but is modified (1) to indicate which of the benefits listed in their table have been confirmed by the HCRC experience and (2) to include additional benefits documented from the HCRC experience. Table 16-1 is therefore an extension and confirmation of that published by Åstrand and Rodahl.

For example, the first entity listed in the table which has been confirmed by HCRC experience is *muscle mass* shown by an X, in the original table, to increase. The fact that an increase in muscle mass has been confirmed by the HCRC experience is notated by a (C) adjacent to the X. Later in the table under the heading "heart rate," the Åstrand and Rodahl table contains a question mark (?) under "De-

Table 16-1. EFFECTS OF TRAINING ON ORGANS AND ORGAN FUNCTIONS (ÅSTRAND AND RODAHL, 1977)*

ORGAN OR FUNCTION	INCREASE	DECREASE	NO EFFECT	REFERENCES
Locomotive Organs				
Strength of bones and ligaments	X			Ingelmark, 1948, 1957; Viidik, 1966; Tipton *et al.*, 1974; Booth and Gould, 1975
Thickness of articular cartilage	X			Holmdahl and Ingelmark, 1948
Muscle mass (hypertrophy)	X(C)	?	X	Marpurgo, 1897; Siebert, 1929; Vannotti and Pfister, 1934; Man-i *et al.*, 1967; Hollmann and Hettinger, 1976; Jansson and Kaijser, 1977; Saltin *et al.*, 1977
Number of muscle cells	?		X	Gonyea *et al.*, 1977
Muscle strength	X(C)			Clarke, 1973; Hollmann and Hettinger, 1976
ATP, creatine, phosphate, muscle	X			Palladin and Ferdmann, 1928; Yakovlev, 1958
PFK action in muscle	X		X	Gollnick and Hermansen, 1973
SDH action in muscle	X			Holloszy, 1973; Saltin *et al.*, 1977
Myoglobin	X			Whipple, 1926; Holloszy, 1973
Potassium, muscle	X			Nöcker *et al.*, 1958
Capillary density, muscle	X			Vannotti and Pfister, 1934; Vannotti and Magiday, 1934; Petrén *et al.*, 1936; Brodal *et al.*, 1977; Saltin *et al.*, 1977
Arterial collaterals, muscle	X			Schoop, 1964, 1966
Circulation				
Heart volume	X(C)		X	Roskamm *et al.*, 1966; Reindell *et al.*, 1967; Ekblom, 1969
Heart weight	X			Siebert, 1929; Thörner, 1949; Liere and Northup, 1957
Capillary density, heart	X			Petrén *et al.*, 1936
Coronary collaterals	?			Eckstein, 1957; Tepperman and Pearlman, 1961
Blood volume, total hemoglobin	X			Deitrick *et al.*, 1948; Taylor *et al.*, 1949; Hollmann and Venrath, 1963; Miller *et al.*, 1964; Sjostrand, 1967; Saltin *et al.*, 1968

(continued)

Table 16-1. *(Continued)*

ORGAN OR FUNCTION	INCREASE	DECREASE	NO EFFECT	REFERENCES
Alkali reserve			X	Åstrand, 1956
Hemoglobin concentration			X(C)	Åstrand, 1956
Plasma protein concentration			X	Åstrand, 1956
Cardiac output rest			X(C)	Åstrand, 1956
Submaximal work	X(C)	?	?	Freedman *et al.,* 1955; Frick *et al.,* 1963; Tabakin *et al.,* 1965; Andrew *et al.,* 1966; Ekblom *et al.,* 1968; Saltin *et al.,* 1968; Rowell, 1974
Maximal work	X(C)		?	Ekblom *et al.,* 1968; Saltin *et al.,* 1968; Rowell, 1974; Barnard, 1975
Heart rate, rest		X(C)		Steinhaus, 1933
Submaximal work		X(C)		Christensen, 1931; Clausen, 1976
Maximal work		?(C)	X	Robinson and Harmon, 1941; Knehr *et al.,* 1942; Ekblom, 1969
Stroke volume, rest	X(C)			Ekblom *et al.,* 1968; Saltin *et al.,* 1968
Submaximal work	X(C)			Åstrand and Rodahl, 1977
Maximal work	X(C)			Åstrand and Rodahl, 1977
ā-v̄O$_2$ difference, rest			X	Åstrand and Rodahl, 1977
Submaximal work	?		?	Åstrand and Rodahl, 1977
Maximal work	X		X	Åstrand and Rodahl, 1977
Oxygen uptake, rest			X(C)	Åstrand, 1956
Given work load		X(C)	X	Åstrand, 1956
Maximal work	X(C)			Robinson and Harmon, 1941; Knehr *et al.,* 1942; Taylor *et al.,* 1949; Ekblom *et al.,* 1968; Ekblom, 1969; Saltin *et al.,* 1968; Pollock, 1973
Blood lactic acid, rest			X	Åstrand and Rodahl, 1977
Given work load		X(C)[14]		Åstrand, 1956; Ekblom, 1969
Maximal work load	X	(C)[15]		Åstrand, 1956; Gollnick and Hermansen, 1973
Local blood flow, working muscle submaximal	?			Eisner and Carlson, 1962; Rohter *et al.,* 1963; Rowell, 1974; Clausen, 1976
Arterial blood pressure, rest		X(C)	X	Åstrand, 1956
Submaximal work		?(C)	?	Ekblom, 1969; Tabakin *et al.,* 1965; Frick *et al.,* 1963; Boyer and Kasch, 1970; Kilbom, 1971; Choquette and Ferguson, 1973; Clausen, 1976
Maximal work	?	X(C)	?	Ekblom *et al.,* 1968; Ekblom, 1969

Respiration

ORGAN OR FUNCTION	INCREASE	DECREASE	NO EFFECT	REFERENCES
Lung volumes, adults			X	Åstrand, 1956
Lung volumes, adolescents	?		?	Åstrand, 1956
Pulmonary ventilation, rest			?	Åstrand and Rodahl, 1977
Submaximal work		X		Åstrand and Rodahl, 1977
Maximal work	X			Ekblom *et al.,* 1968
Tidal air, rest	?		X	Åstrand and Rodahl, 1977
Submaximal work	?		X	Åstrand and Rodahl, 1977
Maximal work	?		?	Åstrand and Rodahl, 1977
Respiratory rate, rest		?	X	Åstrand and Rodahl, 1977
Submaximal work		?		Åstrand and Rodahl, 1977
Maximal work	X			Åstrand and Rodahl, 1977
Diffusing capacity, rest			X	Anderson and Shephard, 1968; Reuschlein *et al.,* 1968; Saltin *et al.,* 1968
Submaximal work			X	Åstrand and Rodahl, 1977
Maximal work	X			Åstrand and Rodahl, 1977

Miscellaneous

ORGAN OR FUNCTION	INCREASE	DECREASE	NO EFFECT	REFERENCES
Body density	X(C)			Skinner *et al.,* 1964, Pařízková, 1973
Serum cholesterol concentration		X(C)	X	Golding, 1961; Björntorp, 1970; Altekruse and Wilmore, 1973; Lopezs *et al.,* 1974; Pyörälä *et al.,* 1971
Serum triglycerides		X(C)[1]	X(C)[1]	Skinner *et al.,* 1964; Fox and Haskel, 1967; Altekruse and Wilmore, 1973

* From Astrand, P. O., and K. Rodahl. *Textbook of Work Physiology,* 2nd ed., pp 394–396. McGraw-Hill, New York, 1977, by permission.

ORGAN OR FUNCTION	INCREASE	DECREASE	NO EFFECT
Myocardial oxygen utilization defined by (HR $\times$ SBP $\times 10^{-2}$), as a function of work load			
At rest		X(C)	
At submaximal loads		X(C)	
At maximal loads		X(C)	
Coronary blood supply	X(C)		
Ratio of exercise work load to cardiac work (Conditioning Index)	X(C)		
Myocardial contractility and ejection fraction	X(C)		
Symptoms and signs of myocardial ischemia (angina pectoris, ST-segment depression, arrhythmias)			
At rest		X(C)	
At submaximal loads		X(C)	
At maximal loads		X(C)	
Systolic blood pressure			
At rest		X(C)	
At submaximal loads		X(C)	
At maximal loads		X(C)	
Diastolic blood pressure			
At rest		X(C)	
At submaximal loads		X(C)	
At maximal loads		X(C)	
Cardiac-peripheral feedback systems[2]			
Preload normalization[3]	X(C)		
Afterload normalization[4]	X(C)		
Plasma electrolyte normalization[5]	X(C)		
Catecholamine stimulus to heart	X(C)		
Contractility normalization[6]	X(C)		
Cardioacceleration normalization[7]	X(C)		
Anaerobic threshold[8]	X(C)		
Patient nutrition knowledge	X(C)		
Caloric intake		X(C)	
Body weight		X(C)	
Per cent body weight as fat		X(C)	
Plasma high-density lipoprotein (HDL)			X(C)[9]
Plasma total cholesterol/high lipoprotein ratio			X(C)[10]
Fasting plasma glucose			
If already* normal			X(C)
If already* elevated		X(C)	
Fasting serum iron			X(C)[11]
Fasting hemoglobin			X(C)[12]
Fasting red blood cell count			X(C)[13]
Number of medications required		X(C)	
Psychological disorders			
Anxiety level		X(C)	
Depression		X(C)	
Hypochondriasis		X(C)	
Fears		X(C)	
Psychasthenia		X(C)	
Coronary-prone characteristics		X(C)	
Self-confidence regarding activities	X(C)		
Sexual problems		X(C)	
Smoking abuse		X(C)	
Alcohol abuse		X(C)	
Nonprescribed drug abuse		X(C)	
General			
Vocational conditions			
1. Likelihood of returning to work	X(C)		
2. Time to return to work		X(C)	
3. Effectiveness returning to work	X(C)		
4. Time lost from work due to illness		X(C)	
5. Tax-ratable income	X(C)		
6. Household work productivity†	X(C)		

(continued)

Table 16-1A. (*Continued*)

ORGAN OR FUNCTION	INCREASE	DECREASE	NO EFFECT
Monitoring of patient (signs and symptoms)			
During rehabilitation program[15]	X(C)		
Rehabilitation follow-up[16]	X(C)		
Quality of life			
Social activity levels†	X(C)		
Interest in current affairs†	X(C)		
General feeling of well-being†	X(C)		
Enjoyment of family†	X(C)		
Enjoyment of friends†	X(C)		
Morbidity[16]		X(C)	
Mortality[17]		?	

* Indicates condition at initial evaluation, i.e., prior to rehabilitation program.

† Self-reporting by patients.

[1] Fasting serum triglycerides were found to remain unchanged across the entire population studied. However, those with abnormally elevated triglycerides are found to exhibit reductions. The closer to normal, the greater the probability that the values will approach 100 mgm/dl at exit.

[2] Cardiac-peripheral feedback systems refer to those physiological mechanisms that integrate cardiac and peripheral functions. Normalization increase means that the mechanisms, when disordered, approach or reach normalcy.

[3] Preload refers to central venous volumes and pressures, which affect, for example, the Starling curve. Diuretics are often used to reduce preload. Exercise conditioning tends to normalize preload from both directions.

[4] Afterload refers to aortic blood pressure re the left ventricle, and pulmonary arterial pressure re the right ventricle. It represents the load against which the ventricle must expel blood. Pharmacologically, it is controlled by arterial antihypertensives to reduce afterload, and by vasoconstrictors to increase afterload. Exercise-induced conditioning tends to normalize preload from either direction.

[5] As renal, pulmonary, muscle, and blood functions normalize, electrolytes tend to normalize. Also, nutritional management is involved, e.g., potassium supplements and sodium restriction.

[6] Contractility improvement is implicit in the situation where the same exercise load, requiring an equivalent cardiac output, occurs at a lower heart rate. Moreover, the elimination of drugs such as quinidine and beta-blocking agents will reduce the negative ionotropic effects of those medications. Moreover, studies show that ejection fractions at rest and with exercise or isometric stress normalize.

[7] A new decrease in heart rate at rest and at all levels of exercise intensity occurs with exercise conditioning. This is associated with a decrease in cardioaccelerator and an increase in cardiodecelerator functions. Moreover, there is a normalization of acceleration and deceleration about the lower basic rate.

[8] Anaerobic threshold, the point during an increasing exercise intensity at which anaerobic muscle metabolism increases with respect to aerobic metabolism. An increase in blood lactic acid and a tendency to acidosis develop. Exercise conditioning extends this point to higher exercise intensity levels.

[9] The cross-population evaluation of HDL demonstrates a small but significant increase in HDL following exercise conditioning as compared to preconditioning. However, there is a poor or negative correlation with exercise conditioning, total cholesterol, and triglycerides.

[10] The total-to-HDL cholesterol ratio shows a small, but significant, cross-population increase with the comparison of exit to entry values. The correlation with exercise conditioning is low or negative, as it is with plasma lipoprotein changes.

[11] Fasting serum iron is found to be low in approximately 12% of individuals entering the HCRC program. These are corrected by nutritional supplementation rather than by exercise conditioning. Indeed, unless an abnormally low fasting serum iron is corrected by nutritional supplements, it will remain low or decrease further. Thus, in those cases where serum iron is normal, no change occurs during rehabilitation. However, in those where it is found to be initially low, it is corrected. In this sense, a rehabilitation *increases* abnormalities of serum iron.

[12,13] The same may be said for hemoglobin, hematocrit, and red blood cell content, i.e., when it is already normal, no significant change occurs with exercise conditioning. If it is low initially, corrective therapy is undertaken to normalize the picture. One interesting variation occurs in a percentage of individuals who suffer from end-stage renal disease and are on hemodialysis. A frequent complication in these patients is a chronic, troublesome anemia which appears to respond to exercise therapy. The mechanism has not been elucidated.

[14,15] As noted in footnote 8, exercise conditioning extends the anaerobic threshold toward higher exercise intensities. Thus, blood lactic acid will be relatively decreased with respect to exercise loads, i.e., as the anaerobic threshold is extended, the lactic acid levels are reduced.

[16] Morbidity: Studies now underway but not completed suggest a significant reduction in premature mortality comparing life tables of the Texas Heart Institute (10 years, 20,000 cases) and HCRC data up to 41 months and 506 cases.

[17] A pilot study of 50 HCRC patients, in which hospital and physician visits, medications used, and days of illness prior to and subsequent to rehabilitation were studied, shows approximately a 50% reduction in overall costs associated with these markers of morbidity. The data from this study are being finished for publication at the time of preparation of this book.

305

crease" and an X under "No Effect." The HCRC experience finds that the heart rate is decreased at maximal as well as at rest and submaximal loads; therefore, the (C) is adjacent to the ?. The table is then extended beyond the Åstrand and Rodahl list under the heading, "Additions to the Åstrand and Rodahl List."

The data supporting the responses of patients to comprehensive cardiovascular rehabilitation are contained in the preceding chapters of this book. It is important to note that this modified and extended Åstrand and Rodahl table is qualitative in the sense that the table shows responses only as increase, decrease, or no change. Again, the original Åstrand and Rodahl (1977) table dealt virtually entirely with the responses to exercise alone. The data demonstrated in this book are largely quantitated and include not only the responses to exercise, but also to the interactions of medical, psychological, and nutritional practices, i.e., comprehensive cardiovascular rehabilitation.

The remainder of this chapter deals with many of the listings of Table 16-1 in more detail and also with the broader perspectives related to cardiovascular rehabilitation.

HOW BENEFITS ARE ACHIEVED

General Organization of the HCRC Comprehensive Cardiovascular Rehabilitation Program

The program is structured around four major areas: (1) General medical management, (2) exercise management, (3) psychological management, and (4) nutrition and diet management. A physician-physiologist director, together with other physicians (associates and residents), manages the medical and exercise components. The exercise activities are under the direct supervision of specialized nurses directed by a physician in a manner simulating a coronary care or intensive care unit. All are certified in advanced life support. The psychology component is headed by a Ph.D., licensed psychologist trained in counseling and clinical psychology. The nutrition component is headed by a registered dietitian (R.D.) with a Master's degree. There is, in addition, a general and business office. All components are directed and directly supervised by the licensed physician-director. The operations involve a staff of ten full-time equivalents as well as rotating students and residents. Also, a sports medicine physiologist (Ed.D.) serves as a general consultant, assures quality control of bicycle ergometry, and assists patients in obtaining and maintaining home exercise bicycle ergometers.

Patients are referred by (1) their cardiologist or attending physician, (2) the Texas Rehabilitation Commission (TRC) through the system of the Commission's local medical consultants (physicians appointed by the TRC), and (3) industries and insurance companies, which referrals are coordinated through the patient's attending physician. Appropriate records detailing the patient's prior medical history are obtained prior to the initial evaluation. The initial evaluation consists of a detailed medical history, also incorporating the past history records obtained from the referring physician and from hospital records as well.

A physical examination is performed together with a spirometric measure of pulmonary function, a resting 12-lead electrocardiograph supplemented by hyperventilation, and frequently by a Valsalva maneuver. A fasting SMAC-20 with serum iron and HDL is obtained. An exercise tolerance test (see Chapters 2, 3, 4, and 5) is performed using sign/symptom limitation. Also, a psychological evaluation (see Chapters 7 and 8) and a nutritional evaluation (see Chapters 9 and 10) are made.

The results of this initial evaluation are then compiled and reviewed in order to reveal medical problems, the initial therapeutic exercise prescription, psychological and nutritional disorders; i.e., a detailed, composite picture of the patient is developed in order to provide individualized as well as group therapy.

The therapy (rehabilitation) program consists of prescribed, monitored, progressive exercise for 30 minutes on a bicycle ergometer preceded by calisthenics and warm-up, and succeeded by cool-down and relaxation (see Chapters 2 and 3). These exercise sessions are conducted three times per week until the Conditioning Index indicates that the patient has achieved an optimal level of exercise tolerance. This averages 13.8 weeks. No more than eight patients exercise in one group with two nurses and a physician supervisor in order that appropriate individual monitoring can be achieved. Appropriate life support facilities are available.

Each patient, either before or after exercise, attends and participates in a group session three times per week. On one of the days, the discussion is concerned with medical and exercise subjects. The objective is that patients understand how the appropriate body systems operate at rest, with physical effort, and under adverse circumstances. These include the cardiovascular, respiratory, blood, and neuromusculoskeletal systems predominantly. They learn the mechanisms by which exercise improves the functioning of the bodily systems, how to interpret signs and symptoms, the actions of medications, the effects of such factors as dynamic isotonic versus isometric efforts, climatic conditions, the limits imposed by their prevailing exercise tolerance, and the efforts and metabolic costs of various vocational, recreational, and social activities, including sexual activities.

On another of the three days each week, the group is under the direction of the psychologist. The purposes and activities are discussed in Chapters 7 and 8. On the third of the three days, the group is under the direction of the nutritionist. The objectives and structure of these sessions are described in Chapters 9 and 10.

The group sessions each last ten weeks. Thus, there are ten in medical-physiological subjects, ten in psychology, and ten in nutrition. Each of these sessions occupies 90 minutes. The patient is in group-structured activities for two and one-half hours, three times per week, i.e., seven and one-half hours per week. Thus, there is an average of 42 exercise sessions, 10 group medical-physiology, 10 group psychology, and 10 group nutrition sessions for a total average of 72 hours of group rehabilitation activities. In addition, virtually all patients require individual counseling with the psychologist and nutritionist and medical examinations with appropriate counseling or therapy (see General Medical Management, p. 321, and Management of Medications, p. 317). On the average, these individual requirements demand 37 hours of staff time.

When indicated medically, other tests such as Holter monitoring, nuclear ventriculography, echocardiography, x-rays, and clinical laboratory procedures are conducted.

At the time the patient obtains the optimal leveling out of the Conditioning Index (see Chapters 2, 3, 4, and 5, as well as preceding sections of this chapter), the patient is exited. This process consists of a collation of the historical events occurring after the initial medical history was obtained; a modified, as appropriate, physical examination; a repeat spirometry, 12-lead electrocardiograph, and exercise tolerance test; and an exit psychological and nutritional evaluation. It should be noted that nursing assessments are made a part of the records of the patient from the initial evaluation, through the rehabilitation program, and including the exit evaluation.

The entire professional staff meets at least weekly to conduct a detailed evaluation of the status of each patient. Records are kept in a computer file and displayed to the staff. Thus, the coordination of physician, nursing, psychologist, and nutritionist information is obtained. Progress and problems are assessed, and a plan for the week is made. The entire staff or components thereof meet more frequently as required.

Use is made of videotapes for both instruction and entertainment during exercise sessions, and instructional videotapes are utilized during group sessions in medicine-physiology, psychology, and nutrition. An array of written material in each of these fields is also given to the patients to improve their informational base and as workbooks.

As the patient is nearing the exit, a prescription for a home bicycle ergometer is provided with a recommendation that the patient prepare for maintaining the home-exercise prescription. The patients are already familiar with the use of the bicycle ergometer; hence, transition problems are minimal. Again, the home bicycle ergometer is regarded as preferable to other forms of maintenance exercise for reasons developed elsewhere in this book.

Occasionally, patients must be away from home during the program and after exit. The HCRC preference for these occasional times when the patient is away from home is to substitute stair climbing for the bicycle ergometer. It should be recalled that maintenance of the conditioning effect requires an exercise intensity level sufficient to provoke an appropriate double product (see also Chapters 2, 3, 4, and 5). In most cases the patient is well beyond an exercise intensity level whereby walking can be substituted for his/her prevailing therapeutic load. Thus, walking uphill or running are the only practical substitutes when the bicycle ergometer is not available. Experience indicates that stairs are usually readily available, the exercise load can be standardized, and stairs are protected from adverse weather. This substitution method for the bicycle ergometer is well accepted by patients for the *occasional* need; thus, compliance and maintenance are assured.

The patient then returns for a brief follow-up visit one month after exit since unanticipated questions usually occur to the patient after leaving the closely structured, guided program, and a delay of one month has been found to be optimal. Routine follow-up visits are scheduled semiannually thereafter.

Careful, detailed records are maintained in order to reveal variations in the patient's condition or performance. Formal reports are routinely given to the referring physician and patient after the initial and exit evaluations and after each follow-up visit. In addition to the routine reports, the HCRC maintains a liaison with the referring physician to coordinate changes of medications, and so forth. These collected data are also used for program evaluation and research purposes to better understand the benefits, or lack thereof, of the methods utilized and how to improve them. It may also be noted that the comprehensive cardiovascular rehabilitation center is an excellent teaching laboratory in clinical medicine, physiology, psychology, and nutrition. Students and residents alike report that their rotation through the center is highly valuable and unique.

The following section of this chapter provides more detailed summary and conclusions as to how the benefits are achieved with respect to each of the components and some general conclusions regarding cardiovascular rehabilitation.

Exercise

Few would argue that cardiovascular rehabilitation relies to a major extent on exercise. Indeed, many feel that it is the keystone, if not the only basis, of cardiovascular rehabilitation (AMA, Council on Scientific Affairs, 1981). Although exercise is a major component of the HCRC program, it should be evident that it must be well coordinated with medical, psychological, and nutritional components to be optimally effective.

For reasons described in Chapter 2, dynamic, isotonic exercise using the bicycle ergometer was chosen at the outset of the HCRC program as the standardized method for exercise therapy. There are three major reasons for having chosen one standardized exercise mechanism in contrast to an array of methods. One reason is technical, i.e., the bicycle ergometer permits a quantitative exercise prescription that is repeatable and can be sustained for the amount of time required to evoke the desired response and, at the same time, allow reliable monitoring of physiological and clinical signs

and symptoms, and response is independent of body weight. A second reason relates to compliance. It is adaptable to a pleasant, comfortable, convenient clinic and home environment as compared to exercises outside of the home environment. Most patients do not wish to become devoted joggers or runners three times a week, indefinitely. The third reason relates to the effectiveness of prospective and retrospective analyses of the results of exercise on human performance. Many experiences reported in the literature demonstrate that comparing multiple types of exercise stimuli or interventions leads to major problems in arriving at conclusions regarding stimulus-response relationships or evaluation intervention trials. Few, if any, exercises or exercise machines designed to provide physical effort are either purely dynamic, isotonic, or purely fixed, isometric. Walking, jogging, and running involve inertia, i.e., accelerating the body mass. Machines designed for body building (e.g., Nautilus), called variously isokinetic or variable resistance, involve significant isometrics. A well-designed bicycle ergometer minimizes inertia (see Chapter 6).

Exceptions to the use of the bicycle ergometer for therapeutic exercise were limited to those who could not utilize the bicycle. These exceptions involved less than 1% of the HCRC patients in which cases the treadmill was utilized. Upper arm ergometry, i.e., the use of a bicycle ergometer turned upside down or a specially designed arm crank ergometer, is useful when leg exercises are impractical, e.g., in amputees or those with spinal cord injuries. To date, the HCRC has not significantly involved itself with such patients. From work published in the literature, it is apparent that upper arm ergometry exercise can be effective in producing a conditioning effect; however, the time and number of triweekly sessions required to achieve a plateau are significantly extended (Blocker and Cardus, 1983).

It has been established and generally accepted that, to be optimally effective, therapeutic exercise should be conducted three times per week at an intensity essentially defined by perceived effort modified by clinical signs and/or symptoms not affecting the patient's perception of effort (see below). Exercise tolerance is determined by the prevailing clinical (medical) status, the state of physiological conditioning, medications, psychological stress, intercurrent infections, and an array of other day-to-day variables such as sleep disturbances, unusual physical activities conducted outside of the program, temporary absence from the program, and so on. The duration of each exercise session has been set at 30 minutes at a *constant,* prescribed bicycle ergometer load (see Chapter 6, Ergometry). The 30-minute constant-load exercise session is preceded by calisthenics, which also serve as a warm-up procedure, and is followed by cool-down on the bicycle ergometer and a recumbent, relaxation session.

Blood pressures are taken prior to the warm-up, calisthenic sequence and at least twice during the 30-minute constant-load bicycle exercise session (at 10 minutes and 20 minutes), or more often if the response to exercise (signs and symptoms) suggests. The blood pressure recorded as *resting* is that obtained after cooldown and the 5-minute recumbent relaxation period. The reason is that the first blood pressure, i.e., prior to warm-up and calisthenics, is usually not resting. Patients often hurry to join the exercise group after driving to the Center, often with stress. It has been found that the postexercise, postrelaxation blood pressure is lower than the preexercise level and more closely represents the resting pressure obtained in conventional ways. It should be emphasized that the cool-down procedure, whether in exercise tolerance testing or in therapeutic exercise, is highly important. The patient is, at that time, vulnerable to hypotension as the peripheral-resistance-sustaining effect of muscular exercise is reduced, leaving only the vasodilatory influences.

The HCRC operates five exercise groups per day, each group containing no more than eight patients. This maximal number is defined by the ability of the Center to adequately monitor each patient via telemetry (electrocardiograph and pulse rate), blood pressure, and other clinical signs and symptoms. It may be noted that the optimal time of day to achieve exercise conditioning appears to be in the morning. Those who attend the "after-five (P.M.)" sessions require an average of 1.5 weeks longer to achieve a plateauing of the Conditioning Index, and their initial blood pressures and heart rates tend to be higher. This difference has been observed in two ways. (1) The same individuals have on occasion switched from the after-five to morning sessions when their working conditions, holiday, and so on, made it possible. (2) It is assumed that, over the three years that an after-five group has been operating, other variables will have tended to equate. The exception is that those in the after-five group have tended

to be those who are well enough to have returned to work, whereas the more ill and deconditioned have tended to attend the morning groups. It is reasonable to assume that this difference should produce an earlier achievement of the Conditioning Index plateau rather than the delayed one which is observed. It is probable that the delay in the after-five group is due to the fact that at the end of the day they are more fatigued, and the integrated stresses of the day result in a higher heart rate, blood pressure, and double product, hence a lower training effect margin. At the time patients are exited and given a home-exercise prescription, it is recommended that they exercise in the morning prior to breakfast and going to work or beginning their daily routine.

As noted in Chapters 1, 2, and 3, the level of exercise load that patients are prescribed while undergoing rehabilitation is for the purpose of stimulating an array of cardiovascular and metabolic processes. The exercise level must be high enough to provoke the so-called training or conditioning effect. Too little will be ineffective; too much, hazardous. The initial exercise evaluation is the exercise tolerance test conducted prior to beginning the therapeutic exercise sessions. The standard exercise tolerance test chosen was the Balke protocol because its steps are closely related to increments of metabolic load, and therefore the usual or "normal" response is a relatively linear rise of heart rate and systolic pressure to each step of the test. Moreover, the test is relatively easier for the patient and staff than other tests, and responses on the treadmill can be compared to those on the bicycle ergometer. The initial exercise tolerance test not only assists in setting the initial therapeutic exercise load but also provides the staff with knowledge of that patient's response to a symptom- and/or sign-limited maximal exercise load.

The exercise tolerance test and the therapeutic exercise load intensity are therefore, in effect, perceived maximal efforts. The end-point of the exercise tolerance test is essentially as far as the patient perceives that he can go in three-minute steps. The therapeutic exercise intensity is as much as the patient perceives that he can undertake for 30 minutes. The only exception to that of limit by perceived maximal effort is when and if the monitoring staff, physician or nurse, decides on clinical grounds (signs or symptoms) that the work load must be otherwise limited.

Borg (1967) had developed scales or ratings

of perceived effort in healthy and athlete populations. He scaled the ratings of perceived exertion from very, very light to very, very hard. He recognized that as exercise conditioning developed, subjects found that they could sustain increasing levels of physical effort with relatively lower rating of perceived effort, i.e., a given level of physical effort became easier as conditioning developed. Moreover, the rating of perceived effort was directly and linearly related to heart rate. Furthermore, the correlation of perceived effort and heart rate varied with age as well as with conditioning. Later, Gutmann *et al.* (1981) studied perceived effort in patients who had undergone coronary artery bypass surgery before and after exercise rehabilitation. They reported that perceived exertion also correlated well with heart rate and that perceived exertion rating shifted to higher heart rates with conditioning in such patients.

The HCRC experience (Peterson and Anderson, 1983) demonstrates that, by examining heart rate, systolic blood pressure, double product, and Conditioning Index, perceived exertion correlates better with double product and Conditioning Index than heart rate alone. As may be noted from the case studies reported in Chapter 3 and grouped data reported in Chapters 4 and 5, heart rate, blood pressure, and double product each varied with respect to work load intensity on a day-to-day basis and in overall trends.

Patients in the exercise conditioning sessions are exercising at essentially maximal perceived effort, i.e., from hard to very hard on the Borg scale unless modified by the monitoring staff on clinical grounds. This in turn is more highly correlated with double product than with heart rate or systolic blood pressure alone. The Conditioning Index is the ratio of exercise level undertaken by the patient to the induced double product (HR $\times$ SBP $\times$ 10^{-2}). It is found that the Conditioning Index (see Chapter 3) is highly sensitive to day-to-day changes in the patient's perception of the prescribed work level and to the double product. For example, a patient may find that a given work load is hard on one day, and very hard the next day when he/she is under more stress, has an upper respiratory infection, has had a poor night's sleep, and so on. This is reflected in a higher double product and a lower Conditioning Index. The overall trend for this patient is, however, that the work level, that is perceived as hard, steadily increases. Also, the average double product remains relatively unchanged as the tolerated work load increases. The overall result is, as detailed in Chapter 4, that the average increase in sustained work load, perceived as hard, is about threefold at the time the Conditioning Index plateaus or becomes asymptotic, while the average double product increases 10 to 15%. Thus, the Conditioning Index does not, on the average, increase percentagewise as much as the exercise tolerance, the difference being about 10 to 15%. The Conditioning Index, therefore, represents the correlation coefficient between exercise tolerance and perceived maximal effort, i.e., hard on the Borg scale.

From time to time it has been suggested that isometric efforts be substituted for dynamic or isotonic exercise (Carú and DePonti, 1979). The arguments in favor of the use of isometrics are (1) that isometrics produce a higher heart rate and systolic pressure and, thus, double product for a given $\dot{V}O_2$ Max than dynamic or isotonic exercise, (2) that the cardiac output is higher with respect to $\dot{V}O_2$ Max with isometric work, and (3) that a hand grip, for example, is less expensive and involves no body motion compared to a bicycle ergometer. It is interesting that the linear relationship of $\dot{V}O_2$ to cardiac output, heart rate, and blood pressure holds for isometric as well as for isotonic effort, except that isometric effort produces higher levels of cardiac output, heart rate, and blood pressure for a given oxygen consumption.

It may be noted that it is a misnomer to refer to isometric effort as work since no movement is involved, i.e., work = force $\times$ distance. Therefore, isometric effort is usually measured as the per cent of maximal voluntary muscle contraction such as hand gripping or squeezing. Studies have shown that when the muscle tension reaches 50 to 60% of maximal, blood flow to the muscle ceases due to the choking off or throttling effect on the vasculature; hence, the muscle must then operate anaerobically.

There are four major arguments against the use of isometrics for cardiovascular rehabilitation: (1) Because of the throttling and cessation of blood supply to the muscle, endurance is short as fatigue and pain develop. (2) Isometric testing is relatively insensitive for the diagnosis of coronary insufficiency (Carú and DePonti, 1979). (3) The subject cannot sustain an elevated double product long enough to induce a satisfactory training or conditioning effect. (4) Its use, due to the insensitivity and high rate of rise of heart rate and blood pressure, may be difficult to measure and dangerous.

These comments on isometrics are relevant to cautions given the HCRC patients regarding pushing, pulling, or lifting weights, except for brief periods and with regard to estimated maximal contractions. The patients are warned that isometrics not only are an unsatisfactory method for cardiovascular conditioning, but may be dangerous, especially for hypertensives or those with signs or symptoms of myocardial ischemia with effort.

Patients frequently wish to know about walking, jogging, or running as means of achieving or maintaining the conditioning effect. This author's comments to patients who ask about jogging develop somewhat as follows:

"Attacking jogging or running may be akin to attacking religion; however, with that risk in mind, it is my opinion that walking will not effectively maintain your Conditioning Index unless your prescribed work load is at, or below, 300 kpm·min^{-1}, a low work load and soon exceeded. Virtually everyone in the HCRC experience has exceeded 300 kpm·min^{-1} within the first one to three weeks. In my opinion, jogging and running are contraindicated for the majority of our patients for several reasons. (1) They cause repeated mechanical stress and impact forces on the thin, fragile cartilage of the joints of the extremities. An informal survey of orthopedists in Houston was met with the consensus that joggers and runners, as, for example, professional football players, develop their degenerative arthritis earlier in life. Moreover, the average age of patients in the HCRC program is in the fifties. (2) Patients must leave the comfort and air-conditioning of their homes at inappropriate hours and subject themselves to the Houston weather which is often very hot and very humid. In other parts of the country, it also may be hot and humid at times and cold or freezing at other times. (3) It is difficult to maintain a steady work load of known intensity. (4) It is much easier to use a bicycle ergometer in an air-conditioned home while watching the news or reading the paper or a book. (5) Patients can have confidence that the exercise load is reasonably known, and repeatable pulse rate and blood pressure are more easily taken if desired. (6) It is expected that the overall long-term compliance will be higher using a bicycle ergometer."

It is explained, however, that walking is not contraindicated since it is a pleasant way to visit the neighborhood, does tend to provide relaxation for many, and burns a few calories.

However, other forms of exercise may be contraindicated depending upon the level of workload tolerance that has been achieved through conditioning. These same considerations apply to vocational counseling regarding physical efforts involved in various jobs. There are many excellent sources of information relating jobs with physical requirements.

It would appear that the metabolic cost of virtually everything people do has been measured, with particular emphasis on sexual activity. About 70% of the HCRC patients complain of reduced libido and about the same percentage of men complain of impotence. Most investigators (Hellerstein and Friedman, 1970; Zohman et al., 1971) agree that dealing with sexual problems represents a significant aspect of comprehensive cardiovascular rehabilitation. The HCRC experience is similar to that of other centers, except perhaps that the HCRC has engaged in a systematic effort to reduce medications that are also known to influence libido, impotence, and premature ejaculation (Papadopoulos, 1980). Also, the film available from Burroughs Wellcome entitled "Sex and the Heart Patient" is shown to all patients, except for the section of the film dealing specifically with medications since the film was developed primarily for physicians. Individual and group counseling, as well as physiological conditioning and reduction of medications, have, as reported by patients, significantly reduced complaints and impotence. Certainly, one of the benefits is the reassurance that comes with knowing that the usual physical effort associated with sexual activities is 300 kpm · min^{-1} more or less and that the patient's exercise tolerance has exceeded that level.

Another question patients ask, which concerns recommended exercise activities outside of those prescribed within the rehabilitation program, is the role that outside exercise plays in burning calories and thus assisting weight loss. It is explained that the loss of 1 lb of body weight involves the dissipation of approximately 3,500 kilocalories and that walking 3 mph for 1 hr uses about 180 kilocalories; thus, about 19 hr of walking 3 mph would be required to lose a pound of body weight, which could be replaced by a few handfuls of peanuts. It is emphasized that, while restriction of calories is the most effective method for weight loss, exercise is a good supplement, especially since its effects integrate over months and years. Moreover, exercise, contrary to usual public opinion, often suppresses appetite.

The nutritionist computes the caloric balance for patients with regard to their weight and other factors in order to achieve ideal weight goals and practices. The assumption is made that, under basal metabolic conditions, the body produces 1 Kcal/Kg of body weight/hr (Consolazio, 1963). There are, however, exceptions to that generally utilized relationship. One exception is that a larger proportion of the body weight of obese people is low-metabolizing fat. Thus, an obese person will tend to use fewer calories with respect to body weight than a lean person. The most direct and reliable way of measuring caloric utilization is to measure O_2 consumption ($\dot{V}O_2$ and CO_2 production [$\dot{V}CO_2$]) and compute respiratory quotient (RQ) during exercise tolerance testing. A less direct way, but one usually used, is to estimate the per cent body weight as fat by anthropometric measures and to correct to an equivalent lean body mass. The so-called Mayo Clinic normogram (Consolazio, 1963) should then be corrected for excessive body weight. At the HCRC markedly obese people are tested using the Beckman Metabolic Cart in order to better manage obesity (Toshiko et al., 1983).

Two other factors, not previously covered per se in this book, deal with long-term follow-up and compliance and the question of secondary prevention relative to reduction of risk factors. Both are, of course, interrelated. The overall experience with dropouts, i.e., patients ceasing to attend the program once started, has been 12% due to psychological and logistical (e.g., moving away from the city) problems and only 3% due to intervening health problems. Once having completed the program, the HCRC has experienced an overall maintenance rate with respect to continuation of regularly prescribed exercise and attending follow-up evaluations of 76%. This unusually low recidivism rate is, we believe, due to continued emphasis during the program of the importance of maintenance by informing and demonstrating to the patient how and why rehabilitation methods work to their benefit, and how the benefits will decline if maintenance is not regular and long-term. Moreover, the purchase of a home bicycle ergometer is recommended and prescribed. Again, the bicycle ergometer appears to be superior to other home-exercise forms in long-term maintenance. Increasingly, insurance companies are allowing reimbursement for prescribed bicycle ergometers.

There is a third benefit that is apparent, though less than satisfactorily quantitatively demonstrated at present. This benefit relates to the mechanisms by which the heart and the so-called peripheral physiological functions are interrelated to provide for an optimally functioning whole body. This subject might be referred to as the mechanism by which homeostasis is maintained over wide ranges of metabolic functions of the body, such as going from rest to exercise, from supine to upright, under emotional and physical stress to sleep and relaxation, from satiation to hunger, from adverse to comfortable climates, from health to illness.

The American Physiological Society has for more than five decades included an organization of its members called the Circulation Section. At a meeting of the Circulation Section in 1949, Dr. Henry C. Bazett, who was then president-elect of the American Physiological Society and who was one of my principal mentors while I was a medical student at the University of Pennsylvania, said (paraphrased): "Listening to the presentations of this group, one would think that the body's periphery, and all that it contains, exists only to serve the heart." It is clear that the heart is but the source of energy to move the blood among the various organs that supply and utilize the blood's contents in proportion to the demands of the body as a whole. However, the heart could not long function adequately were it not connected to the other functions of the body ("the periphery") through an intricate and complex system involving both feedback and control mechanisms. Examples are the so-called pre- and afterload constituted by the venous (pre) and arterial (after) blood pressures and volumes which are part of the controls of cardiac function, the humoral, electrolyte and gas-related contents of the blood as they enter and leave the heart, the innervation of the heart, and so on. Were these not present and operating effectively, the heart would not effectively serve the "peripheral" needs. The heroic Barney Clark's experience with an artificial heart, which was devoid of such controlling influences, exemplifies the need for highly sensitive and optimally functioning mechanisms that tie the heart to the body's demands.

Many status post–myocardial infarction and heart surgery patients enter a comprehensive cardiovascular rehabilitation center with many of these control and feedback mechanisms in disorder. Indeed, most patients receiving medications that affect these complex mechanisms, or who have an array of clinical dysfunctions, also suffer from disorders of the cardioperipheral interacting mechanisms. The causes of the disorder are multiple: disease, deconditioning, medications, disordered nutrition, and psychology. A statement often made at the HCRC is that "if one doubts that the brain is connected to the heart, we recommend that he work in the Center for one week."

It is evident that the hypotension so often seen in cardiac patients normalizes as the Conditioning Index rises. Likewise, hypertensive levels also tend to normalize. Preload adjusting medications and diuretics are less often needed and can usually be discontinued. Simply by observing their contraindication list and reported undesirable side effects, it is clear that adrenergic blocking agents markedly block important feedback mechanisms. After all, that is primarily their rationale for use. It has been proposed that a significant benefit of physiological conditioning brought about by exercise is an increase in hemoglobin and/or hematocrit and thus an increased oxygen-carrying capacity. The HCRC study, as a cross-population study involving uniform and standardized exercise protocols, does not confirm that proposed benefit.

A perusal of the modified Åstrand and Rodahl table presented earlier in this chapter should leave little doubt that exercise-induced physiological conditioning tends to normalize and improve a large array of peripheral mechanisms which, together with the improvement in heart function, permit an average threefold increase in exercise tolerance in patients with an array of significant health disorders. The need for further research to better elucidate the entire array of cardiac and "peripheral" functions and their interactions is evident.

In summary, with regard to exercise, the HCRC plan predetermined that one mode of exercise would be standardized and applied to all patients—the stationary bicycle ergometer. The exceptions were only those patients who could not operate a bicycle ergometer. There were many practical and technical or tactical reasons for this decision. The major strategic reasons were that only in this way could the responses to exercise be analyzed without the problem that has plagued so many other programs, i.e., nonstandardized, difficult to quantitate, exercise stimuli. In other words, exercise is the stimulus to a complex set of physiological responses. If important characteristics of the stimulus vary from patient to patient or from time to time, the responses will be difficult or impossible to relate back to the stimulus. The second major strategic reason is that the bicycle ergometer should be the most appropriate vehicle for achieving compliance with long-term home-exercise prescriptions so that large numbers of patients will maintain their exercise. Conversely, many fewer patients will continue to jog or run, and walking is simply inadequate to maintain conditioning. A statistically satisfactory population of patients who have completed the HCRC program has been analyzed. The mean increase in exercise tolerance for men was from 211 kpm · min^{-1} (SD 93) on admission to the program to 596 (SD 125) on exit, i.e., a 282% increase. This almost threefold increase, for a population that contained a high proportion of patients with high-grade disease who were seriously disabled, elevated them from average level of exercise tolerance, which is low marginal for vocational and recreational activities, to a level well in excess of that required for all but the highest physical effort in vocational and recreational activities. Some patients reached exercise tolerance levels in excess of 1,000 kpm · min^{-1}.

From a clinical and scientific point of view, this almost threefold average increase in exercise performance was associated with only a relatively small increase in heart rate (about 15%), systolic blood pressure (about 7%), and double product (about 12%). Thus, while the cardiac output, regardless of the degree of conditioning, remains quantitatively and directly proportional to exercise intensity and oxygen consumption of the body, with essentially the same proportionality (Åstrand and Rodahl, 1977), the heart is providing a proportionately higher cardiac output with a markedly lower (about 12%) increase in heart work and myocardial oxygen consumption. Thus, the heart has apparently become significantly more efficient in that it can perform its job of pumping blood to the body's tissues at a much lower work load itself and a much lower oxygen demand. Thus, in effect, a heart with an impaired coronary circulation can pump a larger cardiac output with the same impairment of coronary perfusion. This benefit then reduces the signs and symptoms of myocardial ischemia associated with physical effort.

Moreover, a further benefit is achieved in that the heart rate at rest and at all levels of exercise, within the limits of exercise tolerance (now increased about threefold), permits a larger beat-to-beat and time-integrated coronary perfusion because coronary blood flow occurs predominantly during diastole, which is extended inversely with the heart rate. There is evidence also that this improved perfusion favors subendocardial areas of the heart which are usually in highest jeopardy (see Chapter 3).

The statistics of improvement of exercise tolerance for women are percentagewise about the same as for men, except that the mean increase in exercise tolerance is from an initial level of 154 to an exit level of 379 kpm · min^{-1}, i.e., 246%. The other changes noted for men apply to women as well (see Chapters 2, 3, and 4).

Another indicator or marker for the progress of training or conditioning in patients was developed at the HCRC and termed the Conditioning Index. Simply, it is the ratio of the amount of exercise the body is performing (such as on a bicycle ergometer) to the amount of work the heart performs to provide the cardiac output demanded by the exercise as measured by the double product. This ratio, therefore, is

$$\text{Conditioning Index} = \frac{\text{Bicycle ergometer work load (kpm · min}^{-1})}{\text{Heart rate} \times \text{systolic blood pressure} \times 10^{-2}} \times 10^2$$

It was anticipated and has been demonstrated that this ratio is valuable for several purposes. It allows the rehabilitation center to track the progress of the conditioning effort and to identify the impact of a number of everyday factors that impede or enhance the conditioning process. Thus, it provides a valuable aid to medical, psychological, and nutritional management. Moreover, it is a reliable indicator of the level of exercise tolerance that a patient can achieve in a rehabilitation center and thus indicates when the patient should be exited and placed on a home maintenance exercise program. Moreover, it is valuable for the patient in that he can be shown a quantifiable indicator of achievement, and it illustrates to the patient the day-to-day factors that can affect exercise tolerance, a feeling of well-being, and perceived exertion.

The major factors that modulate the conditioning effect, and the patient's perception of difficulty in performing a level of exercise, i.e., the Conditioning Index, are (1) psychological stress, (2) medication variations, (3) intercurrent infections, and (4) additional physical exertion. It is an excellent way to demonstrate why a patient, or all people for that matter, may

have good days and bad days and, moreover, how to achieve more good than bad days—or at least understand why they occur. Longer term trends in the Conditioning Index are valuable indices of long-term disease trends. A declining trend suggests a declining clinical status; a maintained or even slowly climbing Conditioning Index suggests health maintenance and even further improvement.

Thus, properly provided and monitored exercise therapy not only results in significant improvements in exercise tolerance with reduced symptoms and signs of myocardial ischemia, but it provides a firmer basis for medical, psychological, and nutritional management. In effect, an exercise stress test or a therapeutic exercise prescription, which is said to be symptom-sign limited, is really limited by what may be called maximal perceived effort, or by signs and symptoms that the monitoring observer regards as limiting, rather than as perceived by the subject. The therapeutic exercise load is therefore lower than the exercise tolerance test limit. In other words, unless the monitoring observer limits the exercise level on clinical grounds, the exercise load is limited by the extent to which the subject or patient can tolerate the exercise, usually described as maximal fatigability or leg pains; the subject states that he just cannot go further. As noted earlier, Borg (1967) defined a scale of perceived effort ranging from very, very light (numerically 6) to very, very hard (numerically 20). The maximal perceived effort utilized by the HCRC in exercise tolerance testing is very, very hard, while exercise therapy is from a perception of hard to very, very hard, but at very, very hard, the exercise level is reduced.

Experience indicates that the exercise intensity at which to start a patient in a therapeutic conditioning program corresponds to 60% of the maximal double product reached in the initial exercise tolerance test, *or* at a level defined by limiting clinical signs or symptoms, whichever is lower. This starting difference, i.e., lower than the highest level reached in the initial treadmill exercise tolerance test, is (1) because the patient will usually do better on the treadmill at the initial exercise tolerance test than on a bicycle ergometer with which the patient is usually less efficient; (2) because the duration of a therapeutic exercise session is 30 minutes, compared to exercise tolerance test steps of three minutes each. After the patient has experienced one to three or four bicycle ergometer sessions, he is usually able to achieve adequate efficiency, and the exercise load can be increased. Experience indicates that the load can then be increased about 10%. After this initial "break-in" period, the therapeutic exercise load is adjusted as required to achieve an optimal conditioning trend which will continue to increase until a limit is reached. Everyone, including an Olympic athlete, will have a limit of exercise tolerance that relates to his physiological or pathophysiological limits. This limit may relate to the heart's limited capacity to increase cardiac output, or to the pulmonary system's limit to exchange physiological gases between the blood and ambient air, or to neuromusculoskeletal conditions, and so on. Thus, for example, the ultimate limit of exercise tolerance of a "cardiac patient" may be a coexisting COPD rather than the heart's improved capability to pump blood. In other words, the patient's heart may define the limit of his exercise tolerance at the time he begins the program, and as his cardiovascular conditioning improves, the limit may then become his ventilatory capacity.

An essential role of the staff in prescribing and monitoring therapeutic exercise intensity is to prescribe an exercise load adequate to provoke a *double product* (heart rate $\times$ systolic blood pressure $\times 10^{-2}$) sufficient to provoke the training or conditioning effect within the limits of safety. The double product represents the myocardial work and its oxygen demand to generate a cardiac output required by the body's exercise load. In other words, a primary purpose of prescribing skeletal muscular exercise is to induce exercise for the heart and other physiological systems involved in the training or conditioning process.

As conditioning proceeds, the double product, provoked by a given body exercise intensity, declines. Since the ratio of cardiac output to the body's exercise (metabolic) load remains essentially constant, the decline in double product with respect to body exercise implies that the heart is providing cardiac output at a lower metabolic cost, i.e., becoming more efficient. Conversely, the lesser myocardial oxygen demand implies that the individual can accomplish greater exercise intensity with the same or lower myocardial oxygen supply. Conversely, a person with a limited myocardial oxygen supply can accomplish greater physical effort before reaching his limit. The relationship of double product (heart work) to body work

therefore provides a quantitative guide to the conditioning process (see Chapters 2, 3, and 4).

1. *Exercise tolerance* perceived as "hard" or as limited by signs and symptoms of myocardial ischemia $= E.T._{(H)} =$ prescribed bicycle ergometer work in kpm $\cdot$ min^{-1}.
2. *Double product* maintained within the limits of effectiveness and safety $= D.P._{(Eff)} =$ heart rate $\times$ systolic blood pressure $\times 10^{-2}$ at the prescribed ergometer load.
3. *Conditioning Index* (C.I.) $= \dfrac{E.T._{(H)}}{D.P._{(Eff)}}$

The Conditioning Index therefore represents the coefficient relating exercise tolerance to heart work and myocardial oxygen demand as represented by the double product. The Conditioning Index rises as conditioning proceeds but, of course, has a limit. Indeed, an Olympic athlete's conditioning or training reaches some limit. That limit is recognized as the Conditioning Index levels off or asymptotes. In the everyday life of the patient undergoing rehabilitation, the Conditioning Index does not rise in a smooth manner but has its ups and downs with, however, an upward trend.

This simply means that the prescribed exercise load on a given day, which is synonymous with the patient's exercise tolerance at that time, is determined by the double product at which the patient perceives that he is working at maximal effort or as modified by the monitoring staff. As conditioning develops, the exercise level is increased progressively, using the same criteria, until the Conditioning Index *trend* levels out. The Conditioning Index, then, is the coefficient relating double product to exercise tolerance, i.e.:

$$ET_{(Max)} = DP_{(Mod)} \times CI_{(Max)}$$

As demonstrated in Chapters 3, 4, and 5, many conditions will affect the progress of the conditioning effort and the exercise load to be imposed on a patient on any given day. Chapter 3 contains case studies which demonstrate the most common factors that cause the exercise monitoring staff to modify the prescribed exercise load. The major factors are emotional stress, medication changes, intercurrent illnesses, associated interruptions of the regular three days/week schedule, outside physical or emotional activities resulting in fatigue, and sleep disorders including sleep apnea. Because, in the daily lives of patients in a rehabilitation center, these factors that affect exercise tolerance do commonly occur, the Conditioning Index and exercise prescription level do not usually increase in a smooth upward manner, but are up and down with an upward trend. The Conditioning Index trend is usually S-shaped as in Figure 2-1. These ups and downs are regarded by patients as good days and bad days. Anderson *et al.* (1983), using a mood-rating scale (0 – 10, where 0 is the poorest or worst mood) on a daily basis, found a high inverse correlation with double product at a given exercise load, thus, a direct correlation to Conditioning Index. It is important for the patients to learn the causes of their good days and bad days. In the HCRC experience, this represents a type of "biofeedback" in the sense that, as the patient goes through the program, he learns to control and reduce the factors that cause bad days and to increase the factors that cause good days.

The staff monitoring the patient on a day-to-day basis sees the good days expressed as a lower double product for a given perceived effort and the bad days as a higher double product and/or a higher perceived effort for the same exercise load as occurs on the good days. For example, a patient may, on the good day, find 450 kpm · min^{-1} as the maximal perceived effort (hard on the Borg scale), while the next day, 450 kpm · min^{-1} may be too much, i.e., very hard on the Borg scale.

In Chapter 5 it was demonstrated that some patients exhibit unusual blood pressure responses to exercise. Three general types were described, i.e., the systolic hypertensive response, the diastolic hypertensive, and the fall of both systolic and diastolic pressure, i.e., the decompensatory type (Peterson *et. al.,* 1983). The systolic hypertensive response is associated with an early shift from the aerobic to the anaerobic response to exercise. In such patients, the monitoring staff is alerted. The HCRC policy is to avoid exercise loads that cause the systolic pressure to exceed 200 to 210 mm Hg, rises of diastolic pressure exceeding 10 mm Hg, or a decompensatory decrease exceeding 20% of the usual values. Individual consideration is given to each patient with regard to underlying pathology. Cerebrovascular vulnerability could modify the specific pressure-change policy guides. The diastolic hypertension is usually associated with hypercapnia which, in turn, is associated with COPD or pulmonary congestive failure, the severity of which might alter the decision. In other words,

the staff monitoring exercise sessions must be alert to the clinical status of all patients, to signs and symptoms with clinical significance, and be able to make appropriate decisions with regard to exercise load or other supportive therapy, if necessary.

In a comprehensive cardiovascular rehabilitation center, the physician, nurses, psychologist, and nutritionist meet, as necessary, to review patient status, using the Conditioning Index, double product, and exercise load as guides to manage the patient medically (e.g., adjusting medications), psychologically (e.g., becoming alert to stressful problems and helping the patient learn to manage the stress), and nutritionally (e.g., noting weight, nutritional demands, and so on). Briefly, exercise therapy – related parameters become useful guides to general medical, psychological, and nutritional management of the patient, in addition to the other broader objectives of a comprehensive rehabilitation effort.

After the patient has reached the practical limits of the rehabilitation effort, i.e., when the Conditioning Index has leveled out, the patient is exited at the level of exercise load achieved at that time. An exit exercise tolerance test provides a comparison with the initial exercise tolerance test and is used to set maximal limits. The patient has already learned that he/she must indefinitely maintain a therapeutic exercise program on a three-times-per-week basis. The patient has been shown how deconditioning will recur as rapidly as conditioning was achieved if the therapeutic exercise is not maintained regularly. Virtually all HCRC patients have obtained bicycle ergometers for home use.

It has been found by experience that it is important to have a follow-up meeting with each patient one month after being exited because the patient finds that a number of questions occur after he leaves the structured, guided program. Routine follow-up then is scheduled semiannually. At the one-month follow-up, the patient simply repeats, in the Center, the exercise procedure that he was following on the last day he was in the program. To do that, the patient joins a group that is in session on the day of the one-month evaluation. Following that, a conference with the patient deals with the questions that have accrued.

The exit exercise tolerance level, the exit Conditioning Index, and the exit double product remain as useful guides to interpret long-term follow-up trends. For example, although warned to the contrary, some few patients have sought to exceed or test, by exceeding, the work load prescribed on exit. The Center may then receive a call from the patient or family member to report that the patient tried to exercise at a higher than prescribed exercise load, developed angina pectoris, took a nitroglycerin tablet, became lightheaded, and was forced to lie down. It is explained that the patient exceeded his exercise tolerance, thus raising his double product to a degree that produced myocardial ischemia, and that because he stopped exercising suddenly while also taking a nitroglycerin tablet, his blood pressure fell and he became faint. Moreover, he may have also pushed his double product up until he decompensated as well. One such experience usually reinforces the counseling the patient had received regarding limits while in the program.

Management of Medications

There has been a debate about the relative merits of so-called medical management versus surgical management of patients with coronary artery disease. What is usually meant by medical management is, to a large extent, management utilizing pharmacological agents under clinical conditions. Indeed, there has been a virtual avalanche of new cardiovascular medications introduced within the last decade or two, and the avalanche shows little sign of abating. As the earlier intensity of the debate has subsided, patients tend to be managed by both increased utilization of surgery and of medications. Neither has diminished; both have grown.

An interesting parallel exists regarding the role of comprehensive cardiovascular rehabilitation relative to the use of medications and surgery in the treatment of cardiovascular disease and its related disorders. This section concerns the relative benefits of medication and comprehensive cardiovascular rehabilitation. The question is: To what extent can comprehensive cardiovascular rehabilitation reduce or eliminate such commonly used pharmacological agents as beta-blocking, specific antiarrhythmic, antianginal, antihypertensive, psychotropic, and the more recent calcium-channel–blocking medications?

In Chapter 4 it was reported that the average number of prescribed medications patients were taking on entry to the HCRC program was 6.4 (range, 0–18), including 86 specific generic medications above the 5% level, i.e.,

those with less than a 5% frequency were excluded. Those excluded were drugs not usually associated with the treatment of cardiovascular diseases or their commonly associated disorders (for example, antibiotics and eyedrops). At exit from the program the average number of such medications patients were taking had dropped to 3.1 per patient, i.e., 52%. In 31% of patients, all medications were discontinued.

It has been found that psychotropic medications can be eliminated in 85% of those who had been prescribed such drugs on entry into the program. These include the tricyclics and an array of other antidepressants, tranquilizers, and sedative agents. The reason is clearly that they are no longer needed because depression, anxiety, and sleep disorders are reduced or eliminated.

It has been demonstrated that in 76% of patients with hypertension or to whom antihypertensive drugs were prescribed to reduce afterload, antihypertensive medication could be withdrawn or significantly reduced as blood pressure (resting and with exercise) normalizes. It has been demonstrated that antiarrhythmic and antianginal medication may be eliminated or significantly reduced as both manifestations of myocardial ischemia are reduced or abolished.

The role of beta-blocking agents is of special interest because they were the most frequently prescribed and because of the recent multicenter clinical trials. It has been widely reported that overall these trials demonstrated significant benefits (up to about 25%) regarding reduced mortality and increased survival. What is the justification for reducing or discontinuing beta-blocking drugs in 81% of cases?

At the Thirty-Second Annual Scientific Session of the American College of Cardiology in March, 1983, a symposium was held involving Drs. Curt Furberg, James T. Willerson, and Elliot Rapaport and chaired by Dr. Peter L. Frommer, who at the time of the trials was the Acting Director of the National Heart, Lung and Blood Institute (NIH). At that symposium, the latest thinking, as represented by those analysts, considered the results of the trial (Furberg), the mechanisms that might explain the results (Willerson), and the application of the results to clinical practice (Rapaport).

Briefly, regarding analyses of the study data, it was noted that at least five criteria need be considered: (1) the *statistical power* of the data since multicenters and subgroups were involved in the overall results, (2) *biological ex-*

Table 16-2

TRIAL	CONTROL GROUP MORTALITY	INTERVENTION GROUP MORTALITY	RELATIVE BENEFIT	ABSOLUTE BENEFIT
A	4	3	25%	1/100
B	20	15	25%	5/100

planation of results in that results should ideally be explainable, (3) that *dose-response* relationships be identifiable, (4) that there be *consistency* within the overall trial centers being compared, and (5) that there be replication of the findings. It was stated that the multicenter trials, using different drugs, different doses, different patient mixes, and different periods of follow-up, left much to be desired in each of these five categories. A further caution was voiced regarding the principles of hypothesis testing, in that the analyses were essentially *post hoc,* i.e., it was difficult to know whether analyses were developed to fit the data collected or were developed prior to the data collection.

Another consideration presented at that symposium was the *relative versus the absolute* benefit of treatment. The model example used (Table 16-2) portrayed two hypothetical trials, trial A and trial B. In other words, in trials A and B the relative benefits were the same, i.e., a 25% difference in mortality, yet essentially it requires the treatment of 100 to significantly prolong the life of one in trial A, while the treatment of 100 significantly increases the life expectancy of five in trial B.

The findings reported by pooling the data of the many separate trials and the many subgroups of patients demonstrated benefits reported as 2.6%, with standard deviations and distribution of significance with regard to the many separate trials. The propranolol study is used as an example, since it was most extensive in the clinical trials and the one most prescribed to incoming HCRC patients:

Propranolol Study

$$\frac{\text{\% change of}}{\text{2-year mortality}} = \frac{\begin{array}{c}\text{\% mortality of} \\ \text{control} - \text{\% mortality of} \\ \text{intervention group}\end{array}}{\begin{array}{c}\text{\% mortality of} \\ \text{intervention group}\end{array}} \times 100$$

$$= \frac{9.8 - 7.2}{9.8} \times 100 = 26.5\%$$

Regarding mechanisms, Dr. Willerson emphasized that the mechanism(s) responsible for the reported benefits were, at present, speculative. He discussed many possible mechanisms and concluded that, in his opinion, the two most likely were

1. The reduction in heart rate and systolic blood pressure response to stress and exercise induced by beta-blocking agents.
2. The antiarrhythmic response of beta-blocking agents induced by inhibition of catecholamine effects and/or other antiarrhythmic effects such as exhibited by class I antiarrhythmics.

Regarding the use of beta blockers clinically, it was noted that the trials left questions with regard to dose-response criteria. Dr. Rapaport expressed doubt that significant effects of beta-blocking agents were due to cell-membrane–stabilizing effects since the usual dosages used clinically are too low to bring about that effect. He cautioned against the possible intrinsic sympathomimetic effect. He urged caution regarding the criterion of cardioselectivity of different beta-blocking agents in that probably no beta blocker currently prescribed in the United States is purely a beta-I blocker without having beta-II–blocking effects as well, which affect bronchodilator dilatation, insulin production, and peripheral vasomotor activity. He also noted the high exclusion rate which occurred in the clinical trials and which was estimated to be as high as 75% of all considered subjects, due to administrative problems, age, and medical contraindications to the use of beta blockers. The contraindications were listed as chronic obstructive pulmonary disorders, congestive heart failure, symptomatic sick sinus syndrome, high-grade AV block, insulin-dependent diabetes, renal failure, peripheral vascular disease, psychological depression, and severe left ventricular dysfunction without heart failure.

By contrast, the experiences noted in Chapters 3, 4, and 5 were nonexclusionary; the same exercise protocol and "dose-response" criteria were applied to all patients, which included all of the conditions for which beta blockers were contraindicated. All patients without selectivity have shown improvements as noted in earlier chapters of this book. Moreover, in all patients from whom previously prescribed beta blockers were systematically withdrawn during the rehabilitation program, not only was there a further increase and not a decrease in exercise tolerance, but also there was not a return of arrhythmias after withdrawal. Indeed, arrhythmias declined as the Conditioning Index increased, and there was a mean improvement of more than two exercise tolerance stages utilizing the Balke protocol (treadmill) or its bicycle ergometer equivalent after beta-blocker withdrawal.

It should be emphasized that withdrawal of beta blockers *must* be carried out carefully and stepwise, i.e., as a weaning process. If patients on clinical doses of beta-blocking agents are withdrawn abruptly, a rise in heart rate and blood pressure occurs (see Chapter 3). The resulting abrupt rise of double product and its associated increase in heart work and myocardial oxygen demand, and the decrease in coronary blood supply associated with the increased heart rate, may be hazardous to the patient. The manufacturer and distributors of these drugs warn of the dangers of too sudden withdrawal. The Conditioning Index is a useful guide for phased withdrawal. At the HCRC a system of "titrated" withdrawal based on the Conditioning Index has been valuable in monitoring the results of decreasing beta-blocking agents and knowing when the effects of the drug are effectively gone. The same may be said for most, if not all, antiarrhythmic and antihypertensive medications, i.e., withdrawal should be phased.

It is concluded from the 53-month HCRC experience with patients taking usual prescribed clinical doses of propranolol, timolol, metoprolol, nadolol, and atenolol that (1) beta-blockers can be safely withdrawn, (2) the heart-rate– and blood-pressure–lowering effect of exercise conditioning is greater than that induced by the usual clinical doses of beta-blocking agents, (3) the exercise tolerance is improved over that achieved with the usual clinical doses of these medications, (4) the antiarrhythmic effects of the medications in their usual clinical doses are at least reproduced by exercise conditioning, (5) comprehensive cardiovascular rehabilitation does not have the contraindications of beta-blocking medications and is thus more widely applicable, and (6) as a corollary to (5) above, the undesirable side effects of beta blockers are eliminated, such

as, in addition to the contraindicated conditions, loss of libido, impotence in men, poor temperature regulation, lassitude and tiredness, and diarrhea.

There are both similarities and differences in the actions of exercise conditioning and of beta blockers. Both attenuate the rise in heart rate and systolic blood pressure that accompanies exercise or physical effort of any type and that accompanies psychological stress. They both lower resting heart rate and arterial blood pressure as well. Both also reduce or abolish arrhythmias. One of the major differences is that effective exercise conditioning results in a greater reduction in heart rate, systolic blood pressure, and, thus, double product than do the usual clinical dosages of beta-blocking medications. Moreover, there is on the average a two- to three- stage improvement in exercise tolerance with exercise conditioning than with beta-blocking medications. At least some of the improved exercise tolerance may be associated with the reduced myocardial contractility or ionotropic properties attributed to beta blockers in clinical use, i.e., a greater increase in cardiac output can be achieved by the heart.

Obviously, further research is needed, which may uncover the common mechanisms that cause both similar and different effects of pharmacological agents and exercise together with psychological and nutritional management.

Many fascinating observations have been made regarding the function of the heart following obstruction of the coronary blood supply to the heart, for example, increase in the density of adrenergic receptor sites in the myocytes of the affected area of the heart (Mukherjee *et al.,* 1982), increases in cyclic AMP associated with increased instability of cardiac tissue (Wallenberger *et al.,* 1969), and changes in Purkinje's fiber characteristics and increased influx of calcium (Mukherjee *et al.,* 1979) and catecholamines (Mathes *et al.,* 1971). How these and other important underlying mechanisms are related to the effects of both pharmacological agents and of exercise conditioning offers fruitful fields of research.

At present, little can be said regarding calcium-channel blockers, except that their relative role regarding cardiovascular rehabilitation is poorly documented as yet. It can be stated with confidence, however, that some patients do not do well regarding functional capacity on calcium-channel blockers and do better when the drugs are reduced or discontinued.

Another unanswered question relates to long-term effects on morbidity and mortality. The beta-blocker clinical trials report, as noted above, an overall reduction in two-year mortality (propranolol study) of 9.8% in the control group to 7.2% in the intervention group over 30 months. It should be noted that different centers involved in the clinical trials included different criteria for myocardial infarction, sudden and instantaneous death, and were made up of populations with differing severity of disease; moreover, follow-up times varied greatly. It also appears, though not statistically analyzed at the time (March 1983), that the benefits may be widening, i.e., that the difference in the control and intervention group mortality was increasing favorably.

The HCRC data are currently being evaluated in cooperation with the Texas Heart Institute study referred to in Chapters 11 and 12, which involves about 10,000 individuals for ten years and about 20,000 patients for lesser periods. The propranolol trial is currently reported for two years and includes about 1,800 controls and 1,800 in the intervention group. The HCRC study, to date, has only 101 from the first two years of the program but now followed for an average of 36 months (who *have completed* the program *and maintained* their exercise prescription at home) with a gross, overall mortality rate of 6.2%. Excluding those dying of causes unrelated to cardiovascular disease, the overall mortality is 5.7%. It is *emphasized* that these HCRC data must be regarded with caution. It is evident that mortality statistics and the interpretation of data are complex, and further study is necessary before firm conclusions are drawn with regard to the benefits of cardiovascular rehabilitation on life-span. Such studies are underway and will be reported when completed.

In summary, many patients when first seen for the initial evaluation have been treated for cardiac failure and angina pectoris, i.e., poor ventricular function and ischemia. Frequently, such patients have been prescribed furosemide to reduce preload, usually together with a potassium supplement, a digitalis medication to improve ventricular contractility, and an antihypertensive such as prazosin to reduce afterload. Further, they have also been given one or more long-acting antianginal medications (by mouth and/or by skin) and sublingual nitroglycerin as needed. It is not unusual for patients also to be taking a beta-blocking agent and/or a

calcium-channel–blocking agent, and a class I antiarrhythmic as well. Moreover, the patient also may be taking aspirin and/or dipyridamole, and a variety of anti-inflammatory agents for postcardiothoracic surgery and musculoskeletal disorders, and psychotropic (antidepressant, antianxiety, soporific, and so on) agents. It is not unusual that the patient also may have been prescribed other antiarthritic agents and an antiuricemic drug. When hypertensive, antihypertensives; when hyperglycemic, insulin or an oral antihyperglycemic or severely restricted diets. Some patients are also on warfarin. An important role of a rehabilitation center is to attempt to reveal any significant acute medication problems as soon as possible. Common ones are hypokalemia, especially in patients taking digitalis preparations, sometimes at toxic levels, digitalis and quinidine interactions, blood glucose levels, and so forth. Usually a careful history, physical examination, the electrocardiograph, the exercise tolerance test, and laboratory analysis of the blood (the HCRC normally obtains a fasting SMAC-20 plus HDL cholesterol and serum iron as a part of the initial evaluation) will reveal most medication problems. These routine studies may be supplemented by obtaining blood levels of medications such as digitalis and quinidine, and of prothrombin time with control when indicated. It should be emphasized that hypokalemia itself, and more so with digitalis, may exacerbate existing serious arrhythmias.

The cardiovascular rehabilitation center offers the opportunity for close, frequent monitoring of medication problems, which can supplement the attending physician's overall role in managing the patient. Moreover, medication problems can and do influence the course of rehabilitation itself. It has been demonstrated that comprehensive cardiovascular rehabilitation can benefit the patient by allowing most, if not all, medications to be discontinued or at least substantially reduced. Changing medications should be done carefully, with clinical and monitored indications and certainly with the knowledge and approval of the referring physician. As noted above, the HCRC experience to date is associated with a safe and apparently beneficial reduction of the use of medications of the order of 50%. It is evident that the effect of such a reduction on the cost of health care could be very substantial if such practices were general. It is estimated by the

American Heart Association that the cost of medications for patients with cardiovascular disease exceeds $3 billion per year.

The HCRC has also been conducting a study of the use of 24-hour Holter monitoring as a method of increasing the effectiveness in managing the use of medications in patients under the close scrutiny of a comprehensive cardiovascular rehabilitation program. Three purposes are intended. One purpose is to ascertain the extent to which the pulse-rate–lowering effect of exercise-induced conditioning, often in the setting of coexisting changes in drug utilization, is maintained or sustained over a 24-hour period, including not only an exercise therapy session, but also the other daily activities of the patient. A second purpose is to ascertain the extent to which the effects of reduction or removal of medications are sustained over the 24-hour period. The third purpose is to provide a more rational time sequencing of medications, and perhaps exercise as well, over the 24-hour period. The traditional, or usual, way of prescribing medications, for example three times daily, is morning, midday, and evening. The selection of the time is often left to the patient. It is reasonable to assume that the occurrence of conditions for which the medications are prescribed may vary considerably from the arbitrary time the drugs are taken and at which time peaks and valleys of blood concentration occur. Thus, relating the time of taking of medications more closely to the occurrence of conditions requiring the medications is a rational approach to demonstrate the HCRC experience, emphasizing the variations of internal stress, physical activity, and other conditions that significantly influence heart rate, blood pressure, arrhythmias, angina pectoris, and other physiological and clinical variables.

Although this project, appropriately utilizing 24-hour Holter monitoring, has been underway for less than one year, the results are already encouraging though not yet of a sample size to be reported quantitatively. It is most evident that the reduced heart rate seen after physiological conditioning extends throughout the 24-hour period. It is also evident that the reduction or discontinuance of medications does not result in unexpected effects at other times of the 24-hour period, and it appears that adjusting medication times can better cover conditions such as arrhythmias and angina pectoris when adjusted to times of maximum need rather than an arbitrary three times/day, for example.

Last, the role of a comprehensive cardiovascular rehabilitation center in assisting in medications management also emphasizes the need for careful patient monitoring under the close supervision of a knowledgeable physician.

General Medical Management

When a patient is referred to a dedicated, comprehensive cardiovascular rehabilitation center, stimulated with virtually maximal perceived physical exertion and closely monitored three times per week for a period averaging 12 to 14 weeks, it is likely that there has never before been a period of that patient's life involving such close observation for such an extended period of time. The experiences of the HCRC demonstrate that there are many consequences of this intense three- to three-and-one-half-month interaction between the staff and the patient. Moreover, that patient is followed semiannually for as long as possible. This prolonged period of intensive interacting with a multidisciplinary staff, armed with a detailed history of the patient's medical, social, and vocational history together with a detailed initial evaluation at the Center, provides a major benefit to the patient and the referring or attending physician that could be obtained in few, if any, other circumstances.

One aspect of this situation is that the cardiovascular rehabilitation center is, in a sense, an effective screening center for the patient's referring or attending physician. It is essential that a comprehensive cardiovascular rehabilitation staff understand enough about clinical cardiology and cardiothoracic surgery, as well as general clinical medicine and pharmacology, to play its role, as well as having expertise in exercise physiology, clinical and counseling psychology, and nutrition and dietetics.

Most physicians are well aware that patients, particularly those with cardiovascular disease who are postoperative, post–myocardial infarction, or not postinfarction or postsurgery but are symptomatic, virtually live in fear and uncertainty. The patient and his physician alike have a problem in this regard. Some patients hesitate to call the physician due to denial, fear of what the physician will say, economic concerns, or simply not wishing to bother the doctor. Some patients call the doctor with every irregular heartbeat or twinge anywhere in the body. The structure of the rehabilitation center offers security and an opportunity to explore the significance of the multitude of concerns and symptoms that virtually all patients have. In turn, the rehabilitation center provides the referring or attending physician with better insight as to the status of the patient and more professional information regarding his/her response to the patient's calls or lack thereof.

After becoming acquainted with the HCRC, most referring physicians are satisfied to rely upon the Center for providing day-to-day primary medical care, in addition to the rehabilitation effort itself. In turn, this provides the rehabilitation center with a more sensitive knowledge of how patients' day-to-day health and emotional conditions affect the rehabilitation effort. Indeed, the types of things that affect the rehabilitation process, which have been described in this book, could not have been determined had the HCRC been unable to, in effect, have the whole patient during the rehabilitation process.

Primary care usually involves the evaluation and treatment of simple, common infections, especially the seasonal or epidemic upper respiratory infections and flu, complications of the sternal wound, or of the coronary vein graft harvest site, monitoring of prothrombin time, blood glucose, adjusting of medications, and the variety of primary day-to-day ailments afflicting any general population. Many patient complaints are born out of uncertainty and fear, and hence subside after the patients have been in the program.

A major benefit to the patient of a rehabilitation program is the achievement of a better understanding of how the body works, why the rehabilitation efforts work, and reassurance that death is not about to occur with each PVC, pain, or ache. Especially reassuring is the self-demonstration that the patient can undertake known physical effort without danger. The patient learns the why and extent of his/her limits and how to recognize and live with them.

Moreover, the cardiovascular rehabilitation center staff must be able to ascribe appropriate significance to the entire spectrum of disorders, signs, and symptoms presented by the population of patients in the rehabilitation program and its follow-up sequence. Thus, in addition to being a rehabilitation center, it is also a primary health care center, and in dealing with specific problems in the province of comprehensive cardiovascular rehabilitation, it is a secondary and tertiary health care facility.

The comprehensive cardiovascular rehabilitation center, with close attention to the patient, frequently reveals diseases and functional disorders that would not likely have been revealed, at least as early in their course or natural history. The identification of sleep apnea and anemia of various etiologies, for example, is not uncommon. Others relatively common are chronic obstructive pulmonary disease associated with asthma (often induced by exercise, and exacerbated by beta blockers and other medications), chronic bronchitis, and emphysema associated with a long history of smoking. Peripheral vascular disease and the sequelae of former cerebrovascular accidents or the specter of TIAs often complicate the picture of a patient referred with a primary history of coronary heart disease. Disorders of the musculoskeletal system are common, especially arthritis. Between 30 and 38% have complaints associated with arthritis, low-back syndrome, or other orthopedic disorders. The spectrum of coexisting disorders seen at the HCRC extends from Hansen's disease to myasthenia gravis, from atelectasis to Zimmerlin's atrophy.

As already noted in various chapters of this book, regularly occurring medical afflictions, in addition to the heart disease itself, are

Significant depression and/or anxiety disorders	84%
Hypertension (moderate to severe)	31%
Sleep disorders including sleep apnea	28%
Diabetes or abnormally elevated serum glucose	26%
Chronic obstructive pulmonary disease	13%
Serum iron deficiency	12%
Anemia	9%
Coexisting occlusive peripheral vascular disease	4%
Coexisting stroke sequelae	4%
Medication-management problems, associated with an average of 6.4 medications per patient	

A comprehensive cardiovascular rehabilitation center, treating patients with cardiovascular diseases, an array of associated and unrelated disorders, and involving the adjustment of medications, *must* be staffed by competent people and *must* be operated virtually like an intensive care facility. It must be under the direct and close supervision at all times of an appropriately trained and licensed physician. Conversely, in this author's experience, it should not be argued that a cardiovascular rehabilitation center can be run safely or effectively without careful, continuous monitoring.

Psychological Disorder Management

From the outset, the Houston Cardiovascular Rehabilitation Center was planned and staffed to provide professional, psychological expertise and practice. It was anticipated that the disabilities of most, if not all, patients would contain a significant component of psychological disorder. Moreover, it was anticipated that the large majority of these problems would be situational rather than pathological. Hence, a psychologist rather than a psychiatrist was recruited. However, this was with the understanding that if psychopathology were revealed, or if situations requiring psychiatric expertise developed, that psychiatric involvement would be provided. In fact, psychiatric consultation has been necessary in only a half-dozen cases over four years of operation.

If anything, the HCRC experience has strengthened the conviction that psychological disorders and psychological, emotional, and behavioral issues are critical aspects of successful rehabilitation. Just as the exercise therapy undoubtedly is psychologically and emotionally therapeutic, so too, adequate attention and care to patients' psychological and emotional status contribute to their performance in exercise and to their compliance with the exercise program. Examples of the interactions between psychological/emotional factors and physiological parameters were presented in Chapter 8. These examples clearly show that psychological stress has detrimental effects on patients' physiological responses to exercise, hence, on progress in exercise, and that the resolution of stressful situations contributes to progress in conditioning, largely by the removal of the stress-induced impediment.

The psychological test data reported in Chapter 8 support the following conclusions about the importance of psychological/emotional issues in rehabilitation patients, and about the benefits that result from the inclusion of an active psychological treatment program. Most patients entering the HCRC program exhibit symptoms of anxiety and depression. Interviews of these patients support the idea that in the majority of cases, these emotional symptoms are reactive with respect to the patient's health status. These situational disorders are significantly reduced, if not eliminated, during involvement in comprehensive cardiovascular rehabilitation. The coronary-prone (type A) pattern typifies slightly more than 50% of entering patients, and a smaller proportion

exhibit this pattern to a marked degree. Thus, psychological treatment in cardiovascular rehabilitation should not be based on an assumption that most patients exhibit the coronary-prone personality pattern. Rather, psychological treatment should be broadly focused on improving coping with emotional stress, whatever the source. For patients who entered the program exhibiting the coronary-prone pattern, the strength of the coronary-prone characteristics was moderated to a significant degree. There are indications, in the HCRC data, that early referral to a comprehensive cardiovascular rehabilitation program following a major medical event is prophylactic with respect to preventing more severe and fixed situational emotional reactions that tend to develop when the sources of fears, anxieties, and depression are not adequately identified and addressed in time.

The HCRC's experience in treating the psychological/behavioral/emotional complications of cardiovascular disease has confirmed the initial premise that psychology is the discipline of choice in this setting. Of all the mental health professions, psychology is uniquely qualified to meet the needs of rehabilitation patients and of a rehabilitation center. Psychologists are trained in the delivery of therapeutic services, in the use of interview and psychometric diagnostic procedures, in theories and principles of behavior, motivation, and behavior change, and in research methods. Thus, the psychologist plays a central role in many facets of a rehabilitation center. Nationally, there has been a steady increase in the interrelationships between the field of psychology and the field of clinical medicine, both as partners in practice and in research. The National Heart, Lung and Blood Institute now has a Behavioral Medical Branch to encourage, evaluate, and support research proposals relating the behavioral, clinical, and basic sciences. The American Heart Association and many of its affiliates have increasingly recognized the importance of interrelating the traditional clinical and basic medical science with behavioral science. The comprehensive cardiovascular rehabilitation center offers a valuable laboratory in this fertile area.

Nutrition Disorder Management and Secondary Prevention in Rehabilitation

Cardiovascular rehabilitation has, of course, two objectives. One is to reduce or abolish the disabilities and morbidity associated with already manifest cardiovascular disease. The other objective is to impede or halt the otherwise progressive nature of the major underlying cardiovascular disease, atherosclerosis. A major portion of the literature relating nutrition and cardiovascular disease concerns nutrition-influenced risk factors for atherosclerosis (Stamler, 1983). The role of nutrition and dietetics in reducing disability and morbidity and their role in secondary prevention through risk-factor reduction are perhaps identical or at least overlapping. Obesity is disabling and also regarded as a risk factor, although its power as an independent risk factor is debatable and probably not as strong as hyperlipidemia. The correction of obesity and that of hyperlipidemia are both in the province of nutrition and dietetics. Diabetes is both a disability-producing illness and a risk factor for atherosclerotic disease. The combined efforts of effective exercise-induced conditioning and proper nutrition have been shown to improve the diabetic state, often to the degree that previously insulin- or oral hypoglycemic-dependent diabetics can be controlled by exercise and diet.

To the extent that sodium intake exacerbates hypertension, which is a disease or at least a disorder, and is also an atherosclerotic risk factor, the control of sodium intake is in the province of nutrition and dietetics.

The role of nutrition in general health maintenance and energy balance already covers a wide field and as yet is not fully exploited. The role of dietary elements such as copper and zinc in hyperlipidemia is undergoing a resurgence of interest and research.

Katz stated, "Atherosclerosis is a distinct entity—it is not inevitable, nor is it irreversible. Rather it is preventable and, at least to a point, curable. . . . Further, atherosclerosis is a metabolic disease, the byproduct of an habitually unbalanced diet, excessive in total calories, empty calories, total fats, saturated fats, cholesterol, refined carbohydrates, salt. . . ." (Katz, *et al.,* 1958). If these statements are valid, no comprehensive cardiovascular rehabilitation program should exclude the professional nutritionist and dietitian in a prominent and effective role.

Recently, Stamler (1983) has reviewed the evidence for the 1958 statement in the light of twenty-five years of further research, epidemiological trials, animal experiments, and clinical studies. Stamler draws eight major conclusions from his analyses:

(1) With nutritional survey methods of adequate validity to distinguish one person from another within a population, dietary lipid intake of individuals is significantly and independently related to serum cholesterol of individuals and to long-term CHD risk. Thus, these data from within-population epidemiologic research are complementary and consistent with data from cross-population studies, as well as animal-experimental findings on the important role of dietary lipids in the etiology of epidemic atherosclerotic disease.

(2) The recent resurgence of research on fractions of serum total cholesterol, i.e., on serum lipoproteins, has yielded data complementing and refining —not contradicting—the extensive data on the interrelationship between diet and serum total cholesterol. Long-standing dietary recommendations for prevention of CHD remain valid. Based on the extensive positive experiences of Mediterranean and Far Eastern countries, as well as on controlled experiments in man and animals, these recommendations emphasize moderate reduction in total fat, marked reduction in saturated fat and cholesterol, moderate (not marked) increase of polyunsaturated fat, moderate increase in complex carbohydrates and fiber (from vegetables, fruits, whole grain products, legumes), foods of low caloric density to assist in avoiding or correcting obesity while assuring a high intake of all essential macro- and micronutrients, and avoidance of high intake of sodium and alcohol. When these recommendations are followed, the entire lipid-lipoprotein spectrum is influenced favorably.

(3) The assertion that diet recommendations to influence serum cholesterol and CHD risk are ineffectual is not in keeping with findings from cross-population and within-population epidemiologic studies, controlled experiments in man, and mass public health experience (national and international) during the last 10–15 years.

(4) Dietary cholesterol in the amounts consumed by hundreds of millions of people in the industrialized countries significantly influences serum total cholesterol, cholesterol-bearing lipoproteins, and CHD risk. The assertion that people in general, including apparently healthy people, need not be concerned about dietary cholesterol and foods high in cholesterol (e.g., eggs) is at variance with a vast array of scientific data on man and animals.

(5) Both massive sets of research data and realistic considerations of practical nutritional guidance for individuals, families, and populations compel the conclusion that attention to nutrient and foodstuff composition of the habitual diet—including its lipid composition—is a cornerstone of the effort to achieve improved eating habits, and thereby prevention and control of overweight and of hypercholesterolemia.

(6) Reduction of all fats—without attention to composition of the diet—is not a scientifically sound or practically realistic approach to achieving

sizable improvement in serum cholesterol-lipid-lipo-protein levels for populations of "western" industri-alized countries. To achieve such changes, attention must be given to lipid composition of the diet, partic-ularly to sizable reduction in saturated fat and cho-lesterol intake, plus attention to type of carbohydrate used in place of fat.

(7) The decisive lipid nutritional recommenda-tions for the general population for CHD prevention are low saturated fat and low cholesterol intake. High intake of polyunsaturated fat is not one of the recom-mendations, and has not been for years. The "issue" of high polyunsaturates is in essence a non-issue.

(8) Extensive evidence is available indicating both the efficacy and safety of the nutritional recommen-dations for prevention of the atherosclerotic diseases. Assertions about possible dangers of these recom-mendations are not buttressed by data, but rather are hypothetical, hence are not a sound basis for judg-ment about applying available knowledge to control epidemic disease and improve life expectancy with better health.

As detailed in Chapters 9 and 10, the HCRC program has undertaken, from its outset, to integrate registered dietitians (RDs) who are professionally trained with at least a master's degree in nutrition. There has been a close working relationship between The University of Texas Health Science Center's program in nutrition and dietetics and the HCRC.

The major objectives of the nutrition com-ponent of the HCRC rehabilitation program are to

1. Establish desirable food consumption patterns
   a. 10 to 15% of consumed calories from protein
   b. 30% of consumed calories from fat (10% saturated, 10% polyunsaturated, 10% monounsaturated)
   c. 55 to 60% of consumed calories from carbohydrate, with emphasis on com-plex carbohydrates
2. Decrease sodium intake
3. Increase fiber intake
4. Achieve and maintain ideal weight
5. Deal effectively with specific disorders re-lated to diet or supplements, e.g., dia-betes, hyperlipidemias, low serum iron, diet-related anemias, and so on

These objectives relate to reduction both of disabilities and of risk factors.

In the HCRC experience, 64% of patients have been found to be clinically obese, i.e., >20% over their ideal weight, and 14% have

been morbidly obese, i.e., ≥ 100 pounds or 100% over their ideal weight. Thirty-six per cent of individuals have, prior to referral to the HCRC, already achieved their ideal weight. As shown in Chapter 4, the mean weight loss for all patients was 4.3 lb for men, 6.3 lb for women, and 4.7 lb for all. Since this weight loss occurred in the 64% who were more than 20% overweight, and was corrected for the 36% who were not initially overweight and maintained their ideal weight during the program, the aver-age weight loss for the overweight was 14.5 lb for men, 10.7 lb for women, and 12.9 lb for all. This weight loss occurred over an average dura-tion of 13.8 weeks or, on the average, close to the goal of 1 lb per week. Further correction for the morbidly obese brought the average weight loss for the nonmorbidly obese to the program goal. On the average, those closest to their ideal body weight on entering the program came closest to achieving their ideal weight by the time they exited the program. Follow-up data demonstrate that 76% of those initially be-tween 20 and 50% over their ideal weight at entry had achieved and were maintaining their ideal weight by at least one year from entry into the rehabilitation program.

The general experience of most, if not all, programs concerned with treating the morbidly obese has been discouraging. The HCRC expe-rience is no exception. Since 14% of the HCRC patients were in this category and their weights were pooled with the overall data exhibited in Table 4-1, N, the data are skewed. Moreover, their average weight loss during the program averaged only 7.4 lb, thus skewing the exit data as well. There was a poor correlation of weight loss in this subgroup to any other variable ex-hibited in Table 4-1; indeed, some gained weight in the program.

Mary W. Schanler (see Chapter 10), for two years prior to joining the HCRC, had headed a facility devoted exclusively to treating mas-sively obese individuals. The data from that facility (Rose General Hospital, Denver, Colo-rado) demonstrated almost universal failure to achieve long-term benefits. Weight losses of 100 lbs, for example, would be regained in one month upon leaving the program. It is believed that the general lack of success in this distinct subgroup of obesity is associated primarily with psychological disorders. There does not appear to be a single, underlying disorder, however. Rather, excessive eating appears to serve as a generalized method of coping with psychological distress, albeit a maladaptive method, highly resistant to intervention.

Methods involving hospitalized isolation-starvation, the use of gastric stapling, and team approaches involving psychiatry, nutrition, and medical expertise achieve only transient, if any, success in general. The HCRC is not a facility devoted exclusively to the treatment of obesity. Yet a significant number (i.e., more than in the general population) of patients referred for cardiovascular rehabilitation, with manifest cardiovascular disease and related disorders, also are morbidly obese. There have been, weightwise, enough isolated cases that have responded that a policy to exclude such patients has not been adopted. Indeed, the achievement of increased exercise tolerance and Conditioning Index of this subgroup has been significant, although the scatter is larger than the standard deviation of the pooled data. Among men and women, the morbidly obese appeared in both the highest and lowest percentile of exercise tolerance and Conditioning Index achievement.

In summary, with regard to weight, more than one third of referred patients have achieved an ideal weight prior to entering the HCRC program. Of the approximately two thirds of those over their ideal weight, those who were between 20 and 50% over their ideal weight at entry, achieved their ideal weight within one year. The closer the patient was to ideal weight on entry, the more likelihood there was of achieving ideal weight within the approximately 14 average weeks in the program. The exceptional, distinct subgroup of the obese was the morbidly obese, which achieved little overall success in weight loss. However, there were isolated successes in weight loss, and significant overall gains in exercise tolerance and Conditioning Index.

The other nutrition-related variables of interest both with regard to disability and to risk factor reduction are considered below, under the heading of Secondary Prevention.

SECONDARY PREVENTION

As noted earlier, a comprehensive cardiovascular rehabilitation center has two, interrelated objectives: (1) the reduction or abolition of the disabilities and morbidity associated with already manifest cardiovascular diseases, and (2) secondary prevention through the reduction of risk factors. Insurance companies are often criticized because their reimbursement policies are for the treatment of already established health afflictions and illness but generally exclude reimbursement for primary and secondary prevention, with such notable exceptions as immunization or treatments for potential complications of illness or surgery. It should be understood that insurance companies, especially the commercial companies and Blue Cross/Blue Shield, are in the business of selling insurance and underwriting risk (see Chapters 14 and 15). Few, if any, insurance company physicians or executives would argue against the value of prevention. The issue is that the customer, the purchaser of insurance, is as yet unwilling to pay the costs (premium) for preventive measures. It is not simply a question of cost alone, but also a question of cost:benefit. There is uncertainty of the cost-effectiveness of screening an entire population for risk factors. Furthermore, the cost-effectiveness of reducing risk factors as a means of reducing the incidence and prevalence of disease and its progress, in contrast to diagnosing and treating an individual after signs and symptoms of disease develop and a diagnosis of a treatable illness is made, has not been demonstrated. The major prospective trials in prevention have been conducted by corporate endeavors, or by government-funded studies.

Herein lies another major benefit of comprehensive cardiovascular rehabilitation in that although insurance reimbursement is for the treatment and rehabilitation of manifest, diagnosed health afflictions, in so doing, the risk factors that do exist in that patient are revealed, and the treatments for disability are the same as they would be for risk-factor reductions. Thus, in effect, secondary prevention is instituted under the reimbursable policies of disability treatment and will benefit patients to the extent that prevention does influence long-term morbidity and mortality (Alderman *et al.,* 1981; Amsterdam, 1981; Dustan, 1981; Gotto, 1981; Stamler, 1983).

Moreover, herein lies another opportunity to evaluate the impact of risk-factor reduction on the natural history of industrialized man's most common death- and disability-causing disease.

As reported in other sections of this chapter, and other chapters of this book, the cross-population statistics regarding risk-factor reduction, at least in the HCRC patient population, are gratifying with respect to some risk factors and disappointing with regard to others. To the extent that physiological conditioning and exercise tolerance induced by exercise are risk factors, the benefits of comprehensive cardio-vascular rehabilitation enhanced by medical, psychological, and nutritional management are major. Earlier in this chapter (see "Management of Medications") a brief discussion of mortality statistics was undertaken. Shaw (1981) also presents recent data on the benefits of exercise on mortality. Also, Chapters 11 and 12 deal with mortality in general in cardiovascular disease. The HCRC experience demonstrates significant improvement in exercise tolerance in virtually every patient who completed the program and an overall improvement of essentially threefold. Some start from an exercise tolerance limited to little more than the resting state to exit at the level of a fit college student. The exit level of exercise tolerance and Conditioning Index was maintained overall in 72% of patients followed for four, three, and two years.

To the extent that hypertension is a risk factor, 31% of patients entering the HCRC program suffered from moderate to severe hypertension, with a history of at least five years of hypertension. All exhibited a fall in both systolic and diastolic pressure both at rest and with respect to exercise load. Seventy-one per cent at exit or within six months of exit had blood pressures which were well controlled on reduced or no medications. Also, an average of 71% of those followed for almost five, four, three, and two years have maintained favorable blood pressure levels (see Chapter 5).

To the extent that smoking is a risk factor (Hartz et al., 1981), 61% of prior smokers had already stopped. Of the remaining 39%, 82% stopped or reduced their smoking to under one-half pack of cigarettes per day while in the program. Of the remaining, 18% of those who still smoked on exit were similar in many ways to the morbidly obese in that smoking apparently served as a coping device which was highly resistant to intervention. The benefits regarding smoking cessation have been gratifying, although disappointing with regard to the hard-core, recalcitrant smoker. Overall, 61% of smokers, being faced with evidence of a life-threatening disease, stopped smoking prior to entry into rehabilitation. The remaining 39% had obviously found it difficult to stop even after a heart attack, heart surgery, angina, and arrhythmias, thus representing a distinct subset. Of these, the rehabilitation program was successful in 82% of cases, leaving a further distinct subset of about 5% who did not stop or substantially reduce smoking after both the im-pact of the knowledge of, and suffering related to, manifest cardiovascular disease and comprehensive cardiovascular rehabilitation. Follow-up to four years has demonstrated that 11% of those who had stopped or reduced smoking below one-half pack per day either resumed or increased their smoking.

To the extent that body weight is a risk factor, the problem is similar to that of smoking and has been discussed above.

Although, as Stamler (1983) points out, the evidence shows that nutrition-related risk factors are correlated with atherosclerosis, much remains to be learned about how to achieve better results in lowering these risk factors. The subject of nutrition-related disorders is interesting in that, although few people entering a rehabilitation program claim confidence in their knowledge about psychological, deconditioning, and medical disorders, many proclaim that they have a self-satisfying understanding of the principles of nutrition. When patients are informed that the comprehensive cardiovascular rehabilitation program includes nutrition counseling, the statement, "Oh, I know all about nutrition and diets," is often heard. Indeed, a few patients refuse to become involved in nutrition counseling even when they are presented with evidence of having nutritional disorders. Thus, an assessment of nutrition knowledge is a part of the initial evaluation prior to entering the program. Table 4-1 illustrates the fact that the level of nutrition and dietary knowledge is fairly low on entry but is significantly improved by the program. The scaled rating increased, on the average, from 58 to 79% of expected nutrition-dietary knowledge. As noted, there is a poor correlation between the need to know, i.e., having nutritional disorders, and the knowledge. Nevertheless, in all cases of diabetes who were compliant with both exercise and nutrition therapy, an improvement in the diabetic status occurred. Twenty-six per cent on entry exhibited elevated fasting blood glucose, and 18% were being treated with insulin or oral hypoglycemic agents. Although the overall statistics (Table 2-1) demonstrated a normal level of fasting blood glucose at entry and exit, with no significant difference, those with elevated blood sugars normalized, and the need for insulin or oral hypoglycemic agents was decreased. Although the study is still underway, it is of interest to note that it appears that following an acute myocardial infarction, and more evidently following heart surgery, there is an elevated fasting serum glucose which may resolve spontaneously after a few months. Others have also noted an improvement in what apparently is diabetes with exercise therapy (Gonzalez, 1979). The nature of this phenomenon remains to be defined.

To the extent that cholesterol, triglycerides, and the total cholesterol/HDL cholesterol are risk factors, the overall statistics are that significant, but small, reductions in total plasma cholesterol levels occur. HDL cholesterol increases overall, but is poorly correlated with physiological conditioning measures. The ratio of total to HDL cholesterol drops a small, but significant, amount and is also poorly correlated with physiological conditioning. The overall statistics exhibit an insignificant rise in fasting blood glucose, yet individuals with elevated glucose levels exhibit a significant drop with exercise conditioning. These problems with cross-population statistics are discussed in Chapter 4 and serve to illustrate the need for improved nutrition and dietetic technology to apply the knowledge that nutrition-related disorders increase disability and atherosclerosis risk factors, in order to achieve better results.

To the extent that psychological stress (as differentiated from stressors) and the so-called coronary-prone characteristics are risk factors, the picture is more encouraging. Chapters 7 and 8 provide the basis for and the demonstration of the fact that coping with stress, reduction of coronary-prone characteristics, and the reduction of depression, anxiety, denial, and hypochondriasis are achievable in a comprehensive cardiovascular rehabilitation center. Thus, disability, morbidity, and secondary prevention objectives are achieved.

Although ill-defined in population studies, it is evident that individuals are more or less sensitive to certain substances that in the sensitive ones constitute risk factors, for example, coffee and arrhythmias, alcohol and cardiomyopathy, smoking and Buerger's disease, and so on. A comprehensive cardiovascular rehabilitation program serves to identify and usually to effectively reduce or eliminate the use of these substances.

Also, although ill-defined, so-called iatrogenic risk factors are generally recognized, e.g., the prescription of medications which may increase one or another risk factor while benefiting other medical problems. Oral contraceptives, beta-adrenergic blocking agents, and intermediate adverse reactions are examples. It has been suggested that physician-patient interactions may increase risk factors. The best example is physician enforcement of unnecessary physical activity restrictions.

A family history of cardiovascular disease has been demonstrated and is generally regarded as a risk factor. It is uncertain as to the extent to which this relationship is genetically determined and/or to what extent it is influenced by the life-style of families. The HCRC patients are reminded that obesity is often higher in children with obese parents; overeating is often a family matter with the admonishment of the parent to the child, "Now clean your plate." Smoking appears to be greater with children of parents who smoke, and so on. Studies have shown that of the various influences on life-style, the family physician and pediatrician may have a major impact on changing life-style. Parents and their children apparently take more seriously the views of their physician (another iatrogenic effect) than those of schools and media. While all are important, a comprehensive cardiovascular rehabilitation program can provide an intensive, documented approach to life-style modification for patients, hence, for their families and friends' families. Self-reporting of patients indicates that this sharing occurred frequently among the HCRC patients.

In summary, the cross-population study of HCRC patients has demonstrated that the following risk factors are favorably influenced. Also, Chapter 15 speaks to this from an insurance physician's point of view.

RISK FACTOR	SIGNIFICANT CHANGE
1. Physiological deconditioning	Decreased***
2. Smoking abuse	Decreased***
3. Hypertension	Decreased***
4. High-density lipoproteins (HDL)	Increased**
5. Nutritional deficits	Decreased***
6. Hypercholesterolemia	Decreased**
7. Hypertriglyceridemia	N.C.
8. Total cholesterol/HDL ratio	Decreased**
9. Diabetes severity	Decreased**(*)
10. Obesity and % body weight as fat (except in morbid obesity)	Decreased***
11. Psychological stress and coronary-prone characteristics	Decreased***
12. Negative iatrogenic and specific hazardous substance effects	Decreased*
13. Negative general life-style patterns	Decreased*

It is evident that the effects of comprehensive cardiovascular rehabilitation on these risk factors has not been uniform quantitatively or qualitatively. Those affected to a high quantitative and statistical significance are noted by ***, those of statistical significance but of relatively low quantitative level by **, and those primarily qualitative by *. Cross-population analyses, such as that of the HCRC data, require careful subgroup analyses to improve understanding of the statistics. Correlation and related cluster analyses demonstrate that on the one hand the small but statistical increase in total cholesterol to HDL and % body weight as fat is not correlated with physical conditioning as might be expected, but is correlated with weight reduction. On the other hand, although there is no statistically significant quantitative change in fasting plasma glucose in the overall population, there is a significant reduction in abnormal glucose metabolism in diabetes. The size and characteristics of the subgroup are insufficient to alter the picture of the population as a whole.

With these caveats, it is nevertheless evident that a comprehensive cardiovascular rehabilitation program favorably affects cardiovascular disease risk factors.

INDICATIONS FOR CARDIOVASCULAR REHABILITATION: WHY, WHEN, AND HOW

A perusal of Table 16-1 and the quantitative extent of benefits described in this book indicate that comprehensive cardiovascular rehabilitation may be advocated for all patients who are (1) post–myocardial infarction, (2) post–heart surgery (coronary or valve repair), (3) with known coronary artery disease (symptomatic or not, postinfarct or not) and with brady- or tachyarrhythmias, (4) with cardiomyopathies of known or unknown origin, (5) with occlusive peripheral vascular disease, and (6) with hypertension. Moreover, when such afflictions are accompanied by other disabling medical, psychological, and nutritional disorders, the value of rehabilitation is even greater.

It may be concluded from the HCRC experience, as demonstrated by cases presented in Chapters 3, 4, and 5, that there are few contraindications. The AMA lists the following: "Unstable angina pectoris, severe ventricular dysfunction manifest by a drop in systolic blood pressure or limited cardiac output in response to exercise, or severe dyspnea at low work loads, active cardiomyopathy or myocarditis in the previous year, uncontrolled hypertension, complex dysrhythmias, second and third degree A-V block, uncontrolled atrial fibrillation, substantial cardiomegaly, hemodynamically relevant valvular or congenital heart disease—as well as important noncardiac illnesses, orthopedic, pulmonary, gastrointestinal, and other systemic diseases, particularly the following: recent pulmonary embolism, anemia, uncontrolled metabolic diseases (e.g., diabetes mellitus, uremia, thyrotoxicosis), and transient febrile illnesses."

As the HCRC has developed, no procedures have been considered with more seriousness, care, and caution than acceptance and treatment of patients with conditions that have been listed as contraindications for exercise. Prior to the AMA document (Council on Scientific Affairs, 1981), the American Heart Association (1975) prepared a document containing an even more extensive list of contraindications and reasons for discontinuing, temporarily reducing, or deferring physical effort. If the 1975 AHA list had been strictly adhered to, a major number of patients treated, with significant benefit and no untoward events, would have been rejected. Two key words used in both the AMA and AHA documents are *uncontrolled* and *unstable* with an implied condition of downhill or failing. As noted elsewhere in this book, the HCRC has been structured to be, as closely as possible, a critical care facility with at least one physician and two to three nurses, trained and experienced in critical care, in close attendance at all times. Moreover, monitoring includes continuous, telemetered electrocardiographs with alarm systems, careful watching of clinical signs and symptoms, blood pressure, and a standardized system of providing exercise and assigning criteria for unusual or abnormal responses. In addition, a system for resuscitation and advanced life support is closely and readily available, and the Center is adjacent to the several hospitals of the Texas Medical Center. Also, as noted elsewhere, after more than 30,000 hours of exercise therapy and 2,500 sign/symptom-limited exercise *stress* or tolerance tests, there have been no incidents that could have been related to the use of exercise.

The approach to treating individuals, a considerable number of whom fall into the categories of those on the AMA and AHA contraindication lists, has been slow, careful, monitored, recorded, and analyzed. In each case, the patient and referring physician have been aware of the higher risk that the patient is in, not necessarily resulting from exercise application, but because of the serious nature of the illness. As experience developed and results were certainly more positive than negative, more confidence accrued, and as the number of patients with serious illness treated with benefit developed, it can be said that there are more indications for, than contraindications to, trying comprehensive cardiovascular rehabilitation. This author highly recommends an excellent article by Warren (1982) on sudden death. To be sure, a candidate for sudden death is a candidate for sudden death. It has yet to be shown, in this author's opinion, that *properly* and carefully applied exercise, monitored by experienced professionals, has hastened the death of such candidates. Conversely, it has been demonstrated that many, if not most, can be significantly benefited.

Cautious conservatism is an ancient dictum of medicine, defined by the Hippocratic Oath. The history of medicine is replete with examples of customary and usual practices initially defined more by caution than by experience. As experience, technology, and science develop, previous attitudes and practice patterns change. Some contraindications and indications, as well, become established; others are discarded or changed, to wit: the change from the practice of strict, extended bed rest for myocardial infarction, followed by a prolonged and sedentary convalescence, to early ambulation and an early return to activity.

As has been demonstrated, patients with severe ventricular dysfunction have been selected for comprehensive cardiovascular rehabilitation by the HCRC, and, as documented in Chapters 3, 4, and 5, these included patients with high-grade coronary artery disease, patients who had suffered multiple infarctions, and cardiomyopathies secondary to coronary heart disease, alcoholism, postinfection, and of unknown origin. Of those who were compliant and were gradually reconditioned while being carefully monitored, *all* showed significant improvement. The improvements were exhibited in several ways. Their exercise tolerance increased. Their ejection fractions increased. There was both global and regional improvement in ventricular wall motion, while initial exercise tolerance tests were accompanied by decompensation or the patient was so severely ill that the test could not be taken. The exit tests did not exhibit decompensation unless the intensity of exercise load was pushed beyond the rehabilitation improvement.

One case example is presented in Chapter 3 (Patient #041) to illustrate the point. This patient, after a series of myocardial infarctions and aortocoronary artery bypass surgery, was "totally and permanently disabled." He could not do more than stand on the treadmill for an initial exercise tolerance test. Initially, he could no more than sit on the bicycle ergometer. His resting ejection fraction was 18%, and he was in incipient congestive heart failure. With careful and gradual exercise and psychological therapy, he was able to achieve 350 kpm · min^{-1} on a bicycle ergometer for 30 minutes; he was able to complete stage III of the exercise treadmill tolerance test; and his ejection fraction had increased to 38% at rest with a slight, but insignificant, rise with stress. He returned to work. This required seven months rather than the average 14 weeks.

At the other end of the scale, a patient (#221, Chapter 3) entered the program with cardiomyopathy of unknown origin. His entry ejection fraction was 20% at rest, his heart was markedly dilated, and he could not complete stage I of the initial exercise tolerance test. On exit, after 8 weeks, he could undertake 900 kpm · min^{-1} of exercise on a bicycle ergometer for 30 minutes without symptoms. His heart size was normal, his ejection fraction was 56% at rest increasing to 67% with stress, and he was able to complete stage IX of the treadmill exercise tolerance test. Thirteen per cent of patients referred to the HCRC, in whom ejection fractions were measured, had ejection fractions estimated to be less than 35% on entry. On exit, none was less than 35%, all had improved, and 62% of the 13% noted above had achieved resting ejection fractions of 50% or greater. A study is now underway comparing prerehabilitation ejection fractions with postrehabilitation ejection fractions, together with other criteria such as exercise tolerance, cardiac output, stroke volume, double product, Conditioning Index, angina, arrhythmias, and so on. This study unfortunately is not far enough along to report at the time of writing this book. Obviously, it is a complex subject including validating some of the estimates of ejection fraction that were reported on past medical records simply as "poor," and so on. As indicated in Chapters 11 and 13, and from the HCRC experience as well, a patient may have a "normal" fraction at rest, e.g., >50%, but not exhibit an increase with stress. The ejection fraction and stroke volume may not be directly correlated, and functions such as regional wall dysfunction are important. An *impression* may be provided, however. Patients whose ejection fractions are relatively normal at rest (>50%), even though they may or may not increase with stress during a nuclear ventriculogram test, will usually not exhibit a decompensatory response on an exercise tolerance test (see Chapter 5). On exit from the rehabilitation program, with an average of a threefold increase in exercise tolerance, the resting ejection fraction may not have changed, but the stress ejection fraction will usually have increased. The lower the resting ejection fraction is, on entry, the more likely it is to increase percentagewise. For example, both patients #041 and #221 cited above doubled, or more than doubled, their resting ejection fractions. There is much to be learned; however, it may be said that with diligent monitoring, and careful progression of therapeutic exercise intensity, poor ventricular function per se should not be regarded as a contraindication. Indeed, patient #041 was in incipient congestive heart failure on entry into the program. Patients, as documented in Chapters 3 and 4, with atrial fibrillation, an array of complex arrhythmias, and all but complete AV blocks have been accepted and have improved. Also, as documented in this book, patients with an array of the coexisting disorders listed in the AMA document have been treated at the HCRC. Thirteen per cent also have had significantly impaired pulmonary function related to COPD. Although less improvement (average, 11% in vital capacity, 12% in $FEV_{1.0}$, and 26% in $FEV_{25-75\%}$) occurs in proportion to exercise tolerance, it is clear that COPD per se, even with 25 to 35% of normal values associated with severe emphysema, does not contraindicate cardiovascular rehabilitation, *again,* if judicious clinical judgment, careful monitoring, and gradual conditioning are used. There have been no recent pulmonary embolism cases referred. Nine per cent of patients have had anemias, some relatively severe; 18% have had clinical diabetes. The anemias have improved by treating the anemias; the diabetic patients have improved apparently due to the comprehensive cardiovascular rehabilitation. With regard to orthopedic problems, the only contraindication has been whether or not the patient can exercise. The HCRC offers a rotation for the physical medicine/rehabilitation residents in the Baylor College of Medicine program. They report the rotation as highly valuable because of the interaction of cardiovascular disorders and physical disorders, i.e., neuromusculoskeletal. As noted in Chapters 3 and 16, it is almost impossible to exclude people from a rehabilitation program with intercurrent infections since most acquire at least

one febrile episode during the average 14-week period. Again, judicious clinical judgment must be used. The policy that if their temperature is under 100° F and if they do not exhibit a clinically apparent potential for more serious illness, or if their past medical history so indicates, they are allowed to exercise. Again, the Borg rating, double product, and Conditioning Index are used. If the patient has an upper respiratory infection or seasonal flu that is not clinically severe, or if exercises and the load are found to be very hard or very very hard, the load is reduced until it is just hard. In 53 months in more than 500 cases, no untoward event has occurred. Of course, unstable angina is a contraindication, and the HCRC experience indicates that a persistent, significant ST elevation at rest or with exercise has a poor prognosis.

The experience of the HCRC, scrutinized by the referring physicians of the community now numbering about 125, a staff including at least two and as many as four physicians and three experienced nurses, is such that the list presented in the AMA document is one that can be modified to be less restrictive. There is a major proviso, however, in agreement with another recommendation of the AMA report to the effect that a physician must be in charge, present, and supervising a rehabilitation program at all times. The AMA article calls the need "critical" and the HCRC experience confirms that opinion. It may also be noted that the AMA list is less restrictive than an earlier American Heart Association list of contraindications. Moreover, initial contraindications are based upon caution and may be extensive. As experience and technology advance, there should result a cautious review of contraindications.

Again, there are far more indications than contraindications for comprehensive cardiovascular rehabilitation. In questionable cases, a conference between the referring physician and the rehabilitation center physician usually will serve to triage a given patient and the facts of the case at that time. As in most medical situations, the quality of the institution and the experience of those involved are appropriate criteria.

In addition to the question of medical contraindications that would keep patients from undertaking qualified, comprehensive cardiovascular rehabilitation, there are practical matters of logistics, competing priorities, and motivation. Even with patients of physicians who are advocates of a comprehensive cardiovascular rehabilitation center, patients are reluctant to accept the physician's advice or reject it entirely. Some patients are anxious to return to work and feel well enough to do so. In addition, many of these feel that they can exercise, practice stress and nutrition management, stop smoking, and so forth, on their own. In other words, if there are no significant sense of disability, strong demands to protect a job, and a person who feels that he can handle most situations on his own, there is little the physician can do to change the patient's mind. Houston physicians, for example, see and treat patients from great distances. The HCRC has had enthusiastic patients travel over 100 miles to and from the Center thrice weekly. They were patients who had significant problems and they responded well, but they found it a logistical problem of significance. Others find traveling a half hour in a congested city too much to bear. And, of course, in regions where there are no cardiovascular rehabilitation centers, the physician, although a proponent, is forced to do what he can from his office.

Some patients express the view that after their infarction or after their surgery they are cured and believe that they can, without loss or jeopardy, return to their former life-style. A prior chairman of the Houston Chapter of Mended Hearts, a nationwide organization whose members have undergone heart surgery, told me that he thought it remarkable that so many members strongly believed that their coronary artery bypass surgery had "cured" them of their disease and that they would have no more trouble with their heart. A variously reported percentage of post–coronary artery bypass patients whose grafts occlude, or who undergo progress of the native disease, suffer recurrent angina pectoris, arrhythmias, and other manifestations of myocardial ischemia. These patients are apparently at greater surgical risk after having had the initial surgery. Moreover, a significant number of patients with high-grade coronary artery disease are not candidates for surgery due to the diffuseness or location of the occlusive lesions. The more fortunate patients, who feel well, are not depressed or anxious, are without fear, are at their ideal weight, have normal blood lipids, have stopped smoking and reduced alcohol and coffee consumption, and are compelled to return to their vocation as soon as possible, are least likely to be motivated to undertake the commitments of a rehabilitation program. If also the physicians of such patients are not advocates of a structured, comprehensive cardiovascular rehabilitation program, the patients are less likely to be so motivated or even have the option presented to them.

The referral pattern, therefore, tends to be that those most likely to be referred to, and successfully complete, the program are those who are patients of physicians who are advocates of comprehensive cardiovascular rehabilitation and who have not recovered their functional capacities as they or their physicians had expected or hoped. The two primary ingredients then are physician advocacy and patient receptivity.

As noted elsewhere, the HCRC has experienced a growth of referrals largely on the basis of building a reputation with individual physicians based upon individual experience with patients. The benefits are reported to the referring physician by the HCRC physician, and the patient himself reports how he perceives his benefits to the physician as well. That physician then increases his referrals and the process becomes iterative—the number of physician advocates in the community grows, and, therefore, the referral growth rate increases.

However, even as the growth rate increases, the underlying limit to growth continues to be physician advocacy, in turn related to demonstrated benefits and patient receptivity. Without physician advocacy, the patient who would benefit is less likely to find his way into a structured rehabilitation. Although self-referred patients are not accepted without their physician's approval, the HCRC experience demonstrates that benefited patients tell other patients, who then suggest to their physicians that they be referred for cardiovascular rehabilitation.

One purpose in preparing this book is to increase the number of physician advocates by demonstrating the benefits that can be achieved for their patients. Another is to better define the array of patient conditions that can be benefited. It is also hoped that increasingly the utilization of comprehensive cardiovascular rehabilitation will be regarded as a first step in many cases where coronary artery bypass surgery currently might be considered as the first step.

Regarding the question of when, it is increasingly the experience of the HCRC and other rehabilitation centers that most patients can undertake ambulatory, comprehensive cardiovascular rehabilitation in from three to five weeks following an uncomplicated myocardial infarction, coronary artery bypass, or cardiac valve surgery. With regard to nonoperable, but manifest, coronary artery disease, symptomatic or not, the program should be undertaken as early as the patient is able. The same is true for ectopies or arrhythmias associated with increased risk, even though workup has demonstrated no more than early or low-grade coronary artery disease. As demonstrated, ectopies are significantly reduced and often disappear with appropriate rehabilitation procedures.

It is an impression of the HCRC staff, although not tallied, that at least 50% of patients volunteer the statement, "I wish my doctor had referred me here much earlier." As noted elsewhere, referral to a rehabilitation center is often the last resort in a patient who has not done well with all other approaches. Moreover, patients do better, reach their Conditioning Index plateau earlier, and remain more compliant during and after the program if they are referred early after their acute event — infarction or surgery. Their motivation and receptivity are high. Without rehabilitation, they tend to turn to discouragement, resentment of the health care community, or a resignation to the fact that nothing will help.

Again, this author is encouraged by the as yet small but definite trend to consider comprehensive cardiovascular rehabilitation in many situations where previously the first recommendation would be surgery. Moreover, cardiovascular rehabilitation is an excellent follow-up to surgery and does improve the outcome.

There is the wide question of the applicability of the benefits of exercise, stress, and nutritional management of the population as a whole for the purposes of primary prevention of cardiovascular diseases, improved productivity, quality of life, and "wellness." Again, the answer must be yes, but a qualified yes. One example is the Air Force experience. Several years ago proponents of the view that all Air Force officers should jog or run on a regular basis were able to obtain Air Force acceptance to the extent that a regulation directive was issued. There was, however, no provision made for medical supervision or limit-setting. A number of problems developed, including unexplained sudden deaths that might have been related to exercise periods. At that time, this author was a member of the Air Force Scientific Advisory Board, and Chairman of that Board's Aeromedical Biosciences Panel. At the direction of the Secretary of the Air Force, the

program was reviewed and the regulation was abolished, not because the advocates of exercise were wrong, but because there was no appropriate involvement of the Air Force Surgeon General's office, thus, of Air Force physicians generally. Hence, Air Force personnel were exercising without overall medical supervision. An example of the converse is the Tenneco Corporation, which has undertaken a major program to provide a health and fitness program for their employees. In their example, the corporate physician required that all employees over 41 years of age or who had a medical history of cardiovascular disorders, including hypertension, undertake an exercise tolerance test prior to entering the corporate program.

It is this author's opinion that Dr. Edward J. Bernacki, the Tenneco Corporation Medical Officer, has instituted generally useful criteria. The age of 41 is, of course, arbitrary, while a positive medical history is evident. Moreover, as repeatedly emphasized in this book, a cost-effective program for a well population is quite different from a cost-effective program for patients with manifest cardiovascular disease, including a significant percentage of patients who are quite disabled and candidates for sudden death. Programs for well populations do not require the intensive and costly monitoring that the ill population requires. The close precision of exercise prescriptions based upon day-to-day considerations is not as significant in programs for the well population. The close interaction of a staff of physicians, nurses, psychologists, and nutritionists is not as critical. Conversely, a well-population program, after initial evaluation of participants, can be planned on a population, rather than on an individual, basis and not be closely monitored and supervised.

SOCIOECONOMIC ASPECTS OF CARDIOVASCULAR REHABILITATION

As noted in Chapter 1 and in this chapter, cardiovascular rehabilitation, as represented by what is done in its name, is highly pluralistic. Indeed, there are few parallels in the field of health care generally, and probably none in the traditional armamentaria for treating patients with manifest cardiovascular diseases. Although exercise is generally identified as a therapeutic component of cardiovascular rehabilitation, the types of exercise that are advised and utilized range from walking, jogging, running, wheeled bicycling, and use of the bicycle ergometer and treadmill, to swimming, tennis, calisthenics, and use of general exercise machines such as those built by Nautilus, which combine weight lifting with dynamic body motions. It has been difficult to obtain quantitative responses to exercise because of the diversity of types and uses of exercise protocols. One study (Sivarajan *et al.,* 1981) of patients still hospitalized for acute myocardial infarctions was divided into an exercise and a control group, and the study showed no statistically significant differences between the two groups regarding physiological conditioning measures. It would appear from the study that the intervention group did not receive an exercise stimulus to provoke a response that would differentiate the two groups. This is different, of course, from concluding that provocative exercise does not produce benefits. The National Exercise and Heart Disease Project (NEHDP) (Naughton, 1978) and the MRFIT project have been criticized (Walker, 1983) as not providing appropriate differentiations between control and intervention populations. Thus, both cross-population studies in individual rehabilitation programs and large, multicenter, large-population trials have difficulties in demonstrating effects. Furthermore, exercise alone is not the only variable in the exercise studies since state of health, medications, and psychological and nutritional conditions vary widely within the population. Moreover, exercise programs have been applied to both well populations desiring primary prevention and body building and ill populations desiring rehabilitation and secondary prevention. The responses of the two groups to similar protocols will differ, and when mixed protocols are used, the results are certain to be difficult to sort out. Similarly, multicenter, multipopulation clinical trials of the effects of beta-blocking agents leave unsettled questions, again due to varying criteria of selection of populations, characteristics of the populations, and methods utilized. The manifestation of this general multivariable stimulus, multivariable population, multivariable response state of the literature is confusion in the minds of the public, the health professions, and those who are asked to pay the costs of cardiovascular rehabilitation. In spite of this confusion, however, there is a general belief that exercise is better than being sedentary, that good nutrition is better than bad nutrition, that psychological stress management is better than anxiety and depression, that good medical management is

better than poor medical management. The well and diseased population have undertaken exercise as never before and demand guidance from the health professions. In turn, the health professions demand to know their role. To respond to these demands, the American Medical Association (Council on Scientific Affairs, 1981) has issued a report concluding with the statements:

1. Exercise training *can* improve the *objective* and *subjective* rehabilitation of *some* patients with coronary heart disease and result in increased functional capacity.
2. *Physician direction* and supervision of exercise programs are *critical* to the proper assimilation of these services into the health care system.
3. *Exercise testing is important for prescribing and then monitoring exercise rehabilitation programs* in such patients and may provide prognostic information. *Serial testing may help to individualize the length of the exercise program.*
4. While rehabilitation programs *appear* to provide many *subjective* benefits to the cardiac patient, they have not yet been shown to improve survival.
5. Cardiac rehabilitation should be considered one of the treatments for coronary heart disease *complementary to drug therapy or surgery.*
6. *Further studies that examine the long-term benefit of the different types of exercise programs are indicated.*

(*Note:* The emphasis by italics in the concluding statements is that of this author.)

That report, published in 1981, is a thoughtful report representing the majority opinion of a group of well-informed, experienced individuals. As with most dynamic fields and, indeed, in keeping with Conclusion No. 6, it is the current opinion of this author that those recommendations need updating. From the information presented in this book, Conclusion No. 1 should be revised to read: Exercise training *does* improve objective and subjective functions, *quantitatively and qualitatively, in virtually all patients who can safely exercise appropriately and under careful professional supervision,* and results in increased functional capacity. Conclusion No. 2 should remain unchanged. Indeed, physician direction and supervision are even more critical if No. 1 is to be redrafted as recommended by this author. Number 3 remains correct; however, it could be revised to read that a properly structured exercise therapy program, including monitoring, does provide continuous exercise testing. This is important in differentiating the patient who undertakes unmonitored exercise therapy and is brought in for periodic exercise tolerance testing from the patient in a program in which continuous monitoring (essentially continuous exercise tolerance testing) is a part of the therapeutic program. Number 4 should be revised to read: While rehabilitation programs *do provide many quantifiable objective and subjective benefits,* they have not yet been shown *conclusively* to improve survival. Number 5 should be revised to read: Cardiovascular rehabilitation should be considered *in all patients with coronary and other forms of cardiovascular disease as an adjunct to, and often can reduce or replace, drug therapy. Moreover, in appropriate cases it should be utilized prior to undertaking surgery. Also, it should be considered a follow-up adjunct to surgery.* Number 6 remains valid.

The tone and specific wording of the six AMA recommendations reflect the uncertainties of the time and compromises of the members of the Council in drafting the conclusions. Although noted in the body of the report, the recommendations did not specifically call for inclusion of more than exercise as the basis of cardiovascular rehabilitation. Thus, another recommendation should read, in effect, that optimal cardiovascular rehabilitation programs include effective psychological, nutritional, and medical management components. The list of contraindications to exercise should be more limited, especially if the rehabilitation program is, as recommended, directed and closely supervised by a physician. Conversely, as the list of contraindications shortens, the number and type of conditions appropriate for rehabilitation increase, and the word "some" in Conclusion No. 1 becomes "most." It is apparent that the criteria for the application of surgical and medical treatments have broadened as more experience with better techniques has been utilized. The same is true for comprehensive cardiovascular rehabilitation.

As more experience and better techniques have developed, and the benefits of comprehensive cardiovascular rehabilitation have been better defined and quantitated, the socioeconomic impact of the field can be better defined as well. The referral base, mainly physicians, for cardiovascular rehabilitation becomes better informed, and several consequences should follow.

1. The qualifications for effective comprehensive cardiovascular rehabilitation programs will become better defined, and the present pluralism will decrease, while standardization of programs will increase.

2. It will be more evident to the health care community, the health insurance underwriters, and the public at large that it is more effective to undertake cardiovascular rehabilitation in a comprehensive manner in centers dedicated to rehabilitation, in contrast to do-it-yourself approaches under the general guidance of the physician in an office practice.

3. As cardiovascular rehabilitation becomes better standardized, with less pluralism including office practice, more patients will undergo more standardized exercise with more careful monitoring, and with the additional benefits of integrated medical, psychological, and nutritional management. Thus, the array of benefits that have been ascribed to cardiovascular rehabilitation will become quantitatively and statistically demonstrated to either occur or not occur and the underlying mechanisms will be better understood. The long-range impact of the field on morbidity and mortality will more rapidly and assuredly be established. In short, the iterative process by which the cost-benefit considerations define practice patterns will accelerate.

4. Those who wish to undertake the development of cardiovascular rehabilitation facilities will be at less risk of failure, since referral patterns can be better predicted, costs and revenues can be better defined. Conversely, the present situation, in which centers that have been specialized or devoted solely to cardiovascular rehabilitation have generally struggled to survive with many failures, will ease with acceptance and standardization.

Among the many economic issues associated with cardiovascular rehabilitation is one that concerns the manner in which it is influenced by proprietary interests. Health care providers have traditionally been physicians operating their own practices individually or in groups often assisted by professional management experts who were employed by the physician(s), and nonprofit hospitals whose boards of directors represented the community, governmental agencies, church, and academic institutions. Hospitals have also employed professional management groups.

Both physician and hospital operations are undergoing significant, changing trends. Investor-owned corporations have been buying existing hospitals and building new hospitals and managing them on behalf of the corporation at an accelerating rate. These are termed proprietary hospitals. Increasingly, investor-owned corporations are also buying and building clinics that provide ambulatory health care, especially primary and emergency care. Providing health care as a profitable business is attracting the attention of investor groups and their financial advisors.

Currently, there are several companies that are marketing cardiovascular rehabilitation using one of two general formats. One such format is contracting with, for example, one or more cardiologists to operate a cardiovascular rehabilitation program in their offices whereby the billing for services is under the name of the physician or physician group. The company may supply the equipment, provide one or more nurses, and manage the operation for a fee. Another format is to place a rehabilitation operation in a hospital and operate it for a fee from the hospital.

A key factor(s) in such proprietary operations is the policy(ies) used by third-party insurers for reimbursement. The current Medicare regulations mandate that "non-physician personnel are employees of either the physician, hospital, or clinic conducting the program and their services are 'incident' to a physician's professional services." Most other insurance reimbursement policies, in principle, have the same requirements and at present do not preclude reimbursement for the two types of proprietary rehabilitation services described above, namely, that a proprietary company is operating the rehabilitation program in the name of one or a group of physicians or a hospital.

The question that must inevitably be raised is the extent to which the physician or physician group engaged primarily in general, internal medicine, or cardiology practice can be responsible for the direction and supervision of the rehabilitation effort. In the case of the hospital, to what extent does the hospital require physician direction that is responsible to the hospital? After all, the billing for rehabilitation services is in the physician's or the hospital's name; the billing party is responsible for the quality and safety of the service it provides. The AMA Council report (Council on Scientific Affairs, 1981) notes that physician direction and supervision are "critical." The recent Medicare regulation on cardiovascular rehabilitation mandates control by the billing party. All American Heart Association affiliates and the American College of Cardiology guidelines for standards and quality of cardiovascular rehabilitation emphasize the importance of physician direction and supervision.

How can a physician or group of physicians, busy with their clinical practices, undertake to truly direct and closely supervise the comprehensive cardiovascular rehabilitation of *their* patients? Indeed, how can even the usual group of physicians provide enough patients to support a comprehensive cardiovascular rehabilitation program at an appropriate fee structure while, at the same time, all parties derive "profit margins"? The same questions may be raised concerning a hospital contracting with a third party unless careful quality control and economic considerations are undertaken.

With regard to hospitals undertaking comprehensive cardiovascular rehabilitation, it is generally conceded that the trend of insurance reimbursement policies is to shift reimbursement for ambulatory services from hospitals to lower cost free-standing facilities whenever appropriate. It appears to this author that in most cases the free-standing cardiovascular rehabilitation center is more cost-effective than the hospital-based equivalent. Hospital overhead is usually higher than that of a free-standing center providing the same services and utilizing the same space and equipment. In metropolitan areas where there are multiple, increasingly competitive hospitals, it is unlikely that the hospital will obtain referrals from physicians affiliated with another hospital. Thus, both because of higher overhead and fewer referral sources, the hospital-based facility is likely to be faced with a higher cost per patient than the free-standing center.

The proprietary contractor serving either a hospital-based or the usual limited physician, physician group, or clinic appears to further compound the issue.

However these issues become resolved, the requirements that a rehabilitation center optimally be devoted to rehabilitation, be comprehensive, and be closely directed and supervised by a licensed, appropriately trained physician remain and are unlikely to change.

A further socioeconomic factor related to cardiovascular rehabilitation is its role in vocational guidance and disability determination. In past times businesses paid less attention to health care and disability costs than today, as these costs have risen to the point that they represent a substantial part of the cost of doing business. It is estimated that so-called fringe benefits represent about one third of payroll itself, and in some industries are nearing or exceeding 50%. Those percentages have attracted the attention of business leaders. They frighten everyone, and the demand to reduce these costs is a national issue. Cardiovascular diseases and accompanying disorders represent the largest cause of vocational disability (see Table 1-2). Therefore, reduction of cardiovascular disease disabilities should be a major goal of business and government leaders. It is evident that comprehensive cardiovascular rehabilitation can play a significant role in reducing disabilities, in returning people to work sooner, more effectively, and with fewer absences due to illness. Thus, both health care and disability costs are reduced. Since fringe benefits are finite, more of the benefits can be directed to retirement and other more desirable benefits than illness and premature disability.

Four examples from the HCRC experience may be used to exemplify the potential of cardiovascular rehabilitation in this regard. The Texas Rehabilitation Commission is the state agency charged with the responsibility of providing physical and mental restoration for the disabled who fulfill eligibility criteria. Until 1979, that agency had not utilized cardiovascular rehabilitation to any significant extent. Indeed, there was little knowledge within the agency of its existence.

Discussions with agency representatives emphasized the extent of cardiovascular disease as a cause of vocational disability. It was learned that although a large number of potential clients were cardiovascular disabilities, less than 5% of all clients handled were in that category. The reason was that the counselors and their supervisors believed that essentially the only treatment was surgery, at a cost too high for the agency to bear. An arrangement was made with the agency to provide workshops for the counselors and their supervisors of the rationale for cardiovascular rehabilitation and of potential benefits. During the succeeding two years more than 100 clients completed the program, and of those, 96% were returned to work. A significant number had not worked for a year or more. This rate of successful case closures was done at a favorable cost compared to other types of traditional rehabilitation such as spinal cord and neuromuscular disorders, closed head injuries, and mental retardation, wherein costs per case are relatively high, and success rates are relatively low. The demonstration of cost-benefits of comprehensive cardiovascular rehabilitation has encouraged the Texas Rehabilitation Commission to establish a special counselor and support budget to increase the number of clients referred

for cardiovascular rehabilitation. A new counselor handbook has been issued statewide to better prepare counselors in the field of cardiovascular diseases and diagnostic and therapeutic techniques, with an emphasis on cardiovascular rehabilitation.

The second example is that of a large, heavy-metal manufacturing company, which had noted not only the increasing cost of disability insurance premiums but also the relatively large number of employees on total and permanent disability. An agreement between the company and the unions representing the employees called for a review of all employees collecting disability payments, which were approximately 60% of the wages or salaries earned at the time of disability. Those who were disabled due to cardiovascular afflictions were reviewed. A significant number were declared eligible for work, and appropriate jobs were found for them. Those who were appropriate for cardiovascular rehabilitation were so referred. The company has made it known that the so-called "back to work program" has reduced the company's disability premium payments by about one million dollars per year. Moreover, the rate of application for total and permanent disability declined, since often the process resulted in a change of job unfavorable to the employee.

A study (see Chapter 15) of disability revealed several interesting facts. (1) Only one in seven employees who are declared totally and permanently disabled by their physician qualifies for Social Security disability. Thus, the employee's physician represents a greater advocate of the employee's disability than Social Security. It may be argued that this advocacy may be a well-meaning disservice since unnecessary unemployment and idleness can and does produce more disability than had existed. Alcoholism, sedentary life-style, obesity, and depression accompany idleness, which cannot be coped with. (2) Often the manager or foreman in a company responsible for the productivity of his division and the corporate officer responsible for the cost of disability are not the same and view disability differently. The production responsibility disfavors employees who are not optimally productive and may encourage disability.

The third example is a large company which has undertaken a health and fitness program for approximately 3,000 employees to improve health and productivity and to reduce absenteeism and disabilities. This company provides a structured system of regular exercise, nutrition, psychological, and medical counseling. This company is utilizing some principles developed by the HCRC to track physiological conditioning. Those who develop cardiovascular disease and disorders appropriate for comprehensive cardiovascular rehabilitation are referred as early as possible. Detailed data are being collected to demonstrate the long-term effects of this program.

The fourth example is a working relationship with two companies that handle disability insurance. Able disability counselors employed by the insurance company review the claims, and those that appear suitable for cardiovascular rehabilitation are referred by the insurance carrier for rehabilitation.

Each of these is an example of an organization with economic interests in reducing vocational disability and returning people to gainful employment. This reduces the cost of the products of the involved industries; the state agency is able to fulfill its mission more effectively and, indeed, return more money to the tax rolls than is paid for rehabilitation; the insurance companies believe that by reducing unnecessary disability, their costs and ultimately the premiums they must charge in a competitive field are reduced.

GENERAL SUMMARY

Development of Cardiovascular Rehabilitation

The historical development of comprehensive cardiovascular rehabilitation represents the melding of many disciplines and experiences. Physicians learned that appropriately early ambulation benefited the patient more than unnecessarily prolonged bed rest. Physiologists revealed the mechanisms by which exercise improved exercise capacity through improved cardiovascular, muscular, and other bodily functions in the normal, usually young, and athletic subjects. Exercise physiology was then applied to patients with manifest cardiovascular abnormalities, and formalized exercise procedures were developed for both diagnosis (exercise stress or tolerance tests) and therapy whereby the malfunctioning cardiovascular system would undergo improvement.

There are significant differences between the young, healthy subjects of the exercise physiologist and the older, unhealthy patients of the physician-physiologist. The type of exercise, the criteria for defining the intensity, duration, and frequency, monitoring requirements, con-

traindications, and so forth, are more complex and of greater importance when exercise is applied to ill and disordered patients as compared to healthy people. Indeed, safety requirements are quite different. There are limiting and even life-threatening abnormalities of the physiological systems such as the heart, vasculature, blood, neuromusculoskeletal, and respiratory organs.

In addition to pathophysiological disorders that limit the patient's exercise tolerance and the response to exercise therapy, the patient is also more likely to suffer from psychological disorders that also affect exercise tolerance and wellness in general. Moreover, the patient's medications, while prescribed to improve one or another situation, frequently cause other maladjustments of significant physiological mechanisms. The undesirable side effects of medications add to disability as well as relieve disability. Furthermore, patients more often than healthy people suffer from an array of other health afflictions and nutrition-related disorders.

Cardiovascular rehabilitation is a field attempting to establish its place within the health care community in conjunction with traditional medicine with its accelerated use of a growing number of drugs, and with surgery which has undergone a dramatic growth in the treatment of cardiovascular diseases.

This sorting-out process within the field of cardiovascular rehabilitation, as well as between cardiovascular rehabilitation and the more established medical and surgical treatment practices, is indeed complex, and to many it is confusing. The bottom line of health care has its parallel in business. In business the financial statement is the ultimate *demonstration* of cost-effectiveness, and the major benefit is called profit to the investor. In medicine the ultimate *demonstration* is also cost-effectiveness or cost-benefit. The profit, equivalent to profit in business, is benefit to the patient. The cardiothoracic surgeon's goal is to *demonstrate* benefits and, it is hoped, cost-benefits, that cannot be achieved as well by other means. The clinician oriented to the optimal use of pharmacological agents strives to *demonstrate* that the use of drugs (often called conservative treatment) accomplishes benefits not achievable by other means. Indeed, debates have raged between those representing the medical and those representing the surgical approach to the treatment of patients with cardiovascular disease. The advocates of cardiovascular rehabilitation also have sought to *demonstrate* that the use of exercise and the integration of psychological, nutritional, and medical management with exercise therapy can provide benefits that are not achieved by other means. Indeed, comprehensive cardiovascular rehabilitation can be demonstrated to reduce and often replace the need for drugs and surgery. This is not to claim that cardiovascular rehabilitation should or can replace other forms of medical care or surgery. Optimally, cardiovascular rehabilitation should become an important partner of both the medical and surgical care of patients. The bottom line is the *demonstration* of the merits and benefits of all forms of therapy.

The proponents of cardiovascular rehabilitation have had many problems in achieving clear and acceptable *demonstrations* of the benefits of their field. There are several major reasons: (1) The number of variables is very large and interactive. (2) One of the variables is that cardiovascular rehabilitation programs differ in their structure and practices. The field exemplifies virtually the extremes of pluralism. (3) The majority of practicing physicians believe that they can provide comprehensive cardiovascular rehabilitation as part of a busy office practice by simply instructing the patient to get enough exercise, don't worry, and eat right. This, indeed, may be one end of the spectrum of the pluralism of cardiovascular rehabilitation that has made the demonstration of benefits difficult. (4) Large-scale trials, e.g., MRFIT, have been plagued by the problems associated with variable exercise protocols, variable patient mixes, and in the end by the fact that the controls and intervention groups were apparently not distinctly different enough in their life-styles to provide a clear *demonstration* of differences. (5) The stability and operations of centers devoted to cardiovascular rehabilitation are determined by referrals and by reimbursement policies of health insurance underwriters—commercial, nonprofit (Blue Cross and Blue Shield), and tax supported (Medicare). Referrals are limited by two different beliefs: On the one hand, the belief by some that cardiovascular rehabilitation can be as effectively delivered from the physician's office desk, and on the other hand, the belief of others that the benefits of cardiovascular rehabilitation have not been adequately demonstrated. Reimbursement policies have been restrictive since the insurance companies have not had clear *demonstrations* of benefits or, more par-

ticularly, of the practices by which benefits are obtained; for example, psychological and nutritional services. The inventors of the phrase "Catch-22" or the "vicious cycle" might have used cardiovascular rehabilitation as an example. (6) Because of the lack of enforced guidelines and standards, the field has been further complicated by the entry of providers of varying quality and background. As one insurance company executive put it, "As I see it, everything from fat farms to massage parlors are requesting reimbursement under the banner of cardiovascular rehabilitation." Conversely, it is difficult, if not illegal, to prescribe medications or practice cardiothoracic surgery without a license, guideline standards, and adequate training.

This book has been planned to provide the reader with the concepts and experiences of a well-known cardiologist who understands both the medical and cardiological point of view, and who is closely associated with one of the nation's most active cardiothoracic surgical programs (see Chapters 11 and 12). Moreover, this book has been planned to provide the reader with the concepts and precepts of a well-known insurance company physician and officer. This insurance company physician has also been a pioneer in the development of a preventive health program in his company (see Chapters 14 and 15). These two authors provide both an up-to-date understanding of the fields of cardiology, surgery, and insurance and a basis with which to place comprehensive cardiovascular rehabilitation within the perspective of the fields of cardiology, cardiac surgery, and insurance. Virtually all patients referred for cardiovascular rehabilitation have cardiological and/or surgical histories. The substance of that history should be understood.

The subject of nuclear ventriculography has also been included within this book because it is an exciting and increasingly valuable tool to evaluate the functions of the heart walls and the movement of blood through the heart and lungs. An array of functions can currently be obtained in no other way, except by cardiac catheterization involving contrast ventriculography and selective angiography, which is invasive, involves greater risk and discomfort, and is an order of magnitude more expensive. This field is changing so rapidly that it is likely that the next edition of Chapter 13 is overdue as this book is being printed. Ventricular wall motion can be correlated to coronary artery disease distribution and, in turn, differentiate segmental from global malfunction associated with both coronary disease and cardiomyopathy. End-diastolic and end-systolic volumes and ejection fractions can be obtained, as well as other important data. It is often the method of choice to follow up an equivocal, questionable, or positive exercise stress test and assists in validating the effects of cardiovascular rehabilitation.

The central focus of the book is to demonstrate the benefits of comprehensive cardiovascular rehabilitation and the means by which these benefits are achieved, drawing principally upon the experience of the Houston Cardiovascular Rehabilitation Center.

Principles and Practices of the HCRC

The HCRC was initiated in September of 1978. At the time of writing of this book, more than 700 patients had been referred to the HCRC, of which 506 (71%) had completed its program of *comprehensive* cardiovascular rehabilitation. It is termed "comprehensive" because it includes medical, psychological, and nutritional management as well as exercise therapy and integrates each and all. As a result of patient load, including follow-up visits, more than 2,500 standardized symptom- and/or sign-limited exercise tolerance tests had been performed, and more than 30,000 hours of standardized exercise therapy had been achieved by patients. Moreover, the data from 272 of these patients who had completed the program and had been exited for more than one year were subject to careful scrutiny and statistical analyses for reporting quantitative data. Because of the known problems of *demonstrating* benefits due to variability of therapeutic approaches, e.g., types of exercise, involvement of psychological, nutritional, and medical (including medications) therapies, the HCRC was planned to provide a standardized exercise format, with standardized monitoring procedures and with standardized criteria for prescribing exercise intensity and for deciding end-points for exercise therapy, i.e., in lieu of an open-ended program. Psychological and nutritional methodologies were standardized, and careful medical management was integrated into the system so that medication effects could be managed, and the impacts of intercurrent as well as coexisting health disorders could be identified and related to the response to the rehabilitation procedures themselves. The results of these 53 months of experience, therefore, have added significantly

to our understanding of the benefits, or lack thereof, and in large measure of the mechanisms responsible for patient responses to the practice of a center entirely devoted to comprehensive cardiovascular rehabilitation.

In other words, methodological variability, which has made analyses of cause and effect difficult, was reduced by standardization as much as deemed possible, while provocative yet safe exercise levels were provided. Initial symptom- and/or sign-limited exercise tolerance testing using the Balke treadmill protocol was used because that protocol relates protocol stages to metabolic load steps and because it has advantages for the patient and monitoring staff. This information, together with a detailed knowledge of the patient's medical history and current medical as well as psychological and nutritional status, provides a standardized approach to determining the initial level of therapeutic exercise intensity. From that time until exit from the program (average duration, 13.8 weeks), the patient's exercise intensity is adjusted to provide a double product (DP = heart rate $\times$ systolic blood pressure $\times$ 10^{-2}) which is adequate to provoke the so-called training or conditioning effect, yet not so high as to be hazardous. Double product correlates with heart work and myocardial oxygen consumption. This therapeutic level of double product correlates closely to the Borg rating of hard. A relationship, developed at the HCRC, to track conditioning and the factors that influence it is termed the Conditioning Index (CI) where:

$$CI = \text{Exercise intensity (kpm} \cdot \text{min}^{-1}) \div DP \times 10^2.$$

Thus, exercise intensity, double product, and Conditioning Index all have similar scales.

The standardized therapeutic exercise method utilizes a stationary bicycle ergometer, except on the rare occasions when it was impossible for a patient to sit on a bicycle and use his legs. This method was selected in order to standardize the therapeutic exercise protocol, obtain quantitative reproducible and verifiable work loads that are essentially independent of body weight, optimize acceptability to the patient and thus compliance, reduce climatic and other extraneous effects, and, of course, optimize monitoring of signs and symptoms. Continuous telemetered ECG data, blood pressures, and clinical signs and symptoms are routinely recorded before, during, and after exercise. Exercise sessions are scheduled for each patient on a three times per week basis. The work-load intensity, double product, Conditioning Index, signs, symptoms, medications, coexisting medical, and psychological and nutritional conditions are interrelated and reviewed weekly or more frequently, if indicated.

Regular group-therapy sessions parallel the exercise therapy, including medical-physiology, psychological, and nutritional sessions. Individual medical, psychological, and nutritional evaluations and counseling are provided as necessary.

Thus, the patient, during his tenure in the comprehensive rehabilitation program, is indeed receiving comprehensive cardiovascular rehabilitation. This intensive and extensive experience with ambulatory patients is replicated in few other circumstances in the health care field.

Exit from the program is scheduled when the Conditioning Index plateaus. At this point the patient has reached the optimal, if not maximal, level of exercise tolerance achievable, except perhaps over a long period. The patient, on exit, is encouraged to obtain a bicycle ergometer for home use in order to maintain the condition achieved during the program. The home bicycle ergometer can be ordered as a prescription, which is increasingly recognized for reimbursement under health insurance. Routine follow-up, except for a one- and three-month brief procedure, is then semiannual. The details of the principles and practices summarized above are provided in Chapters 2, 3, 4, 5, 6, 7, 8, 9, 10, and in this chapter as well.

Benefits of Cardiovascular Rehabilitation

Table 16-1 lists 118 functional responses to exercise itself and to the added integration of medical, psychological, and nutritional management as undertaken in comprehensive cardiovascular rehabilitation. That table is basically a composite of the work of many investigators, extended and, where possible, confirmed by the HCRC experience. A perusal of that table will reveal that the listed benefits carry no quantitative assessment but are simply categorized as increase, decrease, or no effect. Moreover, there are question marks associated with some relationships. Further perusal of that list indicates that 95 of the listed functions, which are not accompanied by ?, have benefited from exercise. Eighty of the ninety-five listed functions benefited have been confirmed by the HCRC experience. Again, the list is qualitative. Chapters 3, 4, 5, 8, 10, and 16 contain quantitative results mainly drawing upon the HCRC experience.

From the patient's point of view, the most significant benefit is an improvement in functional capacity; the greater the improvement, the greater the benefit. This is, of course, of major interest to the physician as well, since the most frequent patient complaint is an unsatisfactory capacity for desired physical activity. A significant improvement of exercise tolerance is associated with an increased capacity for vocational and recreational activity and an improvement of wellness or a feeling of well-being at rest and while being active. Wellness correlates with exercise tolerance or functional capacity. In turn, wellness correlates with the Conditioning Index. The Conditioning Index is, in effect, the correlation coefficient between double product (which correlates with the perception of exertion at a given exercise intensity) and the exercise intensity itself.

The exercise conditioning intensity level is set at 60% of the maximal work load and double product achieved in the initial exercise tolerance test using a treadmill and the Balke protocol with three-minute steps, and carried to a symptom- or sign-limited maximum. The initial exercise tolerance test limit, therefore, on the Borg scale is very, very hard and no longer tolerable, or limited earlier if contraindicating signs and/or symptoms appear, i.e., whichever is lower. This initial therapeutic work load (exercise tolerance for 30 minutes) is increased from a mean level of 211 to 596 kpm · min^{-1}, i.e., 282% at exit (men); 152 to 379 kpm · min^{-1}, i.e., 246% for women; and 199 to 548 kpm · min^{-1}, i.e., 275% for all, as a result of standardized, structured, and monitored exercise, supplemented by medical, psychological, and nutritional management. The exercise tolerance stage reached on entry averaged essentially stage III, and on exit just above stage VI. Thus, in an average period of fourteen weeks the mean exercise tolerance, which was marginal for office jobs and minimal recreational efforts, rose essentially threefold to that verging on the requirements of heavy industry and hard tennis.

Poor exercise tolerance may occur in well or in diseased and ill people. In well people it is purely physiological deconditioning. In individuals with cardiovascular disease, to the extent that it is reversible, it is also physiological deconditioning but with further limits caused by pathophysiology, drug effects, psychological stress, and fatigue, due, for example, to sleep disorders. Thus, exercise tolerance, before, during, or after satisfactory cardiovascular rehabilitation, is not a constant. Rather it may vary from day to day in what are regarded as "good days" and "bad days" by patients. Thus, reconditioning is not a smooth, upward process, but it has its ups and downs. These ups and downs are marked by changes in the Conditioning Index, which therefore has been found to be highly valuable in optimally managing the patient during his rehabilitation program. Indeed, it provides valuable feedback to the patient as well in his structured efforts to learn and attentuate those factors that cause bad days and amplify those factors that cause good days. The net result of this process is an average increase in exercise tolerance of about threefold. *That is a significant demonstrated benefit!*

A common set of signs and symptoms, not associated with well people in poor condition, but associated specifically with heart disease, are angina pectoris, ST-segment depression with effort or stress, and arrhythmias that may increase or even decrease with physical effort or mental stress. Another demonstrated major benefit of comprehensive cardiovascular rehabilitation affecting functional capacity is the suppression of angina pectoris, ST-segment depression, and arrhythmias. Moreover, in most cases, these markers of myocardial ischemia disappear at levels of physical effort that had formerly provoked them. Indeed, they often do not appear again at all levels of physical effort within the patient's daily schedule. In effect, they disappear unless the patient overexerts himself, but he learns his limits in a rehabilitation program.

Figure 2-2 illustrates the reasons in principle. Physiological conditioning, or the so-called training effect, not only results in an increased exercise tolerance, but is accompanied by a decrease in heart rate and blood pressure at rest and a decrease in the rate at which heart rate and systolic blood pressure rise with increasing levels of work intensity (see also Figures 5-17, 5-18, and 5-19). Thus, heart rate and systolic blood pressure, and their product, the double product (DP), are lower at rest and at all levels of achievable exercise intensity. The DP represents the heart work load and correlates directly with myocardial oxygen demand. Hence, reducing the DP reduces myocardial ischemia. It would be expected, therefore, that an individual could exert more physical effort without provoking effort-induced angina pectoris and arrhythmias after he became conditioned than before. It might also be expected that when the individual reached a level of physical effort

which resulted in the same heart rate and systolic pressure (i.e., DP), the angina and/or arrhythmias would recur. Indeed, this has been thought to be true. Figure 2-1, however, implies, and the data presented in Chapters 3, 4, and 5 demonstrate, that the levels of angina pectoris, arrhythmias, and ST-segment depression also *decrease with respect to the double product.* Thus, the ischemia-lowering effect of conditioning is more than achievement of higher exercise tolerance for the same double product. The most likely explanation is the fact that conditioning results in an increased myocardial oxygen *supply,* and the most likely explanation is that coronary perfusion within the heart wall occurs mainly during diastole, because during systole the coronary vasculature is throttled by the force of myocardial contraction. As heart rate decreases, diastole is prolonged to a greater degree than systole, hence, beat-to-beat and time-integrated coronary perfusion increases. The heart rate reduction associated with conditioning, therefore, not only reduces myocardial oxygen demand but also increases oxygen supply.

It has been demonstrated (see Chapters 2, 3, 4, 7, 8, and 16) that emotional stress per se results in an increased double product, thus reducing the Conditioning Index and exercise tolerance. Moreover, symptoms of anxiety, depression and difficulty in managing mental stress are among the chief complaints of patients. Therefore, effective stress management results in improved exercise tolerance and therefore constitutes a beneficial feedback, since improved exercise tolerance reduces depression and anxiety. The net effect then of combining exercise conditioning and psychological stress management appears obvious. Indeed, as demonstrated in Chapters 3 and 8, effective stress management plays a significant role in improved physical and mental performance, capacity, and wellness. Thus, other significant *demonstrated benefits* develop.

No one would argue that if the need for taking medications could be reduced or abolished, *another major benefit* could be attributed to comprehensive cardiovascular rehabilitation. Indeed, that benefit is demonstrated in Chapters 3, 4, 5, and 16. The average patient entering the HCRC has been found to be taking 6.4 different medications. After comprehensive cardiovascular rehabilitation, the average patient is taking 3.1 medications—a reduction of 52%. The medication most replaceable by rehabilitation is the beta blocker since it is prescribed principally to lower heart rate and blood pressure, i.e., as an antianginal, antiarrhythmic, antihypertensive agent. These same effects are produced by effective physiological conditioning. Moreover, as shown in Figures 5-17, 5-18, and 5-19, the effects are greater than those achieved with the usual clinical dosages of beta blockers. Furthermore, there are virtually no contraindications to properly prescribed and monitored exercise, unless the patient cannot exercise, whereas the contraindicators to pharmacological beta-blocking agents are many (see Chapter 16, Management of Medications). Indeed, in the multicenter beta-blocker trials, the majority of potential subjects were rejected on the basis of having conditions contraindicating the use of beta-blocking agents. Most other medications usually can be reduced and occasionally discontinued as well. Another major *demonstrated* benefit!

As demonstrated in Chapters 3, 4, and 5, blood pressures, both systolic and diastolic, at rest and at all achievable states of exercise intensity, are reduced. Hypertension is better controlled and in many patients is controlled without the need for antihypertensives. Furthermore, the hypotension often associated with poor ventricular function and accompanying heart disease tends to normalize. Moreover, there is a normalization of many physiological factors involved in the complications of heart disease. Preload, afterload, ventricular contractility, and ejection fraction are normalized, and the point of exercise intensity at which the anaerobic threshold is reached is extended with its beneficial effects on acidosis. Abnormal blood glucose levels and frank diabetes are improved.

It would seem apparent that if it were well known and understood that comprehensive cardiovascular rehabilitation could essentially triple exercise tolerance, reduce or abolish angina pectoris and arrhythmias, reduce or abolish hypertension, reduce or abolish the need for medications, and improve many coexisting medical problems, virtually all patients with an unsatisfactory exercise tolerance, symptoms and signs of myocardial ischemia, hypertension, and other disorders requiring medications would be referred to qualified centers devoted to providing comprehensive cardiovascular rehabilitation.

There are, moreover, additional benefits as listed in Table 16-1, which further contribute to improved health and functional capacity

and to secondary prevention as well. To the extent that deconditioning, hypertension, hyperlipidemia, smoking, mental stress and coronary-proneness, obesity, diabetes, and certain iatrogenic factors are risk factors for atherosclerotic cardiovascular disease, the risk of disease progression is reduced, since all of these factors are changed in the direction of reduced risk. Since most pharmacological and surgical procedures do not cure the disease but rather are palliative, it would seem that the physician and surgeon would be even further interested in comprehensive cardiovascular rehabilitation.

Cost Benefits of Cardiovascular Rehabilitation

It may be hoped that the health care community at large, and those who purchase its services, will come to understand that an optimal mix of therapies currently available should be utilized. Obviously the traditional medical care of patients and an ever widening array of medications, surgery of the heart, vasculature, valves, and conducting systems, and comprehensive cardiovascular rehabilitation each and all have their place. Cardiovascular rehabilitation will further improve the patient who has undergone surgery, and it will supplement the ongoing care of the attending physician. Which therapy is exclusively best under all circumstances is a complex issue; each has a place, and their places are interrelated.

Anyone who has attempted to persuasively demonstrate cost-benefits of individual forms of health care in the highly complex health care field learns quickly how difficult it is. Everyone is concerned about the rapidly escalating costs of health care, and many private and public sector agencies, frustrated in attempts to assign cost-benefit analyses to particular diagnostic or treatment methods, are being forced simply to place caps on overall health care.

In this book (see Chapters 1 and 16, "Socioeconomic Considerations"), a few subjects relative to economics are considered. The Texas Rehabilitation Commission must consider cost-benefits not only with the various causes of disability, cardiovascular disease being the largest, but across all courses of vocational disability treatment. That Commission has been impressed not only with the cost-benefits of cardiovascular rehabilitation in getting clients with cardiovascular disease back to work, but also in comparison to the cost of getting other types of disabilities, e.g., neuromusculoskeletal conditions, back to work. As business finds the "fringe benefit" package no longer a fringe, but representing from one third to one half of payroll costs, a more careful look at disability and health care costs that bleed monies from retirement funds is being taken. Employee benefits are finite, and unnecessary disability costs associated with a small proportion of a company's employees are increasingly regarded as an area to control more tightly. Since cardiovascular disease – related disorders are the largest cause of vocational disability, it is obviously the area to concentrate on *if* disability can be reduced with appropriate cost-effectiveness. *This book attempts to demonstrate the fact that disability can be reduced effectively and at favorable cost.*

Another area considered is that of the hospital versus the free-standing (i.e., outside of a hospital) facility in the care of ambulatory patients not requiring a hospital bed or other immediately available hospital services. It is argued that a free-standing comprehensive cardiovascular rehabilitation center has several economic advantages over the hospital-based center, namely, less overhead and a larger patient-referral base, both of which affect utilization and fixed costs. It is contended that the trend nationally is to move services out of hospitals that need not be performed in hospitals. It is difficult to take large hospital – health care centers apart after they have been established, especially in view of the two-part reimbursement policies such as Medicare A and B, and Blue Cross/Blue Shield which tend to encourage hospitals as a base for virtually all services. Undoing an elaborate and extensive process that has been underway for more than twenty years is economically and politically difficult.

The role of the proprietary or investor-owned and -managed segments of the health care system is increasing. The significance of this trend is debated on many general terms. Specific questions, however, are raised with regard to certain proprietary approaches to market cardiovascular rehabilitation. The questions relate to quality control, safety, and economics. One currently expanding and aggressive proprietary approach is to contract with one or a group of physicians in private practice to provide equipment and nursing and management personnel to operate a cardiovascular rehabilitation service in their office or clinic. Insurance reimbursement policies generally require that the billing be in the name of the physician(s). It is implicit that the physician is directly responsible for the service for which he bills. Moreover, the AMA, American Heart Association affiliates, and the American College of Cardiology have issued guidelines emphasizing that a qualified, licensed physician *must* be in direct and supervisory control of cardiovascular rehabilitation. The AMA recommendation labels the need as "critical." The HCRC experience confirms that position. The question arises as to the role of the physician(s) in the case of the type of proprietary operation which contracts for the operation and management of cardiovascular rehabilitation. Can or will the physician(s), busy with their regular practices, take the time to properly direct and supervise the rehabilitation services for which they are billing? Again, there is the question of utilization. There are few, if any, individual physicians or even groups of four or five, who can refer enough patients to their own rehabilitation service, monitor them, and direct the service, and still maintain a satisfactory patient load in their regular practice. Few cardiologists are likely to refer patients to another practicing cardiologist in order to achieve rehabilitation for their patients.

The other mode of marketing proprietary rehabilitation centers is similar, except that the facility and personnel (except for the physician) are contracted to a hospital. Again, the same questions arise. If the hospital bills for the services, can the hospital afford also to provide close physician direction and supervision? The variables in both types are overhead costs, patient load and revenues, and profit, not only for the physician but for the proprietary operation as well.

The Future Role of Cardiovascular Rehabilitation

It is evident from virtually all points of view that comprehensive cardiovascular rehabilitation is an unusual type of medical practice. It is currently highly pluralistic in structure, practice, and quality; however, the trend is for standardization of quality, structure, and practice. Benefits have been difficult to demonstrate; however, as standardization occurs, demonstration of benefits becomes easier and more quantitative. Its role alongside the more traditional methods of treating patients medically and surgically has been difficult to define; however, its role is becoming more evident as the benefits are more clearly demonstrated. The socioeconomics of health care and reimbursement for its services, in general, have been unfavorable to cardiovascular rehabilitation. In this case too, a sorting-out process is under way which should favorably affect cardiovascular rehabilitation as its benefits are clearly demonstrated. Insurance carriers are increasingly making adjustments to policies favorable to comprehensive cardiovascular rehabilitation.

The nation's physicians, in the public's mind, are held responsible for advising their patients on matters of appropriate health care. The public continues to view the physician as the authority. Thus, the physician has a major opportunity to present his views and have them accepted and followed as perhaps in no other human interaction. The public, as never before, is now aware that cardiovascular diseases and their associated disorders are the afflictions most likely to cause disability and death. Thus, the public is more receptive than ever to having their physicians' advice as to what can be done to help avoid or slow these most common, progressive diseases (primary prevention), and if they have developed to the point of producing symptoms and hazardous signs, what best to do to reduce or abolish their disabling sequelae (rehabilitation), and prevent further progress (secondary prevention). The physician has a broad spectrum to choose from: the use of medications, the use of surgery, and the use of comprehensive cardiovascular rehabilitation. Optimization of the use of these treatment modalities is an important issue. It is hoped that this book will assist the physician in his role.

REFERENCES

Alderman, M. M., and Stanback, M. E. Preventive cardiology: The state of the art. *Cardiovasc. Rev. Rep.*, **1981**, *2*, 7.

Altekruse, E. G., and Wilmore, J. H. Changes in blood chemistries following a controlled exercise program. *J. Occup. Med.*, **1973**, *15*, 110.

American Heart Association Affiliate Publications *Guidelines for Cardiac Rehabilitative Centers.* The Greater Los Angeles Affiliate, Los Angeles, 1981. *Guidelines for Comprehensive Cardiovascular Rehabilitative Centers.* The Texas Affiliate, Austin, 1983. *Guidelines for Organization and Operation of Cardiac Rehabilitation Programs.* The Nation's Capitol Affiliate, Washington, D.C., 1981. *Organizational Guidelines for Myocardial Infarction Rehabilitation Programs.* The North Carolina Heart Association, Inc., Chapel Hill, 1974.

American Heart Association. *Exercise Testing and Training of Individuals with Heart Disease or at High Risks for Its Development: Handbook for Physicians.* American Heart Association, New York, **1975**.

Amsterdam, E. A. Controlling cardiovascular risk factors: A realistic guide to changing bad habits. *Mod. Med.*, **1981**, *49*, 60.

Anderson, M. P.; Peterson, L. H.; and Carter, A. R. Moods, hassles, and responses to exercise in cardio-

vascular rehabilitation. Presented at annual meeting of the American Psychological Association, Anaheim, California, **1983**.

Anderson, T. W., and Shephard, R. J. Physical training and exercise diffusing capacity. *Int. Z. Angew. Physiol.*, **1968**, *25*, 198.

Andrew, G. M.; Guzman, C. A.; and Becklake, M. R. Effect of athletic training on exercise cardiac output. *J. Appl. Physiol.*, **1966**, *21*, 603.

Åstrand, P. O., and Rodahl, K. *Textbook of Work Physiology* (2nd. ed.). McGraw-Hill, New York, **1977**, pp. 394–396.

Åstrand, P. O. Human physical fitness with special reference to sex and age. *Physiol. Rev.*, **1956**, *36*, 307.

Barnard, R. J. Long term effects of exercise on cardiac function. In, Wilmore, J. H., and Keogh, J. F. (eds.) *Exercise and Sport Sciences Reviews*, Vol. 3. Academic Press, New York, **1975**, p. 113.

Bjorntorp, P. Metabolism in patients with ischemic heart disease and obesity after training. In, Pernow, B., and Saltin, B. (eds.) *Muscle Metabolism During Exercise.* Plenum Press, New York, **1970**, p. 493.

Blocker, W. P., Jr. and Cardus, D. (eds.) *Rehabilitation in Ischemic Heart Disease.* S. P. Medical and Scientific Books, Chicago, **1983**.

Booth, F. W., and Gould, E. W. Effects of training and disuse on connective tissue. In, Wilmore, J. H., and Keogh, J. F. (eds.), *Exercise and Sport Sciences Reviews*, Vol. 3. Academic Press, New York, **1975**, p. 83.

Borg, G., and Linderholm, H. Perceived exertion and pulse rate during graded exercise in various age groups. *Acta Med. Scand.* (Suppl.), **1967**, *472*, 194.

Boyer, J., and Kasch, F. Exercise therapy in hypertensive men. *JAMA*, **1970**, *211*, 1668.

Brodal, P.; Ingjer, F.; and Hermansen, L. Number and density of capillaries in the quadriceps muscle of untrained and endurance-trained men: A quantitative electronmicroscopical study. *Am. J. Physiol.*, **1977**, *232*, H705–H712.

Carú, B., and DePonti, C. Isometric stress test in coronary patients. In, Rossi, P. (ed.) *Functional Evaluation and Rehabilitation of Cardiac Patients.* Year Book Medical Publishers, Chicago, **1979**, p. 47.

Choquette, G., and Ferguson, R. J. Blood pressure reduction in "borderline" hypertensives following physical training. *Can. Med. Assoc. J.*, **1973**, *108*, 699.

Christensen, E. H. Beitrage zur Physiologie schwerer korperlicher Arbeit. *Arbeitphysiol.*, **1931**, *4*, 1.

Clarke, D. H. Adaptations in strength and muscular endurance resulting from exercise. In, Wilmore, J. H. (ed.), *Exercise and Sport Sciences Reviews*, Vol. 1. Academic Press, New York, **1973**, p. 73.

Clausen, J. P.: Circulatory adjustments to dynamic exercise and effect of physical training in normal subjects and in patients with coronary disease. *Prog. Cardiovasc. Dis.*, **1976**, *18*, 459.

Consolazio, C. Frank; Johnson, Robert E.; and Pecora, Louis J. *Physical Measurements of Metabolic Functions in Man.* McGraw-Hill, New York, **1963**.

Corr, P. B.; Witkowski, F. X.; and Sobel, B. E. Mechanisms contributing to malignant dysrhythmias induced by ischemia in the cat. *J. Clin. Invest.*, **1978**, *61*, 109–119.

Council on Scientific Affairs. Physician-supervised exercise programs in rehabilitation of patients with coronary heart disease. *JAMA, 1981, 245,* 146.

Deitrick, J. E.; Whedon, G. D.; and Shorr, E. Effects of immobilization upon various metabolic and physiologic functions of normal men. *Am. J. Med., 1948, 4,* 3.

Dustan, H. P. Controlling cardiovascular risk factors: Tricks (and traps) in managing hypertension. *Mod. Med., 1981, 49,* 117.

Eckstein, R. W. Effect of exercise and coronary artery narrowing on coronary collateral circulation. *Circ. Res., 1957, 5,* 230.

Ekblom, B. Effect of physical training on oxygen transport system in man. *Acta Physiol. Scand.* (Suppl.), *1969, 328,* 9–45.

Ekblom, B.; Åstrand, P. O.; Saltin, B.; *et al.* Effect of training on circulatory response to exercise. *J. Appl. Physiol. 1968, 24,* 518–528.

Elsner, R. W., and Carlson, L. D. Postexercise hyperemia in trained and untrained subjects. *J. Appl. Physiol., 1962, 17,* 436.

Emery, Gordon A.; Wilmore, Jack H.; Morton, Alan R.; *et al.* The effect of beta-adrenergic blockade on obtaining a trained exercise state. *J. Cardiac Rehabil., 1983, 3,* 25.

Fox, S. M., III, and Haskell, W. I. Population studies. *Can. Med. Assoc. J., 1967, 96,* 806–811.

Freedman, M. E.; Snider, G. L.; Brostoff, P.; Kimelblot, S.; and Katz, L. N. Effects of training on response of cardiac output to muscular exercise in athletes. *J. Appl. Physiol., 1955, 8,* 37.

Frick, M. H.; Konttinen, A.; and Sarajas, H. S. S. Effects of physical training on circulation at rest and during exercise. *Am. J. Cardiol., 1963, 12,* 142.

Froelicher, V.; Jensen, D.; Atwood, J. E.; *et al.* Cardiac rehabilitation: Evidence for improvement in myocardial perfusion and function. *Arch. Phys. Med. Rehabil., 1980, 61,* 517–522.

Golding, L. Effects of physical training upon total serum cholesterol levels. *Res. Q. Exerc. Sport, 1961, 32,* 499.

Gollnick, P. D., and Hermansen, L. Biochemical adaptations to exercise: Anaerobic metabolism. In, Wilmore, J. H. (ed.) *Exercise and Sport Sciences Reviews,* Vol. 1. Academic Press, New York, 1973, p. 1.

Gonyea, W.; Wrickson, G. C.; and Bonde-Petersen, F. Skeletal muscle fiber splitting induced by weight-lifting exercise in cats. *Acta Physiol. Scand., 1977, 99,* 106.

Gonzalez, Elizabeth Rasche. Exercise therapy "rediscovered" for diabetes, but what does it do? *JAMA, 1979, 242,* 1591–1592.

Gotto, A. M., Jr. Controlling cardiovascular risk factors: How to lower lipids with drugs and diet. *Mod. Med., 1981, 49,* 90.

Gutmann, M. C.; Squires, R. W.; Pollock, M. L.; Foster, ter, C.; and Anholm, J. Perceived exertion—Heart rate relationship during exercise testing and training in cardiac patients. *J. Cardiac Rehabil., 1981, 1,* 52.

Hartz, A. J.; Barboriak, P. N.; Anderson, A. J.; Hoffmann, R. G.; and Barboriak, J. J. Smoking, coronary artery occlusion and nonfatal myocardial infarction. *JAMA, 1981, 246,* 851–853.

Hellerstein, H. K., and Friedman, E. H. Sexual activity and the post coronary patient. *Arch. Intern. Med., 1970, 125,* 987.

Hollmann, W., and Hettinger, Th. *Sportmedizin—Arbeits-und Trainingsgrundlagen.* F. K. Schattauer Verlag, Stuttgart, **1976.**

Hollmann, W., and Venrath, H. Die Beeinflussung von Herzgrosse, maximaler O_2-Aufnahme und Ausdauergrenze durch ein Ausdauertraining mittlerer und hoher Intensitat. *Der Sportarzt., 1963, 14,* 189.

Holloszy, J. O. Biochemical adaptations to exercise in aerobic metabolism. In, Wilmore, J. H. (ed.) *Exercise and Sport Sciences Reviews,* Vol. 1. Academic Press, New York, 1973, p. 45.

Holmdahl, D. E., and Ingelmark, B. E. Der Bau des Gelenkknorpels unter verschiedenen Funktionellen Verhaltnissen. *Acta Anat., 1948, 6,* 309.

Ingelmark, B. E.: Der Bau der Schnen wahrend verschiedener Altersperioden und unter wechselnden funktionellen Bedingungen I. *Acta Anat., 1948, 6,* 113.

———: Morpho-physiological aspects of gymnastic exercises, *FIEP-Bull., 1957, 27,* 37.

Jansson, E., and Kaijser, L. Muscle adaptation to extreme endurance training in man. *Acta Physiol. Scand., 1977, 100,* 315–324.

Katz, L. N.; Stamler, J.; and Pick, R. *Nutrition and Atherosclerosis.* Lea & Febiger, Philadelphia, 1958.

Kilbom, A. Physical training in women. *Scand. J. Clin. Lab. Invest., 1971, 28* (Suppl. 119).

Knehr, C. A.; Dill, D. B.; and Neufield, W. Training and its effects on man at rest and at work. *Am. J. Physiol., 1942, 136,* 148.

Liere, E. J. van, and Northup, D. W. Cardiac hypertrophy produced by exercise in albino and in hooded rats. *J. Appl. Physiol., 1957, 11,* 91.

Lopezs, A.; Vial, R.; Balart, L.; and Arroyave, G. Effect of exercise and physical fitness on serum lipids and lipoproteins. *Atherosclerosis, 1974, 20,* 1.

Man-i, M.; Ito, K.; and Kikuchi, K. Histological studies of muscular training. *Res. Phys. Educ. 1967, 11,* 153.

Marpurgo, P. Uber Aktivitats-Hypertrophie der willkurlichen Muskein. *Virchows Arch., 1897, 150,* 522.

Mathes, P., and Gudbjarnason, S. Changes in norepinephrine stores in the canine heart following experimental myocardial infarction. *Am. Heart J., 1971, 81,* 211–219.

Medicare, Part B Newsletter, February 3, **1983.** Physician Medicare News Letter #139, Cardiac Rehabilitation Programs, Dallas, Tx.

Miller, P. B.; Johnson, R. L.; and Lamb, L. E. Effects of four weeks of absolute bed rest on circulatory functions in man. *Aerospace Med., 1964, 35,* 1194.

Mukherjee, A.; Bush, L. R.; McCoy, K. E.; *et al.* Relationship between beta adrenergic receptors numbers and physiological responses during experimental canine myocardial ischemia. *Circ. Res., 1982, 50,* 735–741.

Mukherjee, A.; Wong, T. M.; Buja, L. M.; *et al.* Beta adrenergic and muscarinic cholinergic receptors in canine myocardium. Effects of ischemia. *J. Clin. Invest., 1979, 64,* 1423–1428.

Naughton, J. The national exercise and heart disease project: Development, recruitment and implementation: exercise and the heart. *Cardiovasc. Clin., 1978, 48,* 205–222.

Nöcker, J.; Lehmann, D.; and Schleusing, G. Einfluss von Training und Belastung auf den Mineralgehalt von Herz und Skelettmuskel. *Int. Z. Angew. Physiol.,* **1958,** *17,* 243.

Palladin, A., and Ferdmann, D. Uber den Einfluss der Trainings der Muskeln auf ihren Kreatingehalt. *Hoppe Seylers Z. Physiol. Chem.,* **1928,** *174,* 284.

Papadopoulos, C. Cardiovascular drugs and sexuality — A cardiologist's view. *Arch. Intern. Med.,* **1980,** *140,* 1341–1345.

Pǎřizková, J. Composition and exercise during growth and development. In, Rarick, G. L. (ed.) *Physical Activity, Human Growth and Development.* Academic Press, New York, **1973,** p. 97.

Peterson, L. H.; Spence, D. W.; and Bernacki, E. The ratio of exercise intensity and the heart rate–systolic blood pressure in exercise stress testing and physiological conditions; the Conditioning Index. *J. Am. Coll. Cardiol.* (In press).

Peterson, L. H., and Anderson, M. P. Borg scale, the heart rate–systolic pressure product, wellness and mood. **1983** (In press).

Petrén, T. Die Totale Anzahl der Blutkapillaren im Herzen und Skelettmuskulatur bei Ruhe und nach langer Muskelubung. *Verh. Anat. Ges.,* **1936,** (Suppl. Anat. Anz., 81).

Pollock, M. L.: The quantification of endurance training program. In, Wilmore, J. H. (ed.) *Exercise and Sport Sciences Review,* Vol. 1. Academic Press, New York, **1973,** p. 155.

Pyörälä, K.; Karava, R.; Punsar, S.; *et al.* A controlled study of the effects of 18 months' physical training in sedentary middle-aged men with high indexes of risk relative to coronary heart disease. In, Larsen, O. Andree, and Malmborg, R. O. (eds.) *Coronary Heart Disease and Physical Fitness.* Munksgaard, Copenhagen, **1971.**

Reindell, H.; Konig, K.; and Roskamm, H. *Funktionsdiagnostik des gesunden und kranken Herzens.* Georg Thieme Verlag, Stuttgart, **1967.**

Reuschlein, P. S.; Reddan, W. G.; Burpee, J.; Gee, J. B. L.; and Rankin, J. Effect of physical training on the pulmonary diffusing capacity during submaximal work. *J. Appl. Physiol.,* **1968,** *24,* 152.

Robinson, S., and Harmon, P. M. The lactic acid mechanism and certain properties of the blood in relation to training. *Am. J. Physiol.,* **1941a,** *132,* 757.

Rohter, F. D.; Rochelle, R. H.; and Hyman, C. Exercise blood flow changes in the human forearm during physical training. *J. Appl. Physiol.,* **1963,** *18,* 789.

Roskamm, H.; Reindell, H.; and Konig, K. *Korperliche Aktivitat und Herz und Kreislauferkrankungen.* Johann Ambrosius Barth, Munich, **1966.**

Rowell, L. B. Human cardiovascular adjustments to exercise and thermal stress. *Physiol. Rev.,* **1974,** *54,* 75.

Saltin, B.; Blomqvist, G.; Mitchell, J. H.; *et al.* Response to submaximal and maximal exercise after bed rest and training. *Circulation,* **1968,** *38* (Suppl. 7), 1–78.

Saltin, B.; Henriksson, J.; Nygaard, H.; Andersen, P.; and Jansson, E. Fiber types and metabolic potentials of skeletal muscles in sedentary man and endurance runners. *Ann. N.Y. Acad. Sci.,* **1977,** *301,* 3–29.

Schoop, W. Bewegungstherapie bei peripheren Durchblutungsstorungen, *Med. Welt,* **1964,** *10,* 502.

——— Auswirkungen gesteigerter korperlicher Aktivitat auf gesunde und krankhafveranderte Extremitat-

sarterien. In, Roskamm *et al.* (eds.) *Korperliche Aktivitat und Herz und Kreislauferkrankungen.* Johann Ambrosius Barth, Munich, **1966,** p. 33.

Shaw, Lawrence W. Effects of a prescribed supervised exercise program on mortality and cardiovascular morbidity in patients after a myocardial infarction. *Am. J. Cardiol.,* **1981,** *48,* 39–45.

Siebert, W. W. Untersuchungen uber Hypertrophie des Skelettmuskels, *Z. Klin. Med.,* **1929,** *109,* 350.

Sivarajan, E. S.; Bruce, R. A.; Almes, M. J.; *et al.* In-hospital exercise after myocardial infarction does not improve treadmill performance. *N. Engl. J. Med.,* **1981,** *305,* 357.

Sjostrand, T. (ed.): *Clinical Physiology.* Svenska Bokforlaget, Stockholm, **1967.**

Skinner, J. S.; Holloszy, K. O.; and Cureton, T. K. Effects of a program of endurance exercises on physical work. *Am. J. Cardiol.,* **1964,** *14,* 747.

Stamler, J.: Nutrition-related risk factors for the atherosclerotic disease—present status. *Prog. biochem. Pharmacol.* (Karger, Basel), **1983,** *19,* 245–308.

Stein, R. A. The effect of exercise training on heart rate during coitus in the post myocardial infarction patient. *Circulation,* **1977,** *55,* 738.

Steinhaus, A. H.: Chronic effects of exercise. *Physiol. Rev.,* **1933,** *13,* 103.

Tabakin, B. S.; Hanson, J. S.; and Levy, A. M. Effect of physical training on the cardiovascular and respiratory response to graded upright exercise in distance runners. *Brit. Heart J.,* **1965,** *27,* 205.

Taylor, H. L.; Henschel, A.; Brozek, J.; and Keys, A. Effects of bed rest on cardiovascular function and work performance. *J. Appl. Physiol.,* **1949,** *2,* 223.

Tepperman, J., and Pearlman, D. Effects of exercise and anemia on coronary arteries of small animals as revealed by the corrosion-cast technique. *Circ. Res.,* **1961,** *9,* 576.

Thörner, W. Neue Beitrage zur Physiologie des Trainings. *Arbeitsphysiol.,* **1949,** *14,* 95.

Tipton, C. M.; Matthes, R. D.; and Sandage, D. S. In situ measurement of junction strength and ligament elongation in rats. *J. Appl. Physiol.,* **1974,** *37,* 758.

Toshiko, K.; Bruce, R. A.; Hossack, K. F.; *et al.* An evaluation of the Beckman metabolic cart for measuring ventilation and aerobic required during exercise. *J. Cardiovasc. Rehabil.* **1983,** *3,* 38.

Vannotti, A., and Magiday, M. Untersuchungen zum Studium des Trainiertseins. *Arbeitsphysiol.,* **1934,** *7,* 615.

Vannotti, A., and Pfister, H. Untersuchungen zum Studium des Trainiertseins. *Arbeitsphysiol.,* **1934,** *7,* 127.

Viidik, A. Biomechanics and functional adaptation of tendons and joint ligaments. In, Evans, F. G. (ed.) *Studies on the Anatomy and Function of Bone and Joints.* Springer-Verlag OHG, Heidelberg, **1966,** p. 17.

Walker, W. J. Changing U.S. life style and declining mortality—A retrospective. *N. Engl. J. Med.,* **1983,** *308* (editorial).

Warren, J. V. Critical issues in the sudden death syndrome. *Baylor College of Medicine, Cardiology Series,* **1982,** *5,* 6.

Whipple, G. H. The hemoglobin of striated muscle, 1, Variations due to age and exercise. *Am. J. Physiol.,* **1926,** *76,* 693.

Wilhelmsen, L.; Sanne, H.; Elmfeldt, D.; *et al.* A controlled trial of physical training after myocardial infarction. *Prev. Med.,* **1975,** *4,* 491.

Wilmore, Jack H.; Eroy, Gordon S.; Morton, Alan R.; *et al.* The effect of beta adrenergic blockade on submaximal and maximal exercise performance. *Cardiovasc. Rehabil.,* **1983,** *3,* 30.

Wollenberger, A.; Krause, E. G.; and Heier, G. Stimulation of 3', 5'-cyclic AMP formation in dog myocardium following arrest of blood flow. *Biochem. Biophys. Res. Commun.,* **1969,** *3,* 664–670.

Yakovlev, N. N. Problem of biochemical adaptation of muscles in dependence on the character of their activity. *J. Gen. Biol. USSR* (Eng. trans.) **1958,** *19,* 417.

Zohman, L., and Tobis, J. *Cardiac Rehabilitation.* Grune & Stratton, New York, **1971,** pp. 164–166.

INDEX

349

Coronary thrombosis. *See* Diagnosis of cardiovascular disease

Corticosteroids. *See* Surgery as a treatment for coronary heart disease

Counseling, predischarge after ACB. *See* Surgery as a treatment for coronary heart disease

Creatine kinase isoenzyme assay. *See* Nuclear medicine

Death, sudden, 329–330

Decreased mortality in patients with myocardial infarction, 189, 305

Denial, psychological, 100–101, 122

Depression, psychological
  alcoholism, 125, 126
  definition of, 99–100
  premorbid depression, 106, 125
  psychological test results
    entry profile, 139–141
    entry-exit changes, 143–144
  reactions to cardiac events, 99–100
  situational, 118, 124–125
  treatment, 120–121
  tricyclic antidepressants, 127–128

Diabetes, 7, 147, 154, 324, 327–328. *See also* Glucose metabolism disorders

Diagnosis of cardiovascular disease. *See also* Cardiovascular rehabilitation, medical management; Insurance, assessment of insurance risk, insurance medical examination; Organization and structure of a cardiovascular rehabilitation center
  acute myocardial infarction, 189
  aneurysm, left ventricular, 183
  angina: pectoris, 174, 175, 192–193; Prinzmetal's, 175, 187; refractory, 186; unstable, 174, 175, 193
  atherosclerosis, 185; regression of, 185
  atrioventricular node, 186–187
  bundle branch block, left, 179
  claudication, 189
  corneal arcus, 174
  coronary spasm, 173
  coronary thrombosis, 173
  ear crease, 174
  ectasia, 182
  hypertension, 252, 253
  hypotension, exertional, 69–88, 192
  infarction: myocardial, 173, 184, 193; of normal coronary arteries, 184; silent, 173
  intracavitary thrombi, 181
  left bundle branch block, 179
  left main disease, 179
  left ventricular aneurysm, 183
  mitral regurgitation, 182
  multivessel disease, 179

  muscle dysfunction, papillary, 182
  myocardial failure, 190
  myocardial infarction, 173, 175, 184, 189, 193; acute, 189; of normal coronary arteries, 184; nontransmural, 175; ruled out, 193; subendocardial, 193
  papillary muscle dysfunction, 182
  peripheral vascular disease, 189
  poor distal vessels, 215
  poor left ventricular function, 213
  Prinzmetal's angina, 175, 184, 187; vasospastic, 184, 187
  radiographic changes, 175
  refractory angina, 186
  silent myocardial infarction, 173
  spasm, coronary artery, 184, 186
  thrombi, cardiac, intracavitary, 181
  thrombolysis, 183
  thrombosis, coronary, 173
  unstable angina, 193
  vasospasm, 175
  ventricular fibrillation, 194
  ventricular tachyarrhythmias, 202
  ventricular tachycardia, 202

Dialysis patients with end-stage renal disease and cardiovascular rehabilitation, 65

Diet, 147, 150, 154–157, 165–170
  dietary goals for United States, 155
  goals for therapy for cardiovascular patients, 154–157
  guidelines for specific hyperlipoproteinemias, 156
  implementation of principles for cardiovascular recommendations, 165–170
  recommended composition, 155–156
  recommended intake for cardiovascular patients, 160–161
  risk factor for cardiovascular disease, 147, 150

Diltiazen. *See* Medications

Dipyridamole (PERSANTINE). *See* Medications

Disabilities associated with cardiovascular disease
  contributors to, 5–10
  prevalence, incidence, 9
  reduction following cardiovascular rehabilitation, 336–338. *See also* Benefits of cardiovascular rehabilitation

Disorders coexisting with cardiovascular disease. *See also* Cardiovascular rehabilitation, medical management
  age, 22
  alcohol abuse, 125, 126
  anemia, 8, 22, 322
  anxiety, 22, 323
  blood acid-base disorders, 8
  blood electrolyte disorders, 8
  case reports, 26–56
  clotting/bleeding disorders, 22. *See also* Surgery
  depression, 22, 322, 323
  disorders of glucose metabolism including diabetes, 7, 8, 22, 62, 322